HANDBOOK OF ETHNOGRAPHY IN HEALTHCARE RESEARCH

T0386346

This handbook provides an up-to-date reference point for ethnography in healthcare research. Taking a multi-disciplinary approach, the chapters offer a holistic view of ethnography within medical contexts.

This edited volume is organized around major methodological themes, such as ethics, interviews, narrative analysis, and mixed methods. Through the use of case studies, it illustrates how methodological considerations for ethnographic healthcare research are distinct from those in other fields. It has detailed content on the methodological facets of undertaking ethnography for prospective researchers to help them to conduct research in both an ethical and safe manner. It also highlights important issues such as the role of the researcher as the key research instrument, exploring how one's social behaviours enable the researcher to 'get closer' to his/her participants and thus uncover original phenomena. Furthermore, it invites critical discussion of applied methodological strategies within the global academic community by pushing forward the use of ethnography to enhance the body of knowledge in the field.

The book offers an original guide for advanced students, prospective ethnographers, and healthcare professionals aiming to utilize this methodological approach.

Paul M.W. Hackett is professor in ethnography at Emerson College, Boston, USA, a visiting professor in health research at the University of Suffolk, UK, and a visiting scholar at the Royal Anthropological Institute in London. He has developed the declarative mapping sentence out of his research which is concerned with the categorial understanding that humans have of their world and how such understanding underpins and facilitates behaviour, drawing upon several branches of psychology, philosophy, anthropology, and research methods. His publications include around 20 books and articles in leading journals.

Christopher M. Hayre is a senior lecturer at Charles Sturt University in New South Wales, Australia. He has published both qualitative and quantitative refereed papers in the field of medical imaging and brought together several books in the field of medical imaging, health research, technology, and ethnography.

HANDBOOK OF ETHNOGRAPHY IN HEALTHCARE RESEARCH

Edited by
Paul M.W. Hackett, PhD, and
Christopher M. Hayre, PhD

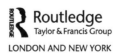

LONDON AND NEW YORK

First published 2021
by Routledge
2 Park Square, Milton Park, Abingdon, Oxon OX14 4RN

and by Routledge
52 Vanderbilt Avenue, New York, NY 10017

Routledge is an imprint of the Taylor & Francis Group, an informa business

British Library Cataloguing-in-Publication Data
A catalogue record for this book is available from the British Library

Library of Congress Cataloging-in-Publication Data
Names: Hackett, Paul, 1960– editor. | Hayre, Christopher M., editor.
Title: Handbook of ethnography in healthcare research / Edited by
Paul M.W. Hackett and Christopher M. Hayre.
Description: Abingdon, Oxon; New York, NY : Routledge, 2021. |
Includes bibliographical references and index. |
Identifiers: LCCN 2020028624 (print) | LCCN 2020028625 (ebook) |
ISBN 9780367336332 (paperback) | ISBN 9780367336349 (hardback) |
ISBN 9780429320927 (ebook)
Subjects: LCSH: Medical anthropology–Research. |
Medical anthropology–Moral and ethical aspects. |
Medical anthropology–Social aspects.
Classification: LCC GN296.5.B47 H36 2021 (print) |
LCC GN296.5.B47 (ebook) | DDC 306.4/61–dc23
LC record available at https://lccn.loc.gov/2020028624
LC ebook record available at https://lccn.loc.gov/2020028625

ISBN: 978-0-367-33634-9 (hbk)
ISBN: 978-0-367-33633-2 (pbk)
ISBN: 978-0-429-32092-7 (ebk)

Typeset in Bembo
by Newgen Publishing UK

*Dr. Christopher M. Hayre would like to dedicate this book to his supportive wife Charlotte
and his daughters Ayva, Evelynn, and Ellena. Love to all.
Professor Paul M. W. Hackett would like to thank Jessica whose support makes it all possible.*

CONTENTS

CONTRIBUTORS

Tine Aagaard, University of Greenland, Greenland.

Haris Agic, PhD, in Medical Anthropology Health and Society, Development Leader for Society, Culture and Arts at Study Promotion Association, Studiefrämjandet, Stockholm, Sweden.

Ditte Andersen, Senior Researcher at VIVE, The Danish Center for Social Science Research, Copenhagen, Denmark, den@vive.dk.

Maria Louise Bønnelykke, Department of Culture and Learning, Aalborg University.

Alicia Carlson, Video Production Manager, Office of Marketing, Emerson College, Boston, MA, USA.

Michelle M. Doucette, Independent Public Health Researcher, University of Greenland.

Antonella Fabri, Business Anthropologist, Caleidoscopio Ethnographic Research, University at Albany.

Gillie Gabay, College of Management Academic Studies, School of Behavioral Science and Psychology, Israel.

Jeff Gavin, Senior Lecturer in Department of Psychology at the University of Bath.

Jonathan Glazzard, Professor of Inclusive Education, Carnegie School of Education, Leeds Beckett University, Leeds, UK.

Martina Grimaldi, Lecturer in Cultural Anthropology and Ethnology, University of Bologna, Alma Mater Studiorum, Italy.

Deirdre Guthrie is an ethnographic consultant and research advisor for the Wellbeing Project based in Paris.

Paul M.W. Hackett, Visiting Professor of Health Research Methods, School of Health Sciences, University of Suffolk; Visiting Scholar, Royal Anthropological Institute; Professor of Ethnography, School of Communication, Emerson College; Honorary Fellow, Department of Philosophy, Durham University.

Steve Hagelman, Ethnographic Research Inc.

Graham Hall, Professor of Applied Linguistics, Northumbria University, UK.

Anne Harris, VC Principal Research Fellow, RMIT University, Melbourne, Australia; ARC Future Fellow School of Education, Australia; Director, Digital Ethnography Research Centre, Melbourne, Australia; Creative Agency Research Lab, Melbourne, Australia.

Hira Hasan, Department of Applied Anthropology, University of North Texas, USA.

Christopher M. Hayre, Senior Lecturer, Diagnostic Radiography, Charles Sturt University, New South Wales, Australia.

Julia Hecking, Mount Holyoke College, South Hadley, Massachusetts, USA.

Immy Holloway, Professor Emeritus of Health Research, Bournemouth University, UK.

Áine M. Humble, Professor, Family Studies and Gerontology Department, Mount Saint Vincent University, Halifax, Nova Scotia, Canada.

Cathrine V. Jansson-Boyd, Anglia Ruskin University, Cambridge, UK.

Stacy Holman Jones, Professor and Director in Centre for Theatre and Performance, Monash University, Australia.

Michael Klingenberg, Senior Lecturer in Adult Nursing, Leeds Beckett University, UK.

Bettina Kolb, Lecturer, Department of Sociology, University of Vienna and Department of Health Science and Social Work, Carinthia University of Applied Science, Villach, Austria.

Laura Lorenz, Visiting Research Scholar, Heller School for Social Policy & Management, Brandeis University, Massachusetts, USA. llorenz@brandeis.edu.

Elizabeth Lynch, Associate Professor, Department of Preventive Medicine, Rush Medical College, Chicago, IL, USA.

Taylor Malone, School of Communication, Emerson College, Boston, USA.

Ruth Montgomery, Andersen Independent Public Health Researcher, University of Greenland, Greenland.

Anke Plagnol, Senior Lecturer in Behavioural Economics City, University of London, UK.

Elise Radina, Professor of Family Science and Social Work, Miami University, Oxford, OH, USA.

Melinda Rea-Holloway, Ethnographic Research Inc.

David Resnik, National Institute of Environmental Health Sciences, National Institutes of Health, National Institutes of Health.

Karen Rodham, Professor of Health Psychology, Staffordshire University, UK.

Jessica Schwarzenbach, Independent Researcher, Massachusetts, USA.

Tamira Snell, Insights Lead at Nordic Health Lab and Associated Partner at Copenhagen Institute for Futures Studies.

Ruth Strudwick, is a diagnostic radiographer and an associate professor in Diagnostic Radiography, University of Suffolk, Ipswich, UK.

Susan Squires, Professor, University of North Texas, USA.

Jonathan Tummons, Associate Professor and Deputy Head of School, School of Education, Durham University, UK.

Tom Vine, Associate Professor, University of Suffolk, Ipswich, UK.

ACKNOWLEDGEMENTS

The editors would like to thank all of the authors who have contributed to this book for their commitment, hard work, and determination. It has been a pleasure to work with you and to bring together this collection of chapters. We believe that these demonstrate the continued importance of conducting ethnography for health research. We have personally found this to be an exciting and enriching project, which we hope readers will enjoy and utilize.

FOREWORD

Ethnographic vision

Professor Shane Blackman

Ethnography has become more popular as a research method and research councils such as the ESRC and AHRC, and government departments including Health and Social Care, Work and Pensions, and Education have actively sought data from ethnographic studies. This is evident from the varied contributors within this Handbook. Increased popularity, of course, does not mean increased acceptance. The *Handbook of Ethnography in Healthcare Research* does not set out to replace, oppose, or critique positivism in healthcare, or to demonstrate that ethnography has the answers. It explores new agendas in ethnographic research in healthcare. The chapters highlight that qualitative methods are both exploratory and produce outcomes which are generalizable and of high value for patients, doctors, nurses, and all professionals within healthcare. Ethnography seeks to be inclusive through access to experience to offer rich data both inside and outside clinical settings, through participant observation, conversational interviews, personal documentary evidence, digital ethnography, and the researcher themselves.

The ethnographic studies here reveal that fieldwork can be dynamic yet also boring; the accounts bring forth a range of contradictory, oppositional, and pleasurable experiences through encounters with anger, frustration, guilt, irony, and humour. Recognition of these different lived experiences of people of different ages, social classes, sexualities, and ethnicities enable us to address healthcare issues from a variety of stand points, where ethnographic interventions deliver positive results in understanding and through sharing knowledge. A number of the chapters here recognize that ethnographic studies may be positioned in opposition to the dominant positivist model operated within health sciences. There is also recognition that the rise of ethnographic studies, to some extent, has been held in check by the status of biomedical science and its hegemonic position. Yet during the Coronavirus pandemic of 2020 we have seen research uncomfortably coexist between science and politics, delivered online as a daily furor defined by accusation, blame, censorship, and lack of transparency. Science has been used for political purposes whether it has been allowed to offer answers or not permitted to speak. Ethnography is familiar with politics, decolonization, critical questioning, and "fired up" accusations; throughout its long history ethnography has sought out what is uncomfortable to enhance the understanding that all research depends on the subjective understanding of trust.

Ethnography is established though relationships and it can fall apart quickly when respect is not its top priority. This approach is more than a research method used to collect qualitative empirical data, it is about empathy, conflict, and interpretation, and as Clifford Geertz (1973) explained, ethnography is where the researcher and the researched are engaged in applying imagination. In this book we see that ethnographic studies are achieved through relationships and intimacy—there is care and sensitivity both in the research practice of fieldwork and in the writing of the research itself as a publication. The attraction and value of the ethnographic studies in this book is that they are personal stories of journeys lived through fear, shame, anxiety, self-realization, triumph and disaster, and even laughter.

What marks ethnography out as a research method is usage of the field diary, whether hand written or electronic, audio or visual. From the moment they are in the field the researchers are actively recording, interpreting, writing, and constructing the text. From its beginning, ethnography has been understood as both interdisciplinary and beholden to no discipline. All ethnographers know that they are standing on the "shoulders of giants." Over a hundred years ago, the method was first used in the discipline of anthropology by key figures such as Franz Boas (1858–1942) and Bronislaw Malinowski (1884–1942). In (1916: 418) Malinowski said that, "I found the lack of philosophical clearness on matters connected with ethnographic and sociological field work a great setback." In 1915, Robert Park set out the urban fieldwork manifesto of the Chicago School of Sociology and from the 1920s ethnographic research techniques to collect and analyze data were professionally taught and systematically organized at Chicago, for example, Palmer's (1928) *Field Studies in Sociology: A Student's Manual.* Pre-dating such academic development was Harriet Martineau (1838), who could be considered an ethnographic primer and who not only prioritized first-hand observation but also teaching ethnography when she said in the Advertisement of her book, "The best mode of exciting the love of observation is by teaching 'How to Observe.'"

Ethnography is both a method and research technique, and a methodology that is a philosophy of method. Ethnographic methods are focused on being open and sharing experiences. This can advance knowledge. Ethnographers enable the data to speak back, to question the research and the researcher. This may mean allowing the participants to collect data, do analysis, and take part in coproduction of texts. Within qualitative research the researcher is always part of what is happening. Sometimes the researcher tries to minimize their involvement, but at other times they may guide participants to engage with ideas. Trying to pigeonhole ethnography is not what ethnographers do.

Speaking on fieldwork, Malinowski (1926: 127) states: "Open air anthropology, as opposed to hearsay and note-taking, is hard work, but it is also great fun." The assertion that research can be fun still remains a taboo topic because an ethnographic approach involves immersion within, and an investigation of, a social world which can be painful and emotionally upsetting for all. Self-awareness is important in ethnography because, as the researcher, you are directly learning about people's experiences and feelings. Formally this is described as reflexivity, where you show sensitivity towards your research subjects and also reflect on what is your role in speaking with them. In all the chapters of this book, we see that in order to conduct successful ethnographic fieldwork, the researcher is required to be responsive and flexible to the needs of the research subjects and to build positive contact on a constant basis to enable data to be forthcoming.

The aim of ethnography in healthcare is to observe behaviour within a clinical, natural, and everyday setting or context to discover the meaning and value people put into their actions and ideals. Ethnography is alive to the real opportunities of dynamic fieldwork encounters and experiences: we see here that researchers need to be prepared for surprises! An ethnographic vision enables research to offer something new, alternative, or different from what was anticipated or expected, so the researcher should be prepared to improvise. Therefore, flexibility within research design and fieldwork management are the markers of a sophisticated and receptive researcher who is aware of the changes within the setting at the level of theory and methodology.

References

Blackman, S. (2010) 'The Ethnographic Mosaic' of the Chicago School: critically locating Vivien Palmer, Cliff ord Shaw and Frederic Thrasher's research methods in contemporary reflexive sociological interpretation. In Hart, C. (ed), *The Legacy of the Chicago School of Sociology*. Kingswinsford: Midrash Publishing: 195– 215.

Geertz, C. (1973) Thick Description: Towards an Interpretive Theory of Culture. In *The Interpretation of Cultures*. London: Hutchinson, pp. 3–30.

Malinowski, B. (1916) Baloma; The Spirits of the Dead in the Trobriand Islands. *The Journal of the Royal Anthropological Institute of Great Britain and Ireland*, 46(Jul–Dec): 353–430.

Malinowski, B. (1926) *Myth in Primitive Psychology*. London: Kegan Paul.

Martineau, H. (1838) *How to Observe Morals and Manners*. London: Charles Knight.

Palmer, V. (1928) *Field Studies in Sociology: A Student's Manual*. Chicago: University of Chicago Press.

Park, R. E. (1915) The City: Suggestions for the Investigation of Human Behavior in the City Environment. *American Journal of Sociology*, 20(5): 577–612.

PART I

Introduction

1

INTRODUCING ETHNOGRAPHY AND ITS RATIONALE FOR HEALTHCARE PRACTITIONER USE

Christopher M. Hayre and Paul M.W. Hackett

Introduction

This introductory chapter sets the scene for this book volume and introduces ethnography as a methodology to the reader. As we will come to acknowledge, the use of ethnography is well-established for researchers within a range of health settings. For example, in the author's own discipline, diagnostic radiography, the rise of ethnographic approaches is providing greater clarity into the professional practices of diagnostic radiographers and the care experienced by patients undergoing medical imaging examinations. Whilst the prospective chapters in this book are from experienced researchers and academics who have undertaken ethnographic studies within health settings, there are also examples outside the healthcare setting, which provide unique contexts that can be transferred into clinical environments. In this introductory chapter, we begin by discussing what ethnography is, focusing on its methodological purpose and how, for healthcare professionals, it can uncover central phenomena previously undocumented. Next, the authors reflect on the virtues of undertaking ethnography as experienced researchers, whilst importantly reflecting on our own journeys of pursuing ethnography as both a research methodology and an enlightenment in our own professional conduct.

What is ethnography?

Ethnography is regarded as a methodological tool that "gets close" to a particular group and/or sub-group to uncover cultural phenomena. Historically, it has its roots in British social anthropology, whereby researchers went out to study foreign cultures, and in American Sociology (from the Chicago school), whereby observation was used to explore urban industrial society. These schools of thought aimed to provide an overarching objective: that of cultural description (Brewer, 2000). Since then, the rise of ethnography has been identified in many academic disciplines, notably business, sociology, criminology, education, politics, and healthcare. In short, it is generally accepted that ethnography offers exploratory researchers an opportunity to uncover the social reality of individuals and groups in order to better enhance our understanding of their social world (Hammersley & Atkinson, 2007).

In Chris Hayre's work, the rationale for using ethnography was due to an immediate disconnect in diagnostic radiography practice. For example, the pedagogical principles and practices offered at his higher education institution (as an undergraduate radiography student) were seen to be dichotomous with what was practiced in the clinical setting. Looking back, he remained inexperienced as a student radiographer. He was "learning by doing," and as he continued to observe the clinical environment, he would replicate the social practices by conforming to cultural norms. As he developed and became more competent as a student radiographer, leading to gradation and then becoming a practitioner, he began to appreciate the complexities around the diversity of diagnostic radiography practice, but importantly, how this disconnect was also influenced by workplace cultures.

Deciding to embark on a PhD remained a key driver for the first author in order to enlighten his own practice and understand the observed behaviour of clinical work. In response, ethnography provided an opportunity to study a culture (of radiographers in this case) within their own settings (Hobbs & May, 1993; McGarry, 2007) and, not forgetting the primary purpose, in order understand why a dichotomy existed between principles professed within the higher education setting when compared to the day-to-day practices of diagnostic radiographers. Hobbs and May (1993) agree, stating that ethnography enables researchers a way of telling it like it is, by learning and then describing the culture observed and looking at the actions of individuals. Further, Denzin (1997) reminds us that researchers aim to unveil the participants' interpretation and then draw from their own conclusions by using many alternate incidences in order to understand the cultural perspective. These former tenets remained high on the agenda of uncovering radiographic practices.

For prospective ethnographic researchers reading this book for the first time, we firmly acknowledge that in order to document/uncover findings, researchers need to become part of the culture being studied in order to gain understanding and insight. This typically involves observation, which remains a key method for ethnographers, both historically and contemporaneously. There are alternate forms of observation, which is beyond the scope for this introductory chapter, but we direct readers to the following texts (see Roth, 1962; Spradley, 1980). Looking back, participant observation remained an important method in the first author's own research, enabling him to observe and listen to what was being said and ask questions as an insider (as a diagnostic radiographer himself) (Hayre, 2016). This is important when it comes to utilizing ethnography as a methodology of choice because it is the observed behaviour that should be examined in its natural state and undisturbed by the researcher as much as possible (Hammersley & Atkinson, 2007). We also suggest that when considering ethnography, observation is carried out over a period of time that not only meets the aims and objectives of the study but also ensures that the behaviour of others is not linked to the researcher's presence in the field. For example, Wolcott (1999, p. 49) reminds us that "people can sustain an act or maintain their best image only so long." This is commonly regarded as the Hawthorne effect, whereby the presence of the researcher alters the behaviour of those studied. It is, however, accepted that over a longer period of time this fades, and thus the "real" behaviour begins to emerge (Nieswiadomy, 2002). In short, for the first author, ethnography offered a valued insight into a specific culture underexplored within his own profession, diagnostic radiography, which subsequently expanded the evidence base and at the time of writing this chapter influenced transnational policy for the radiographic profession. In short, our view is that ethnography has the ability to add value to all healthcare disciplines and expand the existing body of knowledge and, importantly, challenge commonly held beliefs and viewpoints of practice.

What is ethnography? Ethnography is a methodological tool that can offer prospective ethnographic researchers the opportunity to critically engage with contemporary healthcare practices and also provide the opportunity for innovation and change within a health discipline, which is well evidenced in this book volume.

The virtues of ethnography in healthcare settings

The editors will now comment on the virtues ethnography offers when it comes to researching within the healthcare environment. Because of its increasing use amongst healthcare practitioners to gain deeper insight of either practitioners' or patients' perspectives, Hammersley (1992, p. 35) terms it "practitioner ethnography" following its recent uses amongst vocationally based disciplines, such as practicing healthcare professionals. Further, as a healthcare professional, reflection remains an essential tool. Reflection is often used to gain perspective on a clinical situation, patient interaction, and the practice/application of new knowledge, for instance. It is also central when renewing our professional registration in order to demonstrate continuous professional development as healthcare professionals. In addition, the methodological practice of ethnography is not wholly dissimilar: the engagement of reflexivity enables ethnographers to critically reflect on their interactions with peers, participants, colleagues, the research environment, and the generation of new knowledge when in the field. Further, the association between reflection (as a healthcare practitioner) and reflexivity (as an ethnographer) offers similar opportunities and virtues whereby the unification of such practices can help develop a greater appreciation and understanding of self-management. For example, by undertaking and pursuing ethnography as a research methodology, we are not simply implementing a research strategy that ends upon leaving the research field, but instead one that continues and develops, involving workplace interactions coupled with the management of potential hostile situations, while we, importantly, remain ethically mindful of our own positionality within the context of the social world around us.

When ethnographic researchers consider their methods in healthcare contexts, with the overarching aim of ascertaining "what people say they do and what they actually do," researchers typically align to social constructionism and interpretivism in order to help obtain new knowledge and understanding through cultural exploration of a particular context (Brewer, 2000). For example, interpretivism identifies and searches for patterns of descriptive meanings, helping to understand the participants view. Constructionism is a form of interpretive research (Taylor, 2002), which states that meaning is not discovered but constructed (Crotty, 2005). Constructionism can be formed from our everyday experiences, our history, our use of language, our knowledge, and our social action, which are all interconnected and, over time, lead to shared meanings (Brewer, 2000). Whilst these are commonly utilized and generally accepted as ethnographic norms, we urge ethnographers to critique whether positivist methods can be used to help uncover the social world, depending on the research questions posed. For instance, Hayre and Blackman (2020) recently identified the combination of both interpretivist (observation) and positivist (X-ray experimental) methods within a single ethnographic methodology. After philosophically grappling with the ideological disconnect, the emergent discourse presented offers what the authors term "an umbrella strategy." The acceptance and/or acknowledgement of positivism within ethnography is rarely discussed nor evidenced within healthcare literature. Further, for Hayre and Blackman (2020), there was a genuine recognition and acceptance of the philosophical challenges (and even juxtaposition) for the healthcare professional and the researcher. However, after critical reflection, discussion, and recognition of what the purpose of ethnography is (ethnos – "a people" and -graphy, meaning "writing"), this reminded us that ethnography focuses on writing about a group and/or a sub-group of individuals being studied, regardless of philosophy. Thus, because positivism remains central to the practices of optimizing X-rays clinically, it was helpful to include positivist approaches as part of the culture being researched.

Thus whilst for most ethnographic researchers there remains firm use of qualitative methods, which typically involves observation, interviews, focus groups, and examination of written documents and/or diaries (and remains the general consensus throughout this book), we do welcome the utilization of positivist approaches, which can draw on a range of research philosophy within contemporary ethnographies. Chapters 8 and 11 in this book recognize the integration of quantitative methods in order to support or refute phenomena. In order to provide an example of the aforementioned approach, the following was deemed appropriate in the work by the first author:

1) Participant observation: Used to observe contemporary radiographic practices and note "what the radiographers did."
2) In-depth semi-structure interviews: Explored key themes derived from the clinical observations and uncovered deeper meanings into "what had been seen."
3) X-ray experiments: To reflect on specific radiographic phenomena observed and contribute X-ray findings with "what had been seen" and "what had been said" regarding specific phenomena.

The above methodological strategy arguably demonstrates an emancipation of research methods and philosophy within the diagnostic radiography setting. Inductive and hypothetical-deductive approaches are becoming well-established in health disciplines (Henwood, 1996) in order to study the effectiveness of clinical and person-centredness (Mellion & Tovin, 2002). This remained central to the ethnographic journey of the first author, which may resonate with authors transnationally in their respective health disciplines. In short, one of the key virtues of ethnography resides in its versatility to be applied in a number of health contexts and to encompass an array of research strategies depending on what the research seeks to uncover.

Summary

This chapter sought to provide two key introductory messages. First, we provide a definition to ethnographic research and explore how the first author came to consider and adopt this methodological approach for his own research. As identified above, a key driver behind this selection resulted in the dichotomy of pedagogical principles and the observed behaviour of healthcare professionals as a student radiographer. These experiences help contextualize the utility in which ethnography offered a professional community the ability to uncover professional practices that resonated with the discipline as a whole. Second, we sought to provide some key attributes that ethnography offers. For example, not only do we feel that ethnography provides a toolkit for researchers, but it can also provide academics with the virtues of upholding professional excellence throughout an academic career. Finally, we have argued that whilst qualitative methods are typically aligned to ethnographic approaches, the health disciplines offer a wide range of methodological (and philosophical) opportunity that engages positivist traditions in order to help discern the social world around us.

References

Brewer, J.D. (2000) *Ethnography*. Buckingham: Open University Press.

Crotty, M. (2005) *The Foundations of Social Research – Meaning and Perspective in the Research Process.* London: Sage.

Denzin, N.K. (1997) *Interpretive ethnography*. Thousand Oaks: Sage.

Hammersley, M. (1992) *What's Wrong With Ethnography*. New York: Routledge.

Hammersley, M. and Atkinson, P. (2007) *Ethnography Principles in Practice,* 3rd Ed. New York: Routledge.

Hayre, C.M. (2016) Radiography Observed: An Ethnographic Study Exploring Contemporary Radiographic Practice. PhD Thesis. Canterbury Christ Church University.

Hayre, C.M. and Blackman, S. (2020) "Ethnographic mosaic approach for health and rehabilitation practitioners: an ethno-radiographic perspective." *Disability and Rehabilitation*: 1–4.

Henwood, S. (1996) "Managing quality in diagnostic imaging departments." *Radiography*, 2 (2): 111–117.

Hobbs, D. and May, T. (1993) *Interpreting the field – Accounts of ethnography*. Oxford: Oxford University Press.

Mellion, L.R. and Tovin, M.M. (2002) "Grounded theory: a qualitative research methodology for physical therapy." *Physiotherapy Theory and Practice,* 18 (3): 109–20.

McGarry, J. (2007) "Nursing relationships in ethnographic research: what of rapport." *Nurse Researcher,* 14 (3): 7–14.

Nieswiadomy, R. (2002) *Foundations of Nursing Research*. 4th Ed. Prentice Hall: Upper Saddle River, USA.

Roth, J.H. (1962) "Comments on secret observations." *Social Problems*, 9 (3): 283–284.

Spradley, J.P. (1980) *Participant Observation*. New York: Holt, Rinehart & Winston.

Taylor, S. (2002) *Ethnographic Research*. London: Sage.

Wolcott, H.F. (1999) Ethnography – A Way of Seeing. Altamira Press: Oxford.

PART II

Ethical considerations

2

ETHICAL CONSIDERATIONS IN ETHNOGRAPHY[1]

Jessica Schwarzenbach and Paul M.W. Hackett

Introduction

Other chapters in this book address aspects of ethics which apply to the practice of qualitative research within a healthcare setting. However, this chapter utilizes a slightly different approach by containing largely anecdotal reports from the authors' personal experiences. In this chapter the term *consideration(s)* signifies the application of continuous and careful thought. As a consequence of this perspective, the chapter addresses many ethical features of the actual practice of qualitative interview research and constructs a body of cautionary advice for future investigators.

The healthcare industry embodies a unique set of power differentials between medical researchers and those who seek medical assistance. Often research is conducted in a situation where outcomes are uncertain and patients are especially vulnerable to feelings of fear and confusion. Medical care professionals are often perceived by those undergoing physical and mental care as experts who inherently possess greater knowledge (and thus power) as well as influence due to their familiarity not only with the illness itself but with the language and operations of the healthcare establishment. Ethical awareness of this power differential between researcher and patient is codified through written laws and regulatory bodies such as institutional review boards (IRBs), the Belmont Report, the American Psychological Association (APA), the British Psychological Society (BPS), the British Medical Association (BMA), etc., but even when following ethical guidelines and with the best of intentions, well informed researchers may cause unwitting discomfort to subjects through naïve or careless behavior. Although participants must review and sign informed consent documents before interviews, situations may develop that the researcher and the participant do not anticipate. This chapter offers some insight into how notions of trust as well as the researcher's honesty regarding his or her own biases are paramount when negotiating with a participant regarding the sharing of information and some of the unexpected emotional responses that may affect the research findings.

Ethicality

The term ethics is a complex concept, yet it is often oversimplified through definitions referring to notions of right and wrong behavior. The Ancient Greeks used the word *ēthikos* to pertain to moral character, which was interrelated with the term *ēthos*, a reference to custom. Thus, ethics encompassed the moral principles of an individual or group. As a qualitative researcher, numerous choices must be made. We must attempt to understand our motives and prejudices, how our backgrounds affect our decisions, and what information we retain and what we disregard. We must also respect and protect the participants' trust in us whilst safeguarding the use of their information in a way that transcends desires for sensationalistic data. Consequently, researchers must proceed cautiously. Often what seems to be an intuitive and sensitive research methodology may develop into a complex process imbued with difficulties that could affect the credibility of the research project.

Research design

The success of an ethically sound qualitative research project rests upon the strength of its research design. The research design refers to the process of managing all aspects of the study including the context, materials, and procedures and how these will be utilized to potentially answer the research question(s). In qualitative research the investigator constructs the research design after assessing various arrangements of the investigation's components in an attempt to generate the most informative responses from participants. Many inaccurate outcomes in otherwise well thought out research projects arise through design flaws, tempting some researchers to conceal these imperfections in their final results and reports.

Within the authors' experiences, ethnographic or qualitative researchers sometimes value the significance of good research design less than quantitative researchers. Research design is central to quantitative enquiry as quantitative researchers choose appropriate experimental designs in order to allow identification of the effects of specific experimental (independent) variables upon other specific outcome (dependent) variables (or combinations of these variables) whilst reducing the effects of background confounding variables. The authors believe that qualitative researchers would benefit by spending as much time and effort upon the careful study of research design as their quantitative counterparts. In qualitative research, attempts are not made to partition the effects of independent variables upon dependent variables as interest lies in how respondents experience events and understand the circumstances that impact their lives. However, methodically designed qualitative research may help the investigator avoid unreliable conclusions.

Emergent design model

In contrast to following a clearly organized guideline, the researcher, when utilizing the emergent design model, is allowed the flexibility to respond to what *emerges* from the data as the research progresses. Emergent design originated within grounded theory and with its open-ended format has become popular among novice qualitative researchers. However, the emergent process is difficult to undertake successfully. To understand the complex aspects of human experience, investigators must be able to assemble evidences and descriptions from participants' actions and interactions while they are discussing the situation/phenomenon being explored. Often inexperienced investigators embrace emergent design as they enjoy the excitement of not knowing in what direction unexpected data will lead them.

One of the defining tenets of emergent design is the permission given to the investigator to ask diverse questions of participants during the interview process, resulting in the collection of dissimilar data from participants in the same study. The second author experienced an example of an unheeded emergent design flaw when he was recruited into an ongoing longitudinal medical research project. This study had been running for a number of years when several questions were added to the research instruments. Unfortunately, none of the investigators had considered how these additional questions related to the instruments previously employed in the study. The new questions were developed from the results of the questionnaires' previous administrations and were thus assumed legitimate. Therefore, the responses to the new questions were thought to be directly commensurate with the old information, presupposing a continuity of understanding to develop from the study's different phases. However, the new questions and procedures differed from previous stages in subtle ways and the new responses, whilst yielding interesting information, were distinct enough from the earlier research to be noncomparable. For example, a question asked during the later phase of this study inquired how youth respondents felt about the importance of family in their health regimens. This question had been developed because during the initial research stages a question had requested respondents to talk about the people they considered to be important to them. All respondents mentioned their families, whilst some respondents also mentioned people outside their families. However, in the new round of the research, questions were not asked about non-family members. Thus, the results from different stages of the research were neither cumulative nor directly comparable. Conclusions from the different stages of the research made only partial sense in regard to the investigation of the importance of families.

Without doubt, different questions asked at different times to the same people or to different persons within a particular time frame may become problematic. Sometimes an interviewee will present unforeseen information that may perturb the investigator who had not thought to include this type of data. This situation may confuse the examiner as to what to do next. Sometimes unique and serendipitous data may prompt the researcher to re-contact participants to gain further information about unanticipated developments. Yet reconnecting with former interviewees may strain the trust between respondent and researcher. These previously interviewed participants have already given precious time to help answer your research questions. Creating extra demands upon participants in order to make newly discovered data more comparable may aggravate the researcher/subject relationship and affect the quality of a study's results. Unfortunately, even for the seasoned researcher, emergent design with its tangle of unique and incomparable data may become exasperating and disorderly.

The lack of regulatory codes of practice within emergent design may create additional hardship for the inexperienced investigator. If in-depth interviews are employed, the researcher may have trouble controlling the amount of information contained within the myriad of responses from new participants. Furthermore, novice researchers may have difficulty ignoring data that could uniquely inform dissimilar features of the research questions. An investigator new to this research approach may thus become overwhelmed by the amount of cumbersome and confusing data. A methodology that helps keep a research project on course amongst the multiple opportunities and ambivalences of the emergent design model is a mapping sentence. A mapping sentence is a tool used in Facet Theory that offers an adaptable framework in a declarative mapping sentence format (See Chapter 8, The Declarative Mapping Sentence as a Framework for conducting Ethnographic Health Research). The declarative mapping sentence provides a structure within which the interaction between researcher and participant may be defined and also offers a method for interpreting subjects' responses.

Interviews

Central theories inherent to qualitative inquiry recognize that all research is value-laden, that the research context is shaped by the research project, that multiple realities need to be taken into account, and that investigators explore their frequently unrecognized personal biases. Thus, qualitative research can be rife with ambivalence and uncertainty. Another fundamental aspect of qualitative methodology is the desire to explore the "why" underlying quantitative studies.

Researchers who are new to qualitative research often assume that talking to people and writing up results is a more personalized and sympathetic way to understand human complexity than other research designs. However, neophyte researchers are often unaware that talking intimately with people about their significant concerns may generate complicated relational issues that require a sense of moral responsibility. Respondents' viewpoints, fears, and opinions must be treated with utmost consideration whether you concur with them or not: trust between researcher and participant is of the utmost importance.

There is an assortment of interview techniques available to qualitative researchers, yet interviewers must be aware that their chosen style may affect the quality of the interview process. The most commonly utilized types of interviews are structured, semi-structured, and unstructured formats. A structured interview, with questions organized beforehand, is the least complicated procedure for the investigator to code and write up as the exchanges with respondents can be more easily arranged for comparison. However, all interview styles, along with the technology used (telephone, recording, video, Skype, in-person, etc.) influence the interview data. Even the inclusion of props or the setting in which the interview takes place (the participant's home, your office, an institution, a café, etc.) may affect the data emerging in the conversation.

The second author has experienced uncomfortable situations while collecting healthcare data, i.e., receiving verbal abuse from bystanders or from the subjects themselves. He was verbally attacked by an interviewee who used expletives to state the uselessness of healthcare research. The author had to make a great effort to continue the interview to its useful conclusion. He has also been bitten by an aggressive dog and another time had a trouser leg torn. Whilst these situations may be unpleasant, they are fairly easy to cope with and may be considered learning experiences behooving greater care in the future. However, the second author questions the value of data gathered in these sorts of situations. For example: how much rapport was established with the respondent after her dog bit through his trousers; how much was he able to focus on the content of the interview; and how trustworthy was the information produced by the interview?

Generally, qualitative researchers feel there is more rapport established when conversing face-to-face with a participant, using eye contact and body language to help develop a better understanding of the interview content. However, some participants may feel more at ease when answering questions on written questionnaires or telephone interviews than when meeting a stranger in real time to discuss personal material. The interviewer may also be more comfortable with less direct contact but must be aware that a participant who feels confident and safe is more likely to share information.

An interesting, though challenging, interview style is the *active interview*. Here, the interviewer and respondent are encouraged to co-construct meaning through the creation of a joint narrative. The investigator does not seek impartiality in this style but takes an assertive role to actively stimulate responses from the participant. Both the interviewer and interviewee are considered equal partners in the conversation, which can be liberating but also intrinsically problematic and difficult to accomplish. Conversely, this unconventional interview format may generate data that otherwise would not have emerged.

Data collection

Qualitative and ethnographic researchers are often concerned with the quantity of data their study will require: how many interviews or sort procedures they should conduct. In contrast to the power calculations used in quantitative research, the qualitative researcher has no fixed methodology to establish sample size. The reader must be aware that all types of research have functional restrictions which determine data collection, such as money, time, or other resources available for the project, and most importantly, the interviewee's desire to cooperate.

To avoid some of the errors associated with questions of quantity, the eager qualitative researcher must learn to establish a balance between gathering too much and too little data. Inexperienced researchers must pay attention to tiring participants who may start to repeat themselves during an interview. This is often a symptom of an overlong data gathering session, as are the times when respondents are no longer able to offer novel interpretations to questions. On the other hand, data quality may decline when the researcher hurries through the interview, attempts to adhere to too rigid a time schedule, ends the session before data saturation has been reached, or uses identical criteria to specify the amount of data to be gathered from all participants. A better choice is to realize that different amounts of meaningful information are supplied by different individuals. The researcher must be finely attuned to how long and in-depth a procedure the respondent will accept: the goal is to finish the interview when saturation has been achieved.

The researcher's lack of focus may also negatively impact the amount of interview data collected due to nerves, personal issues, or divided attention while taking notes, etc. Absolute concentration is necessary, and if the plan is to write up the data post-interview, the researcher must be confident about the accuracy of his or her memory. The authors, however, recommend the use of audio and/or video recordings, although such implements in themselves may disrupt the construction of rapport in the research environment. Whilst mobile phones have become ubiquitous, many respondents may feel uncomfortable having their exact words chronicled by these devices. Oftentimes, participants will hesitate to sign their names to the informed consent document which is a necessary part of their agreement to take part in any research project. If the respondents sign but do not consent to the utilization of audio/visual recordings, then the researcher must rely upon note-taking during the interview and post-data gathering recollections. Although video and aural recordings may increase the veracity of what emerged during the conversation, both authors have encountered the capriciousness of recording devices and advise the use of a backup instrument to document a participant. On the other hand, both authors have also experienced occasions when both instruments were unreliable, causing sections of data on a series of interviews to be unintelligible. The most effective protection against these types of difficulties is to take the time to write up your impressions of interviews immediately after each data collection session. If the recorded material is examined promptly and poor-quality data is discovered, researchers may be able to retrieve some of the missing information by writing up the conversation while the dialogue is still fresh in their memory. If more than one researcher is involved, then discussions immediately after an interview may reveal important insights.

Research materials

When conducting an in-depth interview or focus group in qualitative research, the investigator may introduce supplementary objects to generate dialogue and allow participants to experience a hands-on understanding of the topic. There is also the belief that initiating projective stimuli may elicit subconscious responses from the participant to visual or textual materials related to the area of study. The reactions of the participant to the introduced objects may disclose a valid indication of the participant's comprehension or, contrarily, misunderstanding of the research question. The timing of when and by what means auxiliary objects are introduced in an interview may affect the ensuing data collection. Often when researchers use supplementary materials, they believe they are employing similar data gathering procedures with all participants. However, minute irregularities in the researcher's delivery may lead to dissimilar experiences for the respondents.

Research respondents/participants/subjects

When conducting an ethnographical study, researchers carefully choose participants for their specific knowledge (experience or understanding), engagement in certain activities, or relationship to the subject matter of the investigation. In quantitative research, a researcher most commonly selects participants randomly or proportionately to represent a specified population. If an interviewee ceases to participate in a quantitative project, the researcher must be concerned about the non-representativeness of the remaining sample. The missing person's data may distort the ability to generalize from the results (i.e., the sample may become skewed). The lack of a sample's representativeness in ethnographical research is of less concern, yet the loss or absence of a participant will affect the results: the missing data (the singular details, involvement, expertise, understanding, etc.), will be unavailable to the findings. Even if the participant completes a few interviews or activities from a series before disappearing, all data gathered from this participant must be discarded.

Some of the greatest sources of error and concern in qualitative research are issues to do with respondents who wish to create a positive image of themselves. This often subconscious desire to be well regarded by the investigator (and future public) may produce atypical behaviors that may affect the research's validity. The investigator must make great efforts to dispel any doubts regarding the representation of respondents by ensuring the subject's anonymity (if desired) and the confidentiality of the study results. Nevertheless, participants may withdraw from a research project for numerous reasons: being troubled by their interview performance, feeling uncomfortable with the topic of investigation, reappraising what they said, or having doubts about how their thoughts and feelings are going to be used by the researcher. The rapport between participant and researcher often determines the trustworthiness of the data, its interpretation, the results, and the relevance of conclusions. Frequently, while disclosing information during an interview, participants will request that the material discussed be placed "off the record." This is completely permissible, and "off the record" information can still enlighten the researcher's understanding of the situation at hand. The investigator should make every effort to create an interview environment that is pleasant and comfortable: a relaxed and trusting participant discloses more information than a defensive and suspicious participant.

As stated above, healthcare professionals, due to their expertise and medical knowledge, usually possess greater authority than those they attempt to help. However, sometimes when professionals are questioned about their own field, they may perceive an inquiring researcher as intimidating and a power reversal may develop. Therefore, the researcher must always consider the pressures, often unacknowledged, of power relationships influencing a study. Differences between respondent and researcher in age, education, race, areas of knowledge, class, gender, professionalism, etc., may affect how research questions develop, how the interview is conducted, and how the final write-up is assembled. Investigators must realize that what may seem to them a common place matter could appear highly charged to the interviewee. One respondent may find certain questions relevant while another may be affronted by them. Using a field journal is sometimes helpful to record emerging conflictual conditions in order to avoid potential friction.

We, as investigators, must be conscientious about representing participants honestly and respondents must have confidence that we will represent them accurately and in a way with which they are comfortable. Participants generally receive little or no recompense for giving us their time and efforts and are central to qualitative investigations: they must not be used instrumentally. Researchers must cultivate a trust-based relationship with participants and resist misrepresentation that may be construed as harmful or untrue. In attempting to consider all the options discussed above researchers may realize that responsible research means facing difficult conflicting ethical responsibilities.

Anonymity

Participant anonymity, if requested, requires discretion which the neophyte researcher may readily give, especially in sensitive circumstances, however, the investigator must be aware that respondent anonymity means that none of the respondent's expertise, background information, or related primary data (artifacts, images, written material, etc.) will be available for inclusion as the material may hold clues to the participant's identity. To wit, background characteristics of the respondent, including the bases for their comments to be seen as authoritative, will have to be omitted, even when providing verbatim quotations from the transcript. Furthermore, one participant's request for anonymity may affect how all the other respondents in the study are presented. In some studies, named contributors may put at risk the anonymity of those participants who wish to remain unnamed. Thus, when offering anonymity, the researcher must consider that he or she may end up with an entirely anonymous sample.

Sometimes, the assigning of pseudonyms will alleviate respondents' concerns about too extensive a scrutiny into their personal perspectives or public representation. Yet, removing all recognizable attributes in the write-up are not always sufficient anonymity for some participants. Another alternative to soothing a concerned participant about the way he or she will be represented is for the researcher to explain to participants at the commencement of the interview that before the completed report is finalized, subjects may read and edit their own transcriptions to check for data accuracy. This process is called a member-check and is a way for researchers to establish their intentions to represent subjects honestly and to verify the accuracy of the information presented in the study.

Trustworthiness: biases and the member-check

Ethnographers accept the notion of the subjectivity of the researcher and thus the influence of a researcher's bias. Each investigator brings his or her own distinctive experiences, preconceived ideas, and personal outlook to collecting and interpreting data. *Bracketing* is the name given to a method used in qualitative research that strives to reduce these inherent individual biases. As investigators commence a project, they must reflect and declare all the features of their identity that may impact the collection and analyses of data. In contrast to quantitative research with its quest for validity, qualitative enquiry seeks to establish the trustworthiness of the data presented.

A researcher may also attempt to improve trustworthiness through the above-mentioned strategy of the *member-check*. The respondent is given the option to edit the material and return the revised version to the researcher. This process can continue until both researcher and respondent concur that the interview data is represented accurately. Often respondents produce thoughtful corrections that clarify misconceptions. However, participants may discover they no longer support their documented statements and wish to either remove those comments or completely change their stated positions. Some participants told the authors that they wanted to replace ambiguous statements with more confident terminology, others wished to edit their statements such as "It is" to "It might be" to sound less peremptory. Another unintended predicament developed when a respondent perceived a bias in the manner in which the first author represented him in the final report. He challenged the style in which the researcher had documented their conversation. He noticed the interviewer's dialogue was summarized, thus appearing succinct and word perfect, whilst his language was captured verbatim, incorporating all of his grammatical flaws and idiosyncrasies. He believed this manner of presentation could be understood as a strategy to promote the interviewer's point of view over his own. This unintentional effect of the style of her report was a complete surprise to the author. She believed the goal of the report was to present the respondent's thoughts in his very own words and not those of the researcher's. The collected data in her study had been extensive and substantial editing was necessary to make a readable account for publication. The author made the decision to condense her own talk in order to be able to use direct quotations from the participant, thereby capturing the most authentic portrayal of his viewpoint. Sometimes inequity is attributed to interviewers because their language may appear more eloquent than participants due to their understanding of the research topic and their reading of pre-written questions. Yet in this case the author had to acknowledge the respondent's complaint: her representations of interviewer and interviewee were not portrayed in an equivalent manner. Thus, without changing the participant's actual words, a researcher may construct an account differing from what an interviewee might expect: any selection or elimination of data could adjust the perspective of the completed document.

The consideration at the center of the previous example is one that reflects how a recording of ordinary speech differs from participants' expectations of language based upon their experience of novels, films, theatre, etc. Everyday conversation includes all types of utterances, yet eliminating any expression from a transcript may be deemed an alteration of what took place during the interview. For example, even deleting pronouncements such as "you know" which may convey solidarity (Are you with me?), or "ah-huh" an affirmation (I know), or "hmmm," hesitation (I need to think about that) along with any other vocal sounds, repetitions, pauses, etc., may reshape the nature of the dialogue. These types of utterances may communicate mutual understanding, eagerness, doubt, incredulity, reassurance, misgivings, indecision, hostility, acceptance, etc., and are all indicators of researcher and participant rapport.

The inexperienced researcher is best to be apprised of these difficulties associated with the in-depth interview. The authors reiterate that respondents may like to revise data to complement their role in the dialogue. What was intended as a joint scrutinization of the accuracy of particulars may become "participant profile-management" effecting the significance of the collected material. On the other hand, if a researcher declines to offer a *member-check,* the truthfulness of his or her interpretation of the discussed issues may not be supported by the respondent. Not only could the data's credibility be disputed but the study may also lose the benefit of the participant's continued cooperation and insight.

Another difficulty with the *member-check* may occur when a respondent wishes to exit a study after reading the report and that person's data is uniquely significant to the research. The first author experienced this distressing situation in an investigation in which all of the other study participants had enthusiastically examined her interpretations and provided useful criticism. She found the other participants' scrutiny of the data and comments had improved the trustworthiness of her study, confirming to her the positive value of the *member-check*. However, in this case, she was obliged to withhold one participant's unique information from the final report. Thus, when addressing contentious ideas or circumstances, a researcher must realize that an investigation could be compromised if data important to the study cannot be represented due to the concerns of even one participant.

In an attempt to avoid some of these ethical quandaries, a reciprocal agreement between respondent and researcher may be constructed prior to the interview. This contract might specify the sorts (and quantity) of alterations the participant will be permitted to carry out and also state the limits of the role of the researcher. However, being asked to sign this sort of contract before an interview might suggest to respondents that they may not approve of the final presentation of the research: a feeling of suspicion may be introduced and hinder the desired rapport between researcher and participant. If trustworthiness is not achieved, the study will suffer. Qualitative research strives to challenge the participants' thinking in unusual ways through the interview process and to enhance their understanding of the research topic and of themselves. How an investigator emends a written representation ought to be determined by the research questions and the topic of study whilst respecting all participants.

A final *member-check* consideration worthy of mention is again related to contributors' concerns about how they will be regarded by their peers, culture, and families if identified within a study. Most often, providing anonymity assuages these fears, yet allocating false names and removing distinguishable characteristics may not be sufficient. One participant wanted to review how his responses contrasted with the other cases in the study. one requested a gender alteration to further obscure recognition, and one contributor asked for all of her negative statements to be removed so that she would be regarded in a more positive light. Consequently, when a researcher employs the *member-check,* she or he must be mindful that any study, but especially one that could be controversial, may be compromised due to altered or eliminated data affecting the trustworthiness of the results. Another difficulty influencing rapport is that contributors may not understand that some privacy will be sacrificed when permitting an interview. Also, novel topics may emerge in an interview and the respondent may be confronted with unexpected questions about (uncomfortable) issues. Another strain on rapport is when an investigator decides to "go native" (identifying with some, or all, of the cultural traits of the participant) during the interview period, but upon returning to an academic environment, reshapes his or her position with a more scholarly viewpoint.

As the *member-check* may be fraught with difficulties, how else might a qualitative researcher establish trustworthiness in a study? *Triangulation* is a process that attempts to supplement the validity of an analysis, in which at least two other researchers examine the raw data of a study and conduct a separate analysis in order to reconcile or invalidate the researchers' initial conclusions. *Triangulation* may be utilized to decrease inaccuracies, challenge misleading information, and actually produce more in-depth data. However, *triangulation* is not considered to have standardized protocols that reliably test subjective assessments. Moreover, other researchers may have their own agendas when assessing your data, which may, consciously or sub-consciously, influence their evaluation of your interpretations. The difficulty here is to find other investigators with an interest in your topic who have the proficiency and time to make a comprehensive assessment of your findings.

Data conversion, interpretations, and meaning-making

Other significant areas in need of consideration in qualitative research become evident after the completion of the data gathering process. This data may materialize in the form of written notes, video recordings, still images, and audio accounts, etc., all of which must address the research questions and be converted into information that is comparable between data collection approaches. This conversion process is often more difficult than at first thought and may result in multiple inaccuracies. In qualitative research, collected data is usually transcribed into written text through reduction, summarization, and interpretation—all processes which create opportune conditions for making mistakes (especially when a neophyte researcher strives to make the data "fit" the research questions).

Interpretation of a body of material begins with data coding which involves recognizing and extricating the important words, phrases, and significant groupings of text from the transcript. Researchers must analyze the components of data through direct impressions in order to make meaning of the respondent's utterances. However, any process involving interpretation, modification, explanation, reduction, etc., may produce errors in meaning as perspectives of respondent and researcher may differ. To make sense of data requires a particular type of artful interpretation founded upon diligent and methodical inspection. The examiner begins the meaning-making process by citing multiple references within the recorded dialogue, etc., while also noting a participant's intricate efforts and strategies to make sense of the issues addressed by the research questions. The analyst must document characteristics of the interviewee's lived experiences as well as particulars of how his or her reactions were formed within the context of the interview.

There are multiple approaches available when undertaking analyses of textual data, including: discourse analysis, narrative analysis, content analysis, thematic analysis, and grounded theory. A popular method for examining qualitative data is a combination of content and thematic analysis: *content-based thematic analysis*. This procedure is utilized to determine the elements of analysis in the data/content (understood as a participant's explicitly stated narrative in terms of what happened and to whom, when, where, etc., along with attributes of the underlying conceptualizations implicit in the text). These elements arise from the comments, opinions, and ideas recorded in the conversation, as well as the emerging patterns (themes, and subthemes) found in the more descriptive data.

Analysis begins through a close examination of the interview story and a selection of words, sentences, or short paragraphs (sometimes known as *chunks*). The researcher then assigns these *chunks* to specific categories in an attempt to understand and organize the meanings communicated through them. However, the term *meaning* carries multiple levels of understanding. The first author favors a description of the nature of meaning defined in Webster's Seventh New Collegiate Dictionary:

1a: *the thing one intends to convey especially by language:* PURPORT; b: *the thing that is conveyed especially by language:* IMPORT; 2: INTENT, PURPOSE; 3: SIGNIFICANCE; 4a: CONNOTATION b: DENOTATION.

The above definitions illustrate how the term "meaning" can be associated with conveyance, intention, purpose, significance, implication, indication, etc., and can be understood to make known, signify, bring out, suggest, represent, etc. a message of importance, most commonly through language. To construct such an understanding, the researcher must decide how to identify the components or word *chunks* in a text that elucidate that which is important to the respondent. However, there is no one correct way of assigning meaning to significant components of an observation, narrative, etc.

Qualitative research is unique in the research field in that investigators are expected to utilize their intuition and propose knowledgeable impressions when making meaning from research data. Moreover, qualitative research does not consider the researcher's subjective and essential understandings as inaccuracies. Intelligently designed research protocols that are clearly identified and abided by are capable of proffering set limits upon research while curtailing error, misinterpretations, and value judgments. Such protocols include the declarative mapping sentence.

Below, we provide characteristic difficulties confronting a qualitative researcher when making meaning from research data. These details are based upon an analysis conducted by the first author. Her study comprised six in-depth interviews with the resultant audio recordings converted into 140 pages of written text. She went over and over the transcripts to give shape to a working summary of their content. She jotted down comments about each interaction and when she found parts of the dialogues unclear or questioned her own inferences, she asked for advice from another researcher. Ambiguous elements were underlined and annotations reflecting her impressions, interpretations, and revelations were scribbled in the text's margins. Each interview was read once again along with another round of note-taking in order to clarify contrasts and similarities between participants' points of view. She also examined these notes for evidence of whether her interview style had influenced the dialogues. Finally, she developed category headings that seemed to produce a logical and consistent structure to the interviews and placed data under these headings, especially noting both recurrent and uncommon remarks. Despite following a thorough protocol, the first author could not claim unbiased analyses. She also bore in mind that most respondents had talked about their complaints about the service being examined. She realized her efforts to encourage participants to divulge more in-depth particulars about the research question had developed into an underlying feature of the interview process. Furthermore, she was unsure that she had mined all significant messages and meanings from the data. Only after her analyses had been perused by other researchers did she become confident about her interpretation of the data.

Context and external influences upon the research findings

The concept of *context* and its effects upon the research findings is extensive within a qualitative study. The notion includes: the choice of the physical setting of the investigation; the researcher's quest for understanding; broad issues of identity, i.e. the relationship between interviewer and interviewee (their values and thoughts); as well as wider events occurring during the data collection period (the interface between historical, economic, political and cultural forces). Further external influences to be addressed by an investigator include: time of day, time of year, or variations of these; other persons present during data collection; the length of the data gathering period; atmospheric effects (temperature, lighting, noise, etc.). All these features and circumstances may have some impact upon the research findings.

Generalizing from your data

Another ethical consideration bearing scrutiny is when qualitative researchers attempt to use conclusions from a specific project and make these findings relevant to persons other than those investigated in that study. This is applying the process of *generalization* which may be the explicit or implicit aim of practically all research writing. Nevertheless, the qualitative investigator must be reminded that small non-random samples are not representative of a greater population. While conducting qualitative investigations within the medical care industry, researchers may be confronted with circumstances in which a single person alone possesses the knowledge or experience to answer specific research questions. In this type of situation, the in-depth study is the most comprehensive research method available as it allows the investigator to vigorously examine the life story/biography of the selected participant. However, despite the fact that narrative is a formidable agent for substantiating a theoretical standpoint, studies comprised of only a few individuals and their stories are not representative of how other people think, feel, and act. Investigators must be mindful of these sorts of limitations and intelligibly portray these restrictions within the research report.

Conclusion

In this chapter we have attempted to create a conversation around the various ethical concerns relevant to qualitative/ethnographic research. We aspired to draw the reader's attention to numerous and diverse sources of inaccuracies that may complicate the conduction of a rigorous ethnographical investigation. The series of ethical considerations described above are not intended to be an all-inclusive inventory but mere suggestions to kindle interest and understanding of the difficulties inherent within ethnographic inquiry and to encourage discussion among medical care researchers.

Note

1 This chapter is based on a previous chapter, Ethnographic Caveats, Hackett, P.M.W. & Schwarzenbach, J.B., (2015). In P.M.W. Hackett (Ed.), *Qualitative research methods in consumer psychology: Ethnography and culture*. New York, NY: Routledge.

3

ETHICS OF ONLINE RESEARCH WITH HUMAN PARTICIPANTS

Jeff Gavin and Karen Rodham

Introduction

In 2017, we wrote a short think piece on research ethics in the digital age (Gavin & Rodham, 2017). We had been invited to write that article for two reasons. First, our experience of conducting research in the online world. Between us we have worked on projects ranging from: online support for eating disorders, self-harm, and persistent pain to studies exploring dating, sexting, online intimacy, and revenge porn. We have also collected data using various online sources such as public forums; private bespoke forums; social media such as Facebook, Instagram, and Twitter; online dating sites; as well as traditional "pen and paper" surveys disseminated and completed via online platforms, such as Qualtrics. And second, when we first began to use the online world in our research, we quickly realized that ethics panels were (in our opinion) overly anxious about the ethics of doing so. They seemed to struggle to understand this kind of research, not just from a practical but also an ethical point of view. As a consequence, alongside our research, we decided that we ought to write about the ethics of conducting research on (and in) the online world.

What is online research?

Put very simply, we define online research as research which is conducted in or by the Internet or in or by digital social media. The British Psychological Society (2017, p. 3) uses the term "Internet Mediated Research", and broadly defines it as "any research involving the remote acquisition of data from or about human participants using the internet and its associated technologies". So, a researcher may decide to conduct an online study – perhaps running a survey using the online survey platform Qualtrics. Maybe they will prefer to run focus groups with people from all over the world joining in. Maybe they will collect data that they can subsequently analyze – for example, Instagram posts, Tweets, snapchats and so forth. Indeed, the Internet and digital social media present researchers with myriad opportunities to recruit and collect data from a diverse range of participants (e.g. Brownlow & O'Dell, 2002; Roberts, 2015; Skitka & Sargis, 2006), in ways that are often cheaper than traditional methods (e.g., no travel costs, no postage costs). The online environment also allows researchers to observe behaviour and communication (e.g. Kraut, Olson, Banaji, Bruckman, Cohen, & Couper, 2004).

Box 3.1 Illustration of the multi-layered online world, example adapted from Alexander (2008)

A YouTube member uploads a video. Others comment on this video, which is subsequently discovered by other Internet users through social aggregators and search services. These people add comments to the original video entry (which they might link to from their own YouTube, Facebook or Twitter accounts via "liking" or "sharing" the video or "following" the original poster), view the video, and add further comments on YouTube, thus intensifying and contributing further to a networked discussion across multiple sites, with multiple authors and with new text, hypertext, and audio-visual content.

What is wrong with existing research ethics guidelines?

The online world is continually evolving and has multiple layers which bring the potential for unintended consequences. This means that it is impossible for there to be a clear set of all-encompassing rules. Think for a moment about fake news (the intentional presentation of misinformation) and the more recent "deep fake" video examples. A deep fake video consists of manipulated videoclips in which someone else's face is inserted into pre-existing videos frame by frame. As a short aside, the videos are called deep fakes after the Reddit user called "deepfake" who first created them (Guera & Delp, 2018). It is not always easy to recognize fake news and deep fakes are, as is suggested by their name, deeply hidden and almost impossible to determine as "fake". As such, this creates a challenge for future researchers in the form of a philosophical and ethical question: "What is real?" We do not intend to answer this complex question here. Instead we have argued (Gavin & Rodham, 2017) that researchers need to accept that ethics for our digital age requires the development of a different mindset, one that maintains the central ethical mantra of "do no harm" – but does so not through traditional clear cut "if-then" rules and regulations but through the process of solving puzzles. Indeed, just as in "real life", we cannot control for all eventualities; in the multi-layered online world we need to think about different questions: What counts as data? Whose permission do we need to seek to use the data? What data, even if we can see it, might be considered private? How do we define open access? What happens if someone who is a private user links and contributes to a multi-site discussion? Does this then render his or her contribution public? (See Box 3.1) Whose permission do you need to seek? How would you solve this ethical puzzle?

We have already mentioned the difficulties ethics panels have had when assessing our applications for ethical approval. It is also clear that our professional bodies have grappled with similar dilemmas. They have struggled to produce ethical guidelines that can keep abreast of the fast-changing online world. In 2002, the British Sociological Association (BSA) decided that it was more appropriate to put the onus on the researchers themselves, as part of their professional competence, to keep abreast of developments in online research:

> Members should take special care when carrying out research via the Internet. [...]
> Members who carry out research online should ensure that they are familiar with
> ongoing debates on the ethics of Internet research and might wish to consider erring

on the side of caution in making judgements affecting the well-being of online research participants.

(BSA, 2002)

More recently, the British Sociological Association (2017) published their "Statement of Ethical Practice" which has a separate annex entitled "Ethics Guidelines and Collated Resources for Digital Research". Both documents can be downloaded from the Association's "Guidelines on ethical research" website. These two documents, and particularly the annex, offer a more in-depth exploration of the possible ethical issues surrounding online research. But the conclusion is very similar: that the field is fast moving and that there are likely to be unintended, and possibly currently unimaginable, consequences of researching in and on the online world. And, as a result, the researchers themselves, need to be willing and able to engage in an ethically appropriate manner:

> [...] we should remember that 'the fields of internet research are dynamic and heterogeneous [as] reflected in the fact that as of the time of this writing, no official guidance or 'answers' regarding internet research ethics have been adopted at any national or international level' (AoIR, 2012: 2). Aside from ever-changing technological contexts, and the unstable public/private distinction, the AoIR [Association of Internet Researchers] also identifies the complex and unresolved relationship between data and persons: 'Is one's digital information an extension of the self?' The data/person relationship is a central issue for research ethics, as ethics aim to minimise harm, and harm is typically understood in relation to 'persons' (2012: 3, 6–7). This all leads back to reiterating a dynamic, situational, process-based and dialogic approach to ethical digital research; where you anticipate that unforeseen situations, issues, and technologies may arise, and you are prepared to engage in an ongoing way.
>
> *(BSA, 2017, p. 8)*

Similarly, the British Psychological Society's (BPS) second edition of the Internet-Mediated Research Guidelines (2017) recognized that as technology advances, changes, and grows, it extends the opportunities for research whilst at the same time, introduces extra complexities in ways that might not at first be obvious. The second edition BPS Internet-Mediated Research Guidelines (2017) highlight the issues facing researchers and the need for ethical guidelines *not* to be used as a rule book, but as a set of guiding principles. In short, it is not possible to have a set of ethical rules that can deal with all situations. How then, as researchers, do we uphold the essence of our ethical principles when conducting research in and on the online world?

In this chapter we set out to address this question by returning to the three universal principles that underpin the notion of "do no harm" with respect to how we go about conduct ethical research:

- respect for the autonomy, privacy, and dignity of individuals and communities;
- scientific integrity;
- maximizing benefits and minimizing harm

We will structure our chapter according to these universal principles and will share good and bad practices to demonstrate how we can work towards maintaining the overarching goal of ethical research: do no harm to your participants.

Respect for the autonomy, privacy, and dignity of individuals and communities

In the online world, working out what is public and what is private is not straightforward. How do we label different types of information that could become data if we collect it? How can we be sure that someone posting information online knows or expects it to be public? Does it matter if information is posted (and collected for research) on discussion forums, Twitter, YouTube or Facebook? Should researchers be asking themselves the following question: just because we *can* collect online information, *should* we? For example, at the time of writing, the default setting on Qualtrics (a simple-to-use, web-based survey tool) is set to collect data on the precise location of respondents. This is not unique to Qualtrics; many data harvesting software packages for collecting Tweets have the same default setting. Failure to turn off such features means that it is possible to conduct analyses which may reveal people's personal characteristics and potentially their identity, which they may have assumed to be private.

In the UK, the recent introduction of the General Data Protection Regulations (GDPR) published by the Information Commissioner's Office (2018) has highlighted the problem related to collecting data "just because you can". In essence the GDPR is Europe's new framework for data protection laws. The UK Research and Innovation organization (UKRI) has a very useful summary for how the GDPR impacts researchers. One of the requirements of the GDPR is that researchers must have a clear rationale for collecting different types of personal data. Personal data is described as information that relates to an identified or identifiable individual. This could be a person's name or might include other identifiers such as an IP address or a cookie identifier. The key issue here is that if it is possible to identify a person directly from the information being collected and analyzed, then that information may be personal data.

In addition to ensuring that we consider carefully what counts as personal data, the GDPR also introduces the notion of data minimization. This refers to the expectation that only data which is relevant to the research in question will be collected. In other words researchers need to be able to demonstrate that they have appropriate processes in place to ensure that they only collect and hold the personal data they need. In other words, gathering or collecting information just because you can access it is not permissible unless you have clear rationale that links back to your research question. In the same way that researchers must, in effect, seek consent from their ethical bodies to collect data, so too should they seek informed consent from their participants.

Under GDPR, even data collection methods that may previously have seemed straightforward, quite rightly require further thought. For example, if we choose to collect data by means of a quantitative online survey, how can we be sure that a participant who shuts down their web browser has simply decided that they no longer wish to participate or that they have decided to withdraw consent? How can we be sure it is still okay for us to use the data we collected before they shut down their web browser? The BPS (2017) suggests that these kind of potential issues should be anticipated and withdrawal procedures made as clear and robust as possible. One example offered is to display a clearly visible "exit" or "withdraw" button on each page of a survey. If participants were to click on this button they could then be taken to a debrief page and a tick box section asking participants to confirm they are still happy for their data to be included in the study.

For qualitative research there are different considerations. If a member decides they no longer wish to participate and withdraws from the discussion in the same way those participating in a face-to-face focus group have the option to do, what should a researcher do with the data? Omitting that person's contributions is likely to render the other participants' words meaningless. A focus group is, by its very nature, interactive; what one member of the group says will build on the contributions of others. Removing one voice can mean that the whole group discussion is unusable. However, as long as an information sheet is explicit about the process of withdrawal, this issue can be prevented. For example, it is common for those being invited to take part in face-to-face focus groups to be told that they can withdraw from the group discussion itself, at any time, *but* that all contributions they have made up to that point *will* be included in the analysis. The same clause could easily be included in information sheets for online focus groups.

Ethical concern about consent in the context of online studies is illustrated well by the following study where researchers had sought consent from what they considered appropriate sources. In 2008, a team of experienced researchers in the USA published a study based on data taken from the Facebook profiles of the entire cohort of a U.S. university (Lewis, Kaufman, & Christakis, 2008, see Zimmer, 2010 for review). Their focus was on how friendships and tastes develop over time. The researchers had permission from both Facebook and the university in question and had also received ethical approval from the relevant boards. They downloaded each student's name, gender, major, and their network of friends, including who was tagged in their photos. They collected information on tastes, political views, and romantic interests, and inferred students' race from their photos and group membership. Students from the same university were used as research assistants to access this information because, in 2006, Facebook privacy was predominantly based on university networks, and only those in the same network could see your profile. This meant that these research assistant-students had access to the profiles that the researchers themselves could not access.

In accordance with ethical guidelines, permission to use the data was not sought from the users, but the data were anonymized and all identifying information (such as names and identification numbers) removed from the published data. Unfortunately, as regular social media users know, it is not difficult to use indirect means to find somebody on Facebook. In this case the university was identifiable by its unique characteristics (e.g., the number of students, the combination of degrees offered), and from here individual students could easily be identified, particularly if they were in some way unique (such as the only female Latvian law major, to take a hypothetical example). The net result was that participants did not consent to their data being used, and worse, their anonymity was not protected.

Scientific integrity

Ensuring research maintains the principle of scientific integrity means that it "should be designed, reviewed, and conducted in a way that ensures its quality, integrity, and contribution to the development of knowledge and understanding" (British Psychology Society, 2014, p. 9). If a research study is not designed well or is conducted poorly then it is effectively a wasted opportunity. A poorly designed or implemented study will not collect high quality data. As such, it wastes resources (financial, equipment, time) and more importantly devalues the contribution of the participants and, in so doing, affords them a great lack of respect. At worst, such research may lead to inaccurate or misleading information being shared or influencing subsequent research, policy decisions, and so forth, and as such, it can have the potential to cause harm. Researchers must therefore ensure that their work meets high quality, robust scientific and scholarly standards.

Scientific integrity vs participant safety

The underpinning principle of scientific integrity is very clear and unambiguous. However, scientific integrity can conflict with the need to keep participants safe. For example, when conducting qualitative research the actual words used by participants are important. How people say things, the words *they* choose to use when talking about things are important. However, unlike face-to-face interviews or focus groups, collecting text from online sources brings the potential that the extracts could be placed into a search engine and the original interaction or posting identified and with that identification comes the risk that the person's identity could be traced and revealed. For example, the BPS guidelines note that:

> On a legal note, should a person find out that their online posts or traces of activity have been accessed, stored and used as research data, they are likely to have rights under the Data Protection Act to stop these data being processed if they could be linked to them personally. In many cases it is very unlikely that a person will ever find out that their online posts have been used for research purposes. However, this does not preclude the responsibility of the researcher to ensure that maximal anonymisation procedures are implemented (for example, researchers may consider paraphrasing any verbatim quotes so as to reduce the risk of these being traced to source, and participants iden-tified). Here again, the principle of proportionality becomes pertinent: considerations of the level of risk/harm must be weighed up against scientific value, the quality and authenticity of reports of research findings, and possible practical issues too.
>
> *(BPS, 2017, p. 14)*

This then provides us with a clear example of a time when scientific integrity – using the data as it was collected – may be outweighed by the need to ensure participants' confidenti-ality is maintained. This might well involve paraphrasing verbatim quotes in order to reduce the risk that what someone said online can be traced back to them. The paraphrasing would be completed post analysis and so would not impact on the researcher's ability to interpret the data they have collected; it may however, render the report of the study less convincing to the reader (and journal reviewers), perhaps even undermining the epistemological and ontological bases of the study (for example, in the case of Foucauldian discourse analysis or narrative analysis where it is language and the way in which language is used which is central to the analysis).

The decision to paraphrase (or not) also has consequences for replication. We are thinking here of the fact that there is currently a drive towards ensuring research is both open and trans-parent. As such, it is becoming more common for researchers to be expected to deposit their data in an open science repository. What then should we do with qualitative data collected from the online world? If we need to paraphrase it in order to protect anonymity and confidentiality of our participants (who, by the way, if the data was collected from a publicly accessible site, may be unaware that their words have been used in research), should we deposit the paraphrased text or the original text? If we do the latter, we are potentially opening up the possibility that our participants may be identified. If we do the former, the data available for other researchers to analyze is not the actual data that was collected, which defeats the purpose of open science.

A solution used by one of the authors of this chapter (JG) in disseminating his research on online dating is to illustrate his arguments with screenshots of his own (mock) online dating profile (Gavin & Griffin, 2012). Similarly, in a series of recent studies examining the perceived attractiveness of autistic males' online dating profiles, the same author and his colleagues first analyzed the actual profiles of autistic male online daters, and then used this analysis to create a prototypical profile to use (and manipulate) in a number of online experiments (Gavin, Rees-Evans, Duckett, & Brosnan, 2019). As it was considered ethically impossible to use profile photos of real online daters, the researchers used an "average" face comprised of a composite image created by averaging and then combining the shape and colour information of a number of individual facial photographs using specialized software.

In contrast, for our research on images of self-harm posted on a public forum (Rodham, Gavin, Lewis, St Denis, & Bandalli, 2013), creating "mock up" images would have been inappropriate. The images *were* the data, therefore we needed to analyze the images themselves. We took two approaches to maintaining the scientific integrity of our data whilst also ensuring participant safety. During the dissemination phase of this study, we only used images of self-harm that contained no identifying information such as faces or a distinctive background. This rendered them privately public; that is, private in the sense that they contained no identifying information, but public in that anyone could see them (Lange, 2007). Our second strategy was to publish a content analysis of the images without including the images themselves. In each of the cases cited above, ethical and methodological compromises are made in consideration with the specific research questions, type of analyses, and social context of the online site in/on which the research is conducted.

Maximizing benefits and minimizing harm

Maximizing benefit and minimizing harm refers to the aspiration that the research conducted brings the most benefit it can without harming, or, at the very least, minimizing the risk of actual or potential harm as a consequence of data collection, analysis and publication. In short, this process is about "ensuring scientific value (maximizing benefits) and taking steps to protect participants from any adverse effects arising from the research" (BSA, 2017, p. 18).

In whatever social context we as researchers work, we should be mindful and respectful of social structures. The BPS code of human research ethics (2014, p. 10) states: "unwarranted or unnecessary disruption should be avoided unless the psychologist judges that the benefits of intervention outweigh the costs of such disruption". This holds for online research and comes back to the difficulty that sometimes arises in distinguishing between what is considered a private or a public online space by users. It is not necessarily the interventions themselves that are potentially harmful, but their possible scope for compromising the anonymity/confidentiality of participants. Researchers should consider such potential unintended consequences. For example, if researchers enter open access online spaces that are considered private by their users, their presence is likely to be unwelcome, their arrival considered invasive and potentially socially irresponsible. To mitigate this, if the proposed research is highly valued in terms of scientific integrity and potential benefits, then a researcher might feel that joining a group without disclosing that they are a researcher is an appropriate course of action. Doing so will enable them to undertake undisclosed observation and data collection whilst avoiding disrupting the space and causing potential harm perhaps to group cohesion. However, this strategy is not to be taken lightly, for it brings with it potentially serious negative consequence for those being studied. For example, Roberts (2015) shared an example of what happened when an online community learned later that they had been the focus of a research study. One community member commented:

> When I joined this, I thought it would be a support group, not a fishbowl for a bunch
> of guinea pigs. I certainly don't feel at this point that it is a safe environment, as a

support group is supposed to be, and I will not open myself up to be dissected by students or scientists.

(King, 1996, p. 122)

The expectations of those being researched must be considered, anticipated, and taken into account when planning research. This in itself is not straightforward:

Defining a space from the 'outside', based on access, and from the 'inside' based on participants' experience of the social activities taking place ... are two different positions that do not necessarily correspond.

(Bromseth, 2003, p. 73)

Whose perspective about access is correct? How do social media users feel about researchers lurking and gathering data? Hudson and Bruckman (2004) showed that users' expectation of privacy often conflicts with the public setting in which their interactions take place. While they may be interacting in a public space, they behave (and it seems, expect to be treated), as if this is a private space. Conversely, Hargittai and Marwick (2016) have explored the 'privacy paradox' from another angle: when individuals claim to be concerned about privacy whilst their behaviour, especially online, runs counter to these concerns. From this point of view, there is a recognition that even if you personally have concerns and do all you can to maintain your privacy, once something is online it can generate a life of its own. One of their participants sums this up neatly:

On Facebook, I think it's been drilled into me that you just have to assume anything you post is public. You can set your privacy settings at the strictest you want, but you just have to assume that anything you put out there can be made public to the world.

(Hargittai & Marwick, 2016, p. 3746)

What, then, are we as researchers to do about this paradox? As with much of this multilayered online world, there is no straightforward solution. How do we as researchers do the right thing without inadvertently doing the wrong thing? If a researcher announces their presence overtly, it is likely that how that group interacts may change. If a researcher lurks and, in effect, surreptitiously collects data, they run the risk of compromising the group if their presence is subsequently recognized.

Conclusion

At the start of this chapter we posed the question: if it is not possible to have a set of ethical rules that can deal with all situations, how then, as researchers, do we uphold the essence of our ethical principles when conducting research in and on the online world? This is an important question for us as researchers to consider, for the online world has made it both easier and harder than ever to conduct research. The landscape of the online world changes so rapidly that the British Sociological Association (2017) clearly stated that it was not possible to create guidelines that would be able to address all current and future forms of digital research that may become possible. This is an issue picked up by Kosinski, Matz, Gosling, Popov, and Stillwell (2015) who noted that when they were writing their article, the American Psychological Association's website only listed three documents containing guidelines relating to research on the Internet, all of which had been written before Facebook came into being. This inability to keep up with the fast-changing online world means that the onus is on both ethics committees and researchers to approach online research with an open, curious, and pragmatic mind, that at all times has the phrase "*do no harm*" at its centre. In other words, the basic ethical principles underpinning research remain universal: 1) do no harm, 2) respect the autonomy, privacy, and dignity of participants, 3) maintain scientific integrity, and 4) maximize the benefits and minimise the harm of research. What is different is how these principles might be applied in a fast changing, multi-layered context with the high risk of unintended consequences. How the principles are applied and how unexpected happenings are dealt with will rely on the researchers' and ethics committees' ability to act carefully with due diligence with the information they have at that time. In summary, as far as researchers who conduct online research are concerned, we feel that they would do well to heed the words that have been ascribed to Maya Angelou:

Do the best you can until you know better. Then when you know better, do better.

References

Alexander, B. (2008). Web 2.0 and emergent multiliteracies. *Theory into Practice, 47*(2), 150–160.

AoIR, (Association of Internet Researchers) (2012). *Ethical Decision-Making and Internet Research.* Available at: http://aoir.org/ethics/

British Psychological Society (2014). *BPS Code of Human Research Ethics.* www.bps.org.uk/news-and-policy/bps-code-ethics-and-conduct

British Psychological Society (2017). *Ethics Guidelines for Internet-Mediated Research.* www.bps.org.uk/news-and-policy/ethics-guidelines-internet-mediated-research-2017

British Sociological Association (2002). www.britsoc.co.uk/media/24310/bsa_statement_of_ethical_practice.pdf

British Sociological Association (2017). Statement of Ethical Practice. www.britsoc.co.uk/ethics

British Sociological Association (2017). Ethics Guidelines and Collated Resources for Digital Research. www.britsoc.co.uk/ethics

Bromseth, J. (2003). Ethical and methodological challenges in research on net-mediated communication in a Norwegian research context. In M. Sorseth (Ed.), *Applied ethics in Internet research* (pp. 67–85). Trondheim, Norway: NTNU University Press.

Brownlow, C., & O'Dell, L. (2002). Ethical issues for qualitative research in on-line communities. *Disability & Society, 17,* 685–694.

Gavin, J., Rees-Evans, D., Duckett, A., & Brosnan, M.J. (2019). The attractiveness, trustworthiness and desirability of autistic males' online dating profiles. *Computers in Human Behavior, 98,* 18195.

Gavin, J., & Griffin, C. (2012). The technological affordances of online dating sites: A comparative study. 10th Asia Pacific Conference on Computer Human Interaction (APCHI2012), August 28–31, Matsue, Japan.

Gavin, J., & Rodham, K. (2017). Ethical research in the digital age. *Psychology Review,* 2–5.

General Data Protection Regulations: https://ico.org.uk/for-organisations/guide-to-data-protection/guide-to-the-general-data-protection-regulation-gdpr/

Guera, D., & Delp, E.J. (2018). *Deepfake Video Detection Using Recurrent Neural Networks.* 15th IEEE International Conference on Advanced Video and Signal Based Surveillance (AVSS). DOI: 10.1109/AVSS.2018.8639163

Hargittai, E., & Marwick, A. (2016). "What Can I Really Do?": Explaining the Privacy Paradox with Online Apathy. *International Journal of Communication, 10,* 3737–3757.

Hudson, J.M., & Bruckman, A. (2004). "Go away": Participant objections to being studied and the ethics of chatroom research. *The Information Society, 20,* 127–139.

King, S. (1996). Researching internet communities: proposed ethical guidelines for the reporting of the results. *The Information Society, 12*(2), 119–127.

Kosinski, M., Matz, S.C., Gosling, S.D., Popov, V. & Stillwell, D. (2015). Facebook as a research tool for the social sciences: Opportunities, challenges, ethical considerations, and practical guidelines. *American Psychologist, 70*(6), 543–556.

Kraut, R., Olson, J., Banaji, M., Bruckman, A., Cohen, J., & Couper, M. (2004). Psychological research online: report of Board of Scientific Affairs' Advisory Group on the conduct of research on the internet. *American Psychologist, 59*, 105–117.

Lange, P. G. (2007). Publicly private and privately public: Social networking on YouTube. *Journal of computer-mediated communication, 13*(1), 361–380.

Lewis, K., Kaufman, J. & Christakis, N. (2008). The Taste for Privacy: An Analysis of College Student Privacy Settings in an Online Social Network. *Journal of Computer-Mediated Communication, 14*(1), 79–100.

Roberts, L. (2015). Ethical Issues in Conducting Qualitative Research in Online Communities. *Qualitative Research in Psychology. 12*(3), 314–325.

Rodham, K., Gavin, J., Lewis, S., St Denis, J., & Bandalli, P. (2013). An investigation of the motivations driving the online representation of self-injury. *Archives of Suicide Research, 17*(3), 173–183).

Skitka, L.J. & Sargis, E.G. (2006). The Internet as psychological laboratory, *Annual Review of Psychology, 57*, 529–555.

Zimmer, M. (2010). "But the data is already public": On the ethics of research in Facebook. *Ethics and Information Technology, 12*, 313–325.

4

CULTURAL VARIATION IN INFORMED CONSENT FOR CLINICAL RESEARCH PARTICIPATION

David Resnik and Julia Hecking

Introduction

Informed consent is one of the cornerstones of ethical research with human subjects and has occupied a prominent place in numerous guidelines, regulations, and laws ever since its appearance in the *Nuremberg Code* in 1947 (Resnik 2018). Although most people living in Western countries are familiar with the concept of informed consent and would not question its importance, this was not always the case. Indeed, informed consent did not become a standard part of medical practice in the U.S. and other Western nations until the 1960s (Berg, Applebaum, Parker, & Lidz 2001). Also, in some parts of the world the idea that an individual has the right to give his or her informed consent for medical care or research participation is a foreign notion (Macklin 1999). In this chapter, we will examine the ethical and legal basis of informed consent and review the published research on cultural variation in informed consent for clinical research participation.

Brief history of informed consent

For many years, medical practice in Western nations was paternalistic insofar as doctors often made decisions for patients without presenting them with information they needed to know about their condition or their options for treatment. Even when patients were presented with information and options, they often deferred the decision to the doctor. This paternalistic ethic was based on the Hippocratic Oath, which instructs doctors to benefit their patients and protect confidentiality but says nothing about the patient's right to make medical decisions. Informed consent started to become incorporated into clinical practice during the 1960s and 1970s as a result of the Patient's Rights Movement and some influential court decisions related to medical malpractice (Faden & Beauchamp 1986. In *Canterbury v. Spence* (1972), for example, the Federal Appeals Court for the District of Columbia held that physicians have a legal duty to provide their patients with the information that a reasonable person would want to know.

Informed consent for research participation was also not part of standard medical practice in Western nations before the mid-20th century. Doctors often experimented on their patients without telling them that they were conducting research, and they did not clearly distinguish between medical therapy and medical research (Resnik 2018). A notable exception to this norm occurred when U.S. Army physician Walter Reed conducted experiments to determine the cause of yellow fever in the early 1900s. Reed's experiments involved exposing human subjects to mosquitos thought to carry the disease. 33 people participated in these experiments and six died from yellow fever. Reed asked the volunteers to sign an informed consent document prior to participating, which was translated into Spanish for the Cuban participants who did not speak English. Volunteers received $100 in gold for their participation, free medical care, and free burials (if they died). This is thought to be the first instance of the use of an informed consent document in biomedical research (Resnik 2018).

Although the Nuremberg Code, adopted in 1947, emphasized the ethical necessity of informed consent for research participation, many investigators continued to study human subjects without obtaining their consent. For example, participants in the Tuskegee Syphilis Study (1932–1972), which was sponsored by the U.S. Department of Health, Education, and Welfare, were not told that they were in a research study. They were told only that they were receiving treatment for "bad blood." Likewise, subjects in the U.S. Department of Energy's secret human radiation experiments, which took place from the 1930s to the 1960s, were not told that they were participating in research or that they were receiving radiation. Human subjects in the Jewish Chronic Disease Hospital Experiments, which took place in 1963, were not told that they had been injected with liver cancer cells as part of a study of the immune system's response to cancer (Resnik 2018).

Informed consent became a widely practiced standard for research with human subjects in Western nations (e.g. U.S., Canada, U.K., Europe, Australia) in the 1970s, when the National Institutes of Health (NIH) and the Food and Drug Administration (FDA) revised their regulations for the protection of human research subjects (Resnik 2018). In 1981, 16 U.S. federal agencies adopted the revised NIH regulations, which became known as the Common Rule (45 CFR 46). The revisions were based in part on an influential document, *The Belmont Report*, which was written by the National Commission for the Protection of Human Subjects in Biomedical and Behavioral Research (Resnik 2018). *The Belmont Report* articulated three ethical principles for research with human subjects: respect for persons (which requires that informed consent be obtained prior to research), beneficence (which requires minimization of risks and maximization of benefits), and justice (which requires equitable distribution of risks and benefits) (National Commission for the Protection of Human Subjects of Biomedical or Behavioral Research 1979). Other Western nations soon developed laws, regulations, and policies based on NIH and FDA rules. Today, over 130 countries have enacted laws, regulations, or policies for research with human subjects (Office of Human Research Protections 2019).

U.S. human research regulations

The Common Rule requires that informed consent "will be sought from each prospective subject or the subject's legally authorized representative" and "appropriately documented" (Department of Homeland Security et al. 2017 at 45 CFR 46 111a). The Common Rule describes 16 types of information that should be conveyed to subjects during the consent process, including the nature of the research, risks and discomforts, potential benefits, alternatives to research participation, confidentiality protections, additional costs to the subject (if any), the right to refuse to participate or withdraw without reprisal, how to withdraw from a study, and the length of the subject's participation (45 CFR 46.111b and 111c). The Common Rule also requires that consent take place under conditions that minimize the possibility for coercion or undue influence, that subjects receive information that a reasonable person would want to know, that information be conveyed in a language understandable to the subjects, and that subjects not be asked to waive legal rights (45 CFR 46.111a). The Common Rule includes exceptions to the informed consent requirements. An institutional board review (IRB)[1] can waive or alter the informed consent process if it determines that risks to subjects are minimal and it would be impractical to conduct the research without a waiver or alteration (45 CFR 46.111e). An IRB can waive documentation requirements if it determines that risks are minimal and the only record linking the subject to the research is the consent document, or if the risks are minimal and the subjects belong to a cultural group in which signing forms is not norm (45 CFR 46. 117c).

The Common Rule and the FDA regulations are very similar in content and scope. The main difference between these sets of rules is that the FDA regulations include exceptions to informed consent requirements for emergency research in which the subject faces a life-threatening condition for which there is no effective treatment, an experimental treatment is available, the subject is unable to consent, and a legally authorized representative (such as parent, guardian, or next of kin) is not available (Resnik 2018).

International guidelines on consent

The *Nuremberg Code*, which was promulgated by the Council at Nuremberg as a means of judging Nazi doctors and scientists for war crimes, was the first international guideline for research with human subjects. The first principle of the Code states that "[t]he voluntary consent of the human subject is absolutely essential (Nuremberg Code 1949)." The Code also states that the subject must have the legal capacity to give consent and should be able to exercise the "free power of choice, without the intervention of any element of force, fraud, deceit, duress, over-reaching, or other ulterior form of constraint or coercion" (Nuremberg Code 1949. The Code states that the subject should have enough knowledge and comprehension of the research to make a responsible choice concerning participation. The Code does not include provisions for allowing a legally authorized representative to consent for the subject (Nuremberg Code 1949).

In 1964, the World Medical Association adopted the *Declaration at Helsinki*, which has been revised nine times, most recently in 2013 (World Medical Association 2013). The *Helsinki Declaration* states that physicians have a duty to "protect the life, health, dignity, integrity, right to self-determination, privacy, and confidentiality of personal information of research subjects" (World Medical Association 2013). One of the chief ways of meeting this obligation is to ensure that human subjects participate in research only if they (or their legally authorized representatives) have given consent. Consent should be voluntary and free from duress. Subjects should be informed about the "aims, methods, sources of funding, any possible conflicts of interest, institutional affiliations of the researcher, the anticipated benefits and potential risks of the study and the discomfort it may entail, post-study provisions and any other relevant aspects of the study" (World Medical Association 2013). Consent also should be properly documented in writing and witnessed. Subjects should be told that they can refuse to participate or withdraw without fear of reprisal. An ethics committee, such as an IRB, can approve research on identifiable human biospecimens or data that does not involve consent if consent would be impossible or impractical (World Medical Association 2013).

The Council for International Organizations of Medical Sciences (CIOMS), a group established by the World Health Organization (WHO) and United Nations Educational, Scientific and Cultural Organization (UNESCO) in 1949, adopted its *International Ethical Guidelines for Biomedical Research Involving Human Subjects* in 1993. The CIOMS Guidelines were revised in 2016 and renamed the *International Ethical Guidelines for Health-related Research*

Involving Humans (Council for International Organizations of Medical Sciences 2016). The CIOMS Guidelines, like the *Nuremberg Code* and *Helsinki Declaration*, include rules for providing and documenting informed consent. The *Guidelines* also address other relevant consent topics, such as essential information that should be conveyed to the subject, the voluntary nature of consent, freedom of choice, deception, comprehension of information, the capacity to consent, consent by a legally authorized representative, and procedures for modifying or waiving consent (Council for International Organizations of Medical Sciences 2016).

Moral basis for consent

Informed consent is based on three moral principles. The first is the obligation to allow autonomous (i.e. competent) individuals to make their own decisions. This fundamental moral principle, known as respect for autonomy, is supported by several Western moral theories including: natural rights theory (as developed by John Locke and others), Immanuel Kant's moral theory, and John Stuart Mill's harm principle (which says that liberty should be restricted only to prevent harm to others (Faden & Beauchamp 1986; Resnik 2018). Respecting autonomy is also part of what it means to respect persons, according to the authors of *The Belmont Report*. Informed consent enables individuals to make their own decisions concerning research participation. Providing individuals with relevant information about the research helps them to make autonomous decisions pertaining to the participation. Coercion, undue influence, duress, and deception are unethical because they interfere with or compromise autonomous decision-making (Faden & Beauchamp 1986).

The second moral principle is the obligation to avoid harming other people, also known as the principle of non-maleficence (Resnik 2018). The three moral theories mentioned above, as well as numerous others (including natural theory and utilitarianism), the Hippocratic Oath, and *The Belmont Report*'s principle of beneficence imply ethical duties to not harm others. Consent enables researchers to avoid causing harm by helping individuals to protect themselves from harm. If an individual decides not to participate in a study because he or she deems it to be too risky, the potential harm to the individual will not occur, and the researcher will avoid causing harm (Resnik 2018).

The third moral principle is the obligation to promote and maintain trust when engaged in relationships that depend on trust, such as the relationship between a physician and a patient or an investigator and a human subject. Trust is an essential component of research with human subjects since subjects must trust that investigators will protect their rights and well-being. If subjects do not trust investigators, they will not participate in research or they will withdraw from research. Informed consent helps to build and maintain trust by respecting the participant's autonomy and dignity. Informed consent also helps to promote honest and open communication between investigators and subjects, which is also essential for trust. When researchers do not obtain consent, as has happened in abuses of human subjects like those discussed above, trust breaks down. Obtaining consent irresponsibly (e.g. by not following consent requirements) can also undermine trust (Resnik 2018).

Although informed consent has widespread support from different Western moral theories and traditions and is required by various national laws, regulations, and guidelines, disputes still arise pertaining to various topics related to consent, such as: how to obtain consent, what types of information to convey to subjects, how much information to share, the degree of comprehension required for consent to be valid, how much decision-making capacity is required for consent, what constitutes coercion or undue influence, whether people can be involved in low-risk research without consent, and whether opt-out consent procedures are acceptable (Resnik

2018). Many of these disputes stem from underlying disagreements about how to prioritize conflicting moral values or principles, such as the obligation to respect autonomy vs. the obligation to benefit society by advancing human knowledge through scientific research.

Cultural variation in informed consent

While U.S. clinical research informed consent policies emphasize protecting individual rights and autonomy, other countries place more emphasis on community and family-unit decision-making. In these cultures, the concept of "autonomy" is seen in a relational rather than an individual context, meaning that an individual's sense-of-self is influenced by his or her social roles, responsibilities, and connections to the community or family (Clough, Campbell, Aliyeva, Mateo, Zarean, & O'Donovan 2013; Frimpong-Mansoh 2008; Pratt, Van, Cong, Rashid, Kumar, Ahmad, Upshur, & Loff 2014; Sariola & Simpson 2011). In cultures that define their members by their relations to others, the Western formal practice of autonomous informed consent process is viewed as a foreign concept (Cook 2015). This is because the decision-making process usually involves the family and community, not just the individual, and because medical practice may place a higher emphasis on values other than individual autonomy or privacy, such as physician loyalty or compassion. In such cultures, if a patient is invited to participate in a clinical trial, it would be customary for the family to be involved in the decision, while in the U.S., the family or community would not be involved unless explicitly called upon for input (Cook 2015; Macklin 1999; Ruiping 2015). As there has been a significant increase in the last twenty years in international research projects and multinational clinical trials, researchers are increasingly being challenged to adopt new clinical trial procedures that may create a conflict between the investigators' research standards and the ethical values of the culture in which the trial is being conducted.

Methods

To better understand this conflict and how to manage it, we reviewed the literature on cultural variation in informed consent for clinical research. We defined "culture" broadly to include characteristics such as religion, nationality, geographical location, and ethnicity that influence the informed consent processes. To obtain articles for our review, we used an institutional resource that provided access to 268 databases, including Elsevier ScienceDirect, EBSCOhost Premier, SpringerLink, ProQuest Sciences, JSTOR Life Sciences, and MedlinePlus (PubMed).

We conducted our search using the terms, "human subjects," "clinical research," "informed consent," and "nationality." We refined our results year (1990 or later), subject (informed consent), language (English), publication type (academic journals), and availability (full text online). This search identified 1168 results. Results were excluded if they were not clinical research studies (i.e. letters or short commentaries) or not an analysis of a clinical research study, and if they explicitly discussed research in vulnerable populations (prisoners, children, pregnant women, neonates, etc.).

Results

When the Western, individualistic concept of informed consent is applied in non-Western settings, participants may experience confusion and distrust because this concept may be inconsistent with their community values and because they may not be accustomed to making medical decisions without the input of community/familial leaders (Kumar, Mohanraj, Rose,

Paul, & Thomas 2012). To help alleviate ethical tensions due to cultural differences, researchers working in foreign countries sometimes alter the informed consent process of a clinical research trial to better align with the values and practices of the local cultures, while still upholding the rights and autonomy of human subjects. Recently, informed consent practices have been altered in various ways, described below. (See Table 4.1 for examples of studies on cultural variation in informed consent.)

Community consent

To minimize ethical conflicts, many investigators and governments have either encouraged or mandated that researchers gain community-level informed consent from community leaders, elders, or local health organizations (Brear 2018; Dyall, Kepa, Hayman, Teh, Moyes, Broad, & Kerse 2013; McDonald, Benger, Brown, Currie, & Carapetis 2006; Preziosi, Yam, Ndiaye, Simaga, Simondon, & Wassilak 1997; Zion 2003). Community consent is obtained prior to gaining individual participant consent, and generally functions as the researchers' "go-ahead approval" to conduct research in the community; however, it is not a replacement for individual consent, which must also be obtained, according to international guidelines (CIOMS 2002). This practice of coupling community consent and individual consent has been adopted because it acts to respect aspects of both individual and relational forms of autonomy. It respects relational autonomy because seeking community consent follows the structured cultural policies of working with the leaders of a community prior to working with individuals, and it respects individual autonomy because the individual has the final say in whether they wish to participate in research.

It is important to note that this model does not give individuals the free choice to partake in research without the consent of the community, nor does it guarantee that existing community power dynamics will not influence an individual's decision to participate in research. Little research has been conducted investigating individual attitudes about losing the choice of self-determination to participate in research without prior community consent, but substantial work has been conducted investigating influential power structures that may affect an individual's voluntary choice to consent following community-consent.

Although potential research participants may consent in a confidential setting, unequal power relations between researchers and participants and between community leaders and participants may affect a participant's comfort with declining an invitation to participate in a research trial (Gikonyo, Bejon, Marsh, & Molyneux 2008; Brear 2018; Kelly 2003; Zion 2003). Studies have suggested that a participant may feel uncomfortable declining an offer to participate because they may view the community-consent obtained prior to individual consent as an "instruction" or "order" to enroll, or because they may feel that a breach of confidentiality could result in punishment or ostracization by the community (Brear 2018; McDonald et al. 2006; Zion 2003). As it is becoming common to obtain community consent, future researchers may need to add additional educational and confidentiality measures to ensure that this practice does not unintentionally constrain individual agency in the consent decision.

Educational considerations

Research trials conducted in non-Western countries are beginning to enlist local leaders, clinicians, and community members in the research process. These individuals help to run informative meetings, recruit participants, build community trust, translate informed consent documents, and may explain research terms like, "voluntary," "randomized," "placebo," "blind,"

Table 4.1 Examples of research on cultural variation in informed consent for research participation

Study Title & Author	Location	Study Descriptions	Key Concepts
Primary Research			
The Lililwan Project: study protocol for a population-based active case ascertainment study of the prevalence of fetal alcohol spectrum disorders (FASD) in remote Australian Aboriginal communities. (Fitzpatrick et al. 2012)	Australia	Researchers investigated the prevalence of FASD and other health and developmental problems in school-aged children residing in the Fitzroy Valley born between 2002 and 2003.	Participant recruitment occurred through visits to parents/caregivers by "community navigators" (local Aboriginal people working as a part of the research team), during which they would explain the nature of the study and the purpose of the informed consent forms. This was conducted in the participants native language and aided with visuals/pamphlets. Researchers obtained written consent at *three* points during the study: prior to diagnostic interviews, prior to clinical assessment, and prior to sharing management plans for health providers. Ethics approval was sought from groups including the Western Australian Aboriginal Health Information and Ethics Committee, and the Kimberley Aboriginal Health Planning Forum Research Subcommittee.
Engagement and recruitment of Māori and non-Māori people of advanced age to LiLACS NZ. (Dyall et al. 2013)	Australia & New Zealand	This paper described the recruitment process and methods for a longitudinal cohort study (LiLACS NZ) investigating the predictors of successful advanced ageing and wellbeing between members of the Māori tribe, and non-Māori people in the same geographical area. Researchers examined a range of physical, psychological, health, social, environmental, and cultural factors. This study included taking a blood sample. (*n*= 421 Māori, *n*=516 non-Māori)	The researchers enlisted the Rōpū Kaitiaki o Ngā Tikanga Māori (Protectors of the Principles of Conduct in Māori Research) to help oversee the research process and protect indigenous interests by helping to construct questionnaires using the native language/wording, host community recruitment meetings, and ensure that blood samples were handled in line with Māori traditions. Participant-written consent was obtained at each stage of the process (interview, physical, etc.). During informed disclosure, participants were given a pre-planned list of all blood analyses, as well as information on the storage guidelines and potential future research that may use their samples. If a participant's blood was not used, they had the option to request that their blood be returned.

(continued)

Table 4.1 Cont.

Study Title & Author	Location	Study Descriptions	Key Concepts
Audiovisual documentation of oral consent: A new method of informed consent for illiterate populations. (Benitez et al. 2002)	Paraguay	This paper discusses the development of a multi-step informed consent process named, "audiovisual documentation of oral consent" (ADOC) that aurally, visually, and photographically recorded the participants participating in the consent process. The consent was for participation in, "The Guarani Indians Project" (a genetic population study in Guarani people in Paraguay). (*n*=100 total, *n*=42 for those who consented to participate)	As Guarani Indians have traditionally used oral communication, the informed consent documents were read aloud to a group of participants. After given the chance to ask questions, participants were asked to "step forward" to give their consent. These participants were then required to give oral consent in their native language and sign a written consent document with a signature or a fingerprint. This implicit opt-in process was determined to function in line with the Guarani customs, because explicit refusal (opting out/denying consent) is not part of Guarani social customs.

Analytical Research

Study Title & Author	Location	Study Descriptions	Key Concepts
Challenges in informed consent decision-making in Korean clinical research: A participant perspective. (Choi et al. 2019)	South Korea	This study explored the challenges associated with the informed consent decision- making process in an anti-cancer drug clinical trial. Researchers individually interviewed participants to determine the effectiveness and ethicality of South Korea's informed consent disclosure processes. (*n*=21)	It was found that the informed consent documents adhered to the information disclosure guidelines outlined in Article 7 of the Korean Good Clinical Practice Regulations, however, the disclosure of this information varied greatly between participants. On several occasions the informed disclosure occurred *after* consent (written or oral) was obtained. Due to a lack of an opportunity to ask questions about trial, researchers concluded that participants were likely to depend on information from family, friends, or the internet when deciding to participate. Additionally, the informed consent documents averaged at 15 pages long, and were frequently above the relative reading level of the participants.

Table 4.1 Cont.

Study Title & Author	Location	Study Descriptions	Key Concepts
Practical experiences in obtaining informed consent for a vaccine trial in rural Africa. (Preziosi et al. 1997)	Senegal	While conducting a study of a new pertussis vaccine in the Niakhar community in Senegal, researchers evaluated the process for obtaining community and individual consent from parents. Village chiefs were first informed of the study by a field physician, which was followed by presentations to the community by field staff about the study structure, the vaccine, and the principle of randomization. Following this, researchers privately obtained informed consent of the mothers.	Written or verbal informed consent was re-recorded with each subsequent vaccination during the trial. The researchers noted that by having several informative community meetings before the individual informed consent process allowed for easier comprehension of the study and gradual decision-making on the part of the mother. It is important to note that many mothers believed that they had already given consent during the community meetings, so researchers had to explain the concept of individual informed consent to them upon the individual meeting.
The Quality of Informed Consent in a Clinical Research Study in Thailand. (Pace, Emanuel, Chuenyam, & Duncombe 2005)	Thailand	This study investigated the informed consent process in the Thailand branch of the ESPRIT (Evaluation of Subcutaneous Proleukin in a Randomized International Trial) stage 3 clinical study comparing the effectiveness of IL- z plus antiretroviral therapy versus antiretroviral therapy alone reducing the rate of HIV disease progression. The informed consent process was held in two parts: a group discussion (~5–10 participants for 2 hrs) led by trained clinical trial nurses, followed by individual interviews with the physician.	During the group discussion, the protocol was read page by page, and participants were encouraged to ask questions about the trial. The researchers acknowledged that this environment may intimidate the participants, however, they suggested that this approach may reduce the inequality in the environment that is normally shaped by highly paternalistic doctor-patient relationships. The informed consent document was 2,600 words long and included information on the voluntary nature of participation, the right to withdraw, the purpose of the study, the study procedures (randomization and injection schedules), the potential risks/benefits, and alternatives to participation. From a post-informed consent survey, researchers concluded that the participants, "viewed the informed consent process favorably, had a high level of comprehension of all aspects of the study except randomization, and made a voluntary decision to join the study."

and "right to withdraw" to trial participants, using culturally relevant examples and definitions (Clough et al. 2013; Choi, Choi, & Lee 2019). In cultures with an oral tradition or high rates of illiteracy, researchers may even use visual aids or videos to demonstrate these terms (Fitzpatrick, Elliott, & Latimer et al. 2012; McDonald et al. 2006; Preziosi et al. 1997). Overall, this process is designed to provide the participants with the necessary tools to make an autonomous, educated decision to partake in the study. Importantly, when in communities that practice paternalistic medicine, researchers must acknowledge that participants may become more wary of a researcher or a study when they are given much more information than to which they are usually accustomed (Sariola & Simpson 2011). This increased skepticism can be due to a lack of experience with making individual medical decisions, or it may be due to the existing belief that the purpose of the informed consent is simply to legally protect the researchers/sponsors, rather than to give the participants a chance to express their autonomy (Gikonyo et al. 2008).

Another method that has been recently proposed to protect participant rights and aid in participant comprehension is the hybrid approach model. This model explicitly divides the responsibilities of informing the participant and obtaining the participant's voluntary consent between the physician investigator and a neutral third party (Grady 2019). To reduce the potential of investigator-participant power dynamics encroaching on the autonomous decision-making of the participant, a third individual is introduced whose role is to reduce the therapeutic misconception (i.e. mistakenly believing the intent of the study is to provide therapy, not to produce knowledge), help the potential participant access additional information about the study, be present during consent acquisition, and to ensure that the participant understands that their decision to participate is voluntary and that there will be no negative repercussions if they choose to decline an invitation to participate in the clinical study. By splitting up the roles supporting the informed disclosure and informed consent processes, participants may be better informed about the study itself and may be better equipped to consent in a truly voluntary manner (Grady 2019).

Obtaining informed consent

With the goals of building community trust and increasing the involvement of the individual participants in their own decision-making, several investigators have also adopted a multi-step informed consent process in which participants are asked to give consent at multiple stages of a clinical trial, rather than just at the start of the trial (Dyall et al. 2013; Fitzpatrick et al. 2012; Gulbrandsen & Jensen 2010; McDonald et al. 2006). Studies implementing a multi-step informed consent process have concluded that it helps to strengthen community relationships, build investigator-participant trust, and even combat the misconception that the informed consent process exists only to legally protect the researchers (Dyall et al. 2013; Gikonyo et al. 2008; McDonald et al. 2006).

By having participants reconsent multiple times during the trial, researchers are providing participants with additional opportunities to opt-out of a study after initially consenting. Though this may hinder participant retention, this process may provide participants with a chance to reevaluate their decision to participate in the study as they become more educated on the nature of study itself, and as they have more time to reflect on what research participation may mean for them personally. By inserting consent renewals into the study process, researchers relieve participants of the individual burden that comes with choosing to withdraw from a study because they are allowing participants to withdraw from a study by not opting in, rather than by opting out. This slight alteration to the protocol may also be more appropriate when conducting research in vulnerable populations or in communities that tend to avoid explicit actions of refusal, such as the native Guarani communities in Paraguay (Benitez, Devaux, & Dausset 2002).

Another important aspect to consider in the informed consent process is the time between informed disclosure and consent acquisition. As some studies have found that this time window can vary drastically, and that disclosure may not even occur before the investigator obtains participant consent (as found in the investigative work conducted by Choi et al. 2019), it is important to ensure that participants have enough time both to review the aspects of the study to make their own uncoerced, educated decision, as well as enough time to consult community leaders, friends, or family if they so wish (Gulbrandsen & Jensen 2010; Loue, Okello, & Kawuma 1996).

Media of informed consent

In addition to altering the process of obtaining informed consent, it has become common for researchers to alter the medium through which informed consent is obtained. Informed consent in the U.S. is typically obtained through a participant's signature; however, consent can also be obtained verbally, through a fingerprint, or through a combination of the three methods (Benitez et al. 2002). When working in cultures with an oral tradition or in illiterate populations, it may be more appropriate to have participants give verbal consent following a verbal description of the study by the researcher rather than having them sign a written consent form that they cannot read or that is in a language that is not their own. This practice is not only more culturally or socially appropriate, but it also acts to protect the safety of the participants by reducing the chance that they would consent to a clinical trial that may not be in their best interests simply because they may not be able to read and comprehend the consent form.

Conclusions

Our literature analysis revealed that the informed consent process is generally modified in one of four main ways when Western researchers work in a culture with different values pertaining to the clinical research process:

1) Consent of community leaders may be sought prior to obtaining the individual consent of community members.
2) To aid in participant comprehension of the details and nature of research, investigators may alter informed disclosure documents to better reflect the language and concepts commonly used in the culture. They may also enlist local researchers, clinicians, and community members to help design and conduct the informed consent procedures.
3) The informed consent procedure may be modified to reinforce the concept of opt-in participation, give participants more time to discuss their potential enrollment with others, and allow for easier withdrawal from the study.
4) Instead of obtaining informed consent through written documents, researchers may use record consent verbally or through a fingerprint in cultures with an oral history or with high rates of illiteracy.

Overall, these four methods are aimed at reducing influential power dynamics between researchers and participants, ensuring participant comprehension, respecting the values of the community, and reducing the possibility for undue influence, coercion, or exploitation of participants. The analysis and recognition of cultural conflict in research methodology has pushed investigators to become more critical of their own research procedures and informed consent practices. In addition to these smaller project-specific changes, larger, more inclusive national guidelines have been developed in recent years (Roberts, Jadalla, & Jones-Oyefeso 2017). One major recent policy development to the field of culturally sensitive research was the creation of *The Ethics and Governance Framework for Best Practice in Genomic Research and Biobanking in Africa* by the H3Africa Consortium Working Group on Ethics (Yakubu, Tindana, Matimba, Littler, Munung, Madden, Staunton & De Fries 2018). In the hopes of combining the Western individual-centered ethics and African community-centered ethics, policy makers detailed four principles stating that research should 1) be sensitive to local cultures; 2) be beneficial to the community and the global population; 3) involve community consultation; and 4) be respectful, fair, reciprocal, and equitable. These guidelines provide an excellent framework for how foreign researchers can operate in a culturally sensitive manner when conducting research while upholding broader principles of human dignity and rights.

Since bioethics as a discipline has primarily been a Western product, it is important that Western researchers conducting clinical trials in non-Western cultures acknowledge local values and norms so that any implementation of ethical standards is done so in a non-imperialistic manner that will advocate for the rights of the population. Furthermore, by working to create guidelines that act in accordance with the values of various cultural values and regional standards, researchers and bioethicists will be better equipped to discover underlying similarities in ethical reasoning that will aid in the formation of a more universal standard of ethics. This is especially important as the number of international and multinational clinical trials have been steadily rising over the last two decades and is expected to keep growing well into the future.

Acknowledgments

This research was supported by the Intramural Program of the National Institute of Environmental Health Sciences (NIEHS), National Institutes of Health (NIH). It does not represent the views of the NIEHS, NIH, or US government.

Note

1 An IRB is an ethics committee that is responsible for reviewing and overseeing research with human subjects.

References

Adams, V., S. Miller, S. Craig, Sonam, Nyima, Droyoung, P.V. Le, & M. Varner. 2007. Informed Consent in cross-cultural perspective: clinical research in the Tibetan Autonomous Region, PRC. *Culture, Medicine & Psychiatry*, 31(4): 445.

Benitez, O., D. Devaux, & J. Dausset. 2002. Audiovisual documentation of oral consent: A new method of informed consent for illiterate populations. *The Lancet,* 359(9315): 1406.

Berg, J.W., P.S. Appelbaum, L.S. Parker, & C.W. Lidz. 2001. *Informed Consent: Legal Theory and Clinical Practice*, 2nd ed. New York: Oxford University Press.

Brear, M. 2018. Ethical Research Practice or Undue Influence? Symbolic Power in Community- and Individual-Level Informed Consent Processes in Community-Based Participatory Research in Swaziland. *Journal of Empirical Research on Human Research Ethics*, 13(4): 311.

Canterbury v. Spence. 1972. 464 F.2d. 772, 782 D.C. Cir. 1972.

Choi, I-S, E.Y. Choi, & I-H Lee. 2019. Challenges in informed consent decision-making in Korean clinical research: A participant perspective. *PLoS ONE,* 14(5): 1.

Clough, B.A., M.M. Campbell, T.A. Aliyeva, N.J. Mateo, M. Zarean, & A. O'Donovan. 2013. Protocol for Protection of Human Participants: A Comparison of Five Countries. *Journal of Empirical Research on Human Research Ethics*, 8(3): 2.

Cook, W.A. 2015. Questionable informed consent of vulnerable pregnant research participants in South India – What a staff reminder poster does not say. *Nursing Ethics*, 22(2): 264.

Council for International Organizations of Medical Sciences. 2016. International Ethical Guidelines for Health-related Research Involving Humans. Available at: Department of Homeland Security; Department of Agriculture; Department of Energy; National Aeronautics and Space Administration; Department of Commerce; Social Security Administration; Agency for International Development; Department of Housing and Urban Development; Department of Labor; Department of Defense; Department of Education; Department of Veterans Affairs; Environmental Protection Agency; Department of Health and Human Services; National Science Foundation; and Department of Transportation. 2017. Federal Policy for the Protection of Human Subjects. *Federal Register* 82(12): 7149–7274.

Dyall, L., M. Kepa, K. Hayman, R. Teh, S. Moyes, J.B. Broad, & N. Kerse. 2013. Engagement and recruitment of Māori and non-Māori people of advanced age to LiLACS NZ. *Australian and New Zealand Journal of Public Health,* 2: 124.

Faden, R.F., & T.L. Beauchamp. 1986. *A History and Theory of Informed Consent.* New York, NY: Oxford University Press.

Fitzpatrick, J.P., E.J. Elliott, J. Latimer, et al. 2012. The Lililwan Project: study protocol for a population-based active case ascertainment study of the prevalence of fetal alcohol spectrum disorders (FASD) in remote Australian Aboriginal communities. *Journal of Pediatrics and Child Health,* 51(4): 450.

Frimpong-Mansoh, A. 2008. Culture and voluntary informed consent in African health care systems. *Developing World Bioethics*, 8(2): 104.

Gikonyo, C., P. Bejon, V. Marsh, & S. Molyneux. 2008. Taking social relationships seriously: Lessons learned from the informed consent practices of a vaccine trial on the Kenyan Coast. *Social Science & Medicine,* 67(5): 708.

Grady, C. 2019. A Hybrid Approach to Obtaining Research Consent. *The American Journal of Bioethics,* 19(4): 28.

Gulbrandsen, P., & B.F. Jensen. 2010. Post-recruitment confirmation of informed consent by SMS. *Journal of Med Ethics,* 36(2): 126.

International ethical guidelines for biomedical research involving human subjects. 2002. Council for International Organizations of Medical Sciences (CIOMS), World Health Organization, Geneva.

Kelly, A. 2003. Research and the Subject: The Practice of Informed Consent. *Political and Legal Anthropology Review*, 26(2): 182.

Kumar, S., R. Mohanraj, A. Rose, M.J. Paul, G. Thomas. 2012. How "informed" is informed consent? Findings from a study in South India. *Indian J Med Ethics,* 9(3): 180.

Loue, S., Okello, D., & Kawuma, M. 1996. Research bioethics in the Ugandan context: a program summary. *Journal of Law, Medicine & Ethics*, 1: 47.

Macklin, R. 1999. *Against Relativism: Cultural Diversity and the Search for Ethical Universals in Medicine.* New York: Oxford University Press.

McDonald, M.I., N. Benger, A. Brown, B.J. Currie, & J.R. Carapetis. 2006. Practical challenges of conducting research into rheumatic fever in remote Aboriginal communities. *The Medical Journal of Australia*, 8: 511.

National Commission for the Protection of Human Subjects of Biomedical or Behavioral Research. 1979. *The Belmont Report: Ethical Principles and Guidelines for the Protection of Human Subjects of Research.* Washington, DC: Department of Health, Education, and Welfare.

Nuremberg Code. 1949. *Trials of War Criminals before the Nuremberg Military Tribunals under Control Council Law No. 10*, Vol. 2, pp. 181–182. Washington, D.C.: U.S. Government Printing Office.

Office of Human Research Protections. 2019. International compilation of human research standards, 2019 edition. Available at: www.hhs.gov/ohrp/sites/default/files/2019-International-Compilation-of-Human-Research-Standards.pdf. Accessed: June 21, 2019.

Pace, C., E. Emanuel, T. Chuenyam, & C. Duncombe. 2005. The Quality of Informed Consent in a Clinical Research Study in Thailand. *IRB: Ethics & Human Research,* 27(1): 9.

Pratt, B., C. Van, Y. Cong, H. Rashid, N. Kumar, A. Ahmad, R. Upshur, & B. Loff. 2014. Perspectives from South and East Asia on Clinical and Research Ethics: A Literature Review. *Journal of Empirical Research on Human Research Ethics,* 9(2): 52.

Preziosi, M.P., A. Yam, M. Ndiaye, A. Simaga, F. Simondon, & S.G. Wassilak. 1997. Practical experiences in obtaining informed consent for a vaccine trial in rural Africa. *The New England Journal of Medicine*, 5: 370.

Resnik, D.B. 2018. *The Ethics of Research with Human Subjects: Protecting People, Advancing Science, Promoting Trust*. Cham, Switzerland: Springer.

Roberts, L.R., A. Jadalla, & V. Jones-Oyefeso. 2017. Researching in Collectivist Cultures. *Journal of Transcultural Nursing*, 28(2): 137.

Ruiping, F. (Ed.). 2015. *Family oriented informed consent: Eastern Asian and American perspectives*. Switzerland: Springer.

Sariola, S., & B. Simpson. 2011. Theorizing the 'human subject' in biomedical research: International clinical trials and bioethics discourses in contemporary Sri Lanka. *Social Science & Medicine,* 73(4): 515.

World Medical Association. 2013. Declaration at Helsinki, 2013 Revision. Available at: www.wma.net/policies-post/wma-declaration-of-helsinki-ethical-principles-for-medical-research-involving-human-subjects/. Accessed: June 21, 2019.

Yakubu, A., P. Tindana, A. Matimba, K. Littler, N.S. Munung, E. Madden, C. Staunton, & J. DeVries. 2018. Model framework for governance of genomic research and biobanking in Africa – a content description. *AAS Open Res*, 1: 13

Zion, D. 2003. Culture, community and consent: A response to Barrett and Parker. *Monash Bioethics Review,* 22(3): 23.

5

ENCOUNTERING HOSTILITY IN ETHNOGRAPHIC RESEARCH

Christopher M. Hayre and Paul M.W. Hackett

Introduction

The utilisation of ethnographic research and auto/ethnographic accounts is on the rise within the field of medical imaging. Not only do these approaches provided a glimpse into the clinical practice of medical imaging (Hayre, 2016b), they also offer a platform for understanding patient and individual experiences, offering pertinent empiricism and viewpoints previously unseen (Nightingale, Murphy, Eaton, & Borgen, 2016; Barry, 2020). To date, few published works reflect on the use of multi-sited ethnography within the medical imaging environment, whereby more than one research site is compared as part of an overarching research methodology. In response, this chapter reflects on the first author's experiences of undertaking multi-sited ethnography and details encountering a sensitive/hostile situation at one site, which led to the cessation of data collection.

The authors begin by identifying hostile experiences outside of the medical imaging environment, thus strengthening its rationale for discussion in the medical imaging profession (Blackman, 2007; Chomczynski, 2018). We identify the value and need of incorporating emotion within qualitative research and how it remains integral to enhancing the trustworthiness of the qualitative approaches (Blackman, 2007). Next, this chapter provides insight into encountering hostility as an ethnographic researcher within the medical imaging environment. Lastly, discussion around how to best avoid and/or limit hostile encounters in ethnographic research is outlined in order to support prospective researchers in future studies. It is anticipated that this will not only provide methodological insight for encountering hostility amongst the researcher with his or her participants, but, importantly, it will allow researchers to recognise the value in documenting emotion through critical reflexivity. This chapter adds to the existing evidence base by providing a unique lens whereby research encounters may not always go to plan.

Hostility in ethnographic research: an overview

Ethnography is a research methodology that aims to "get closer" to social reality (Hammersley & Atkinson, 1997). Stemming from the Chicago School, it is regarded as the study of culture and is now widely used in many disciplines, such as criminology, business, education, and healthcare. Further, there is recognition that ethnography can encompass quantitative as well as qualitative methods in order to enhance our understanding of the social world around us (Hayre &

Blackman, 2020). Whilst the first author's own work has previously captured original empiricism linked to the professional practices of diagnostic radiographers, there are, however, few works that discuss encountering hostility in medical imaging research. Discussions surrounding hostility are generally accepted outside the field of medical imaging, but few exist within the discipline, which may be linked to researchers shying away from the topic, in particular when having to write about events that may be seen as controversial and/or against the cultural norm (Blackman, 2007). Further, Blackman (2007) affirms that ethnographic researchers may often be reluctant to explore the legitimacy of emotional relationships that occur between the researchers and the researched, attributing to what then becomes "hidden ethnography" (ibid.). However, it can be these "hidden ethnographic attributes" that reinforce the trustworthiness of qualitative research in order to identify and critically examine how studies have been carried out, with any difficulties identified.

In the past, there has been a reticence toward incorporating emotion into methodological accounts. Barter and Renold (2003, p. 100) argue that "emotion is deemed to be epistemologically irrelevant", thus present a strong reluctance of incorporating emotion within reflective accounts. Further, Coffey (1999) reminds us of the potential unwillingness to give realistic accounts amongst younger academics as they try to build and sustain an academic career, with the aim of gaining acceptance within their respective profession. Central to any ethnographic study is, however, the notion of reflexivity, which remains a common tool amongst qualitative researchers whereby critical reflection amongst interactions with participants is captured. Denzin and Lincoln (1998) remind us that "the reflexive turn" in contemporary qualitative research has created a space whereby it is now possible to write the researcher into the world they investigate and reflect on interactions with participants. This remained central in the authors' own research and rationale for reflection on hostile encounters (see Hayre & Strudwick, 2019). In addition, Bourdieu and Wacquant (1992) claim that reflexivity critically examines the power relationships by which the ethnographic researcher is exposed. For example, the origins, biography, locality, and intellectual bias of the researcher are of central importance. Further, this can help provide an audit trail of the research process and support empiricism generated within the field work (Hayre & Strudwick, 2019). Lee-Treweek and Linkogle (2000) consider reflexivity as an opportunity in qualitative sociology to grasp how understanding emotion can contribute to greater academic insight for prospective researchers. This, in turn, for most inductive approaches, may result in socio-cultural events that are unpredictable due to the explorative nature and potential of coming up against a hostile situation within the research environment(s).

As identified above, some negativity surrounds the study of emotion within sociology. It is often associated with a pessimistic lens whereby the examined profession or context is seen inferior to the expected norm. In contrast, and optimistically, it can be seen as a positive attribute by asserting legitimacy of the topic and a critique of the methodological process itself (Kemper, 1990). According to Shilling (2002), the negative nature of considering emotion is because it sits within the realm of subjectivity and is thus regarded as "unscientific". However, it is argued here that regardless of an individual's ontological and epistemological position, considering emotion remains central in qualitative research whereby reflexivity remains an important tool for understanding the researcher-participant relationship(s). This is also something that is generally underexplored in medical imaging research.

Hostility in the medical imaging environment: a multi-sited comparative analysis

Hostility within existing literature has been linked to encounters amongst radiographers and radiologists in the clinical setting (Ehrlich & Coakes, 2020, p. 101). Fortunately, hostility is rarely reported and regarded as unlikely between radiographers and their patients (Lane, 2016), yet this paper offers a research lens whereby hostility can also occur between researcher and radiographic practitioners. Fielding (2011, p. 249) makes the distinction between a hostile environment and sensitive topics. The former is defined as a situation where a research population (or participant) is actively resistant to research and is focused on limiting a researcher's access to data for reasons felt to be important enough to warrant the behaviour (ibid.). In short, it could be argued that it is not the physical presence of the researcher the group defines as a problem, but the topics he/she touches upon and/or the questions he or she asks. This leads some to assume the interconnectedness between sensitive topics and potential for hostility which may arise through ethnographic research.

An illustration of the links between the sensitivity of a research topic and hostility was demonstrated when, as part of a multi-sited study, the second author was engaged in a protracted in-depth qualitative interview with an elderly participant. The interview went well and the interview was concluded successfully. The interviewer also reflected on the interview and noted how he felt an increasing sense of unease as the participant revealed more about the medical conditions they had and especially how these impacted their daily life. Later that day the participant called him at his office and, in a hostile manner, withdrew consent to use the interview and stated the reason being that he had not realised how personal the interview would be. The level of hostility upset the researcher greatly, especially as he felt the interview had been successful and this left him considering his position as a researcher and how influential his presence was when interviews were not only negative but also positive in their outcome.

The ability for an author to reflect on his/her multi-sited ethnography is important in order to enable him/her to identify and apply a "multi-sited research imaginary" enabling the researcher to look across the different research sites and draw on methodological comparisons (Marcus, 1998). Abu-Lughod (2000, p. 264) supports this by recognising the value of undertaking research at multiple sites, whereby one can generate new knowledge that is focused on understanding both emotion and locality whilst engaging with power structures. In response, this positional reflection examines the experiences of one research site whereby hostility was encountered.

In this case, hostility had been expressed towards the second author even before he had entered the interview. Hostility had arisen because the interviews had been arranged by someone else and the participant had not been thoroughly prepared nor informed about the upcoming interview itself. During this case the second author experienced mild hostility, such as the participant not calling her dog away from him when the dog barked and aggressively jumped at him when he met her at her front door. Another dog actually bit and tore his trouser leg and he received no apology from the participant. Perhaps the most hostile reaction the second author met on a doorstep was when he was greeted by a hail of expletives from a participant expressing the fact that he had forgotten about the appointment and that the research seemed a "fucking waste of time" whilst he allowed his dog to bark and snap at the author with bared teeth. In such situations it is obvious that the information that came out of the interviews was structured through hostility and antagonism between the participant and the second author. It was also interesting to note how the medical professionals with which he was working with were not concerned with the impact of the hostility on the data gathered.

Central to gaining access to the field are the gatekeepers in qualitative research who are regarded as a key member of the group, permitting entrance into the field. However, it is important to note that no matter how much help a gatekeeper provides you with getting involved into the social life of others, the identity the researcher creates is crucial for acceptance amongst your participants. Hammersley and Atkinson (1995, p. 83) suggest that researcher's should work on their "impression management" and underscore how carefully it can be created. The more hostile the environment may be, the more sensitive the topic will become and thus the greater should be your concern about the group's perception of your appearance and the more you should be prepared for any possible conflict (Hammersley & Atkinson, 1995). The first author recollects his first impression when entering the research site:

> As I entered the new research site you are always conscious of your first impressions with participants. On arrival, I recollect the unique layout of the department, whereby two general X-ray rooms interconnected the viewing area. In addition, and upon observation, the layout of the X-ray rooms had small lead (Pb) protective screens which radiographers stood behind in order limit their radiological exposure. This small area was unlike any other clinical site where I had undertaken my research whereby I had limited access to the observed clinical practice itself. It was my intention to learn from previous research encounters and remain neutral and ensure I did not ask too many questions or take notes immediately.

The notion that researchers should remain mindful of their positionality when undertaking ethnography in medical imaging research has been identified (Hayre & Strudwick, 2019). It is asserted that when researchers examine their own discipline, they often find themselves with conflicting attitudes to their participants, hence the importance of beginning neutrally and remaining sensitive to the questions or observations posed (ibid.). It is also generally accepted that researchers do not ask questions straight away that are directly related and/or sensitive to the research (Hammersley & Atkinson, 1995). After several hours and upon the first author's observations it was felt that his usual method of note-taking (using a pen and A5 notepad) would not be an ideal form of note-taking. Burgess (1990) reports instances whereby researchers have been required to dash to the toilet to jot down notes. For this author, the case was not dissimilar: due to the tensions experienced, it was necessary to leave the clinical area to record data in order to ensure he captured what was possible (Hayre, 2016a). In short, taking written notes in the immediate vicinity of participants' would have been extremely uncomfortable and intrusive (ibid). Further, although gatekeeper approval, ethical clearance, and consent had been obtained to access and conduct the proposed research, it is important to remember that the ethics of limiting harm and causing distress in fieldwork is not binary, and remains on-going in practice. Tracy (2010) describes how multifaceted the ethical journey is within qualitative research and how the researcher should remain "ethically minded" whilst in their research role. Further, ethics is not just a means, but rather constitutes the universal end goal of qualitative quality itself, whereby procedural, situational, and relational actions, as well as exiting the field remain central (Chomczynski, 2018). Tracy (2010), importantly, acknowledges that good qualitative researchers take care of others, as well as themselves, with the most successful researchers being self-critical of their own research practices and the impact on others. When conducting qualitative research within the area of health, the second author has encountered several situations in which he has been permitted into the homes of participants and has discovered extremely concerning conditions. These have ranged from dirty and unhygienic homes to an elderly person who was essentially living on a dirty mattress on the floor and unable to take care of themselves. In these settings the second author found that the participant welcomed his presence but that relatives of the participant may have felt intruded upon and expressed hostility for agreeing to take part in the research. However, hostility from whatever source is always disturbing and also affects the quality of information gained. In some of these situations the second author was not made aware of what sort of conditions to expect prior to visiting participants and thus became aware of the privileged access he was permitted and also of his ethical duty to patients and their families and to medical professionals. He was encroaching on their lives, and this came with a sense of unease. The second author also felt unease due to the unequal roles of researcher and practitioner. He occupied the former position when working with nurses, general practitioners, surgeons, and other medical staff, whereby he experienced feeling like "an outsider". It is also interesting to note that he has often noticed that medical staff who are active researchers within healthcare and social aspects of health settings have been negativity displayed to researchers due to their non-research active colleagues. Frequently, it feels, as if being a researcher is seen as being a trespasser or an interloper who is meddling within professional practice from a position of not understanding their medical and health roles.

When critiquing the first author's research practices, initial signs of the sensitive nature to the research were identified whereby participants felt uneased by his presence, with some participants commenting: *"are we passing for you?"* and *"are we doing well enough for you?"* Hammersley and Atkinson (2007, p. 91) describe this as the "culture shock" that can put the ethnographer in immediate confrontation with his/her participants. This was the first glimpse into the first author's role and the potential intrusion the he had caused in the clinical environment. Later in the day, a senior radiographer questioned his presence in the department: *"have you nothing better to do than watch us at work?"* This was the author's first encounter of such direct questioning to his presence within the research environment. He immediately felt that his presence was causing direct discomfort to individuals and in order to ensure that he did not cause any additional distress he offered to leave the field. In response, the senior radiographer felt that due to the busy nature of the department, *"it would be a good idea to come back another day"*. The first author decided the leave the field upon his request.

This encounter not only identifies the discontent expressed by the senior radiographer, but, looking back, it is clear that other situational factors arguably facilitated this response. When comparing experiences with other research sites as part of the wider study, there are three areas that warrant further discussion. First, due to the geographical layout of the department the first author was unable to assist and/or help radiographers when appropriate, which he felt had enhanced his relationship with other participants at other sites (Hayre, 2016a). For example, in other environments he could assist with moving patient trolleys/beds, open X-ray doors, and alert radiographers to potential pitfalls and mistakes prior to irradiating patients. These interactions had helped developed trust and gain acceptance amongst participants, thus becoming more aligned with being observed as an aid rather than as a hindrance. Second, as the key research instrument in this study, his position when situated in the viewing room was arguably inferior for data collection. He was limited empirically as he was unable to "get close" to the X-ray room and observe the practices of diagnostic radiographers. This led to the author becoming "ethnographically-isolated" whereby his primary role as an ethnographic researcher was problematic. Lastly, due to the increasingly busy nature of the department and the increased workplace pressures of the general imaging environment, it remained problematic to be helping participants with the increase in workload and thus potentially leading to being viewed as an individual not assisting but merely critiquing "what they do and how they do it". Looking back, methodologically, the response from the senior radiographer was more complex than first identified and was arguably a result from a combination of the aforementioned phenomena, which inevitably led to this encounter.

After reflecting on his impact within this research capacity, the first author decided not to continue in order to prevent any further disruption and/or potentially confrontational encounters. This experience, however, offers a unique insight for prospective researchers whereby not all environments may be suitable for ethnographic research and thus critical evaluation of research sites by researchers prior to entering the field may be necessary in order to limit the abovementioned experience.

Considerations for mitigating potential hostile encounters in ethnographic research

When undertaking ethnography there is an element of unpredictability inherent within the methodology. In response, it is reasonable to expect that for some ethnographers, sensitive topics may lead to hostile/confrontational situations amongst participants. It is generally accepted that in environments that are more hostile than others, close attention to group hierarchy is required. Cialdini (2006) reminds us that the more a group is closed, the more it is usually integrated and hierarchized. This means that when doing fieldwork research, we should respect group hierarchy in trying to win trust and acceptance from its members. We must do this not only because these groups have the ability to "open and close the door" on our research, but it is also crucial for maintaining a sound working environment (Chomczynski, 2018). If a researcher decides not to include a key member in their efforts to become familiar with the group, this can be dangerous for the researcher as well as other people with whom we start to communicate with (Hammersley & Atkinson, 2007; Chomczynski, 2018). In the work by the first author, he felt unable to gain the trust and acceptance within the local radiographic department, and this arguably led to a "closing of the door", but it also demonstrates the importance for ethnographers to become part of the social group and participate in the group's activities, which will encourage acceptance and respect for the cultural norms and rituals of the group. This example, in comparison with other sites, leads to question the impact of merely observing as a participant and not participating within the group. For instance, if the author had helped in the everyday workload (as undertaken at other sites) he may have become accepted by becoming "one of the team" and "part of the social group". Without this, it would seem that my presence was merely critically gazing and doing little to help. However, the author notes how sometimes it is a component of the researcher's role as defined by the protocol to not become part of the staff's working group. Moreover, even when group membership is part of the research design, attempting to join the group may be received as though the researcher was inveigling their way into the team.

Ethnographic research explores the social action and deeper elements of a particular culture, and, as identified above, the relationship of the researcher with his/her participants. Whilst ethnographers try to adopt a variety of roles, they must remain intellectually poised between familiarity and strangeness, whilst socially poised between stranger and friend (Hammersley & Atkinson, 2007, p. 100). Looking back, the first author felt he remained a stranger, which led to the cessation of research in the field due to confrontation. It is important for prospective ethnographic researchers to ensure they find a balance between becoming a friend to participants, yet acknowledge the potential and danger of becoming a stranger in order to prevent hostile encounters.

Conclusion

This chapter sought to reflect on the softer skills associated with ethnographic research. Whilst emotion and hostility are rarely discussed and considered within ethnographic literature, this chapter provides an opportunity for discussing such encounters, such as ones that may lead to the cessation of empirical research. This chapter provided evidence affirming the importance of incorporating emotion with ethnographic research and how it can be used to strengthen the methodological rigor of the qualitative journey itself. Furthermore, through critical reflexivity, it is evident that the researcher, research environment, participants, and gatekeepers all play a pivotal role in limiting the potential for hostile encounters in the medical imaging environment, which prospective researchers should examine and maintain prior to entering the research environment.

References

Abu-Lughod, L. (2000) Locating ethnography. *Ethnography*. 1(1): 261–267.

Barter, C. and E. Renold. (2003) Dilemmas of control. In R. Lee and E. Stanko (eds.) *Researching Violence: Essays on Methodology and Measurement*. pp. 88–106. London: Routledge.

Barry, K. (2020) On the "Flip Side": an autoethnography utilizing professional reflective practice skills to navigate a medical experience as the patient. *Journal of Medical Imaging and Radiation Sciences*. 51(1): 47–53.

Blackman, S. (2007) 'Hidden ethnography': crossing emotional boarders in qualitative accounts of young people's lives. *Sociology*. 41(4): 699–716.

Bourdieu, P. and L. Wacquant. (1992) *An Invitation to Reflexive Sociology*. Cambridge: Polity Press.

Burgess, R.G. (1990) *Studies in Qualitative Methodology – Reflections on Field Experience*. London: JAI press Inc.

Chomczynski, P. (2018) Doing ethnography in a hostile environment: the case of a Mexico community. *Sage Research Methods Cases*. London: Sage.

Cialdini, R.B. (2006) *Influence: The Psychology of Persuasion*. New York, NY: Harper Business.

Coffey, A. (1999) *The Ethnographic Self*. London: Sage.

Denzin, N.K. and Y.S. Lincoln. (1998) *Strategies of Qualitative Inquiry*. London: Sage.

Ehrlich, R.A. and D.M. Coakes. (2020) *Patient Care in Radiography – With an Introduction to Medical Imaging*. 10th edn. London: Elsevier.

Fielding, N. (2011) Working in hostile environments. In C. Seale, D. Silverman, J.F. Gumbrium and G. Gobo (eds.) *Qualitative Research in Practice*. p. 23. Thousand Oaks, CA: Sage.

Hammersley, M. and P. Atkinson. (1995) *Ethnography: Principles in Practice*. London, England: Routledge.

Hammersley, M. and P. Atkinson. (2007) *Ethnography Principles in Practice*, 3rd edn. New York: Routledge.

Hayre, C.M. (2016a) *Radiography Observed: An Ethnographic Study Exploring Contemporary Radiographic Practice*. PhD Thesis: Canterbury Christ Church University.

Hayre, C.M. (2016b) 'Cranking up', 'whacking up' and 'bumping up': X-ray exposures in contemporary radiographic practice. *Radiography*. 22(2): 194–198.

Hayre, C.M. and S. Blackman. (2020) Ethnographic mosaic approach for health and rehabilitation practitioners: an ethno-radiographic perspective. *Disability and Rehabilitation*. 1–4.

Hayre, C.M. and R.M. Strudwick. (2019) Ethnography for radiographers: a methodological insight for prospective researchers. *Journal of Medical Imaging and Radiation Sciences*. 50(3): 352–358.

Kemper, T. (1990). *Research Agendas in the Sociology of Emotions*. Albany: State University Press of New York.

Lane, A.N. (2016) Medical imaging and consent: when is an X-ray assault? *Journal of Medical Radiation Sciences*. 63(2): 133–137.

Lee-Treweek, G. and S. Linkogle. (eds.) (2000) *Danger in the Field*. London: Routledge.

Marcus, G. (1998) *Ethnography Through Thick and Thin*. Princeton, NJ: Princeton University Press.

Nightingale, J.M., F. Murphy, C. Eaton, & R. Borgen. (2016) A qualitative analysis of staff-client interactions within a breast cancer assessment clinic. *Radiography*. 23(1): 38–47.

Shilling, C. (2002) The two traditions in the sociology of emotions. In J. Barbalet (ed.) *Emotions and Sociology*. pp. 10–32. Oxford: Blackwell.

Tracy, S.J. (2010) Qualitative quality: eight "Big Tent" criteria for excellent qualitative research. *Qualitative Enquiry*. 16 (10): 837–851.

PART III

Design and planning

6

THE DOOR-TO-DOOR ETHNOGRAPHER

Recruiting patients and healthcare providers for ethnographic research

Melinda Rea-Holloway and Steve Hagelman

Introduction

If someone asked you if they could spend all day, maybe multiple days, observing you and even filming you, would you be up for it? What if they wanted to observe you at work? What if your line of work had very strict regulations around collecting personal data, the very thing this person, a complete stranger, is asking to do?

It is no wonder that recruiting for healthcare research is a daunting undertaking. Often, it can take longer than the fieldwork itself. This chapter will identify challenges and offer advice on how to mitigate some of these challenges. We will cover the process for recruiting patients outside of the healthcare system and for recruiting healthcare professionals (HCPs) and patients inside healthcare spaces, like private practices and hospitals.

Recruiting patients outside of the healthcare system

Recruiting patients for fieldwork outside of the healthcare system is by far the easier of the two types of healthcare recruits. You only need the green light from one person (and maybe their family) rather than a large, often bureaucratic organization. The primary difficulty is finding the types of patients you need. If you're looking for people with a more common condition like osteoporosis or heart disease it isn't so tough, but it can be a real challenge if you are looking for patients with a rare disease. Also, like any recruit, it becomes more difficult when you begin to stack sampling criteria. It is easy to find someone who has osteoporosis. It becomes more difficult if you're looking for someone with osteoporosis who is also on a certain combination of medications, who is also within a certain age range, and who also has a particular attitude about their condition. All of those are reasonable requests from a client or stakeholder, but in combination, it can make an initially easy recruit far more challenging.

The first step then in recruitment is deciding on the sampling criteria. It is important to consider not only *who* you would like to conduct fieldwork with, but also *where* you would like to observe, *when* you will need to be there, and *what* kinds of things you would like to learn about. Considering each of these before officially beginning the recruitment process is important because it will help frame the types of questions you will want to ask potential participants and will help you identify a sample that will provide a more valid and holistic understanding of the topic of interest. We typically create a screener that includes questions addressing all of the above so we can both find the right participants and schedule fieldwork during a time when we can observe targeted behaviors or contexts. However, it is also important to be flexible during the early stages of the recruitment process. One of the most important elements of an ethnographic approach is induction, and we approach our recruitment with that in mind. We often learn via the screening process about important differences in the who, where, when, and what dimensions that we did not know about or could not have anticipated. When this happens, we adjust our sampling matrix accordingly.

Ethnographers are committed to achieving a sample that reflects the meaningful distinctions between people *and* contexts. For example, when we wanted to understand the insertion of central venous catheters, we made a list of the types of HCPs that inserted them (IV therapy nurses, anesthesiologists, radiologists, ER doctors), but also a list of the types of contexts in which they were inserted (pre-surgery, outpatient surgery, radiology, hospital bedside). We used this list to guide our recruitment and screening process to make sure that we were able to achieve a sample that allowed us to note patterned similarities and differences between the HCPs we shadowed and also between the contexts we observed. When doing fieldwork with patient populations, this attention to context is equally important. We are not only looking to identify differences between patients (health status, age, medication history, etc.), but we are also interested in sampling for variables that may impact their daily lives and experiences of the disease. This might include things like where they live, the type of family or support situation they have, whether or not they have health insurance, and how long they have been living with the disease.

Regardless of who or what you are looking for, it is always wise to build extra time into the timeline for healthcare studies. How much time you'll need will vary on your sample size and how hard potential participants are to find, but you can expect to spend more time recruiting for healthcare research than you would for other types of ethnographic work. If you have a tight timeline (we always do), it can help to start your fieldwork before you have found all of your participants. Starting data collection might even cause you to rethink your sampling criteria. For instance, you might hear about an alternative treatment and want to add a few participants who are receiving it. Even if you don't have a tight timeline, taking an iterative, dynamic approach to sample selection can be beneficial.

Finding participants

Once you are set on what types of patients and contexts you are looking for, the next step is actually finding them. Recruiting for many of our healthcare studies requires using at least a few different sources, particularly for rare or difficult to find patient populations. Regardless of the source, we have found that a couple of things are key to achieving a successful healthcare study recruit: transparency, professionalism, and remembering who the expert is. We try to make our research objectives and processes clear to potential patient gatekeepers, outlining our methods for ensuring confidentiality and protecting patient data, and emphasizing our inductive process aimed at learning from the patient. In fact, over the years, most of the people who we approach about our studies (in healthcare or not) are intrigued by our desire to listen and understand real life. However, especially with vulnerable patient populations, gatekeepers tend to be protective and when recruiting for these types of studies, you must be prepared to fully explain your research plan, your credentials, and your understanding of HIPAA (more on this later).

Sources of potential participants might include:

- *Organizations and groups.* You can sometimes find potential participants through in-person or online support groups or organizations devoted to specific health issues. We have regularly asked organizational contacts and group leaders to spread the word about our research. Even if they just allow you to put up a flyer, that can be a great start. In addition, exploring these groups can also be a form of fieldwork—seeing what people in these groups talk about can be a first step in developing an understanding of your research subject. These groups are particularly valuable resources when looking for patients with rare diseases. We did a study once about people with acromegaly, a condition which effects only around 60 people per million (Holdaway and Rajasoorya 1999). We weren't at all sure that we could find a sample, and if we had tried to use traditional recruiting methods, we'd still be at it. Instead, we snowballed out from a number of acromegaly organizations (in addition to healthcare providers), and in the end, the recruit wasn't nearly as difficult as we thought it would be.
- *Healthcare providers and other professionals.* We have had some success recruiting patients through medical practices or specific HCPs, although this can be more time consuming than other methods for recruiting. We have had the most success via practices who have a relationship with either us (because they have participated in one of our studies in the past) or our client (when we are able to share that information). Due to ethical and privacy regulations, HCPs are usually reluctant to become an intermediary in this process, but they sometimes will share information about our study with patients via flyers hung in their office or handed out to specific patients. They might also be willing to let the ethnographer hang out at the office so that they can explain the study to patients who might be interested in participating. Once, when we were doing a study on schizophrenia and bipolar disorder, we snowballed out from a variety of doctors, nurses, social workers, and case managers to identify not only individual potential participants, but also to help us understand some of the organizations and services that these patient populations might need. This allowed us to not only begin our fieldwork with a better understanding of the needs of these patients, but also gave us additional contacts for potential recruitment.
- *Recruiting companies.* It is always better to find participants yourself, but there are times when you simply don't have enough time or the resources to develop a sample without bringing in a professional recruiter. Recruiting companies who specialize in pairing researchers with patients may be the quickest and easiest way to recruit, but it can also be costly and you run the risk of having a sample of "professional participants," participants who participate in research regularly. This can really work against the goals of ethnographic research, which is dedicated to capturing unfiltered, real life. In addition, we have found that sometimes patients we find via professional recruiters seem to have an idea of what it means to participate in market research, and we might have a harder time establishing an ethnographic dynamic (these participants may look to us to guide the conversation). For these reasons, when we use professional recruiters, we typically don't rely on them as our only source of participants.
- *Networking and snowballing.* Traditional ethnographic sampling always relies on going to a place or group of people that you want to understand, making a connection, and then working out from there to other people and other settings. Once you have identified some of the important variables and contexts for the patient population you want to study, you can target settings or people who might intersect with, or regularly come in contact with the people you are looking for. For example, if you are looking for patients who have breast cancer, you might ask to hang up flyers at a shop that sells wigs or hats designed for cancer

patients. If you are looking for patients who have diabetes, you might meet with a diabetes educator or a bakery that sells sugar-free pastries. Your own social network might be a useful resource in pointing to potential participants too. Reaching out to people you know (or even past participants) and asking who they know with this or that condition or who use this or that medication or product can be a fruitful exercise.

Ethical considerations

Heath care research recruiting requires special and rigorous attention to the protection of the information that you will be collecting. Since you will be collecting personal health information from the moment you start recruiting, you should have a documented plan on what type of personal data you are going to collect and how you are going to protect it. You should be prepared to share this plan with your client and potential participants. Although outside of the scope of this chapter, acquainting yourself with the rules and regulations of HIPAA is a good first step if you're doing research in the United States.

Setting the ethnographic tone with participants

Before you can begin fieldwork, it is important to spend some time setting expectations with participants and laying the groundwork for your ethnographic visit. Most people will have never heard of ethnography, let alone participated in an ethnographic study before and so they will probably have inaccurate assumptions about what it will involve. We have found that taking the time to explain our approach (especially how it differs from a standard interview) really helps to make fieldwork more productive, and also usually helps to transform our participants into much more active partners. Although each ethnographer's fieldwork process will be a little different, there are a few things we always communicate to participants prior to fieldwork:

1. *We explain what we're studying and how we can best learn about it.* We mention some of the things we'd like to observe and talk about but also emphasize that we want them to weigh in on when and where we visit. We acknowledge that we are nosey but try to explain why. For example, when we studied overactive bladder, we knew that it would be important to get a tour of our participants' homes and perhaps even inside their cabinets and dressers in order to see how the condition might impact the material culture of toiletries and clothes. We also knew it would be important for us to be with participants during times when the condition impacted their lives. So, during our initial calls with participants, we explained why this was all important and asked them to think about what might help us understand these impacts. At the same time, avoiding too much detail about the research project and its goals is prudent in order not to sway the participant, so when we have these discussions with participants, we always stress that *they* are the expert. This is a "there are no right or wrong answers" plea to help them feel open and honest with us and to reinforce that we are truly there to learn from them and that we will be following *their* lead on what to explore and talk about.
2. *We ask them not to prepare or change anything in preparation for our visit.* This includes not cleaning their house (which many do anyway), not sending the kids to a babysitter, and not prepping what we want to see (e.g., not laying out their medications on the dining room table before we come). We explain that we are all about real life and that having things as they normally are is essential for our work.
3. *We tell them who is coming (especially if there is more than one person) and that we will be videotaping the visit.* We use cameras so much that it can be easy to forget to mention them, but

not letting participants know ahead of time can come as a very unpleasant surprise. We let them know exactly how the video will be used (mostly to help us remember what we learn) and let them know we will be signing a confidentiality agreement with them regarding these uses.

4. *We outline their compensation.* Some people would happily participate in the research for free. In fact, we have found that money is generally not the primary motivator for many of our research participants, especially health care research participants. Most people like the idea of a captive audience for several hours where they can share their unique experiences and opinions. Some patients find it very cathartic because they may hesitate to share some of their most difficult experiences and deepest fears with their loved ones. We often find ourselves standing at the door after one of these visits, being embraced and thanked for the opportunity. Still, for the corporate work we do, we pay participants an incentive as a way to thank them for their time.

The need for flexibility

As with any kind of in-person research you can expect reschedules and changes of plan, and it is important to keep in mind that this is not necessarily bad. Ethnography is all about trying to capture and understand real life, and let's face it, real life is messy. We give participants a reminder phone call a day or two before the actual visit because things can come up and people can forget. Also, you are sometimes visiting people who are in poor health, and it can be hard to predict when they might feel well enough to have a visitor. Life can be unpredictable for anyone, but it can be especially unpredictable when you have a serious health condition. This need for flexibility will continue into your fieldwork, so adopting the right mindset now can set you up for more productive and less stressful fieldwork.

Recruiting for fieldwork in healthcare spaces

When your research requires you conduct fieldwork in healthcare spaces like clinics and hospitals, additional time needs to be set aside for your recruit, *a lot of additional time* in many cases. This is the most challenging type of recruit we do as a company, and we get many, many more hesitations and outright rejections for these projects than any others we do. There are a few reasons for this apprehension:

- HIPAA is a major concern, often a deal breaker. This can especially be the case for non-HCP gatekeepers. We have found that office managers and receptionists tend to be less likely to hear us out than nurses and physicians.
- The idea of being observed at work is not that appealing for anyone, but especially for those who run the risk of being sued for malpractice.
- You are not asking for agreement from one person but from an entire organization. These days, more and more hospitals and even small practices belong to large health networks or university systems. This means that a practitioner at a given practice cannot give permission without consulting the parent company. Figuring out who to ask within the bureaucratic system can be daunting or even impossible. In addition, within a given practice, there are often dozens of potential participants or "others" that might be impacted by the research and before permission can be obtained, some HCPs may feel the need to get consent from everyone.
- Cameras (and even extra people) are out of place in health care environments (see HIPAA, above).

- HCPs are busy. Too busy (they often think) for researchers. Most are overwhelmed and struggle to keep up with their daily workload, and the thought of adding more to their plate is unfathomable. We should note, however, that it has been our experience that they greatly overestimate how much work we will be!
- The incentives for participating might seem paltry to physicians and the benefit for them might not outweigh the perceived cost. For pharmaceutical-sponsored research, larger incentives might be prohibited because of anti-bribery laws.

So, this type of recruit is an uphill battle, but despite the odds we have done it successfully and repeatedly. It just takes a thick skin and lots and lots of persistence. Here are some tips for making the process a little less painful and a little more productive.

Finding practices

There are healthcare providers all over the country, and identifying practitioners of a certain specialty is as easy as an internet search. We have found that it is best to try to approach a practice in person, but it is rarely practical to visit every potential practice, so you'll likely need to do a mix of dropping in on practices and cold calling via the phone. Either way, it is best to develop a clear plan for not only the initial contact but also for the inevitable follow-ups required. Good old-fashioned record keeping is essential in this regard. Being able to mention previous contacts, who you spoke with, and what was determined sounds easier than it will be in practice. You will likely be contacting a couple of dozen practices for each one that will eventually agree to participate, so keeping track can be a nightmare.

There are also healthcare recruiting companies who can help connect you with HCPs who may be more accustomed to working with researchers. These companies tend to recruit primarily for focus groups, surveys, and qualitative interviews, so they might not have a lot of experience recruiting for ethnographic, in-context work. This can make it a little more challenging, but we have found the recruiting companies are generally willing to help. Still, much like recruiting patients, finding your HCPs through a recruiter runs the risk of getting "professional participants." For this reason, we like to use a variety of methods for recruiting, supplementing with help from recruiters when necessary.

Gatekeeper strategies

Throughout the recruiting process, but especially in the beginning, you should be prepared to talk with lots of gatekeepers whose job it is to keep you from eating up the time of very busy HCPs. It is important to have a script ready for the gatekeepers which should include a brief explanation of the research as well as how it can benefit them and their patients. You won't have a whole lot of time to make your points, so you'll want to make them succinctly. Having a sizeable incentive helps, but you should also stress how unobtrusive the process is and how the research findings might ultimately benefit the practice of medicine and patient care. The fact is that this isn't something that anyone will sign up for unless you talk it up a bit. Ethnography in healthcare spaces requires a lot more salesmanship than they taught us in school and so you might want to brush up on the old ABCs of selling.

You'll also want to have answers ready for common questions and concerns. These include who you are working for, how you are going to protect and use the data, and how you will handle getting their patients to agree to the research. If you get to the point where you are answering these questions, that's a good sign, but you should make sure that you look and sound like you have done this before! Providing a detailed description of your plan to address each of their concerns will go a long way toward building credibility and trust. We have even found that it is sometimes helpful to preemptively address some common concerns.

It is also useful to have some printed materials about you, your organization, and what the fieldwork will look like that can be handed out, faxed, or emailed to the office. Printed information offers decision makers something physical they can look at when they have an extra moment. Asking the gatekeeper if it is okay to provide them with information also gives you a valid reason to follow up with them later about it.

The most important thing about this salesmanship phase is to stay confident. You will get a lot of rejections, and it can be easy to feel defeated. Eventually someone will agree and before you know it, you will have enough willing HCPs to complete a sample. It might be completely exhausting, and failure is a real possibility, but more often than not we've filled our samples, even if we did get bruised and battered along the way.

Ethical and red tape considerations: HIPAA and institutional review boards

Once you get past the gatekeeper and receive buy-in from the decision-maker, you still might have a significant hoop to jump through—institutional review boards. Many healthcare institutions and practices require that all research conducted within their facilities be examined to determine whether it meets standards of merit and that ethical concerns have been addressed. In the United Sates, we can often do observational work in private clinics without having to go through a review board, but we usually need to if we want to do research in a hospital or an academic setting. This can cost time and money and including these costs in your research plan is essential. A single review can be thousands of dollars and doesn't ensure that you will ultimately get permission (or that you will get permission in time for your deadline). Depending on how often the IRB committee meets, applying for approval might eat up a month or more of your timeline. If you need to go through an IRB, most hospital websites have instructions on starting the process, and we'd suggest soliciting advice from or collaborating with your primary contact at the hospital. Although the process can be time-consuming and stressful, we have found that most IRBs are not opposed to ethnographic fieldwork.

Prepping heath care professionals

In order for the fieldwork to go smoothly, it is very important to notify and prepare everyone in the practice on what to expect. Your process might need to be a little more formal and detailed than when you prep individual patients (see earlier in this chapter). You'll likely be working with multiple HCPs and administrative staff, and doing research in clinics and practices has more logistical challenges than observations in people's homes.

You need to find agreement with the organization ahead of time on which HCPs will be a part of the study, which types of patient interactions you will be able to sit in on, and how you will gain patient consent. These all need to be explained to any relevant players prior to the fieldwork, including HCPs and administrative staff. Ideally you will meet with them before they start their work day, either that morning or on a prior day. The last thing you want is for any of the HCPs to show up to work with an unwelcome surprise—an ethnographer with a camera. We learned this the hard way. One time we had secured permission to do fieldwork in a pre-surgery area of a medium-sized hospital. We had gone through IRB approval and had passed through multiple layers of gatekeepers to finally arrive at the hospital on the morning our fieldwork was set to start. We met with our contact in the pre-surgery area who assured us we were good to go. Almost as an afterthought (we were new to this work at the time and pretty naïve), we asked who would be performing the procedure and whether they had any questions about our plan. She looked sort of confused and said, "I'm not sure. You mean you haven't talked to them?" This set off an unfortunate chain of events which ended with us in the office of the Chief of Anesthesiology, being lectured about the relatively low position that anesthesiologists occupy in the hospital's hierarchy and how this oversight was yet another manifestation of the disregard in which they were held. It took us several days of hanging out in the pre-surgery area to convince the anesthesiologists to let us observe them.

Also, keep in mind that you're not the boss. This is their space, and they will guide the fieldwork process too. They will have ultimate say on how everything plays out even if it is not how you usually do things or if it is not ideal for the research. They may have specific rules they want you to abide by or they may require that certain rooms, patients, or subject areas are simply off limits. Chances are, the HCPs will never have done anything like this before, and they may learn as they go what they are and are not comfortable with. Ethnographers have to be sensitive to this and not overstep boundaries. In other words, prepare your HCPs as much as you can, but expect changes once you're there. We have also found that it generally takes about half of a day for HCPs (or anyone we are observing at work) to get comfortable and *natural* with us. Don't get discouraged if at first things seem too buttoned up or if you seem to be excluded from some important contexts. Chances are, after lunch, you might find your HCP loosening up and inviting you into those contexts.

This highlights a very important consideration in doing workplace ethnography. Because it takes longer to build rapport and because there are so many moving parts and so many players, you should always try to stay as long as possible. A few hours definitely isn't enough. Most of what we learn about how HCPs interact with their patients and how they interpret and follow "standard practices" we learn during the later stages of our fieldwork. If we left the practice after a few hours, we would have a very different understanding of how things work. This is especially the case with HCPs that didn't make the initial decision to let you observe them. We were once given permission to observe a team of IV therapy nurses at a regional hospital. The head nurse in charge of the team thought our research sounded fascinating and was happy to agree to participate. The nurses we were going to observe were substantially less enthusiastic about our presence. In fact, the nurse we were assigned to on the first day was openly hostile at the prospect. Although she had agreed to participate, we got the impression that she felt coerced and so we suggested she opt out. After about 30 minutes, she came back, thanked us for being sensitive to her concerns and asked us to explain our research. She ultimately opted back in and allowed us to shadow her on and off for a week. During the first day although she was polite, she was definitely not comfortable. As the second day progressed, she became much more relaxed and even circled back to correct some of the procedural things she had shown us the day before. She explained that she had originally been concerned that we were "grading" her and so she had tried to do things more by the book. After she felt comfortable that we were just trying to learn, she showed us how she really did things and explained the rationale.

The need for flexibility in making connections, scheduling, and rescheduling

When setting up fieldwork dates, it is important to remain flexible. For one, it might take longer than expected to get all the clearance needed to enter the field. Also, if you are studying a very specific topic, e.g., a certain type of patient or a certain type of interaction, you may need to wait until the last minute to schedule a time when the healthcare practice knows they will have that targeted patient or type of interaction. Like most ethnographic research, you'll save yourself a lot of stress if you remain flexible about your fieldwork. You definitely don't want the practice to feel pressured to artificially create the situation you are wanting to observe, so, as in most things, patience is a virtue.

At last, in the field! But the recruit continues

You've recruited your sample, you've prepared the staff on what to expect, and you're in the field, hanging out with the doctor. Everyone is being very nice and accommodating but wait, your recruit isn't done yet! All throughout your day you'll be meeting new people; patients come and go, new HCPs and administrative staff show up, pharmaceutical reps and medical students drop by. It turns out the recruit doesn't end until your fieldwork ends, and you'll find that you'll be explaining yourself and trying to get buy-in all the while you're in the field. You'll want to make sure you bring extra consent forms and have a brief script prepared to explain the research to everyone you meet. You might have a couple of scripts. 1. An elevator speech (one that can ideally be delivered in less than a minute) to someone that you'll be spending time with and actually collecting personal information from. 2. A one- or two-line explanation for people who are there but not involved in the research. You'll find you'll get a lot of quizzical looks from passing patients and providers. Something as simple as "I am hanging out with Dr. X, trying to understand the experiences of people with Y," is fine for non-participants who are just curious.

You'll want a more thorough explanation for the people who are going to actually be part of the research. Key things to include are:

1. What you are doing
2. Why you are doing it (including whether it is for school, for a pharmaceutical company, etc.)
3. What you are going to do with that data
4. What they might gain or lose by participating
5. That they can choose not to participate at any time (and this will not impact their care or job)
6. What you will need from them if they do participate (a signed consent)

Essentially for this longer elevator speech you'll want to cover the basics of your consent form, and more often than not, you'll give this speech when you're asking them to sign it.

The good news is that in-the-field recruiting tends to be the easy part—patients are usually very gracious about researchers sitting in to observe interactions. We once showed up to shadow a gastroenterologist on a day he was performing colonoscopies, and we assumed that it might be difficult to get patient consents on the fly. We were guessing that we might get 50% of patients to agree, given the sensitivity of the procedure. We were shocked to get all but one patient to consent. Most said, "If Dr. G is good with it, so am I."

Although HCPs are hit and miss, it usually isn't the end of the world if one or two don't want you shadowing them. If you've made it this far, this part of the recruit won't be all-consuming, and you'll finally be able to focus on the actual research.

Conclusions

No bones about it, healthcare recruiting is challenging. You'll get a lot of rejections, but it is important to keep going. We've had recruits for healthcare studies last months, but more often than not, with a lot of persistence, we find our sample. No matter how you approach it, it is hard work, but we hope that some of these strategies and approaches can help you achieve fantastic samples.

Reference

Holdaway I.M., & C. Rajasoorya. (1999) Epidemiology of acromegaly. *Pituitary.* 2(1): 29–41.

7

ETHNOGRAPHIC RESEARCH DESIGN

Ruth Montgomery-Andersen and Michelle M. Doucette

Introduction

Intercultural research poses significant and complex challenges for research participants and for the researcher themselves. Issues of particular interest in contemporary intercultural research include ownership of data and the creation of respectful, culturally safe research protocols. This chapter will address topics that can directly influence intercultural research design including: working with(in) Indigenous cultures as an "Other"; understanding language and its influence on design; Indigenous languages and intellectual property; working alongside or under the direction of Indigenous leaders, researchers, community panels, and their influence on design; as well as Culture Bearers' support and guidance and how their influences strengthen the relevance and validity of any community based study. Intercultural research collaboration between Indigenous peoples and non-Indigenous researchers is the primary focus of this book chapter. Researchers motivated to engage in intercultural research must contemplate the impacts of their relationships in respect to being an "Other" scientist, the historical realm of research experiences within Indigenous communities, and the researchers' relationship to the people, the families, the communities, the Elders, and to Culture Bearers. As intercultural researchers we are interested in looking beyond the sharing of knowledge and towards the development of intercultural competencies in the creation of new knowledge. Common challenges facing intercultural research collaborations often include: language differences, lack of exploratory research funding from granting institutions, time constraints, community politics, cultural competence, and a variety of other barriers. Researchers are also insensitive to the needs and requirements of the communities—this is true in many communities around the globe (Gordon, 2014). Throughout this chapter we will reflect on current collaboration practices and share personal examples of research situations we have encountered that can be understood in different ways if we critically examine our experiences in the context of intercultural collabor ation. We hope to challenge each reader to reflect on the purpose of intercultural research, the reason we do research, and how we generate knowledge. Each researcher must reflect on why knowledge is collected or created and for whose benefit? Are we being of service to the communities whose knowledge we are gathering? Is it for their use or is it for our benefit?

We chose to use the term settler, and describe ourselves so, in this article, as it is a term that is accepted by a vast majority of Indigenous communities when respectfully validating non-Indigenous individuals. As non-Indigenous settler researchers we are personally invested, motivated, and driven to articulate what we have learned to help further the discourse for training the next generation of intercultural researchers. In an effort to express our positionality we take a moment to introduce ourselves: Ruth Montgomery-Andersen is a midwife, born in the United States, educated in Denmark, who now lives in Greenland. Ruth's research focuses on childbirth, cultural resiliency, and Greenlandic families. Michelle Doucette is a social epidemiologist with roots in Ontario who has settled in Nunavut. Michelle's research interests are focused on understanding the impact of social determinants of health on population health outcomes, women's experiences of food security, and chronic disease. Both authors of this chapter have chosen to work and live in Inuit communities in the arctic.

Often non-Indigenous researchers that work together with Indigenous communities seek to draw on community member's traditional knowledge and cultural competencies, especially language competencies and ways of knowing (epistemology) which are the unique, intangible, intellectual and cultural property of each community, cultural, or linguistic group. In respectful collaborations between Indigenous communities and non-Indigenous researchers both parties have much to gain. For the communities, there can be economic incentives, policy incentives, resource incentives, and advocacy incentives. Communities may direct research to answer their own questions, develop policy and advocacy platforms, or develop infrastructure and economic development through employment. Researchers stand to gain increased knowledge from these collaborators, and may often act, or be expected to act, as catalyst for translation of research findings to policy and decision-makers. In contemporary intercultural research, Indigenous communities and Indigenous researchers are actively advocating for self-determination in research and demanding Indigenous led research take priority, and co-developed intercultural research to be more tightly managed and overseen. Indigenous communities demand and expect to act as gatekeepers and "gate openers" within their own communities. It is the responsibility of all researchers that work within Indigenous communities, or in intercultural research broadly, to conduct and contribute to research ethically and respectfully in ways that mitigate past traumatization and support the development of trust and mutual knowledge, and that benefit or serve purpose for all members of the collaboration.

Among several contemporary issues in intercultural research, some outlined above, another noteworthy focus in this chapter will be on the shifting understandings of ownership and control of research data, ownership of created data, and ownership pertaining to the creation of research protocols and tools. In the past, researchers notoriously extracted knowledge from Indigenous communities with little regard for the rights of individual communities to own their own data. In contemporary intercultural research, the expectation is that researchers work in collaboration with communities to co-develop research protocols and address or negotiate data ownership agreements specific to each community's articulated needs and desires, however they may be articulated—whether by legislation, policy, practice, or orally conferred.

With the above context in mind, we have organized this chapter to describe and present several issues that intercultural researchers encounter that can be challenging for both communities and researchers to navigate. We will focus on Indigenous communities' self-determination in research and offer thoughts on how researchers may approach intercultural research as allies. We also offer this chapter as a reference that may assist communities in holding intercultural researchers accountable in their practices and approaches.

The chapter is organized to contemplate specific topics that can directly influence intercultural research design, including:

1. Demographics of an Indigenous country, in this case Greenland;
2. A short history of colonization;

3. Indigenous self-determination in research and the challenges of conducting culturally relevant and safe research in Indigenous communities;
4. Culture Bearers, their support and guidance in research design, and their role in data analysis;
5. Language and its influence on research design;
6. Ownership of intellectual data;
7. Co-developed research designs;
8. Working with(in) Indigenous communities as an "Other";
9. Analysis strategies

Demographics

A central tenant of intercultural research is working outside of one's own culture and immersing within another. The authors have had various and rich experiences as intercultural researchers in arctic Indigenous communities, among Inuit. Learning about the cultural, geopolitical, linguistic, and historical context of a place is key to being able to successfully integrate a codeveloped research protocol that is respectful and thoughtful of context.

Greenland Kalaallit Nunaat, meaning "Land of the people", is an autonomous constituent country, socially and politically linked with the Kingdom of Denmark. It is located between the Arctic and Atlantic Oceans, east of the Canadian Arctic Archipelago. Greenland is, by area, the world's largest island that is not a continent, as well as the least densely populated country in the world. Though physiographically a part of the continent of North America, Greenland has been politically associated with Europe for about a millennium. Greenland was a Danish colony until the 5th of June 1953, when the colony Greenland became a Danish county. In 1978 the people of Greenland voted to gain Home Rule and in 1979 Denmark granted Home Rule to Greenland. Self-government was granted on the 21st of June 2009 (Statistics Greenland, 2012).

Greenland has an ethno-cultural history with the Inuit peoples of Alaska, Canada, and Siberia (Gesink, Rink, Montgomery-Andersen, Mulvad, & Koch, 2009). This common history not only pertains to language, but also to relational worldview, spirituality, and cultural traditions (Nuttall, 1992). Greenlanders rely on hunting and fishing as an integral part of life, and elements such as place, including natural and built environments influence their lives and livelihood (Rink, Montgomery-Andersen, Tróndheim, Gesink, Lennert, & Kotalawala, 2012). As with other peoples throughout the world, global warming, climate change, pollution, and changes in ways of life are a part of the reality of the everyday lives of the people of Greenland. These changes directly affect the Greenlandic people and are experienced because of a direct dependence on the land, sea mammals, and in many cases on ice to support their way of life (Ehrlich, 2001; Jorgensen, 2008; Malaurie, 1985).

Greenlanders are not a minority but the majority within their own country, which has a different ethnic makeup to that of many Indigenous communities. Despite this fact, systems of Greenland remain directed towards the needs and beliefs of a Scandinavian or Northern European culture, in many cases making these systems culturally inappropriate for the Greenlanders themselves (Kruske, Kildea, & Barclay, 2006). Intercultural researchers entering co-development research endeavours within Greenland, among Inuit, will need to consider the policy and legislative frameworks that are used to oversee public administration, and in turn authorize, approve, and license research in the country.

Colonization

Colonization in Indigenous communities in the Arctic, and broadly across the global south, has left legacies of oppression, marginalization, neglect, and abuse. Before entering the world of intercultural research it is imperative that researchers understand the particular context of colonization in the community with(in) which they hope to work.

Colonization is one of the major challenges that has influenced which traditions have survived in modern day Greenland. Without tradition, it is difficult for individuals to "interact and feel that they have any influence over their environment, even decades after independence is achieved" (Kruske et al., 2006, Montgomery-Andersen & Montgomery-Andersen, 2014). Families and kinship structures are both products and producers of their own environments and of their social systems (Montgomery-Andersen & Borup, 2012). While the creation and establishment of family is a universal experience, each family and each cultural entity creates the culture and traditions surrounding this experience and is defined by their own cultural norms and value sets (Douglas, 2010; Montgomery-Andersen & Borup, 2013).

Many Indigenous cultures have experienced loss of land, language, cultural practices, and, perhaps most devastatingly, an official identity due to lack of recognition of unique cultural groups and their inherent rights under various regimes of law. The people of Greenland, as well as other Indigenous cultures and communities, have ready-made healthcare and political systems designed to meet the needs of a European, middle class, and predominantly Christian culture (Montgomery-Andersen & Borup, 2013). Through colonialization, they have developed systems to meet the needs of the majority populations of the cultures that have colonized them, such as Australia, Canada, or Denmark.

Indigenous self-determination in research

Self-determination in research is the express desire to define, guide, and realize research priorities that are identified from within communities or population groups, that meet local needs, and that serve local purposes. Novel research with nebulous understandings of purpose and returns to the community itself is not only unnecessary, it is very often harmful. Intercultural researchers must engage meaningfully with communities to ensure research endeavours are directed from within, not from outside.

Challenges of conducting culturally relevant and safe research in Indigenous communities

The challenges of creating and conducting ethical research is not new. Definitions such as validity, trustworthiness, transferability, generalizability, credibility, and dependability, have been used in describing the process to ensure a high standard of scientific knowledge and rigor in data collection and the subsequent analysis of data (Bal, 2004; Graneheim & Lundman, 2004). But there can be a disconnect between the theory of ethics and the reality of the process when conducting research. Inherently, the ethics of research with Indigenous communities have gained attention as an important topic in health sciences, social sciences, and community research projects. Often it is the researchers' attitude to sharing power and influence that is a defining aspect of how studies are conducted and not the understanding that useful outcomes can only be achieved in a collaborative effort with the communities (Rink et al., 2012). Local community meetings, information and discussion, and focus groups ensure that the local community is given access to analysis and the results of the research (Elliott, 2005).

"Although all these elements converge toward a respectful and humanistic approach, the participation of communities at each stage of health research necessitates greater attention to ethical considerations" (Blumenthal, 2011, as cited in Wilson, Kenny, & Dickson-Swift, 2018, p. 190).

Smith (2002) uses other concepts, measurements, and definitions for ethically led research with and for Indigenous communities. She reiterates throughout her book *Decolonizing Methodologies* that in all societies language and identity are in some way intertwined. One of the challenges for the researcher when collecting, analysing and presenting the data, is to not forget that she is analysing text outside of her own context, a context which might not be the correct discourse for understanding (Jasen, 1997; Smith, 2002).

Culture Bearers

As intercultural researchers get to know the social workings of a community and seek to find their place in self-determined research, it is important to begin to build relationships with those within society who are respected knowledge keepers, elders, leaders, and Culture Bearers.

As we know, knowledge is passed from one generation to another by word of mouth in most cultures (Banks-Wallace, 2002). With the expression of thoughts, the writing of literature and poems, and the telling of stories, culture and identity find ways to develop and stay alive. In many close-knit communities there are individuals, families, or groups that have a voiced or an unvoiced influence and an official or unofficial station within the community (Loppie, 2007; Pe-Pua, 2006).

These individuals are the guardians of knowledge and tradition in societies, often considered "Culture Bearers". They exercise influence over traditions, stories, and rituals within the culture and help determine which traditions and stories are protected and perpetuated and which disappear from a society's consciousness (Brown, 1989; Montgomery-Andersen & Borup, 2013). Culture Bearers' support, guidance, and collaboration have an influence on the strength, relevance, and validity of the study.

Language

Intercultural research will necessarily encounter language barriers on many fronts, from unique and diverse dialects to varying approaches to intergenerational transmission of language, recognizing and understanding the unique epistemologies expressed through language and vocabulary, and the ability or inability to translate linguistic/cultural concepts from one language to another.

An example of the use of language can be found in these researchers' experiences in data collection in Greenland. In Greenland, the official language is Greenlandic, thus the language of interview-based research is necessarily Greenlandic. When working with other non-Indigenous researchers it is both expected and common that transcripts are written in either English or, preferably, in Danish, and that the published articles are in English despite research data being collected in Greenlandic.

Often researchers in Greenland have little or no knowledge of the Greenlandic language. In the case of the author of this chapter, she herself and a researcher assistant, have invested heavily to develop Greenlandic language skills and now speak Greenlandic and are capable of undertaking research in the language most familiar to many research participants, a valuable but not always feasible strategy for respectful intercultural research. Even with functional spoken Greenlandic skills, the author often finds it necessary for all transcripts to be written in Danish, and published in Greenlandic, Danish, and English.

It is absolutely imperative in such situations that the researchers employ the use of translation and re-translation as an important part of the research process (Kvale, 1996; Montgomery-Andersen & Borup, 2013). Language expert and Culture Bearer Nuka Møller supports this thought and also suggests that the use of language is connected with historical, political, and social issues: "In all societies language and identity are in some way intertwined, and when working in cultures other than one's own the use and understanding of language is of the utmost importance, even more so in Indigenous societies" (N. Møller, personal communications, 2003–2006).

Language is also a part of the struggle for international acknowledgement of the rights to one's culture and lands, and use of language is connected with historical, political, and social issues (Smith, 2002). Acknowledgement of the rights to one's culture and lands. Intercultural researchers must acknowledge the importance of language not only as a means of communication, but also for creating a safe space for the sharing of knowledge.

Ownership of intellectual data

As highlighted in the introduction, intellectual property rights over linguistic, cultural, and Indigenous data is an emerging area of thought and practice, and it has significant impact on the co-development of research protocols. As an aspect of self-determination in research, communities are now expecting and demanding to be the ultimate owners of their own data generated through collaborative research programs. Navigating this hurdle may require educating Research Ethics Boards, Universities, Institutions, and Funders about the necessity of creating new protocols around data collection, data analysis, data storage, and data warehousing and ownership.

The concept of intellectual property and ownership has been debated in Indigenous communities with focus on the ownership of intellectual data (Elliott, 2005; Loppie, 2007; Montgomery-Andersen & Borup, 2013). It is connected to the discourse on Indigenous rights, ownership of data, and subsequently the ethical protocol for research with and for Aboriginal or Indigenous groups, nations, and cultures (Schnarch, 2004). For example, until recently, the Greenlandic community did not have access to research materials collected in Greenland.

Although there is a theoretical understanding that includes acknowledgement that both the researchers and the local community will own the research results equally, scientists and researchers from other countries and cultures carrying out research and studies among and concerning the Greenlandic people have owned and stored the data that they have collected in and about Greenland in their own countries (Montgomery-Andersen & Borup, 2013). They have paid little attention to Greenlandic laws and regulations that concern the gathering, storing, and sharing of intellectual knowledge with the local communities and that include laws regarding delivering results to the Greenlandic Archives and Groenlandica.[1]

Co-developed research designs

In our experience, co-developed research endeavours are guided by community self-determination and are centred around community priorities, engage several layers of consultation and partnerships as research questions are refined, discuss the distribution of roles and responsibilities collectively, identify/prioritize issues of informed consent, and develop data collection/analysis/dissemination plans that meet the need which initiated the research primarily.

In a small or interconnected society where people know and know of each other, it is important to pay special attention to informed consent, confidentiality, protection of the integrity of the participants, and the protection and the ownership of data. This includes the development of informational material in the language of the participants that is written in easily understandable language and ensures that information is provided both in writing and orally that respects linguistic traditions and improves the process of informed consent. In regard to anonymity, it is often difficult in smaller societies and communities. When anonymity is the goal, it is difficult to decide which details are important to keep anonymous, which details are confidential, and which details are culturally sensitive. Within an Indigenous context it is the community itself, through dialogue within the community and with the researchers, that defines what type of data needs to be shared anonymously (Schnarch, 2004).

This process of co-developing research protocols and considering important issues like informed consent and approaches to anonymity should always be supported by dialogue with Culture Bearers and discussions with research assistants. The ethical validity in the studies is incumbent on supporting and developing stringent concepts of informed consent, voluntary participation, confidentiality, and often the ability for the participants to protect anonymity (Montgomery-Andersen & Borup, 2013; World Medical Association, 2020).

The "Other"

As a researcher working in an intercultural research environment, there are many roles you may be required to navigate: you may be a settler, you may be an ally, but you will always be an "Other". Reflexivity and positionality are practices we have employed and found enormously valuable in our research experiences. Intercultural research where "otherness" is most pertinent to contextualize for the purposes of data interpretation is of the qualitative research tradition.

Contextualizing qualitative research

Qualitative research involves 1) the contextualization of subjective data, 2) giving the reader space to assess the analysis, and 3) the interpretation of the researcher (Graneheim & Lundman 2004). As a researcher researching within one's own arena, one is "situated" both as an insider and as an outsider. This oxymoron creates an arena that goes beyond the mechanics of informed consent and ethical validity of research data. It reaches into the metaphysical realm of understanding the researcher's place within the society, in the locality of the research, and the researcher's place within the scientific hierarchy (Costley, Elliott, & Gibbs, 2010; Haraway, 1988; Montgomery-Andersen & Borup, 2013; Schmaus, 2008).

All empirical materials in qualitative research are complex and require analysis methods that take complexity into account by ensuring that the analysis methods are relevant to the data (Banks-Wallace, 2002). It is important to the data that there is a space to reflect and understand the data within the historical and cultural context, but that also looks at the detail of the data when presented. Within qualitative research, and especially in qualitative health research, we are gathering data that tells a story.

The actor decides which details are added and which are left out. When stories are told to an audience or a researcher, they are included in the recreation of the story. The story is thus developed as a relationship between the storyteller and those who listen. (Montgomery-Andersen & Borup, 2013). Within the process the understanding of the material is developed as an act between the storyteller and the audience (Banks-Wallace, 2002; Huisman, 2008; Montgomery-Andersen & Borup, 2013). This understanding uncovers the choices of the participants (both the conscious and the subconscious), and becomes something real that adds to our understanding of the research materials.

Storytelling is and has been a gathering point activity for the family at weddings, funerals, and births in Greenland. As in many cultures, it has also been a means to protect and propagate traditions (Kleist Pedersen, 2006, Montgomery-Andersen & Borup, 2013). Denzin (1997, p. 32–33) describes the qualitative text as a "cultural representation, a genre in its own right" while Lieblich, Tuval-Mashiach, and Zilber (1998) describe the process of giving stories space and letting a global impression emerge from the text. However, when looking at stories within a cultural context there are three important ingredients for the creation of a story: 1) cultural values and norms, 2) immediate story environment, and 3) historical context (Banks-Wallace, 2002). All three ingredients must be present before a deeper understanding can emerge.

Smith (2002) expresses the importance of listening to stories and the knowledge transferred through stories and tales. E. Skifte (personal communication, 2003–2010) suggested that it is not normal for Greenlandic people to voice opinions unless asked. In the author's experience, Culture Bearers have been elders within the community or people of capacity, both male and female. By asking questions and listening to the answers, new ways of understanding the answers can be uncovered and make it possible to ask questions in another way. With this in mind, a deeper understanding of data cannot be attained without using theories that are based on methods that take Indigenous cultural understanding or cultures other than the European and North American into account (Banks-Wallace, 2002; Montgomery-Andersen & Borup, 2013). Patton states in *The King of Monkeys*, "It is a grave responsibility to ask, it is a privilege to listen" (Patton, 2002, p. 417).

Being the "Other"

We have learned through working alongside or under the direction of Indigenous leaders, researchers, research assistants, Culture Bearers, and Community Panels and Boards that our otherness has an influence on design, analysis, and results. By working alongside Indigenous researchers, we have been reminded that although we are researching within one's own arena, we are gathering information about peoples and communities that we are not culturally connected to. This creates the risk that the passion that drives the research can influence the results in a manner that transfigures from being subjective to being biased.

The authors have lived experience as "others" in our Arctic communities. Dr. Montgomery-Andersen is an African American, neither Greenlandic nor Danish, living in a society dominated by two homogenous cultures, neither her own; Ms. Doucette is a white woman, of mixed ancestry living in Inuit Nunangat. Being an "other" is an ethical dilemma and a methodical challenge that cannot be solved but must be acknowledged by ensuring that there are gatekeepers and gate openers involved and that the participants understand that they have the possibility to withdraw or decline participation at any time during the course of the study.

Again, Smith's (2002) words have a great significance in creating an arena for understanding place. She states that when researching in cultures other than one's own, it is important that researchers "clarify their research aims and think ... seriously about effective and ethical ways of carrying out research" (Smith, 2002). At the same time, as a researcher is it important to know that "all people can learn to center in another's experience, validate it, and judge it by its own standards without need of comparison or need to adopt that framework as their own" (Brown, 1989, p. 922).

Analysis strategies

Intercultural research experiences and co-developed research protocols must contemplate power and influence and how it is employed when research data are interpreted. For example, consider: "who interprets data?", "with what lens?", "for what purpose?", and "how do we validate our interpretations?" These are all important issues to consider before you finalize a research protocol, and may be worth revisiting several times as you move forward and through the research program as well.

Validity, trustworthiness, transferability, and credibility

Qualitative interview conversations are encounters between informant and researcher. The researcher explores and attempts to uncover the informant's views while giving space to the individual's right to structure and frame the concepts of the interviews (Creswell, 1998). This includes a consciousness that, while working and researching together with Indigenous researchers and Research assistants, creates space for dialogue. By ensuring ethical validity of the analysis, the researcher's understanding of his or her "situatedness" (positionality) as a constant. It requires that the researcher should be attentive and interested in regard to the research participants', their social environs, and the researcher's understanding of town space in these arenas.

Montgomery-Andersen and Borup (2013) cite Chamberlain and Barclay (2000):

> It is important to any research process to understand and include historical changes and developments; this can be honoured when the historical and cultural context of the data are kept in sight and used as a way to refine categories during the analysis process (Banks-Wallace 2002; Csonka & Schweitzer, 2004). When recording, structuring, analysing, and interpreting text, one of the research goals is to recreate and reproduce meanings and cultural understandings as the participants have understood it. It is in this process the researcher uncovers the choices of the participants, both the conscious and the subconscious.
>
> *(Chamberlain & Barclay, 2000)*

It is the use of the concepts of validity, trustworthiness, transferability, generalizability, credibility, and dependability that lead the process to ensuring a high standard of scientific knowledge in qualitative studies. During past fieldwork it became evident that personal narratives and storytelling were a scientific tool for testing validity and transferability and, therefore, an integral part of the design of the protocol, and they were used for testing validity during all stages of the research. This included descriptive, interpretive, theoretical, generalizability, and evaluative validity (Kvale, 1989; Montgomery-Andersen & Borup, 2013; Thomson, 2011).

Credibility was heightened by the use of several modes of gathering data, each approach seeking to reflect the focus of the studies (Graneheim & Lundman, 2004; Montgomery-Andersen & Borup, 2013). This included important newspaper articles from the time period; policy papers or press releases could also be included or noted in field notes (Banks-Wallace, 2002). Anthropological and cultural documents can be used together with Culture Bearers' interviews to validate the development of categories during analysis (Altheide, 1987; Bryman, 2004; Montgomery-Andersen & Borup, 2013).

Trustworthiness included several methods throughout the data collection process that helped to support awareness of objectivity and subjectivity and to uncover strengths and weaknesses in the data collection and methods (Altheide, 1996). This included snowballing, the use of gatekeepers, purposeful sampling, going back to the source, and dialogue/conversation mapping notes.

Dialogue mapping is used to map dialogue within focus group discussions or interviews. Mapping is conducted in intervals throughout the process and can be used to support findings and to uncover dynamics within dialogues and interviews. The process is as follows: An

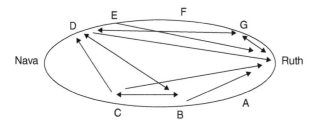

Figure 7.1 Transcription and analysis process

observer should carry out dialogue and conversation mapping during focus group sessions. Dialogue interchange and discussion dynamics were recorded at five- to ten-minute intervals several times during each focus group (Rink et al., 2012). The diagrams depicted in Figure 7.1, together with field notes, were used as support during the transcription and the analysis process (Spradley, 1979). The dialogue/conversation maps can then be used as a support during the analysis process, and used in order to see the dynamics of the discussions or in conversations (Rink et al., 2012, p. 201).

Quotations can be used to create pockets for the voice of the people and communities that are a part of the research. When using a different language from that spoken during the interviews and dialogues, text should be translated back to the original language to ensure the correctness of the translations. This should never be an optional procedure.

Traditional, cultural, and historical knowledge is qualitative knowledge in Indigenous communities and countries. When creating data and knowledge in qualitative processes, it cannot be within a European, Western understanding of "knowledge", whose validation processes are set in a hierarchical structure and educational level. The knowledge of elders and communities is often looked upon as documentation for findings but not as empirical knowledge, thus having no scientific rigor. Indigenous research discourse states the inclusion of community members, elders, and people of capacity as prerequisites for research trustworthiness (Baydala, Worrell, Fletcher, Letendre, Letendre, & Ruttan, 2013; Castellano, 2004; Elliot, 2005; Loppie, 2007; Schnarch, 2004; Smith, 2002).

Interviews and discussion of concepts, interpretations, and language use carry a part of the structure of research with and around the Culture Bearers concept. This does not only support and develop connections to the analysis of collected data, but also in the development of protocols, in decisions related to questions for discussion, and in the analysis of findings. This includes focus groups and discussions and interviews with Culture Bearers (Bird, Wiles, Okalik, Kilabuk, & Egeland 2009; Schnarch, 2004). Culture Bearers are instrumental throughout all phases to heighten the level of understanding of the experiences of participants (Loppie, 2007). Culture Bearers can take part in an ongoing validation process that is conducted while collecting, analyzing, and describing data (Thomson, 2011). Interviews and discussions with Culture Bearers are not anonymous and thus the use of Culture Bearers is a counterweight to the challenge posed by intercultural research not only for the participants but also for the researchers (Loppie, 2007).

As mentioned earlier in the chapter, transcripts of interviews can be used in combination with listening to the original tapes from the interviews and from reading notes from research diaries. In the event that there aren't any Indigenous researchers connected to the project, there should be ongoing discussions with research assistants concerning the analysis and understanding of the translated transcripts to strengthen reliability (Newton Suter, 2012).

To ease finding the correct quotes and information in transcripts, there should be timecodes[2] placed in the transcripts so that the original text can be used and checked during analysis or when selecting quotations (Denzin, 1997).

In the final stages of analysis, a new Culture Bearer is interviewed, this time to discuss findings and to seek to clarify concepts. This supports the theoretical framework of cultural awareness and humility and gives the researcher a chance to step back from their data and analyze the text from outside of their own understanding (Jasen, 1997; Smith, 2002).

Conclusions

As you have read this chapter we have, hopefully, taken you on a journey that explains our perspectives and experiences as intercultural researchers. This is meaningful work, and it is work we continue to try and do better, more respectfully, and more responsibly each day. Any number of forces can act on the movement and settling of humanity amongst new cultures and in new places. Consider large scale motivators for movement like: globalization, climate change, population growth, environmental pressures, or forced migration. We know that people always have, and likely always will, move around and explore our world and therefore we wish to contribute what we can to setting the stage for how we can train the next wave of researchers to consider their role in being stewards of conscious, intentional, respectful intercultural research.

Notes

1 Groenlandica is a national institution that collects, collates, and stores all material that has been published in Greenland, about Greenland, or of Greenlanders.
2 Time codes are points on a tape that tell how long the tape is and how far into the tape the transcriber has come in their transcription of the interview.

References

Altheide, D. (1996). *Qualitative media analysis: Qualitative research methods series 38*. Sage Publications.
Altheide, D. (1987). Reflections: Ethnographic content analysis. *Qualitative Sociology,* 10(1): 65–77.
Bal, M. (2004). *Narratology: Introduction to the theory of narrative*. University of Toronto Press Inc.
Banks-Wallace, J. (2002). Talk that talk: Storytelling and analysis rooted in African American oral tradition. *Qualitative Health Research*, 12: 410–426.
Baydala, L. T., S. Worrell, F. Fletcher, S. Letendre, L. Letendre, & L. Ruttan. (2013). "Making a place of respect": Lessons learned in carrying out consent protocol with First Nations elders. *Progress in Community Health Partnerships*, 7: 135–143. doi:10.1353/cpr.2013.0015
Bird, S. M., J. L. Wiles, L. Okalik, J. Kilabuk, & G. M. Egeland. (2009). Methodological consideration of story telling in qualitative research involving indigenous peoples. *Global Health Promotion*, 16(4): 16–26.
Blumenthal, D. S. (2011). Is community-based participatory research possible? *American Journal of Preventive Medicine*, 40: 386–389. doi:10.1016/j.amepre.2010.11.011
Brown, E. B. (1989). African-American women's quilting. A framework for conceptualizing and teaching African-American women's history. *Signs: Journal of Women in Culture and Society*, 114(4): 921–929.
Bryman, A. (2004). *Social research methods*. Oxford University Press.
Castellano, M. B. (2004). Ethics of Aboriginal research. *Journal of Aboriginal Health*, 1(1): 98–114.
Chamberlain, M., & K. Barclay. (2000). Psychosocial costs for transferring Indigenous women from their community for birth. *Midwifery*, 16(2): 116–122.
Costley, C., G. C. Elliott, & P. Gibbs. (2010). *Doing work based research: Approaches to enquiry for insider-researchers*. Sage Publishing.
Creswell, J. (1998). *Qualitative inquiry and research design: Choosing among five traditions*. Sage Publications.
Csonka, Y., & P. Schweitzer. (2004). Societies and cultures: Change and persistence. In N. Einarsson, J. Nymand Larsen, A. Nilsson, & O. R. Young (Eds.), *Arctic human development report*. Aukreyri: Stefansson Arctic Institute. www.svs.is/AHDR/AHDR chapters/English version/Chapters PDF.htm

Denzin, N.K. (1997). *Interpretive ethnography: Ethnographic practices for the 21st century*. Sage Publications; dx.doi.org/10.4135/9781452243672

Douglas, V. (2010). The Inuulitsivik maternities: culturally appropriate midwifery and epistemological accommodation. *Nursing Inquiry*, 17(2): 111–117.

Ehrlich, G. (2001). *This cold heaven: Seven seasons in Greenland*. Vintage Press.

Elliott, R. (2005). Who owns scientific data? The impact of intellectual property rights on the scientific publication chain. *Learned Publishing*, 18: 91–94. doi.org/10.1087/0953151053584984

Gesink, D., E. Rink, R. Montgomery-Andersen, G. Mulvad, & A. Koch. (2009). Developing a culturally competent and socially relevant sexual health survey with an urban Arctic Community. *International Journal of Circumpolar Health*, 69(1): 25–37.

Gordon, H. S. J. (2014). Building relationships in the Arctic: Indigenous communities and scientists. In G. Fondahl & G. Wilson (Eds.), *Northern sustainabilities: Understanding and addressing change in the Circumpolar world*. Springer. doi.org/10.1007/978-3-319-46150-2_18

Graneheim, U. H., & B. Lundman. (2004). Qualitative content analysis in nursing research: concepts, procedures and measures to achieve trustworthiness. *Nursing Education Today*, 24: 105–112.

Haraway, D. (1988). Situated knowledges: The science question in feminism and the privilege of partial perspective. *Feminist Studies*, 14(3): 575–599.

Huisman, D. M. (2008). *Telling a family: Family storytelling, family identity, and cultural membership* [Unpublished doctoral dissertation]. The University of Iowa.

Jasen, P. (1997). Race, culture, and the colonization of childbirth in Northern Canada. *The Society for the Social History of Medicine*, 10(3): 383–400.

Jorgensen, L. (2008). *Ecological impacts of climate change*. The National Academies Press.

Kleist Pedersen, B. (2006). Children and orality – self reported body and emotional experiences with horror stories. In B. Collignon, & M. Therrien (Eds.), INALCO 2009, Proceedings of the 15th Inuit Studies Conference 5–14. inuitoralityconference.com/art/Kleist01.pdf.

Kruske, S., S. Kildea, & L. Barclay. (2006). Cultural safety and maternity care for Aboriginal and Torres Strait Islander Australians. *Women and Birth*, 19(3): 73–77.

Kvale, S. (1996). *Interviews: An introduction to qualitative research interviewing*. Sage Publishing.

Kvale, S. (1989). *Issues of validity in qualitative research*. Lund: Studentlitteratur Chartwell/Bratt.

Lieblich, A., R. Tuval-Mashiach, & T. Zilber. (1998). *Narrative research : Reading, analysis and interpretation . Applied social research methods series, volume 47*. Sage Publications.

Loppie, C. (2007). Learning from the Grandmothers: Incorporating Indigenous principles into qualitative research. *Qualitative Health Research*, 17(2): 276–283.

Malaurie, J. (1985). *The last kings of Thule: With the polar Eskimos, as they face their destiny*. University of Chicago Press.

Møller, H. (2011). *"You need to be double cultured to function here": Toward an anthropology of Inuit nursing in Greenland and Nunavut* [Unpublished doctoral dissertation]. University of Alberta.

Montgomery-Andersen, R., & I. Borup. (2012). Family support and the child as health promoting agents in the Arctic: The Inuit way. *Rural and Remote Health*, 12(1977): 1–10.

Montgomery-Andersen, R., & I. Borup. (2013). Songlines and touchstones: A study of perinatal health and culture in Greenland. *AlterNative: Journal of Indigenous People*, 9(1): 88–102.

Montgomery-Andersen, R., & S. Montgomery-Andersen. (2014). *"We must be the first example for our children, an example for what they are to become": the caring nature of men*. Grønlandsk Kultur og Samfundsforskning 2012–14. Nuuk, Ilisimatusarfik/Forlaget Atuagkat.

Newton Suter, W. (2012). *Introduction to educational research: A critical thinking approach* (2nd ed). Sage Publishing.

Nuttall, M. (1992). *Arctic homeland - kinship, community and development in Northwest Greenland*. University of Toronto Press.

Patton, M.Q. (2002). *Qualitative research and evaluation methods* (3rd Ed). Sage Publications.

Pe-Pua, R. (2006). From decolonizing psychology to the development of a Cross–Indigenous perspective in methodology: The Philippine Experience. In U. Kim, K. S. Yang, & K. K. Hwang (Eds.), *Indigenous and Cultural Psychology – Understanding People in Context*. Springer.

Rink, E., R. Montgomery-Andersen, A. Koch, G. Mulvad, & D. Gesink. (2013). Ethical challenges and lessons learned from Inuulluataarneq "Having the Good Life" study: a community based participatory research project in Greenland. *Journal of Empirical Research on Human Research Ethics- An International Journal*, 8(2): 110–118.

Rink, E., R. Montgomery-Andersen, G. Tróndheim, D. Gesink, L. Lennert, & Kotalawala, N. (2012). The role of personal responsibility, trust in relationships, and family communication in the prevention of sexually transmitted infections among Greenlandic youth: Focus group results from Inuulluataarneq. In B. Kleist Pedersen, F. A. J. Nielsen, K. Langård, K. Pedersen, & J. Rygaard (Eds.), *Greenland's Cultural and Social Research 2010–12* (pp. 198–208). Ilisimatusarfik/Forlaget Atuagat.

Schmaus, W. (2008, November 6–8). *Two concepts of social situatedness in science* [Contributed paper]. Philosophy of Science Association's 21st Biennial Meeting, Pittsburgh, Pennsylvania. philsciarchive.pitt.edu/view/confandvol/PSA2008ContributedPapers.html

Schnarch, B. (2004). Ownership, control, access and possession (OCAP) or self-determination applied to research: A critical analysis of contemporary First Nations Research and some options for First Nations communities. *Journal of Aboriginal Health*, 1(1). doi.org/10.3138/ijih.v1i1.28934

Smith, L. (2002). *Decolonizing methodologies*. Zed books Ltd.

Spradley, J.S. (1979). *The ethnographic interview.* Wadsworth Cengage Learning.

Statistics Greenland. (2012). *Greenland in Figures.* www.stat.gl/publ/en/GF/2012/content/Greenland%20in%20Figures%202012.pdf

Thomson, S.B. (2011). Qualitative research: Validity. *Journal of Administration and Governance*, 6(1): 78–82.

Wilson, E., A. Kenny, & V. Dickson-Swift. (2018). Ethical challenges in community-based participatory research: A scoping review. *Qualitative Health Research*, 28(2): 189–199. doi.10.1177/1049732317690721

World Medical Association (WMA). (2020). *WMA declaration of Helsinki – ethical principles for medical research involving human subjects.* www.wma.net/policies-post/wma-declaration-of-helsinki-ethical-principles-for-medical-research-involving-human-subjects/

8

THE DECLARATIVE MAPPING SENTENCE AS A FRAMEWORK FOR CONDUCTING ETHNOGRAPHIC HEALTH RESEARCH

Paul M. W. Hackett

Introduction[1]

It was a lovely warm, sunny, spring day in a leafy commuter suburb in south London. The robins, blackbirds, and song thrushes were whistling away, as was the postman as he walked along the lane by the children's park and away from the old corner shop that was run for as long as anyone was able to remember by Mrs. Moffat. Her husband had died some years ago leaving her alone to manage the shop. The postman kept glancing over his shoulder towards the shop as the police were there, some in uniforms, some in suits. Amongst the police was Hercule Poirot, a little French man with impeccable sartorial tastes, a choice of clothes that were however perhaps from an earlier era. In fact, he was Belgian, but due to his accent, hairstyle and moustache, most English people frustratingly mistook him to be French.

The woman's body was lying on its side on the floor behind the counter in the old corner shop near the railway station and Poirot was, annoyingly for the local constabulary, investigating the murder in the corner shop. Mrs. Moffat had been hit over the head by the look of it and, frustratingly for Poirot, the police officers were stomping around seeing only the obvious. But Hercule always saw more; he exercised his little grey cells and went beyond what was immediately apparent. Inspector Japp was content that Mrs. Moffat, the owner of the shop, had been done in by a robber who was up to no good. There had apparently been a little bit of an altercation between the killer and Mrs. Moffat before he had killed her that had resulted in some confectionary, aniseed balls, toffee, and sherbet powder of a variety of colours being knocked to the ground, leaving a rainbow of a commotion on the floor.

"She was obviously serving behind the counter when some young chap came up behind her, hit her over the head and tried to make off with the money", said Japp in the general direction of Poirot. "Mon Amis, if that is the case then why is the cash drawer still closed and the woman dead on the ground with, how do you say, candy all around her" Poirot replied. "The killer was obviously disturbed in the act and had to flee before he could break open the till", Japp replied. "Ah, but it is so easy not to see that which is in front of our own eyes". "What are you going on about, Poirot", Japp said, with no attempt to hide his impatience and irritation. "But if I look closely and I use my little grey cells I can see that there is a small amount, how do you say, a dusting, of sherbet on either side and underneath the poor woman's left leg, but the sherbet is also on either side of the right leg, but not underneath". Somewhat smugly Hercules continued, "and, mon cher, we can see footprints in the sherbet facing towards the woman's body but she is facing into the shop and towards her killer, and yet the blow is to the back of the head". Japp scratched his head, scowled and examined the body. He confirmed what Poirot had said. He turned from the body and back to the great detective. "So what do you make of it then, Poirot? It seems to me as if we have a right strange one here!"

Of course, Poirot did not find the case strange, but appealing and one to which he would have to apply great thought. Poirot liked to exercise his mind and to consider all possibilities and to avoid jumping to the obvious, and often incorrect solution. When conducting ethnographic or other types of qualitative research (Hackett 2015c) we would do well to take a leaf from Hercule's book and not be happy with the simple or obvious answer.

Indeed, there are two goals that I would like my research to achieve and one thing that I want to avoid doing and I think that Poirot, in his detective work, also attempted to achieve these ends. The first thing I would like to achieve is to facilitate a coherent and trustworthy analysis and interpretation of the information I am analysing. The thing that I want to avoid is imposing my own values, beliefs, expectations, understandings, etc., upon the information I have gathered when I analyse my findings. I believe that Poirot too always attempted to meet these goals. The other thing that I would like to achieve through my analysis is to facilitate understanding about the topic of my research that directly relates to research that has already been conducted in the area and for my findings to form part of a cumulative body of knowledge. It may not seem so obvious a goal, but Hercule Poirot also insisted upon employing a great knowledge of previous crime that he constantly called upon. He also a saw himself as building an unsurpassed body of criminal knowledge.

In order to achieve any of the above three aims, I will argue in this chapter that it is imperative that the qualitative research that I undertake is well planned. More than this I will provide a framework for achieving these goals. The framework or template that I suggest using is the declarative mapping sentence (Hackett, (2020, 2019a, b, c, d, 2018a, b, 2017a, 2017a, 2017c, 2016a, b, 2015a, 2014a, 2014b, 2013, 2009a, b, 2006; Hackett & Fisher, 2019a, b; Hackett, Shaw, Boogert, & Clayton, 2019; Hackett & Sovenkova; 2011. Koval & Hackett, 2016; Koval, Hackett, & Schwarzenbach, 2016; Lou & Hackett, 2018a; Schwarzenbach & Hackett 2015).

I believe that Poirot would have appreciated the declarative mapping sentence's organisational and analytic qualities and would have fond pleasure in using its structure to categorise, coordinate, and manage his own investigations and analyses. Alas, we will never know if this is the case, but in the pages that follow I will set out some details regarding how the declarative mapping sentence can be used to plan the gathering and the analysis of ethnographic information. Rather than taking a broad or all-encompassing view of how the declarative mapping sentence can be used within an ethnographic enquiry, I will concentrate on providing an example of its use within thematic content analysis.

Thematic and content analysis using the declarative mapping sentence

When conducting research it is often the case that the researcher is engaging in an information reduction process. By this I mean that he or she is trying to take all of the information and data that has been gathered and reduce this to its more basic or superordinate structure. For example, if a researcher was conducting an investigation into peoples' experiences whilst being in prison, he or she may conduct a series of interviews that ask a selection of participants about their experiences. Alternately, the researcher could choose to use a different information gathering method such as a survey, observations of actual behaviour, and so forth. However, in this example I will stay with the interview procedure for my example. After conducting their interviews, the researcher is likely to have the recording of the interviews transcribed in some way. If the interviews went well it is likely that the transcriptions will form a large amount of information that the researcher will have to decide what to do with in terms of how they will analyse this.

In performing analyses of qualitative data it is common practice to employ some sort of content analysis (Bock & Krippendorff, 2008; Schreier, 2012) or thematic analysis (Smith, 1992, and see also: Drisko & Maschi, 2015; Fonte, Colson, Reynaud, Lagouanelle-Simeoni, & Apostolidis , 2019; Hitge & Van Schalkwyk 2018; Krippendorff, 2018; Neuendorf, 2011; Sclar, Penakalapati, Caruso, Rehfuess, Garn, Alexander, Freeman, Boisson, Medlicott, & Clasen , 2018; Weber, 1990; West, Rudge, & Mapedzahama, 2016 for examples of the use of content analysis in a health and well-being related area of research). Thematic analysis attempts to identify regularities or themes in the data (Braun & Clarke, 2006; Guest, MacQueen, & Namey, 2012). These themes represent the ways in which respondents report thinking, feeling, or acting around the concept being investigated. Themes are identified in the data and are then used to make interpretable the overall body of the collected information that has been amassed. It should be noted that a thematic approach may be used to semantically analyse data through addressing the explicit content of the data. Alternately, a latent approach may be employed in an attempt to identify the underlying assumptions and beliefs that run below the surface of the data. In the former instance the research will attempt to reveal meaning in participants' responses, and in the latter it will reveal the constructs that underlie their utterances and facilitate an understanding of such factors as context. They may, of course, choose to employ a mixture of the two approaches.

Before I go on, however, to describe this form of analysis, I want to make clear that the declarative mapping sentence identifies *facets* as the main aspects of a research area that characterise the behaviour, experience, state-of-affairs, etc., of interest. Facets are then divided into mutually exclusive sub-aspects which are called *elements*. When reading through my description of thematic analysis, it should be kept in mind that, in many ways, themes may be thought of as facets, and codes as elements.

I will now reflect upon thematic analysis in a little more detail. When performing a thematic analysis, the form that the qualitative information takes is usually an interview transcript or observations of behaviour that have been transcribed. Thematic analysis is usually conducted when the researcher is attempting to discover what people think or feel about something—their beliefs knowledge about this entity or what they believe, think is important, or expect in this regard. The sorts of questions that are particularly suitable to thematic analysis are open-ended enquiries such as: How do users of a drug line perceive the counsellors and the service they offer; what are the experiences of people who use an online dating site for individuals who identify their gender in non-binary terms; what do local residents think and feel about changes in the transportation system around where they live; how is the interplay between race and gender portrayed in movies?

In undertaking such an analysis, the researcher scrutinises the data by reading and re-reading it so that he or she becomes over-familiar with the text and is able to identify its common leitmotifs, which should be broad ranging, where they may often embrace deeper meanings than the surface utterances. By common leitmotifs we mean recurring ideas, notions, topics, or configurations of meaning. Becoming over-familiar with data is often just called familiarisation, which is the first phase of any thematic analysis. According to Braun and Clarke (2006, 2012) thematic analysis precedes through five further phases and also goes back and forth between the six steps. During familiarisation the researcher attempts to form an overview of the data and may take notes about the data based upon their repeated reading.

Following this emersion in the data, the second stage involves coding, which usually involves highlighting words, phrases, sentences, etc., and labelling these in a way that describes their content. An example may assist the reader in understanding this process. What follows is part of a fictitious interview with an inmate at a prison:

> "Me, I hate the new system. The way they have changed the dining arrangements. I know since they had that review of the prison, that they have to make some changes. But I think they are doing this for their own ends, you know, giving the job to their brother-in-law's company".

This interview text may be then be coded as follows[2]:

> "*Me,* I HATE THE NEW SYSTEM. The way *THEY* have *changed the dining arrangements*. *I* **know** since *THEY* had that <u>review of the prison</u>, that *THEY* **HAVE TO MAKE SOME CHANGES**. But *I* **think** *THEY* are ~~doing this for their own ends~~, you know, giving the job to *THEY* brother-on-law's company".

Text	Code (element)
hate the new system	NEGATIVE EMOTION
think, know	**Thought**
have to make some changes	ACKNOWLEDGEMENT OF CHANGE
doing this for their own ends	~~Distrust of authority~~
I, me	*Self*
They, their	PRISON AUTHORITIES
review of the prison	<u>Document behind changes</u>
changed the dining arrangements	*Actual changes*

This is a short piece of text and I may be accused of over analysing this. However, this is an illustrative example. It is also possible to criticise my coding for not covering all the possible separately identifiable elements that may be contained in the text. Texts may always be subject to re-interpretation and re-coding. The veracity of a coding rests in its ability to answer the research questions and may be scrutinised through repetition of the analysis by other researchers. Notwithstanding these caveats, in the above example I have highlighted what I consider to be the pertinent parts of the transcription. Each of the colours, underlining and italics represent a different code (or element in the language of the declarative mapping sentence) where each code embodies a thought, belief, characteristic etc., that the interviewee has about the changes in the prison. Codes are initially applied to a text if a characteristic appears interesting or relevant to the research question. If this was the start of a longer interview the researcher would continue reading the text and mark in these colours elements throughout the text that had similar meaning. He or she would also add new colours to text that had an important meaning that was not already coded.

The third phase in thematic analysis involves the generation of themes (facets) from the codes. According to Braun and Clarke (2006), a theme embodies something that is important in regard of the data in relation to the research question. Furthermore, according to these authors, a theme also represents some type of patterning or meaning in the data, where a pattern or a theme may be identified in terms of its prevalence within and across interviews. Braun and Clarke (2006) say that in an ideal situation a theme may be identified as being present a number of times but that a large number of occurrences does not in itself indicate more importance[3]. Themes (facets) are similar to codes (elements) but are broader in their scope and are often made up of multiple codes. If I return to the example of the prisoners' attitudes towards the alterations in their prison, I have identified the following themes:

Code (element)	Theme (facet)
NEGATIVE EMOTION	
Thought	Internal Process
ACKNOWLEDGEMENT OF CHANGE	
~~Distrust of authority~~	orientation/attitude
Self	
PRISON AUTHORITIES	agency
Document behind changes	
Actual changes	focus

I have now gone through the process of identifying codes (elements) and developing themes (facets) from these codes. Having done this, the researcher using a declarative mapping sentence approach arranges the facets (themes) and elements (codes) arranged in a sentence so as to expresses the relationships between the facets. An example of a declarative mapping sentence for the prisoners' experience interview is:

Person (x) being a prisoner, when interviewed about the:

Focus
- document behind changes
- actual changes

Internal process
- felt negatively
- thought

and expressed their:

orientation/attitude
- acknowledgement of change
- distrust of authority

as this related to:

agency
- self
- prison authority

The declarative mapping sentence is read from the start as an ordinary sentence is read. When a facet is encountered (the words in italics) these are not read, but one of the inset hyphenated words (elements) are read from underneath each facet. This is repeated multiple times, changing the permutations of elements read. By doing this the researcher is able to completely describe the prisoner's experiences.

The boundary between facets (themes) and elements (codes) is not rigidly fixed. In fact, the researcher may decide that a code or element is pertinent enough to warrant the status of a theme or facet. On the other hand, she or he may determine that what they originally thought were codes were too nebulous, or on reflection had become irrelevant to understanding the content under enquiry. In this instance, the code or element would be deleted from the theme or facet. How we determine the status of themes (facet) and codes (elements) will depend upon our research questions and how these terms form mutually exclusive categories and are incorporated in the declarative mapping sentence. This activity is linked to step four of Braun and Clarke's (2006) process in which the themes are reviewed and during which the researcher makes sure the themes (facets) accurately represent the data in a way that is useful for the research and by asking how the themes (facets) can be improved. This is achieved by comparing themes (facets) with the original text (data) in an attempt to find omissions and to gauge if the themes actually exist in the data; that is, are the themes (facets) actually what the participant meant. At this stage we may divide facets or themes, amalgamate them, or form new facets.

Step five of the model by Braun and Clarke (2006) requires the forming of precise definitions of, and giving readily understandable names to the themes. However, a theme is defined so as to embody an understanding of the data when taken as a whole along with sympathy for the overall meaning of the research domain. Themes and their names should contain one thought or idea, although a broad theme may be refined by incorporating another term in its name. Finally, the researcher comes to writing up the results. This write-up contains the usual sections found in an academic report. Additionally, it may be useful to include an in-depth section about each theme. Frequencies may be mentioned, but emphasis should be placed upon the meaning of each theme and the relationships between themes, and the researcher should revisit the original research questions and describe how the themes relate to and answer the questions.

By using thematic analysis, or any other form of qualitative analysis that sorts or divides data into themes or sets, a researcher can analyse collections of data of all sizes and through what is essentially a data reduction process, sensitively interpreting meanings that are in the data. It should, however, be remembered that this type of analysis may miss subtle meanings and impose bias through researchers importing their expectations and preconceptions. As well as being used to analyse data, the declarative mapping sentence may also be used to develop research questions, and later in this chapter I will provide examples of this procedure.

Declarative mapping sentences may be used in research that is either inductive or deductive. Inductive research employs an approach in which themes are determined by the data, whereas a deductive approach means that the researcher approaches data analysis with predeveloped themes. Put another way, inductive research develops theory whilst deductive research tests theories. Thus, inductive approaches are essentially exploratory and are especially suited to areas that have not been subjected to research before or very specific research projects such as the one above viewing changes to the prison in question. Conversely, deductive approaches are confirmatory and are employed to test hypotheses that have been developed in previous research.

The example text above about prison experience was very specifically about changes to the dining arrangements. However, if the research had been about experiences of prisons in a more general sense, it may have been appropriate to review previous research into place experience that was developed in the facet theory literature by Canter, (1983), Donald, (1994), and Hackett (1995), and to have performed a deductive study that tested the existing theories within the location of the prison. Facet theory is the theoretical basis for the declarative mapping sentence and is an especially appropriate theoretical source. The facets (themes) that have been discovered to be pertinent in individuals' experience of place are a referent to the sociality/physicality of place, a level of contact with a place, and some form of purposive focus within a place. This framework may then be adapted to the specific characteristics of prison experience.

Keeping the facet structure of the mapping sentence for place experience in mind, after looking at the transcriptions of the full interviews that were (fictitiously) conducted into individuals' experiences of prison, the researcher may notice that it is common for people to mention physical aspects of the prison, for example: the cells in which they live, the place where they eat, the showers, and the social spaces. The researcher may notice the respondents also speak about other people in the prison in terms of them being: other prisoners, guards, or visitors. Finally, the researcher may notice that the respondents often speak about the level or type of connection they have with some parts of the prison and not others. This may take the form of their commenting about the way they directly interact with and have an emotional connection with where they sleep and how they personalise this area, whilst they speak about corridors and eating places as being places they move through and have little emotional linkage with. Through reference to the literature on place experience and this thematic analysis, a declarative mapping sentence could be designed as follows:

Person (x) being a prisoner, reports experiencing the prison in terms of the:

Physical aspects
- Cells
- Social spaces
- Eating areas
- Showers

Which they experience in a:

Level of emotional connection
- More emotional connection
- Less emotional connection

way, and which involve:

Social
- Alone
- other prisoners
- guards
- visitors

In the above example the declarative mapping sentence is being used as a framework to enable the understanding of individuals' experiences of prison and in any write-up of research that used the declarative mapping sentence to facilitate analyses the scholar would state that the declarative mapping sentence was providing a structure within which they were forming their understandings. When using the declarative mapping sentence for prisoners' experiences in custody, the researcher would also use its structure in the presentation of findings and would take each of the facets and present qualitative information, such as verbatim comments and use these to demonstrate the meaning of the facets and their elements and allow the elements to become rich and meaningful.

The declarative mapping sentence for custodial experience may also be developed to allow the inclusion of respondents other than inmates and the recognition that experiences may differ for different people in the custodial setting. To do this a background facet can be included into the first sentence of the declarative mapping sentence that makes the sentence read:

Person (x) being a:

User category
- Prisoner
- Guard
- visitor

reports experiencing the prison in terms of the:

Physical aspects
- Cells
- Social spaces
- Eating areas
- Showers

Which they experience in a:

Level of emotional connection
- More emotional connection
- Less emotional connection

way, and which involve:

Social
- Alone
- other prisoners
- guards
- visitors

By including this background facet, the declarative mapping sentence allows for the researcher to comment on how the responses received from the three different types of prison user either vary or are similar for different types of user. Background facets can take a wide variety of forms. These include demographic and psychological characteristics of participants, features of the place where the research is being conducted, or any other features that systematically differentiate the responses or other types of information that is being gathered in the research.

Designing research using the declarative mapping sentence

It is also possible to use the declarative mapping sentence to design the questions you are going to use in an interview, survey, etc. In this instance, the researcher would read through the declarative mapping sentence that has been designed for your study and choose one element from each facet as you read through (as described in an earlier section). This procedure is repeated several times and each time the sentence is read with a different permutation of elements from all of the facets. An example of this is provided below from the mapping sentence for experience of prisons. If from the physical aspects facet the social spaces element is chosen, from the level of emotional contact facet the less emotional contact element is selected, and if from the social aspects facet the element of visitor is included, the mapping sentence will read as follows:

> Person (x) being a prisoner, reports experiencing the prison in terms of the social spaces which they experience with less emotional connection and which involve visitors.

The researcher may wish to make this sentence into a question that is a little easier to read and a more suitable for using in an in-depth interview whilst still keeping its facet element composition. If the researcher does this the sentence may be turned into the following question:

> Could you tell me about times when you are with prison visitors in the communal area?

In this situation the status of the respondent being a prisoner would be noted.

Having read through the declarative mapping sentence and produced the facet element permutation above, the researcher would read through again and this time select a different facet element permutation. For example, from the physical aspects facet the researcher could select the cell element, from the level of emotional contact facet the researcher could select the more emotional contact element, and the element of alone could be chosen from the social aspects facet. With these selections the mapping sentence would read as follows:

> Person (x) being a prisoner, reports experiencing the prison in terms of the cell which they experience with more emotional connection and which involve being alone.

However, as with the previous example the mapping sentence may be converted into a more simply worded question in the following format:

> What is it like to be alone in your cell?

I hope the process of using a declarative mapping sentence to design questions, or other forms of research instruments, is clear from the above two illustrations. I will not continue repeating facet element permutations in my example, but such repetition of combining different arrangements of facet elements is exactly what the researcher has to do until the research domain, as it is defined by the declarative mapping sentence being used, has been comprehensively addressed by questions, etc.

Why use a declarative mapping sentence in ethnographic research?

There are several reasons an ethnographic researcher may use a declarative mapping sentence in their health and well-being research. One of the most important of these reasons is that by using the declarative mapping sentence the researcher is compelled to explicitly state the characteristics that they believe to be important features of their research. Making such an unambiguous statement is good practice as it guards against data trawling, or simply asking questions with little or no theoretical basis, and hoping something interesting or significant emerges. This is a questionable practice as often this may result in spurious findings to be put forth as valid results. The declarative mapping sentence is essentially a hypothesis for the pertinent aspects of a research domain that the researcher then explicitly and exclusively directs his or her enquiries towards. In research into health and well-being in custodial settings, the researcher using a declarative mapping sentence therefore states after conducting a literature review into the area of prison experience that they believe that the important aspects in this research to be the building, people, and degree of emotional contact. They would then design a study using the mapping sentence's structure and use this structure to analyse the information that came out of the study. This would not only provide substantive information about prison experience but would also allow the researcher to support or refute the declarative mapping sentence as being an accurate portrayal of how participants structure their thoughts and feelings about their custodial experiences.

Conclusions

The declarative mapping sentence has grown out of my qualitative research within the fields of health and well-being research and other applied contexts within the social sciences and humanities.[4] However, the declarative mapping sentence also offers a framework for uniting qualitative and quantitative methods. It is interesting to note Creswell and Clark (2017) comment that thematic analysis offers a strategy for merging the results from quantitative and qualitative research by developing "procedures to transform one type of results into the other type of data (e.g., turn themes into counts) and conduct further analyses to relate the transformed data to the other data" (Creswell & Clark, 2017, p. 70). These authors explain their claims by reference to research by Saint Arnault and O'Halloran (2016) who used a mixed methods approach to study women receiving domestic violence services in Ireland. Creswell and Clark noted how, in this research, the blending of qualitative and quantitative approaches was achieved "through tests quantitatively and a thematic analysis qualitatively, (and in this way) the authors related the survey items of structural and internal barriers to the themes from the interviews" (Creswell & Clark, 2017, p. 188). The declarative mapping sentence provides a framework for achieving such an amalgamation of qualitative and quantitative research procedures and findings.

The declarative mapping sentence may seem like hard work but mapping sentences have been found to provide insight into research areas and if a mapping sentence is used, then the findings from other studies that use a declarative mapping sentence may add up and increase knowledge in that area. This is in line with the assertion by Boyatzis (1998, p. 11) that when conducting qualitative content analysis, "the researcher must interpret the information and themes in a way that contributes to the development of knowledge. This will require some theory or conceptual framework". The declarative mapping sentence meets these requirements and provides a theoretical framework that aids in the development of knowledge. Boyatzis (1998) also stresses the need for research to be in a format that is accessible to other researchers. It is my contention that the declarative mapping sentence translates the themes and other content present in qualitative research into a format that conveys the meaning of the results.

Notes

1 Later in this chapter I will specifically consider thematic analysis and how this form of qualitative analysis is suitable for using within a declarative mapping sentence framework.
2 In this example I am using an inductive approach to the use of thematic analysis in which the codes emerge from the data. More on this and the deductive employment of thematic analysis later in this chapter.

3 In this chapter I have noted that it is possible to blend quantitative and qualitative research approaches and also that it is possible to transform qualitative data into quantitative through noting the frequency of an occurrence. This is a possible way to establish a pattern in the data. However, Lowrie (2015) warns against attempting to count meaning.

4 See, for example: Foxall and Hackett (1994 & 1997 2nd edition); Greggor and Hackett (2018), Hackett (1992, 1993a, b, & c, 1995, 2014, 2015b, c); Hackett et al. (1993, 2018); Hackett and Foxall, (1994, 1995, 1997a, b); Hackett and McCarthy, 2011); Hackett, Sepulveda, and McCarthy (2011); Hackett, St Clair, Gorcos, and McCarthy, (2011); Lou and Hackett, (2018b); Morrison, Burnard, and Hackett, (1991). In this research I have taken a broadly facet theory perspective (Canter, 1985; Hackett & Fisher, 2019a, b) and have used a traditional quantitative mapping sentence.

References

Bock, M.A., & K. Krippendorff. (2008) The Content Analysis Reader. Thousand Oaks, CA: Sage Publications.

Boyatzis, R.E. (1998) Transforming Qualitative Information: Thematic Analysis and Code Development, 1st Edition. Thousand Oaks, CA: Sage Publications.

Braun, V., & V. Clarke. (2006) Using Thematic Analysis in Psychology. Qualitative Research in Psychology, 3(2): 77–101. doi:10.1191/1478088706qp063o

Braun, V., & V. Clarke. (2012). Thematic Analysis. APA Handbook of Research Methods in Psychology, 2: 57–71. doi:10.1037/13620-004

Canter, D. (1983) The Purposive Evaluation of Places: A Facet Approach. Environment and Behavior, 15(6): 659–98.

Canter, D. (ed.) (1985) Facet Theory: Approaches to Social Research. New York: Springer Verlag.

Creswell, J.W., & V.L.P. Clark. (2017) Designing and Conducting Mixed Methods Research, Third Edition. Thousand Oaks, CA: Sage Publications.

Donald, I. (1994) The Structure of Office Workers' Experience of Organizational Environments. Journal of Occupational and Organizational Psychology, 67(3): 241–58.

Drisko, J., & T. Maschi. (2015) Content Analysis (Pocket Guide to Social Work Research Methods) 1st Edition. Oxford: Oxford University Press.

Fonte, D., S. Colson, J. Côté, R. Reynaud, M-C. Lagouanelle-Simeoni, & T. Apostolidis. (2019) Representations and Experiences of Well-being among Diabetic Adolescents: Relational, Normative, and Identity Tensions in Diabetes Self-management. Journal of Health Psychology: An Interdisciplinary, International Journal 24(14): 1976–1992.

Foxall, G.R., & P.M.W. Hackett. (1994 & 1997 2nd edition) Consumers' perceptions of micro-retail design. In, Jenkins, M., & Knox, S. (eds.) Advances in Consumer Marketing. London: Kogan Page. pp. 45–66.

Greggor, A.L., & P.M.W. Hackett. Categorization by the Animal Mind. In Hackett, P.M.W. (ed.) (2018) Mereologies, Ontologies and Facets: The Categorial Structure of Reality. Lexington Publishers. pp. 1–18.

Guest, G., K. MacQueen, & E. Namey. (2012). Applied Thematic Analysis. Thousand Oaks, CA: Sage Publications.

Hackett, P.M.W. (1992) The understanding of environmental concern. Social Behavior and Personality, 20(3): 143–148.

Hackett, P.M.W. (1993a) Consumers' environmental concern values: understanding the structure of contemporary green worldviews. In Van Raaij, F., & Bamossy, G.J., (eds.) European Advances in Consumer Research Volume 1. W Provo, UT: Association for Consumer Research, pp.: 416–427.

Hackett, P.M.W. (1993b) Modeling environmental concern: theory and application. The Environmentalist, 17(2): 12–19.

Hackett, P.M.W. (1993c) Orthodontic treatment: a facet theory approach to the study of personal reasons for the uptake of treatment for malocclusion. Social Behavior and Personality, 21(1): 55–62.

Hackett, P.M.W. (1995) Conservation and the Consumer: Understanding Environmental Concern. London: Routledge Publishers.

Hackett, P.M.W. (2006) Gridworks 2005. Liskard: Diggory Press.

Hackett, P.M.W. (2009a) Experiencing Landscape as a Field of Vision. In Hackett, P.M.W. (2009) Field of Vision. Lochmaddy: Taigh Chearsabagh Museum, and Art Centre.

Hackett, P.M.W. (2009b) Field of Vision. Lochmaddy: Taigh Chearsabagh Museum and Art Centre, Scottish Arts Council.

Hackett, P.M.W. (2013) Fine Art and Perceptual Neuroscience: Field of Vision and the Painted Grid, Explorations in Cognitive Psychology Series. London: Psychology Press.

Hackett, P.M.W. (2014a) Facet Theory and the Mapping Sentence: Evolving Philosophy, Use and Application. Basingstoke: Palgrave McMillan Publishers.

Hackett, P.M.W. (2014b) An Integrated Facet Theory Mapping Sentence Descriptive Model of Contextual and Personal Life-Elements Associated with Students' Experiences of Studying Abroad. Journal of International Students, 4(2): 163–176.

Hackett, P.M.W. (2015a). Classifying Reality, by David S. Oderberg (ed.) (2013) Chichester: Wiley-Blackwell. Frontiers in Psychology, section Theoretical and Philosophical Psychology, 6: 461. doi: 10.3389/fpsyg.2015.00461

Hackett, P. M.W. (2015b) Integrating ethnographic consumer research using facet theory and mind maps. In Hackett, P.M.W. (ed.) Qualitative Research Methods in Consumer Psychology: Ethnography and Culture. Routledge Publishers.

Hackett, P.M.W. (ed.) (2015c) Qualitative Research Methods in Consumer Psychology: Ethnography and Culture. Routledge Publishers.

Hackett, P.M.W. (2016a) Facet Theory and the Mapping Sentence As Hermeneutically Consistent Structured Meta-Ontology and Structured Meta-Mereology. Frontiers in Psychology, section Theoretical and Philosophical Psychology, 7: 471. doi: 10.3389/fpsyg.2016.00471

Hackett, P.M.W. (2016b) Psychology and Philosophy of Abstract Art: Neuro-aesthetics, Perception and Comprehension. Basingstoke: Palgrave McMillan Publishers.

Hackett, P.M.W. (2017a) The Perceptual Structure of Three-Dimensional Art, Springer Briefs in Philosophy. New York: Springer.

Hackett, P.M.W. (2017b) Opinion: A Mapping Sentence for Understanding the Genre of Abstract Art Using Philosophical/Qualitative Facet Theory. Frontiers in Psychology, section Theoretical and Philosophical Psychology, October 2017, 8. DOI: 10.3389/fpsyg.2017.01731

Hackett, P.M.W. (2017c) Commentary: Wild psychometrics: Evidence for 'general' cognitive performance in wild New Zealand robins, *Petroica longipes*. Frontiers in Psychology, section Theoretical and Philosophical Psychology, 8:165. doi: 10.3389/fpsyg.2017.00165

Hackett, P.M.W. (2018a) Declarative Mapping Sentence Mereologies: Categories From Aristotle to Lowe. In: Hackett, P.M.W. (ed.) (2018) Mereologies, Ontologies and Facets: The Categorial Structure of Reality. Lanham, MD: Lexington Publishers. pp. 135–160.

Hackett, P.M.W. (ed.) (2018b) Mereologies, Ontologies and Facets: The Categorial Structure of Reality. Lanham, MD: Lexington Books.

Hackett, P.M.W. (2019a) Facet Mapping Therapy: The Potential of a Facet Theoretical Philosophy and Declarative Mapping Sentences within a Therapeutic Setting, Frontiers in Psychology, section Psychology for Clinical Settings. doi: 10.3389/fpsyg.2019.0122

Hackett, P.M.W. (2019b) Declarative Mapping Sentences as a Co-ordinating Framework for Qualitative Health and Wellbeing Research. Journal of Social Science & Allied Health Professions, 2(1): E1–E6.

Hackett, P.M.W. (2019c) The Complexity of Bird Behaviour: A Facet Theory Approach. Cham, CH: Springer.

Hackett, P.M.W. (ed.) (2019d) Conceptual Categories and the Structure of Reality: Theoretical and Empirical Approaches. Lausanne, Switzerland: Frontiers Media SA.

Hackett, P.M.W. (2020) Declarative Mapping Sentences: Theoretical, Linguistic, and Applied Usages for Qualitative Research. (forthcoming Routledge).

Hackett, P.M.W., & Y. Fisher. (eds.) (2019a) Advances in Facet Theory Research: Developments in Theory and Application and Competing Approaches. Lausanne, Switzerland: Frontiers.

Hackett, P.M.W., & Y. Fisher (2019b) Editorial: Advances in Facet Theory Research: Developments in Theory and Application and Competing Approaches, Frontiers in Psychology, section Psychology for Clinical Settings.

Hackett, P.M.W. & G.R. Foxall. (1994) Consumers' satisfaction with Birmingham's International Convention Centre. Service Industries Journal, 14(3): 369–380.

Hackett, P.M.W. & G.R. Foxall. (1995) The structure of consumers' place evaluations. Environment and Behavior, 27(3): 354–379.

Hackett, P.M.W. & G.R. Foxall. (1997a) Consumers' evaluations of an international airport: a Facet theoretical approach, International Review of Retail. Distribution and Consumer Research, 7: 339—349.

Hackett, P.M.W. & G.R. Foxall. (1997b) The structure of consumers' place evaluations. In Hooley, G., & Hussey, M. Quantitative Methods in Marketing. 2nd Edition. London: Academic Press.

Hackett, P. & L. Jacobson. (1999) The development and validation of an outcome measure of the approach-ability of general practice consultations, Spotlight, 22. March 1999.

Hackett, P.M.W., L. Lou, & P. Capabianco. (2018) Integrating and Writing-up Data Driven Quantitative Research: From Design to Result Presentation. In Hackett, P.M.W. (ed.) (2018) Quantitative Research Methods in Consumer Psychology: Contemporary and Data Driven Approaches. London: Routledge.

Hackett, P.M.W. & K. McCarthy. (2011) A Mapping Sentence for Digital Marketing. In New horizons for Facet Theory: Interdisciplinary Collaboration Searching for Structure in Content Spaces and Measurement, pp. 255–262.

Hackett, P.M.W., J. Sepulveda, & K. McCarthy. (2011) Improving Climate Change Education: A Geoscientifical and Psychological Collaboration. In New horizons for Facet Theory: Interdisciplinary Collaboration Searching for Structure in Content Spaces and Measurement, pp. 219–226.

Hackett, P.M.W., W.C. Shaw, & P. Kenealy. (1993) A multivariate descriptive model of motivation for orthodontic treatment. Multivariate Behavior Research, 28 (1): 166–185.

Hackett, P.M.W., R.C. Shaw, N.J. Boogert, & N.S. Clayton. (2019) A Facet Theory Analysis of the Structure of Cognitive Performance in New Zealand Robins (*Petroica longipes*). International Journal of Comparative Psychology, 32.

Hackett, P.M.W. & Y.S. Sovenkova. (2011) Not all KPIs are equal: understanding the interacting role of KPIs through the use of a mapping sentence. Strategies: The Journal of Legal Marketing, 13(6): 16–17.

Hackett, P.M.W., K.L. St Clair, J. Gorcos, & K. McCarthy. (2011) A mapping Sentence Model for Academic Challenge. In New horizons for Facet Theory: Interdisciplinary Collaboration Searching for Structure in Content Spaces and Measurement, pp. 149–160.

Hitge, E. & I. Van Schalkwyk. (2018) Exploring a Group of South African Psychologists' Well-being: Competencies and Contests. South African Journal of Psychology: Suid-Afrikaanse Tydskrif Vir Sielkunde, 48(4): 553–566.

Koval, E., & P.M.W. Hackett. (2016) Hermeneutic Consistency, Structured Ontology and Mereology as embodied in Facet Theory and the Mapping Sentence, Proceedings of the 15th International Facet Theory Conference.

Koval, E.M., P.M.W. Hackett, & J.B. Schwarzenbach. (2016) Understanding the Lives of International Students: A Mapping Sentence Mereology. In Bista, K., & Foster, C. (eds.) International Student Mobility, Services, and Policy in Higher Education. IGI Global Publishers.

Krippendorff, K.H. (2018) Content Analysis: An Introduction to Its Methodology, Fourth Edition, (2018). Thousand Oaks, CA: Sage Publications.

Lowrie, A. (2016) Ethnography: Textual Methodology. In Hackett, P.M.W. (ed.) Qualitative Research Methods in Consumer Psychology: Ethnography and Culture. Routledge Publishers.

Lou, L. & P.M.W. Hackett. (2018a) Qualitative Facet Theory and the declarative mapping sentence, Contemporary data interpretations: Empirical contributions in the organizational context. Organization 4.1: The role of values in Organizations of the 21st Century.

Lou, L. & P.M.W. Hackett. (2018b) The Facet Theory approach to social research, Contemporary data interpretations: Empirical contributions in the organizational context. Organization 4.1: The role of values in Organizations of the 21st Century.

Morrison, P., P. Burnard, & P.M.W. Hackett. (1991) A smallest space analysis of Nurses' perceptions of their Interpersonal skills. Counseling Psychology Quarterly, 4(2/3): 119–125.

Neuendorf, K. (2011) Content Analysis—A Methodological Primer for Gender Research. Sex Roles, 64(3–4): 276–89.

Saint Arnault, D., & S. O'Halloran. (2016) Using Mixed Methods to Understand the Healing Trajectory for Rural Irish Women Years After Leaving Abuse. Journal of Research in Nursing, 21(5): 369–383.

Schreier, M. (2012) Qualitative Content Analysis in Practice, 1st Edition. Thousand Oaks, CA: Sage Publications.

Schwarzenbach, J.B. & P.M.W. Hackett. (2015) Transatlantic Reflections on the Practice-Based Ph.D. in Fine Art. New York: Routledge Publishers.

Sclar, G.D., G. Penakalapati, B.A. Caruso, E.A. Rehfuess, J.V. Garn, K.T. Alexander, M.C. Freeman, S. Boisson, K. Medlicott, & T. Clasen. (2018) Exploring the Relationship between Sanitation and Mental and Social Well-being: A Systematic Review and Qualitative Synthesis. Social Science and Medicine, 217: 121–34. Web.

Smith, C.P. (ed.) (1992) Motivation and Personality: Handbook of Thematic Content Analysis 1st Edition. Cambridge: Cambridge University Press.

Weber, R.P. (1990) Basic Content Analysis (Quantitative Applications in the Social Sciences 2nd ed). Newbury Park, CA: Sage Publications.

West, S., T. Rudge, & V. Mapedzahama. (2016) Conceptualizing Nurses' Night Work: An Inductive Content Analysis. Journal of Advanced Nursing, 72(8): 1899–914.

PART IV

Interviewing in ethnographic research

9
GETTING DEEP IN THE PAIN
Understanding people through ethnographic research

Antonella Fabri

Introduction

Medical research focuses on the body and illness, often neglecting the mental health of the patient. Conversely, anthropological research, with its emphasis on the ecosystem of the illness, puts the human experience at its core to understand the different implications that accompany illness. Individuals are entangled in a web of intricate meanings and social rules so that anything that concerns the body and health has to be inscribed into a particular social and cultural context. Illnesses have a ripple effect in every aspect of human life (Giarelli 2003).

This article highlights the value of anthropology and the ethnographic method applied to medical research through two case studies. Due to nondisclosure agreements, specifics related to the companies and medical devices cannot be provided. Two different medical companies wanted to find better solutions to improve the lives of people with chronic medical conditions and wanted to know how patients' daily existences were affected by them. One project was conducted in Italy among men affected by prostate cancer, while the other concerned geographic atrophy at varying stages in English patients. In both projects the ethnographies were part of the whole research study and were acknowledged as the most valuable way to learn about these illnesses from the patients' point of views and experiences. Ethnographic research is part of the anthropological endeavor to inquire about the how and the why. When applied to medical issues, ethnography brings forth the way people live with their illnesses, and how they adapt and transform themselves to make their lives more bearable for themselves and their families.

The first case study shows the cultural dynamics created by the introduction of medical devices to several groups of people connected to the patients with prostate cancer. These medical devices had been created to alleviate patients' stress, which was intensified by necessary visits to the hospital. The ethnographic approach applied to this study will reveal the forces at work in the acceptance of new technology, as well as the physical and mental struggles of people with chronic illnesses.

The reason for the creation of the medical devices was to generally increase patients' quality of life and, in particular, to decrease the frequent hospital visits. In theory, the medical devices would offer patients more autonomy and freedom, and free the physicians of routine visits that curbed their time for research, as they themselves expressed.

One of the participants in the patients' forum expressed that one of the downsides of the cancer was the fact that the treatment impinged upon his work, family time, and vacation; he could not travel for a long time or go to places with difficult access to hospitals or other places where he could get treatment. Moreover, all participants voiced their resentment at their hospital experiences, especially at the lack of doctors' attention. The regular visits to the hospital felt to them like a pilgrimage to a place where instead of receiving hope and strength, they often found disappointment. The lack of time devoted to them and the curt, often unsatisfying communication with their primary care doctors, especially after a long time spent in waiting rooms or corridors trying to have a word with their physicians, disheartened many. "I don't enjoy going to the hospital, but at least I might have a chance to see the doctor", said a patient. The respondents talked about their hospital experiences as dehumanizing and humiliating. Not only were they fighting against the viciousness of a tumor, but they often felt isolated in this struggle, lacking emotional support and empathy from the medical personnel in this fight with them.

In both studies, the caretakers' opinion was included as a part of the whole experience with the illness. The main research goal was to place people at the center of the study, dialogically and in a polyphony of voices, to acquire the most comprehensive understanding of these illnesses in order to create medical tools and treatments to improve their lives. On top of fraught communication channels between patients and their doctors, family members and caretakers lamented how difficult it was for them to communicate with their loved ones and how they too felt let down by the medical culture. Some pointed out that their loved ones often came back from doctor's visits more depressed than before they had left home.

As mentioned above, the introduction of the medical tools at the forums and their reception by different groups of people exposed interesting socio-cultural dynamics that recall Foucault's history of medical discourse. Foucault explores the formation of institutions and discursive practices through a critical reading of the history of Western thought. In particular, he traces the origins of medical discourse to the modern era—the 19th century—when the individual is exposed to the reading of doctors and interpreted through the language of positive science. Foucault uncovers the deep meaning of speech and identifies the relations in which individuals are enmeshed. The transition from punishment as a spectacle to a more civilized one, in the 19th century, occurs, according to Foucault, when a process of change into institutions emerges. Medicine and hospitals are part of the institutions that he considers repositories of discourse that punish individuals not publicly any longer but from within, through discursive practices. He underlines that in modern times the punishment is deployed by language and techniques that isolate the patient and expose him to the private, scientific gaze (Foucault, 1989).

Rembrandt's "Anatomy Lesson" recalls Foucault's vision of the body as the subject of discursive practices. In the painting the doctor is surrounded by his students in front of a body while the body is being analysed, dissected. This is the visual image of what Foucault identifies as the medical gaze that makes the individual an object of study, like a corpse, and subjects it to authority of science. It is the representation of an act of domination executed by the doctor, who is on a throne like a judge in the process to proclaim a sentence and transform the body into an abstraction and invisible entity (Barker, 1984, p.75).

The body of the man in the picture signifies the body politics: the way people create institutions—such as the penal and medical systems—and are simultaneously subjected to rules and orders created, in part, by those very same enablers. Thanks to the doctor's gaze, the individual acquires meaning while becoming entangled in the capillary power of the institutions that govern and control their lives (Foucault 1977). The hospital, as an institution, is responsible, according to Foucault, for another kind of normative behavior: the relationship between doctor and patient. As he posits in *The Birth Of The Clinic,* "In the rational space of disease, doctors and patients do not occupy a place as of right; they are tolerated as disturbances that can hardly be avoided: the paradoxical role of medicine consists, above all, in neutralizing them, in maintaining the maximum difference between them, so that, in the void that appears between them, the ideal configuration of the disease becomes a concrete, free form, totalized at last in a motionless, simultaneous picture, lacking both density and secrecy, where recognition opens of itself onto the order of 'essences'" (Foucault 1989, p. 24).

Similar to Foucault's approach to rewrite the history of Western thought, the effort of anthropological analysis is to examine cultural practices and dynamics to shed light on what has not been seen and said before. Thanks to the ethnographic method, anthropology can provide a critical analysis of social practices and reintroduce as actors those who have been excluded from history. Through ethnographies we can learn about those who are marginalized and not represented as a social reality and develop empathy about their conditions.

James Clifford presents a range of analytic issues that define ethnography: "Ethnographic writing is determined at least in six ways: (1) contextually (it draws from and creates meaningful social milieu); (2) rhetorically (it uses and is used by expressive conventions); (3) institutionally (one writes within, and against, specific traditions, disciplines, audiences); (4) generically (an ethnography is usually distinguishable from a novel or a travel account); (5) politically (the authority to represent cultural realities is unequally shared and at times contested); (6) historically (all the above conventions and constraints are changing). These determinations govern the inscription of coherent ethnographic fictions" (Clifford & Marcus 1986, p. 6).

In medical-anthropological research, unlike that of a scientifically minded doctor, the gaze of an ethnographer is focused on the people enmeshed in medical institutions and their practices. Ethnographers linger on people's emotions and behaviors; they watch and listen attentively to nuances and particulars that would be invisible and imperceptible to others. Once data are collected, they are pieced together and run through a critical lens that will offer a better view of the whole picture. Ethnographic accounts are ways to not only hear personal stories, but to understand the multiplicity of voices that surround individuals and grasp the complexity of the human experience. These stories become sources of learning and inspiration for people in the field of medicine who attend to the needs of people with diseases. Aspects and experiences of a patient's life are pivotal for the development of new products and technology in the field of health and medicine.

Ethnographies inform design because they draw from human behavior and needs. Especially in the field of medicine, human-centered research is critical to helping understand the depth of the human experience and deliver successful design innovation. Technology has opened new frontiers to medicine and the research behind it needs to take into account the stories of people who are at the end of the research. Therefore, patients and caretakers are the primary users of new technology that aims to improve medical conditions and quality of life.

The use of technological innovation in the treatment of prostate cancer

In 2016, I had the opportunity to conduct a series of forums on the new treatment options available to patients with prostate cancer who, thanks to recent technological developments, can now administer their own treatment in the comfort of their homes. The companies that were involved in the research process had designed medical devices that were introduced at these forums. They resembled everyday objects as to be carried along by patients and stored away inconspicuously without being immediately recognised as medical devices for serious illnesses. But doctors perceived them as a threat to the health of their patients and their own authority in managing every aspect of treatment. They could not understand the myriad of ways in which going to the hospital to get the treatment constituted a jarring disruption of the patients' lives. Some doctors expressed the feeling that, "the hospital, even if an inconvenience in patients' lives, means safety for them".

The physicians who participated in the ethnography believed the hospital to be the only place that dispenses the best treatment especially to patients exposed to such a big life threatening illness such as cancer. Doctors, soundly in good faith, defended the authority of the hospital by stressing and repeating the concept of safety in connection with this institution. By placing their authority and the validity of the hospital as the safest place for patients above all, they replaced what patients might have known to be their most intimate, safe space—their homes—with a more sterile, utilitarian space: the hospital. The concept of safety during the ethnography was leveraged by doctors as a way to safeguard their position and reaffirm their belief that patients should not be administering the bulk of their treatment unsupervised and in their own homes.

It would be interesting to notice that etymologically, the word *patient* originally meant "one who suffers". The English word comes from the Latin *patiens,* the present past participle of the verb *patior,* meaning "I'm suffering". From its outset then, it is made clear from the language itself that the condition of the patient is one of suffering and being at the mercy of medical institutions. It's the same language that reflects what doctors projected over the patients: patients embody an entity lacking something, presenting a contrast with wholeness and totality. They are dispossessed of authority, knowledge, decisional power, and ultimately health because, from the doctors' point of view, they put themselves at risk by not embracing their superior knowledge.

Although themselves part of the medical sphere, nurses are often considered conduits between patients and doctors. However, during the forum discussions they too criticized the way some doctors approach their relationships with patients, seeing them as failing to relate with those looking to them for comfort and empathy. Some of them said that the language doctors use is incomprehensible, even to them and others who operate in their same field— "they speak 'medicalese' (doctors' language)". Nurses empathize with the patients because they interact with the patients and their caretaker. They can see and feel the patients' pain and relate with their frustration toward doctors and the whole medical system. During the discussion nurses stood by patients and caretakers and comprehended the positive change that new forms of treatments would have introduced in their lives if adopted. In their view, and contrary to physicians' belief, home-administered medicine did not necessarily expose patients to higher risks in most of the cases.

As Foucault elaborates, discursive institutions often rely on the notion of safety to secure and perpetuate their control, "Do not concentrate the study of the punitive mechanisms on their 'repressive' effects alone, on their 'punishment' aspects alone, but situate them in a whole series of their possible positive effects, even if these seem marginal at first sight. As a consequence, regard punishment as a complex social function" (Foucault 1977, p. 23). The doctors in the forum failed to acknowledge the toll that stress, derived from the physical limitation imposed on patients by the hospital, would have on patients' mental health. They further seemed to not hold in high consideration the aggravating fact that each regular visit to the hospital involves several hours of waiting around for the mere ten minutes or so actually needed for the administration of treatment. Granted, this situation is not nearly entirely the fault of doctors, but rather a symptom of the inefficient and, at times, painfully slow Italian medical system.

The discussions I had with each group offered the opportunity to understand culturally mediated views, the embodiment of illness, and the role of objects in the creation of culture. One of the insights we drew from the group discussions was that emotions are overwhelming and isolating. The feelings of shame and inadequacy that, at times, pervade patients create a wall between them and those close to them. A participant voiced this by saying, "I'm made in a bad way…I'm the weak link of the chain".[1] Letting down their guards and allowing emotions to flow was cathartic and revelatory, especially because it's rare that Italian men talk about their feelings so openly. Traditionally, in Italian culture, men who vent their feelings are considered weak or feminine. This is especially true of men in the age cohort represented in this forum.

During the conversation, men felt comfortable expressing their stress at their feeling of inadequacy stemming from the changes occurring in their bodies. Even while some accepted a diminished sense of virility, they still feared the possibility of losing their spouses. For many, the threat of losing their masculinity was the same as losing their identity. One participant, visibly the most relaxed of all of them, said, at the end of the session, "For us men this illness is a big problem. The possibility of losing our masculinity causes a lot of insecurity. You're no longer the strongest one in the family". Many felt that their cancer made them vulnerable, like helpless children: "One feels belittled by it, like a child who needs somebody to take him by the hand and tell him what to do. Life has changed radically for me".

On top of an already complicated relation between patients and doctors, the Italian healthcare system makes interactions between doctors and patients hard, and the system itself is hard to navigate for somebody who is not already within it. Patients and doctors are polarized by a system that is not user friendly, that marginalizes those who should be instead at the center of the services offered by the medical institutions. Patients feel like they deserve better care and attention, while physicians claim to be underpaid, understaffed, and overworked. Thus, doctors, entangled themselves in the spiral of the institution and overwhelmed by the load of work and responsibilities, prefer to stick with the status quo. Changing the way patients would receive treatment would lead to the revision of some medical tenets and the effort to listen to the patient as a suffering human being.

Given the ubiquitous nature of technology in today's society and the momentous improvements it has allowed for in the field of health and medicine, the theories of Michel Foucault and Bruno Latour are valuable lenses through which to examine the cultural meaning of technology as applied to the social life of medicine. While Foucault, In *The Birth of the Clinic,* emphasizes the medical gaze in connection with technology and power (1989, p. 89), Latour, in his work on Actor Network Theory (Latour 2005) analyses the relationship between objects and people. This theory complements the ethnographic process by highlighting the importance of studying the interconnected web of society from the links between people and their role in creating relationships.

Latour emphasizes the connection between science and politics and the importance to understand social processes. He maintains that instead of focusing on single practices and phenomena, objects, ideas, and processes are pivotal forces in creating social situations (Latour 1993). His concept of technology as social circulation offers a critical approach to the role that medical tools play in the context of the forums on prostate cancer, thus allowing us to understand better the position of the people in each group. Medical tools during the discussion conducted were not just objects but had become expressions of relationships and modes of communication, as well as opportunities that could lead to alternatives that create new assemblages and connections. Therefore, as Latour suggests, we should focus more on the relations that objects create rather than on the object itself.

In the specific case of the Italian research study, we could argue that technology, by offering new medical treatments, could turn the seemingly oppositional relationship between doctors and patients into a dialogical one. The ethnographies conducted in Italy show that technology could change medical culture. Medical tools could be viable ways to change not just the medical treatment of cancer, but the lives of the patients. Technological advancements could either continue to be tools at the doctor's disposal or, instead, pivotal for a change of medical systems that shape unequal social relationships.

During the research study, patients were very much in favor of using the new medical devices. They offered the opportunity to restore some sense of normalcy and agency to this new and daunting phase of their life. By the end of the discussion, illness had become a truly collective experience, connecting the respondents to each other, and the medical tools introduced offered the promise of a new self-identity for the patients. These devices and the way they were able to create a bridge between the identity of the respondents as patients and their former, more independent selves, are tangible examples of a human-centered design meant to humanize the health system. The medical devices presented at the forum were not just tools for cancer treatment but objects that encapsulated the opportunity for a path of improvement in the quality of life.

Geographic atrophy

The research on geographic atrophy presented here was conducted in England in 2016. The fieldwork consisted of interviews, observations, and shadowing with six people— four men and two women –between the ages of 50 and 80 and included their family members or caretakers, if available.

Geographic atrophy (GA) is a disease that affects people's sight by consistently narrowing their field of vision, drastically and steadily decreasing their quality of life. People suffering from GA are overwhelmed by a sense of loss and estranged from what was once familiar; they encounter countless limitations and estrangement because the illness entails relearning how to move, act, and be perceived in the world.

Lack of peripheral vision changes the way they walk, read, socialize, and take care of themselves. Once simple tasks like personal hygiene and dressing themselves become major challenges to their autonomy. They find that their need to reorient themselves starts with developing new knowledge and a new perception of the self. Pivotal in this search are objects introduced to help reorganise their world and acquire new bearings. They are confronted with a new perception of fragility and repair, struggling to not be overcome by a sense of mourning for what they have lost and longing for their past world. As their vision narrows, so does their ability to exist and take part in it what they once knew.

The worldview and experiences of those with GA are shaped not so much by what they can see and do, but by the absence of everything they no longer can. The loss of eyesight is lived as a dispossession, as a bereavement that marks the beginning of a transformation. Many patients are determined to embrace their new condition from the outset and start the difficult work of reinventing their new self. Yet it is extremely hard to take care of people with this chronic illness because of its constant degenerative nature and the need to continuously adapt daily routines to its present stage.

The participants in the study did not think of themselves as ill because they said that GA is a condition independent from their health and, hence, not an illness, but more like an injury. I do think that this rationalization somewhat contributed to their ability to keep a positive attitude. GA is embraced by them as something fortuitous, the result of a freak accident not traceable to any particular event, and yet pervasive. As said by one participant: "It's a disability, and not a disease; disability is a limitation, a less able body, while a disease is infectious. Disabled people don't see themselves as disabled but enabled. You adjust in the way you perceive your problem".

One patient realized that GA would increasingly degenerate and he was therefore unfortunately as healthy now as he would ever be. Rationalizing that every year would be better than the next, he chose to adopt a positive outlook towards life, even given its limitations.

Where the sensation of being functional, having a job, and having an identity is part of their "before GA" lives, frustrations and strategies to overcome them exist in the present. JC, an adult male living with GA, expresses this feeling: "Gradually, I got used to it; the frustration lessened after a period of two years. For a while I was frustrated, but I tried to put it in the back of my mind. I was concerned that I wouldn't act properly or that I would fall over, but I don't go out a lot on my own, so I am not so embarrassed".

As in the case of the study on prostate cancer, there are also tools that can help reshape GA patients' personas and symbolize the fractures between an old and new self. While the space around them is changing according to the progression of the illness, the body becomes the main instrument of knowledge that mirrors a mental image of one's past self. In this context, new objects that help people navigate this changed space become a way to regain control and autonomy. For example, one device allowed them to make tea by announcing the arrival of boiling water to the brim of their cup, and a high-tech visor made reading possible once again by enlarging restaurant menus, TV screens, and books.

Memory also played a big part in patients' reorganization of space; people living with them had to be careful to keep everything in the same order as they found it, as to allow their loved ones to be able to navigate in their own space. Clothing was organised by colors to help them match when getting dressed in the morning. Food in the refrigerator and pantry had to follow a strict sense of placement as well. I learned about the almost obsessive connection they had with objects: old ones reminded them of the person they were and new ones of their challenge ahead.

Memory and imagination were the new guides that provided bearings; a new balance between the body and environment contributed to a tactile understanding of space. In these conditions, memory becomes even more important than it was before because it constitutes the solid ground upon which they can build. But memory has another, less utilitarian function as well: that of reminding them how they used to be and who they are now.

Caregivers were also challenged in that they needed to keep a delicate balance between easing the hardships that their loved ones encounter and helping them regain control of themselves. Since GA constantly degenerates the vision, people needed to continuously learn new tricks, to adopt new ways to remember and maintain a positive attitude while trying to not make it harder for their families to have to care for them. During an interview with JC and his wife, who was his primary caretaker but has severe health problems herself, the couple mentioned one episode in which JC banged his head on the kitchen cabinet door because his wife forgot he would be unable to see that it was open. She tried to keep these limitations at the forefront of her mind but it was sometimes hard to keep up with the progress of the illness.

Merleau-Ponty focuses on the relationship between our senses and the world and the way we get to know and sense the world. He says that knowledge is created through perception, through the body's disposition to reality. "Every sensation includes a seed of dream or depersonalization, as we experience through this sort of stupor into which it puts us when we truly live at the level of sensation" (Merleau-Ponty 2012, p. 223). The writing of an individual's experience corresponds to peoples' experience through their bodies, which are the foundation of knowledge for themselves and their listeners. Merleau-Ponty focuses on how the body performs certain functions and routines and how it becomes the center of experience. This approach offered by phenomenology is very useful to understanding people's experience about a new way of learning and adapting to new ways of experiencing reality.

The wife of another participant in the GA research study expressed her sadness while remembering the time that, during a trip to Alaska, they stopped to admire a breathtaking sunset that her husband could not see. Surprisingly to both of us, he said that he didn't feel sad about not seeing it since he could still appreciate it through her. Later I thought back to his words and finally understood what he meant. Vision had been supplemented by other senses, including his wife's; he meant that perception had supplemented another sense and that one can see in different ways. In the words of Merleau-Ponty, "When I see an object, I always feel that there is still some being beyond what I currently see, and not merely more visible being, but also more tangible or audible being, and not merely more sensible being, but moreover a depth of the object that no sensory withdrawal will ever fully exhaust" (Merleau-Ponty 2012, p. 226).

The doctor/patient relationship can be hard also among GA patients. They too often feel uncomfortable talking to doctors. Susan, who belonged to London's high society, now in her mid-70s, confessed that at the outset of the illness she went to an ophthalmologist instead of a doctor to learn more about her condition because the doctor didn't make her feel at ease. Sometime doctors inflict even more frustration on patients than they felt before. Kathy recalled the effect that it had on her the time that her doctor told her she would soon encounter new limitations, "The way I was being told at my last visit: 'You are on the borderline for driving in England', psychologically affected me". Not only is there not enough communication between doctors and patients, but there is also a limiting discrepancy in what is addressed in the sterile, objective environment of the doctor's office and the messier reality that is manifested in real life. Another patient recounted the story of going to the doctor to have new lenses prescribed. The progression of his illness would be measured based on how well he could read letters on a screen across the room, and the doctor would change his prescription accordingly. However, what the patient soon came to realize, was that his vision was vastly different when looking at letters on a lit-up screen than when he would try to see objects in his daily life.

For many of these patients living with geographic atrophy, the future is ridden with anxiety. In Susan's words, "What am I going to tell my daughter, that I am going blind?" Some people are hopeful that new scientific discoveries will bring back their quality of life, if not their vision, "I am positive that there will be a cure in the next couple of years and that's what holds me up … Maybe something magical might happen, that they can find a cure for it. The future is unknown. Everyday can be worse, or totally black".

Conclusions

The two cases discussed in this article show the value of anthropological analysis in the field of medical research. Applied anthropology sheds light on aspects of peoples' experiences and on particular cultural contexts that would be unknown and neglected. The examples provided of the use of ethnography in medical research and human-centered design show the relevance of the use of the ethnographic method for the design and production of technology. From the ethnographic studies emerge the value of collaboration between anthropologists, patients, caretakers, and medical personnel. Such collaboration is the basis for a deep and rich understanding and a driver for innovation. This human-centered approach is more and more utilized by medical research companies to explore and implement new technology that will help those who are affected by an illness to regain autonomy and control of their lives.

Innovation in the medical field leads to the production of devices that generates new relations and new contexts. In the specific case of medical tools whose adoption by patients and doctors has been discussed in the first case study, we have seen how they could open new perspectives and contribute to change in a society where communication between doctors and patients has almost always been absent.

The concept of assemblage derived from Latour's Actor Network Theory offers a path in the search for new opportunities to change old structures and dichotomies such as the oppositional doctor/patient relationship. Latour emphasizes that if we think relationally we can increase the formation of new collaborations and include people who traditionally have been excluded. These collaborations can create cultural change and alternative modes of healing that might efface the demonization of the disease and diminish the isolation of the patient. Moreover, they would be useful in starting new forms of communication between the patients, their family environment, and the medical personnel. In this way, a previously formed assemblage leads to another and from there to new relations and meanings (Puig de la Bellacasa 2011).

Narratives are shaped by social structures and everyday practices. They are texts that lend themselves to critical analysis and to further exploration into the formation of self-perceptions and social dynamics (Good & DelVecchio Good 1981). Culture affects illness; therefore it is important to analyse ethnographies within a cultural context because it gives meaning to all the parts. In the ethnographic accounts, both personal and interpersonal spheres intersect. They reflect the cultural understanding of illness, the language used to talk about it, and the economy and politics that surround the discourse of illness.

The ethnographic approach—capturing embodied experiences—enables a deep understanding of people's representations of memories, emotions, and perceptions of reality. Ethnography is a vehicle of expression of the whole human experience that, as such, is a means to convey embodied experiences and be used in other fields of research.

To conclude, illness is part of a personal narrative that encompasses the single individual, a space where individual and society intersect, and a window overlooking a whole cultural eco-system. Ethnographical accounts of illnesses open up a window onto shared social rules and patterns of behavior and help the narrator to find coherence within the story, a "telos" that projects the subject of the story into the future and beyond their illness. They offer a way to relate to the interlocutor, to empathize with their sufferings, and to spread that knowledge to prompt changes (Friese & Latimer 2019). Hopefully, more ethnographic encounters will open up new terrains for medical improvements and for better, more effective interactions between patients and medical personnel.

Acknowledgement

I wish to thank Teodoro Fabri Upton for his assistance and patience in editing this article.

Note

1 On this topic Giddens observes: "Pride and self-esteem are based on 'confidence in the integrity and value of the narrative of self-identity'. Shame, meanwhile, stems from anxiety about the adequacy of the narrative on which self-identity is based - a fear that one's story isn't really good enough" (Giddens, 1991).

References

Barker, F. (1984) *The Tremulous Private Body*. London: Methuen & Co.

Clifford, J. & G.E. Marcus. (eds.) (1986) *Writing Culture: The Poetics and Politics of Ethnography*. Berkeley: University of California Press.

Foucault, M. (1977) *Discipline and Punish: The Birth of the Prison*. New York: Pantheon Books.

Foucault, M. (1989) *The Birth of the Clinic*. Routledge: London.

Friese, C. & J. Latimer. (2019) 'Entanglements in Health and Well-being: Working with Model Organisms in Biomedicine and Bioscience'. *Medical Anthropology Quarterly*, 33 (1): 120–137.

Giarelli, G. (2003) *Il Malessere della Medicina, Un Confronto Internazionale*. Milano: Franco Angeli.

Giddens, A. (1991) *Modernity and Self Identity*. Stanford: Stanford University Press.

Good, B. J., & M.J. DelVecchio Good. (1981) 'The Semantics of Medical Discourse'. *Sciences and Cultures*, 177–212.

Latour, B. (1993) *We have Never been Modern*. Cambridge, MA: Harvard University Press.

Latour, B. (2005) *Reassembling the Social: An Introduction to Actor-Network Theory*. Oxford: Oxford University Press.

Merleau-Ponty, M. (2012) *Phenomenology of Perception*. New York: Routledge.

Puig de la Bellacasa, M. (2011) 'Matters of Care in Technoscience: Assembling Neglected Things'. *Social Studies of Science*, 41: 85–106.

10

AN ETHNOGRAPHY OF A UNIVERSALLY DESIGNED PLAY ENVIRONMENT

Hira Hasan and Susan Squires

Introduction

While architects have been designing playgrounds for differently-abled children for decades, there is no particular research that has investigated the needs of the children and their families from their point of view. In 2014, a Dallas, Texas based non-profit organization, For the Love of the Lake (FTLOTL) Foundation, became aware that the playgrounds in White Rock Lake Park (WRLP) lacked inclusiveness and accessibility. WRLP is one of the largest parks in Dallas, encompassing over a thousand acres of land and FTLOTL is one of the non-profit organizations working for the park's conservation and maintenance. Flag Pole Hill playground in WRLP constructed in 1998 needed refurbishment and to celebrate its 20th anniversary, FTLOTL committed to incorporating universal design in the playground by undertaking a renovation project. To ensure that the new playground met the community's needs, FTLOTL commissioned a needs assessment to be undertaken by an anthropologist in order to generate insights for an inclusive playground.

The aerial view of the Flag Pole Hill in Figure 10.1 and panoramic view of the Flag Pole Hill playground area in Figure 10.2 shows the play equipment including the slide set, spring bouncers, monkey bars, and bucket swings on a ground covered with woodchips. Abundant trees, benches, and sidewalks can also be seen along with the pavilion in the background.

Literature review

The importance of play

There is consensus in research that play is essential to the healthy growth of a child. Play is not only enjoyable but also crucial to the processes of learning and development (Gleave 2012). Active play—as opposed to passive play opportunities—stimulates healthy activity, provides physical exercise, and builds strength. It leads to perceptual, conceptual, and intellectual development. Integration of cognitive abilities and the development of language also benefit from play (Weininger & Fitzgerald 1988). Occupational therapists use play as a means to help children with disabilities reach therapeutic goals. Play activities are used to achieve treatment objectives such as "fine motor skill development, postural control, and concept development" (Missiuna

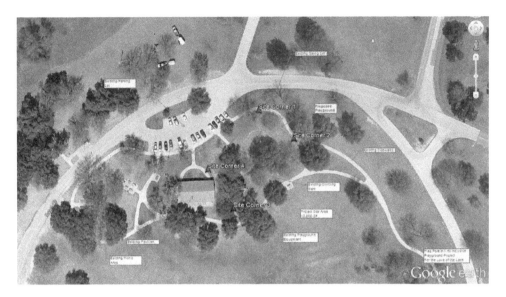

Figure 10.1 An aerial view of Flag Pole Hill playground area, 2015 (Google Earth)

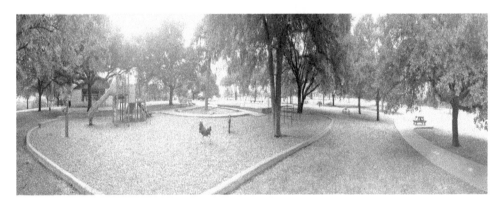

Figure 10.2 Panoramic view of Flag Pole Hill playground area, 2015

& Pollock 1991: 882). Children with physical or neurological challenges spend a considerable amount of time during the day in therapy and in turn need more play opportunities to catch up on what their nondisabled peers engage in. Tai encapsulated the benefits of play for children, including those with disabilities as follows:

1. Brain development, physical development, and health.
2. Building social, emotional, and life skills.
3. Helping to develop awareness for risk.
4. Encouraging children to experiment, generate ideas, practice skills, role-play, invent.
5. Allowing an opportunity for children with disabilities to interact with their peers.
6. Offering opportunities for choice and decision-making.
7. Establishing a critical bond with nature during childhood. (Tai 2006)

Without adequate play opportunities, children with disabilities might acquire secondary disabilities, including diminished motivation, imagination, and creativity, poorly developed social skills, and increased dependence (Missiuna & Pollock 1991). Consequently, play is not just a therapeutic tool in general but also a preventive measure for secondary disabilities.

Playgrounds

Since playgrounds are associated with free play, pleasure, and adventures, a conducive environment, appropriate space, and suitable cultural setting are extremely important. They are places for physical activities as well as places for skill building and social gatherings. Yet, they can also be places where children with disabilities are often excluded from play opportunities. "Universally designed playgrounds offer opportunities for all children to develop physical, cognitive, sensory, and social skills and provide a balance of play experiences to build all these skills" (Landscape Structures 2016). Importantly, playgrounds provide more than equipment, they provide a contextual environment for inclusive play that serve as participatory, socializing, and inclusive spaces. Well-designed playgrounds create a positive atmosphere for all children with varying abilities. The choice to use an anthropological approach to the playground needs assessment was based on its holistic approach that stresses the importance of context that is significant for implementing the concept of inclusion. Descriptors such as "ADA (Americans with Disabilities Act) accessible" and "inclusive/universally designed playgrounds" have become almost synonymous when describing these playgrounds; however, each is quite distinct. Accessible design acknowledges that children with disabilities have access to the playground, but it doesn't take into consideration social integration or other facets of the child's experience. Universal design makes place for children with disabilities alongside their able-bodied peers on the playground. ADA accessible playgrounds meet minimum accessibility standards per the legal framework, whereas a universal design normally meets and exceeds those requirements (Steinfeld 1994).

The anthropology of play

Anthropological studies have found that children have a remarkable and undisputed capacity for learning in general and learning culture in particular. Children's play culture can have its own language, fads and phases, values, and even its own history and geography as seen in the play landscapes children create and recreate for themselves (Casey 2005). Play is an element of culture and society and it fulfills a "culture-creating function" (Huizinga 1949: 71). For anthropology, culture is learned and not inherited. "Anthropologists believe that the most important influence in human development is the ecological and cultural setting within which a child will grow up" (Weisner 2015: 451). Childhood is a time of enculturation where identity formation, social relations, and social actions are learned. Children are a part of society's fabric with their own social and political agency, and play is a fundamental necessity for testing and practicing the roles and responsibilities children will have as adults. It is during this time that the foundations of inclusion can be instilled. Inclusion is embracing diversity, rather than simply tolerating the differences (Ludvigson, Creegan, & Mills 2005). Inclusive play creates a conducive environment by integrating social inclusion with physical accessibility, where usability of equipment doesn't discriminate against abilities.

While much research on play has been undertaken by developmental psychology, their explicit focus on the individual rather than social, cultural, and historical context, along with its experimental methodology can be limiting (Sawyer 2002). Developmental psychologists assume the universality of child development while anthropologists are much more ready to accept that there are cultural differences in play (Sawyer 2002). Nonetheless, play rests at the boundary of psychology and anthropology, and using the insights from both can bring an "ethnographically enlightened psychology and a more cognitively aware anthropology" (Goldman 1998). The work of Brian Sutton-Smith (1981) is such an example. He employed an interdisciplinary research approach towards play as he drew insights from history, cross-cultural studies, psychology, sociology and education. His main findings revealed that the playground is a place that mostly runs itself and needs little intervention from adults.

Using the anthropological perspective to investigate play

Anthropology is an important and relevant research frame to study inclusion and disabilities. As an anthropologist suggested, the purpose of anthropology is to make the world safe for human differences (Benedict 1974). Early anthropology focused on marginalized communities and looked beyond human differences and mitigated the distinctions between "West and the rest," and "us versus the other." The idea of cultural relativity is to accept diverse cultures as being primarily different, rather than being lesser or inferior. Likewise, inclusion is removing barriers between us and the other, able-bodied and differently-abled, and considering disabled as not being less developed than their peers but having developed differently.

However, disability is not merely a physical, psychological, or intellectual handicap but is the social exclusion that takes place due to bodily differences. There is a distinction between embodied limitations and social discrimination where impairment is what we have while disability is what we experience (John & Wheway 2004). Moreover, disability is cultural segregation since people with disabilities may not be able to identify with the general culture and population in general. The differently-abled are often labeled "the other," somehow separate from people who are not considered to have disabilities (Ablon 1995). Ablon identified community's reaction to people with special needs as the disabling force rather than the bodily differences. "Othering" excludes one from full participation in society and prevents one from fulfilling normative roles and results. When one group "others" another group, they perceive them as weaker to make themselves look stronger or better (Foucault 1987). While the process of othering manipulates power dynamics, an inclusive playground has the potential to minimize power relations based on abilities. It imparts a sense of equality among children as all children are provided equal play opportunities.

Universally designed playgrounds incorporate some of the basic concepts of an anthropological framework including diversity, acceptability, and equality. The physical space as well as its socio-cultural construction is designed to facilitate removal of physical and social barriers. The focus is on children, not as isolated individuals, but as members of a rich, dynamic environment in which they are unified on the basis of their similarities rather than their differences. Children internalize their similarities and differences and learn that everyone has different strengths, which makes nobody inferior or superior.

Because the literature on play, childhood, and disability, has identified all three as "experiences," ethnography is a particularly appropriate tool to study the physical, mental, social, and emotional experience in context. Subtle nuances of how differently-abled children use playgrounds can be appropriately explored through ethnographic tools. Ablon's pioneering ethnographic approach to the study of disability helped to move medical anthropology from a disease framework of disability to an ethnographic focus (Kasnitz & Shuttleworth 2004). Ethnography provides an insider's perspective on experiencing disability, especially for children as it enables "… a more organic story to emerge" when studying children with varying abilities (Davis, Watson, & Cunningham-Burley 2008: 235). However, in medical anthropology "impairment-disability is still situated peripherally to the core research issues of illness and healing" (Kasnitz & Shuttleworth 2004: 142). Anthropology's genuine fascination with "the other" can logically inform the field of disability studies, yet this connection has not fully been utilized (Klotz 2003). Diversity of differently-abled children's lives can be explored by ethnographers being reflexive about how these children experience and respond to issues of access (Davis et al. 2008). Therefore, there is a need for further research in the area of disability studies.

Research design

This exploratory, qualitative research project was guided by anthropological theory and methods. Ethnography constitutes one of the primary methodologies in anthropology, which is the detailed and systematic study of human cultures providing their "thick description" (Geertz 1973: 6). An anthropological toolkit was used to investigate what suited parents of children with disabilities and their children's physical and social needs. This research study analyzed core or common needs amongst the participants rather than variations between them. The research findings were initially planned to be incorporated into a new, redesigned playground in 2016.

Goals of the research

The goal of this needs assessment was to generate insights to create a universally designed playground by understanding the perspective of the families who would use the facilities. FTLOTL wanted to know what kind of facilities they should build and what features and equipment were required by families and their children. Research questions focused on:

- What are the barriers to play in the current playground?
- What kind of equipment is preferred?
- What is the opinion about space utilization and the layout of the playground?
- What are the perceived benefits and risks of inclusion in the play area?
- How can the playground overcome these risks and barriers?
- What other aspects should be addressed in the playground?
- What type of events or activities will draw users to the playground?

Sample

The demographics and size of the sample were decided in consultation with FTLOTL. A purposive sampling technique was adopted to ensure that all respondents lived somewhere around the Flag Pole Hill area and represented families having children with varying disabilities, genders, and ages. The resulting sample included fourteen participants in total, each of whom had at least one child with either a physical, social, or intellectual disability within the ages of 2 and 13 years. Owing to the rigorous and challenging recruitment process, later parents from the entire DFW metroplex were considered. Fortunately, in due course, nine out of the fourteen participants were located within the ten-mile radius of Flag Pole Hill. Table 10.1 shows the details of the research participants' profile.

Table 10.1 Details of research participants' profiles

No.	Age (years)	Gender	Disability	Ethnicity	Able-bodied Siblings	Distance to Flag Pole Hill (miles)	Interview medium	Parent interviewed	Interview Duration (minutes)
1.	4.5	Male	Down Syndrome and Autism	Caucasian	none/ only child	1.5	in person	Father	28
2.	5	Female	Down Syndrome	Caucasian	8-year-old sister	2	in person	Mother	32
3.	8	Male	Nonverbal Autism	Half-Hispanic, Half-Caucasian	twin sister	5	in person	Father	54
4.	7	Female	Hemiparesis, Speech delays, Visual field cut, Wears an AFO	Caucasian	5- and 7-year-old sisters	8	on the phone	Mother	32
5.	12	Male	Cerebral Palsy, Epilepsy Blind, Nonverbal Autism	Hispanic	none/ only child	20	in person	Mother	36
6.	12	Female	Nonverbal Autism	Caucasian	twin brother	40	on the phone	Mother	25
7.	4	Female	Nonverbal Autism	Caucasian	2-year-old sister	45 (in Denton)	in person	Father	32
8.	13	Male	Down Syndrome, Seizures, can't walk, had a stroke	Half-Caucasian Half-African American	9-year-old brother	3	on the phone	Mother	50
9.	4	Female	Encephalopathy	Caucasian	8-year-old sister	45 (in Denton)	on the phone	Mother	50
10.	8	Male	Hydrocephalus	African American	27-year-old sister	4	on the phone	Mother	33
11.	7	Male	Chronic Lung Disease	African American	mother was expecting second child	3	on the phone	Mother	26
12.	2.5, 4.5	Male	Autism Spectrum Disorder	Caucasian	both children were autistic	3.5	on the phone	Mother	59
13.	2.5	Male	Social issues and Speech delays	Hispanic	7-year-old brother	5	on the phone	Mother	55
14.	15	Male	Nonverbal, Neurological and Physical issues, Uses braces, walker and or wheelchair	Caucasian	only child	18	on the phone	Grandmother	40

Recruitment

Participant recruitment was the most challenging part of the entire research process and data collection was completed after two and a half months of rigorous effort. Snowballing sampling technique also came in useful as existing interviewees referred other parents, schoolteachers and therapists whom they thought would be suitable leads. An application for conducting this research was submitted to the UNT Institutional Review Board (IRB) in early March of 2015 and was approved in April 2015. A flyer was also designed and distributed in order to reach out to the potential participants. When they were approached, a brief introduction of the researcher and the research project highlighting the benefits of their participation was provided. If potential participants agreed to participate, information regarding the study was verbally provided to them before beginning the interview, specifying that their participation was voluntary, and they could refuse to answer partially or withdraw entirely from the interview at any time without obligation. Participants signed informed consent forms before being interviewed, either in person or via email, depending on the medium through which the interview was conducted. As required by the university, anonymity was maintained throughout the study, and personal identifiers were removed from their interview transcriptions.

Ethnographic toolkit

Data collection tools included semi-structure interview guides and observations.

Interviews

The semi-structured interview guide began with a few general, icebreaker questions while the rest of the interview guide consisted of two parts. The first part focused on the current recreation facilities and concomitant barriers to play, while the second part attempted to ascertain the ideal inclusive play environment as perceived by the parents. The interviews were conducted either in person at a suitable place for the parents or over the phone, depending on what was most convenient for them. Five of the fourteen parents were interviewed in person. All interviews were audio recorded and each interview session lasted for around an hour. Fieldnotes were noted during the interviews and a 500-word personal reflection written after each interview session.

Observations

Anthropological research includes developing an emic perspective by observing the research participants in their natural habitat. Following long-established anthropological approaches, an effort was made to avoid preconceived notions and to gain an insider's point of view of a playground experience. Half-hour to an hour-long observations were conducted at inclusive as well as typical playgrounds in the DFW metroplex in Texas. The observations facilitated and enhanced an understanding of the play environment and adaptive equipment and also made it easier to relate to features or facilities referred to by the parents. In addition to taking fieldnotes and photographs during the observations, online videos of children with disabilities playing in different playgrounds were also watched.

Analysis tools

Interviews were transcribed verbatim and Transcribe.wreally.com, a web application, facilitated this process. The interview transcripts were uploaded to Dedoose (app.dedoose.com), an online encrypted qualitative coding program. Dedoose was used to synthesize the findings into coherent themes and coded to find patterns emerging across them. Figure 10.3 shows a word cloud of themes that emerged in Dedoose after the initial round of coding.

Data analysis

Upon completion of data collection and transcription, the transcripts were coded. Each transcript was read a few times to get a general idea of the parent's viewpoint, and then coded, using a complex, bottom-up, inductive approach. In order to operationalize and contextualize codes, rules for categorization were identified, which ensured that categories were consistent and meaningful. Codes were made distinct so that future references could be made without any ambiguity. Finally, a codebook was created with 82 codes, which were clearly identified. Since this was a qualitative study, data were coded based on both frequency of the ideas and also on their mere presence. Patterns that occurred frequently emerged as major themes, while those not so frequent nevertheless formed part of the research findings. Coding was followed by construction of overarching themes from the emergent categories as major needs were organized into assessment themes and categories. Further content analysis was carried out which was

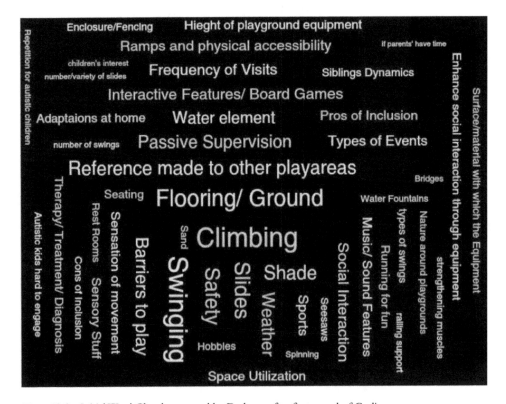

Figure 10.3   Initial Word Cloud generated by Dedoose after first round of Coding

guided by grounded theory (Glaser and Strauss 1967). This facilitated classification of core con-
sistencies in parents' responses about playground usability and in conceptualizing a prospective
framework for the proposed universally designed playground.

Findings

The findings from interview sessions with parents regarding playground usability have been
arranged into themes and subthemes. Overall, interviewees believed a diverse environment
would enrich the playground experience in innumerable ways.

An inclusive environment

Parents wanted an inclusive playground to integrate the principles of equality in play activities so that all children would have equal play opportunities. They hoped that their children
with special needs would feel welcomed, accepted, and treated fairly by their peers. One of the
mothers hoped that one of the benefits of an inclusive playground would be that, "everyone
gets to know each other and recognize that there is big diverse world out there and learn from
each other and grow together." Moreover, parents explained that the true essence of an inclusive environment encompasses diversity of play equipment along with other aspects. Parents
preferred a diverse mix of equipment as the play requirements of each child varied relative to
those of others.

Within the swings category, for example, an entire range was suggested by parents including
adaptive swings, flat swings, platform swings, swings with back support, wheelchair accessible swings, bench swings, swings at a lower level, swings with seats facing each other, bigger
swings, and bucket swings among the options. A range of equipment was also important because
parents had conflicting views. A mother explained that her child "enjoys slides that are not just
straight down. Bumps or twists or stuff like that are thrilling to him." Conversely, a few parents
were not fond of winding slides. A mother specified, "Slides should have wider steps and not
so many curves because kids with braces get caught up in the curves." Thus, equipment needs
of children varied as the disabilities varied. Parents also wanted different heights for various
equipment depending on their child's limitation. Many parents specifically complained about
the limited number of play structures, thus not only variety but also quantity of the equipment
was important for parents.

Capacity building at the playground

Parents hope a playground visit will provide their children with physical and social skill-building
opportunities through interaction with the environment as well as with children of different
abilities.

Physical skill building

Depending on the child's capability, physical exercise was deemed fundamental for a healthy play
experience. Swings, slides, and equipment for climbing, including jungle gyms, monkey bars,
rock-climbing walls, and bridges were undoubtedly the most popular equipment. These were
followed by equipment for spinning, e.g., merry-go-rounds, and for balancing, e.g., seesaws.
A few parents also said that their children enjoyed bouncing on trampolines and spring rockers.
Parents were aware that physical activity on the playground plays a vital role in building strength

and muscles in children. A child using their physical body during play enables them to feel physically confident, secure, and self-assured (Isenberg & Quisenberry, 2002). A mother expounded, "Play therapy is a critical piece of their development…not to mention the physical aspect that builds their strength, and getting out in the sun, they get their vitamin D, fresh air, and all."

An open area for running and sports, within or outside the playground, was a popular demand of the parents. Running away or wandering off was a safety hazard for some children with autism, but for all others it was a source of recreation, which parents encouraged. Some parents suggested playgrounds to have a safe communal area for running where children could fall and not hurt themselves. Despite being aware that playgrounds were not meant for sports, still some respondents insisted on having a safe sports area for soccer, football, basketball, and bat-ball.

Social skill building

Parents considered refining interpersonal and social skills to be one of the benefits of an inclusive environment. Many parents mentioned that their children with different abilities enjoyed social interaction and hoped this playground would provide such opportunities. They opined that their children would gain life lessons including turn-taking, sharing, patience, kindness, and a sense of helping others in such an atmosphere. Parents discussed several types of play activities including team play, parallel play and solitary play that would augment their children's social interaction in the playground. Parents advocated for team play, hence they favored equipment that required the participation of multiple children, like equipment for balancing and spinning, e.g., seesaws and merry-go-rounds, in order to facilitate social interaction. As much as parents of children with autism wanted their children to interact and play with others, they were aware that their children were more comfortable with parallel play. They believed that children learned consciously or subconsciously through parallel play and by observing children next to them. In addition, solitary play was also a means of relaxation for children with autism to internalize the playground experience. Parents of autistic children expressed a need for passive resting areas for solitary play to be incorporated in the playground design. Research has shown that lack of such spaces leads to aimless wandering and aggressive behavior in such children.

Sensory stimuli

Children's engagement in play is dependent upon the stimulation provided by their surroundings. Parents expressed a preference for a sensory-rich playground experience for their children. Tactile, auditory, and visual elements were all deemed essential for sensory stimulation. For example, almost all the parents talked about their children's fondness for water activities, especially in the Texas summer. A sand area was another popular sensory element suggestion. Other tactile elements stated included textured walls and bases. Interactive musical features as well as activities involving music were also popular among parents. Parents shared ideas for making the surroundings visually and aesthetically pleasing for their children, which included the use of vibrant colors; a themed playground concept; benches of different shapes; motivational quotes; and landscaping with ponds, bridges, trees, and ducks. Another common theme expressed by most parents was their child's enjoyment of sensation of movement. One of the mothers shared an explicit portrayal of how her son enjoyed continuous movement:

His happiest times are when he is riding in the car, swinging, but he doesn't get to do that anymore since he is so big for all the swings … we were doing roller skating yesterday and so

I just took him onto the floor of the skating rink and around and around and around [laughing], so he loves movement!

Hence, play structures that induce a strong feeling of movement were thought to be essential for an enjoyable experience. Parents also wanted the playground to be a cognitively stimulating environment and suggested ideas for imaginative play and exploratory play. Imaginative/pretend play was proposed by those who wanted either the play structures or the décor to be designed to trigger dramatic play. A mother shared an observation of her children:

> They would run up the ramp and pretend they were Elsa and building their castle together and then slide down on ice ... my one daughter who has hard time keeping up you know; she could keep up with them [laughing].

Exploratory play was also frequently mentioned, and ideas like integrating games such as scavenger and treasure hunts into the playground equipment were shared. Moreover, respondents suggested integrating interactive features in the play equipment including board games, tic-tac-toe, puzzles, funny mirrors (distorted mirror reflections), interactive features with climbing structures, and speaking tubes or voice pipes.

Nuances of design

Parents emphasized the design of play structures that were suitable for their children and also what caused inconvenience and hindrance during play. Parents frequently mentioned that play should be kept simple and wanted overall equipment in the playground to be easy and intuitive to use. Repetitive play was considered extremely important to engage autistic children and it was suggested having this incorporated in playground activities. Some interviewees' children did not have strong fine motor skills, hence they wanted equipment designed to facilitate a better grip. Parents perceived steps or stairs as hindrances and described how having ramps makes it easier and more practical. Another mother proposed having steps marked with bright colors to guide visually impaired children with autism.

Safety

While parents recognized that play is dependent upon the stimulation that a playground can provide, they were still apprehensive about the heights of the equipment. The cognitive age and physical sizes of a child with special needs may not always be commensurate. Thus, the question therefore arises whether age-segregation of play equipment is required or not. A lot of parents opposed age segregation. A mother whose son was 12 years old and liked to play in an area for 2-to-5-year-olds said, "if there is something that he can participate in, I take him there anyway and nobody cares because he doesn't disrupt anything so I break the rules [laughing]." Conversely, some parents were also cognizant of the hazard of children of varying physical sizes playing together. A lot of parents also mentioned that either their children were too big or too small for the equipment.

Safety was of paramount significance as parents shared many other safety concerns. Taking weather conditions into account for playground visits was the primary safety measure taken by parents, especially with unpredictable Texas weather. Uniform floor surfacing was the biggest concern for all parents and was brought up by everyone during the interview. Wood chips were extremely unpopular and a foamed/soft/padded flooring was suggested. A playground enclosure was also a major safety requirement and a source of peace of mind for most parents, especially for parents with autistic children who tend to wander off. Weather and temperature resistant equipment material was proposed along with curved and smooth finish of play structures. Contrasting the colors of the surfacing with the equipment color was suggested for children with visual impairments and as a way-finding tool. Various other safety measures mentioned included handrails, harnesses and seat belts, regular maintenance, and timely repair of play equipment.

Building community at the playground

Parents shared various facets of playground visits and activities that contribute to building a closely-knit community.

Family outing

Benefits of inclusiveness extended to the family members as visits to playgrounds were considered a recreational outing for the entire family. Parents not only wanted siblings to play together but also wanted themselves to have playful interaction with their children. They wanted their children with disabilities to have fun, yet they didn't want their abled-bodied children to be ignored either. A mother explained, "Having multiple children, a place where all of my kids can kinda play together really and feel that they are not eliminated in any way, on either end of it." Parents wanted the playground equipment to be designed to foster siblings' interaction and to nurture a stronger bond between them. Furthermore, it also made supervision easier for parents.

Community support system

Respondents shared various ideas on how community can provide a support system for them. The playground is not just an area for the children but also a place for parents to socialize, connect, and share their common concerns. Parents of differently-abled children face several challenges in their daily routines and personal lives. Having a child with disabilities can stress the family and even lead to family breakdowns. Special circumstances within the families were prevalent to an extent within the sample. Three out of the fourteen children came from either single, divorced, or remarried families. Such situations within families make it more difficult for parents to cope with their children's disabilities. The support of other parents and community at large would make life better for them. From time to time, parents mentioned that their children could be hard to manage, and a helping hand could facilitate their visit to a playground. Parents described how their playground visits varied if they had other families to accompany them, another person going with them or if both parents were taking the children to the playground together. A few parents also suggested that formation of parent support groups in the playground community would be beneficial and keep the parents connected. Formation of a support network for parents of children with disabilities in the Flag Pole Hill neighborhood would be a morale booster for these families.

Space utilization

Parents believed that appropriate utilization of space and a well-designed layout of the playground is essential. A major consideration for the parents regarding space allocation was that they didn't want their children with special needs to be left out at the periphery of the playground. Most parents believed that the playground should be spread out and not too congested.

They articulated that their children were better at interacting and playing with others if the playground was more spacious. Space was important for children with autism due to their social limitations and for wheelchair-bound children as administrating wheelchairs requires space. Parents were cognizant that they couldn't let their children be on their own but at the same time they wanted them to have a sense of independence for a fulfilling play experience. A mother enunciated that endorsing the concept of independence in the playground would make children "less conscious of being watched" and would not only give them the space they need but also give parents some respite. Most respondents could not leave their children on their own for long on the playground. Even those who allowed their children to be more independent wanted an uninterrupted line of sight for visual supervision. Therefore, the layout of the playground must support and facilitate parental supervision. Parents also discussed space utilization and seating arrangement to encourage social interaction among them. Other ways of building community included support for having different events at the potential playground, as they believed it would be a great way to develop a cohesive community. A few parents even wanted to be involved in the process of building the playground and some also volunteered to offer their services at different stages of the construction.

Surrounding facilities

Support elements and architectural features that would make the playground experience more convenient and pleasant included shade, seating and restrooms (with changing tables) were priorities for almost all parents in this regard. These priorities were followed by ramps, water fountains, trash cans, storage, and a picnic area. Other facilities mentioned included nearby parking, a walking track around the playground for parents to get some exercise while their children play and electrical outlets to charge motorized chairs or scooters.

Recommendations

These recommendations are based on inferences drawn from parents' responses as well as from researcher's own observations for a better play experience.

Building a virtual presence

Nowadays, online representation and social media presence lends more credibility to any venture. Eureka 2 playground, which was being built at South Lakes Park in Denton, maintained a virtual presence.

Figure 10.4 is a screenshot of Eureka 2's website that demonstrates the role of websites in collecting donations, updating the community on the building process, displaying the amount of funds raised, and offering volunteer opportunities, etc. Groups on social media could facilitate networking of parents and lead to the formation of parent support groups.

Input of occupational therapists on design

Many parents throughout the interviews kept referring to how occupational therapy had made a positive impact in their children's developmental growth. The activities that are conducted during therapies could be incorporated in playground structures so that the playground outing is more engaging and at the same time therapeutic. Input from recreational, physical, and occupational therapists may support a more well-informed and well-designed, inclusive play time.

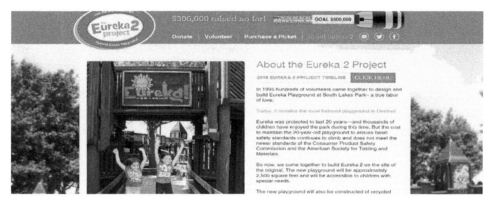

Figure 10.4   Eureka 2 website screenshot

Insights from other playgrounds and play areas

While discussing their preferences for various playground features, parents gave examples of many other playgrounds in Texas and also made references to play areas in malls, specific schools, and in fast food restaurants. Decision makers and designers could keep features and structures of these playgrounds in mind when finalizing the construction plans.

Reference to design guides

The literature review yielded ample design guides of various universally designed playgrounds. For actual design purposes, these readily available design guides can serve as invaluable resources. Success stories of their respective playgrounds can help in making better policy decisions regarding the potential playground.

Retaining and refurbishing some of the current equipment and design

Observations in the Flag Pole Hill playground led to the conclusion that while the existing pieces of equipment were spaced randomly and had worn out with time, nonetheless the playground was not outdated in its equipment design. Installation of new structures and reconditioning of current equipment, along with strategic placement would serve the purpose. The current playground has diverse equipment including interactive as well as sensory features as shown in Figures 10.5 to 10.12.

Playground layout and equipment

Most parents' feedback for the layout was to have the playground structures along the perimeter and some open space and smaller structures in the center. This would facilitate community building as well as provide both periphery and centralized play areas. They wanted the play area not to be congested and a little spread out. Parents shared that they hoped to participate in the playground to enhance their child's experience by helping them use the equipment. Some believed that their children were not comfortable using slides or swings, or climbing or walking across the bridge on their own. Others said that they would like to demonstrate to their children how the equipment was used.

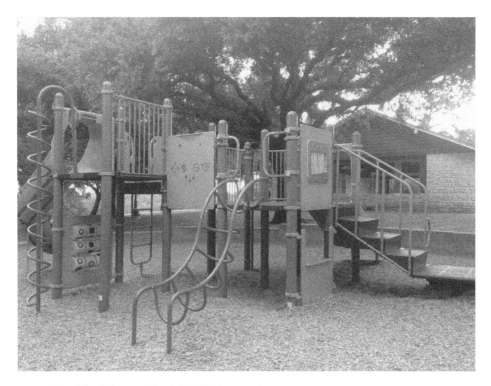

Figure 10.5 The slide set at Flag Pole Hill playground

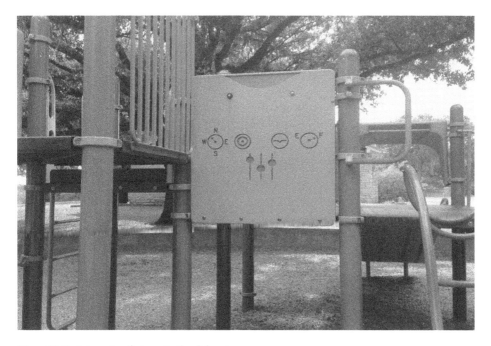

Figure 10.6 Interactive features in the slide set

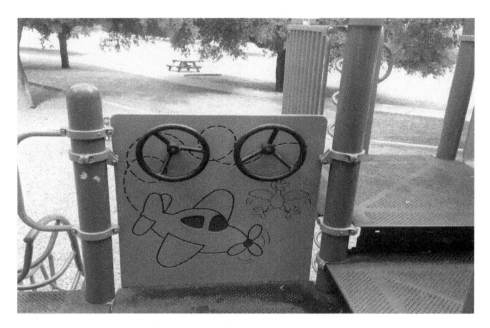

Figure 10.7 More interactive features in the slide set

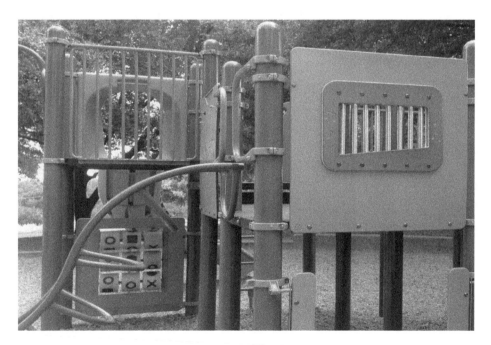

Figure 10.8 Interactive and sensory features in the slide set

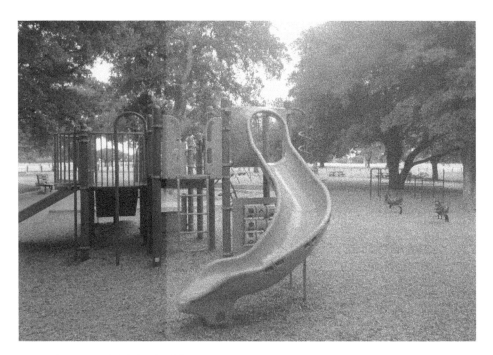

Figure 10.9   Curved slide in the slide set

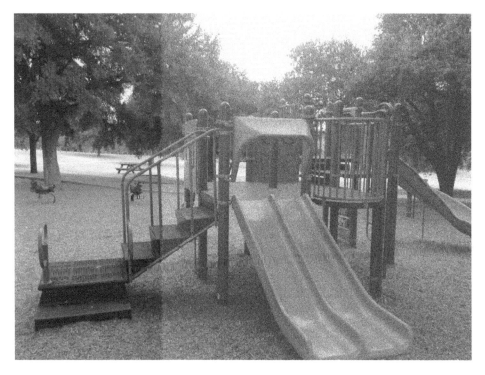

Figure 10.10   Straight-down slides in the slide set

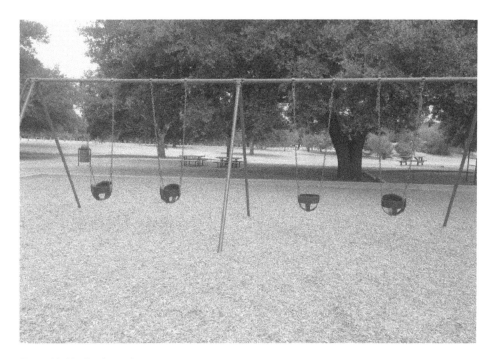

Figure 10.11   Bucket swings

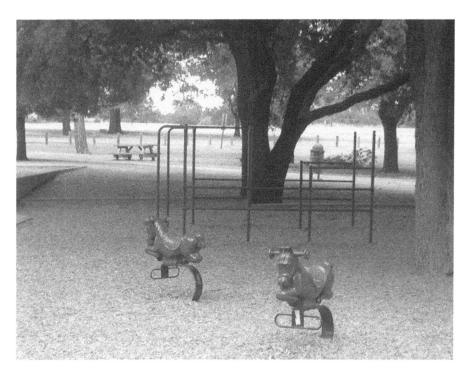

Figure 10.12   Spring bouncers and climbing bars

Volunteer supervision program

FTLOTL has a well-developed volunteer program as it administers Second Saturday Shoreline Spruce Up for the cleanup of White Rock Lake Park. Similarly, volunteer groups can also be formed to assist parents with differently-abled children in the playground, as parents expressed that they desired a helping hand to manage their children on the playground.

Colorful/themed playground

The aesthetic of the playground was an important consideration for the parents. Since most differently-abled children spent their day indoors, a jungle theme would accentuate the out-door play experience. It would also be easier to incorporate the elements of nature within such playground design and equipment. Contrasting the color of the surfacing with the equipment color would result in better vision for children with visual impairments. Similarly, contrasting the color of the fenced perimeter with the surfacing color and marking the change of eleva-tion with different colors would facilitate better visibility. However, color selection has to be done sensibly as dark colors absorb heat and would keep the equipment and the surroundings heated.

Captivating initial visits

Some parents mentioned that they keep searching for different playgrounds to see whether they meet their children's needs and whether their children enjoy them or not. Such comments show that the playground should be designed in a way that captivates children's interest in the first visit or at least in the initial few visits, retains it, and also finds favor with the parents.

Educating the community

Creating a warm and welcoming environment is essential but easier said than done. The majority of visitors to this playground will be able-bodied and might be insensitive towards the minority, i.e. differently-abled children, or genuinely unaware of their condition. To achieve the anticipated goals of inclusion, the entire community, especially children, not only need to be sensitized but also educated about different disabilities. This is not in the scope of FTLOTL alone. However, FTLOTL can try to create awareness in its community and, while redesigning the playground, keep the general attitude of the majority towards disabilities in consideration.

Outcome

After years of research, planning, fundraising, and navigating the city's bureaucracy, in 2018 Flag Pole Hill inclusive playground's construction was completed and inaugurated for public recreation. Figures 10.13 and 10.14 show the playground after the renovation construction took place.

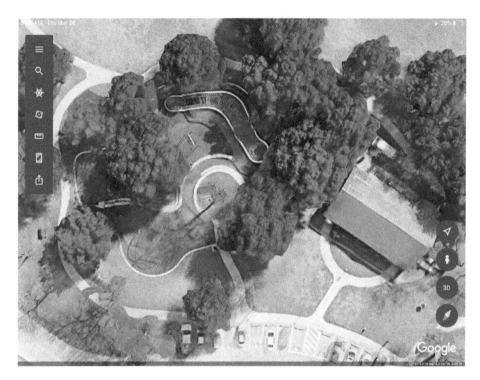

Figure 10.13 An aerial view of Flag Pole Hill playground area, 2018 (Google Earth)

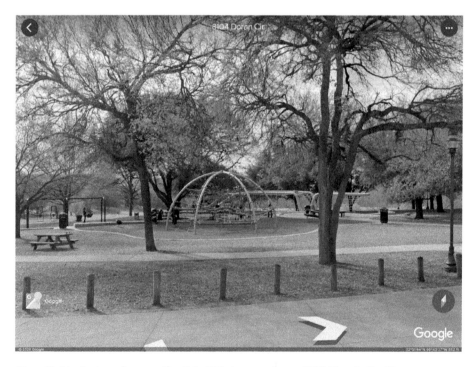

Figure 10.14 A view of current Flag Pole Hill playground area, 2018 (Google Earth)

References

Ablon, J. (1995) Stigmatized health conditions. Social Science & Medicine. Part B: Medical Anthropology, 15(1): 5–9.

Benedict, R. (1974) The Chrysanthemum and the Sword: Patterns of Japanese Culture. New York: New American Library.

Casey, T. (2005). Practical Strategies for Working with Children Aged 3–8. London: Sage.

Davis J.M., N. Watson, & S. Cunningham-Burley. (2008) Disabled Children, Ethnography and Unspoken Understandings. Research with children: perspectives and practices (2nd revised ed.), edited by Pia Christensen and Allison James, eds., pp. 220–238. London: Routledge.

Foucault, M. (1987) Madness and Civilization, A History of Insanity in the Age of Reason. London.

Geertz, C. (1973) Thick Description: Toward an Interpretive Theory of Culture. In Gertz, The Interpretation of Cultures. Selected Essays (pp. 3–30). New York: Basic Books.

Glaser, B., & Strauss, A. (1967). The Discovery of Grounded Theory Strategies for Qualitative Research. Mill Valley, CA Sociology Press.

Gleave, J. (2012) A world without play: A Literature review.

Goldman, L.R. (1998) Child's Play: Myth, Mimesis and Make-Believe. New York: Berg. p. 302.

Huizinga, J. (1949) Homo ludens. A Study of Play Element in Culture (1971 ed.). London: Paladin.

Isenberg, J. & N. Quisenberry. (2002) Play: Essential for All Children. Olney, ML: Association for Childhood Education International.

John, A., & R. Wheway. (2004) Can Play, Will Play: Disabled Children and Access to Outdoor Playgrounds. London: National Playing Fields Association.

Kasnitz, D., & R.P. Shuttleworth. (2004) Anthropology in disability studies. Disability Studies Quarterly, 21(3): 2–17.

Klotz, J. (2003) The culture concept: Anthropology, disability studies and intellectual disability. Paper presented at the Disability at the Cutting Edge: A colloquium to examine the impact on theory, research and professional practice.

Ludvigson, A., C. Creegan, & H. Mills. (2005) Lets Play Together: Play and inclusion evaluation of better play round three. Barnardo's.

Missiuna, C., & N. Pollock (1991) Play deprivation in children with physical disabilities: The role of the occupational therapist in preventing secondary disability. American Journal of Occupational Therapy 45(10): 882–888.

Sawyer, R.K. (2002) The New Anthropology of Children, Play, and Games. Reviews in Anthropology 31(2): 147–164.

Steinfeld, E. (1994) The concept of universal design. Proceedings of the Sixth Ibero-American Conference on Accessibility. Rio de Janeiro (June 19, 1994).

Structures, Landscape. (2016) A Higher Level of Inclusive Play; Ideas for Better Playgrounds for All. Inclusive Play Catalog. Landscape Structures Inc.

Sutton-Smith, B. (1981) A History of Children's Play: The New Zealand Playground, 1840–1950. Philadelphia: University of Pennsylvania Press, pp. 331.

Tai, L. (2006) Designing Outdoor Environments for Children: Landscaping schoolyards, gardens and playgrounds. New York: McGraw Hill.

Weininger, O. & D. Fitzgerald. (1988) Symbolic play and interhemispheric integration: Some thoughts on a neuropsychological model of play. Journal of Research and Development in Education, 21(4): 23–40.

Weisner, T.S. (2015) Childhood: Anthropological Aspects, International Encyclopedia of the Social & Behavioral Sciences, 2nd edition, Vol 3. Oxford: Elsevier. pp. 451–458.

11

TO BE ON A DIET

Ethnography of weight loss between beauty, food, and violence

Martina Grimaldi

Introduction

I conducted my field study in Italy on the patients of nutrition experts and on the experts themselves. I'm interested in the connection between nutrition studies and aesthetics, that is to say between nutrition and beauty stereotypes. As part of my research, I was interested in showing how nutrition theories and dietetics act violently on our bodies.

Secondly, I would like to focus on the agency of individuals, in particular by showing that personal actions are all different and analyzing what the personal motivations that will drive people to act are.

My research focuses entirely on the combination of injunction and appropriation. The methodology I intend to use shows this binomial and it is divided into two parts: the first investigates the injunction side, thus relating to the observation collected during the sessions between nutritionists and their patients, while the latter focuses on the features of appropriation, building on interviews with patients.

The theoretical basis of my research are the studies on incorporation and mostly on its related violence: the major authors to be cited in this field are Maurice Merleau-Ponty (1945) and Drew Leder (1990).

Based on the studies of these two authors, everything that comes into contact with the body, through the senses, sight, touch, and smell is perceived by our body, and indeed incorporated. Incorporation occurs when our body reacts to an encounter with the outside world.

I have applied this theory on two different groups of studies. The first theoretical frame to be discussed is the one relative to analyses on nutrition conducted by the social sciences, in which we find, above all, a "cultural approach" related to food. This approach studies all that surrounds food, for example religion, family relations, nationality, and all the associated symbolisms.

In recent years, food studies have been developed and diversified. There are several studies that question gender in relation to food, such as the research of Susan Bordo (1997), who wrote a very interesting book in which she discusses anorexia, analyzing the reasons underlying the illness by studying these reasons in relation to male power and female submission in the family of the anorexic girl. Counihan (1999) also sought to study nutrition, based on his field research in Italy and the United States, also from a sexual and gender perspective, citing in these studies Adams (2016), who conducted research on the connection between vegetarianism and feminism.

The second theoretical frame is about violence—mostly a symbolic type of violence (Bourdieu, 1998). In this chapter I will expose the methodology I used and the relative problems, as well as the context in which I conducted my research. I will also analyze the data I collected by dividing the analysis into two macro containers: violence and agency.

Methodology

To shed light on my frame of analysis, I needed to use different methodological tools. Next to qualitative methods, I had to employ quantitative tools as well, which I created to be able to better to investigate the Italian situation, little known in France, about nutrition specialists and their patients.

I started doing research to quantify a situation that interests me in Italy.

I first did some research to see if there already was statistical data on the customers of nutrition experts, but unfortunately I did not find anything from the main Italian statistics agencies, such as ISTAT (National Statistical Institute). It was rather complicated to succeed in this research, and I have not managed to find statistics explaining why nutrition topics in Italy are so fashionable and such a daily activity.

Secondly, I focused on understanding the typology of the most consulted specialists and the price of consultations. Since I led my qualitative research in the city of Bologna, I chose to implement the quantitative part in the same city. I then started my observation with the specialist.

In the specialist's office, completely white, there was a ladder in front of the entrance with a small cabin to allow people to undress away from the specialist's eyes. There were two chairs on one side for the patient (or patients) and a desk that separated them from the specialist's chair. On the desk, only a computer, on which the nutritionist wrote when people spoke, and papers with people's files. In addition, there was a higher chair behind the chair of the specialist, on which sometimes came to sit a new specialist to learn how to work with patients.

For the period I was in the office, I was sitting in that chair, behind the back of the specialist; the position took me away from the scene that was unfolding. In the office I had a fixed position, I could not intervene or speak and everything was going very fast. I was simply an observer and my position did not allow me to get closer to patients: at that moment I felt blocked by the specialist.

In any case, even if I could not intervene at all, being able to observe all these meetings was a pivotal step for me in order to realize the complexity of the session and of all these fundamental moments and words to analyze and to have a deeper look into the situation.

During the second phase, I conducted interviews with the patients: I interviewed ten people, eight women and two men. We agreed on a meeting place, choosing public places in a familiar setting, like a café or a park. I wanted to conduct the interviews away from the specialist's office, to have the least possible conditioned conversations—even if it is impossible to be completely free from awe. What I was most interested in in particular during the interviews was, first of all, to guide the discussion on the personal motivations of the patients: I was interested in the therapy process with the specialists, focusing on the point of view of the patient. Motivations mainly interested me, as well as the course of therapy and the relationship with the specialist. In order to do this, I adopted the narrative approach of Groleau, Young, and Kirmayer (2006).

I wanted to allow a free discussion, suggesting small points on which to focus, since, during the interview, there is a construction and a creation of culture. By mutual exchange and speaking, something new will be created and it is this creation that I am also interested in exploring, not only on the answers to the questions I asked.

Methodological issues
The gender dimension

When I started this analysis, I did not want to be interested in one category of patients in particular. I simply wanted to understand why people went to a nutrition specialist and how the meeting unfolded, since it is a growing social phenomenon in Italy at this time. I did not focus on obese, anorexic, or vegetarian patients, and I was not particularly interested in women or men in particular; I tried to be quite open and I decided not to limit myself.

Nevertheless, the observation process was key to understanding that the question of gender could not be omitted. I was able to observe the impact of the gender dimension on my research simply by counting the female and male patients who visited the office during my observation.

Indeed, I saw that, of the 67 appointments, there was a related presence of five single men, 59 single women and three couples (man and woman). We can therefore already understand, from this descriptive statistic, that the science of nutrition is a science that acts especially on female bodies because, like all sciences, it is based on the social and cultural structure of the context in which it is exercised. Consequently, I realized that even if I did not want to shed particular light on this aspect, it is fundamental to understand how to handle this setting more comprehensively.

Language and context

I think that in order to be able to conduct a qualitative research, you have to understand in depth the people you are talking to, and so I decided to conduct the research in my mother tongue: Italian. The understanding of a person is made more simple through language. Can I, therefore, really understand something explained in another language? For me it is very important to also understand all the unsaid, the understated, and that can be understood either through the help of an informant, or in his culture and mother tongue. That is to say, it is incorrect to say that words refer directly to objects, events, etc. Words refer to the way in which we perceive objects and events, how we manipulate them, how we react to them and in general how we consider them (Nadel 1979, 59). It is possible to feel a barrier between us and people who do not speak our native language. I'm interested in getting closer to people and talking with them about my personal experience so I can create a dialogue and then reflect upon it.

When I speak to people in my mother tongue, I realize that my own narrations are different; on the contrary, when I speak in another language I simplify what I say, and I operate at a more superficial level of discourse.

Sometimes, understanding is already complicated enough if we do not know the people with whom we have to speak very well, so I needed to be sure that I could speak in both of our mother tongue and, at the same time, have a shared cultural background behind us.

Italian context

In order to begin the analysis of interviews and observations, one must understand in what context my analysis moves. When I started this work, I did not think that the Italian situation about nutrition studies and their audience was different from the European situation. So, I started doing research to clarify this situation.

In my opinion, this aspect deserves attention because what surrounds nutrition specialists and the fact that it is so common to rely on them is part of Italian politics, economics, and culture. I have used different analytical tools because the world of nutrition specialists and a focus on their studies on the part of patients is a new social phenomenon in Italy and, therefore, there is still much to be studied.

Statistical data

I first looked for statistical data to analyze this phenomenon. The only data I found in terms of quantitative statistics is the frequency of weight control in 2016 and 2017 as seen in figure 11.1.

This is a data set that does not exactly concern the audience of nutrition specialists, but I find that with this resource we can already understand that the interest in weight-related issues in Italy is quite strong. In this graph we see two types of data: the frequency of the weighing of persons over 18 years of age, divided between men and women, and the frequency of weighing divided according to their BMI and, again, by gender.

From this data we can see that 80% of women and 77% of men weigh at least once a year in 2017 and that women weigh more often than men. On the other hand, the statistics that I found are recent, established from 2016. They make it possible to make us understand that the interest carried around weight in Italy is increasing, and that it is different from the other European countries.

A man I met tells me about his nutritionist, saying that she is quiet and open, "Italian way", and that when he is on vacation, the nutritionist allows him to eat all he wants. At the same time, one must be able to understand why Italians—so much linked to good food, to taste, to food-related social settings in the common imaginary—are increasing their control over food and starting to imagine the sphere of "diet" related to weight rather than taste.

Fischler conducted a research project in 2000–2002 with Estelle Masson and Christy Shields about eating habits in Europe and the United States and published the results in the book *Manger. Français, Européens et Américains face a l'alimentation* (2008).

In the second part of the book by Fischler and Masson, we find the work of the team's collaborators who took care of national specificities. Nicoletta Cavazza took care of Italy, and, more specifically, she conducted the investigation in Bologna, the city where I conducted my research. Contrary to what Fischler shows in his investigation, Cavazza argues how "health" and "well-being" replace "fat" in the metaphor of wealth (Fischler, 1998) even in Italy, a country where one always thinks that nutrition is more related to taste than to health. Cavazza explains that keeping fit is a socially valued goal and that in recent years:

> …the relationship between diet and health has become the subject of discussion and controversy among experts; these controversies have been conveyed by the mass media and translated into norms of behaviour.
>
> *(Cavazza, in Fischler and Masson, 2008, 176)*

A mass media analysis is therefore absolutely fundamental for the understanding of the situation.

Media and politics

Mass media analysis is a tool that I employed to start to understand how the media, influenced by Italian politics, are influencing the common imaginations of the Italian people. On the one

Dataset:Aspetti della vita quotidiana - Persone

Misura			per 100 persone con le stesse caratteristiche					
Seleziona periodo			2018			2019		
Sesso			maschi	femmine	totale	maschi	femmine	totale
Tipo dato								
persone di 18 anni e più per frequenza del controllo del peso		almeno una volta a settimana	20.8	26.8	23.9	20.5	25.9	23.3
		qualche volta al mese	23.2	25.5	24.4	23.7	26.3	25
		almeno una volta l'anno	33.2	27.9	30.4	33.2	28.2	30.6
		no, mai	20.2	16.7	18.4	20.3	17.3	18.7
persone di 18 anni e più per indice di massa corporea e frequenza del controllo del peso	sottopeso	almeno una volta a settimana	7.4	24	21.9	14.2	24.8	23.5
		qualche volta al mese	19.3	23.4	22.9	21.6	23.2	23
		almeno una volta l'anno	37.8	32.1	32.8	32.6	30.3	30.6
		no, mai	25.6	18.5	19.4	28.4	19.4	20.5
	normopeso	almeno una volta a settimana	20	27.7	24.5	19.2	26.7	23.5
		qualche volta al mese	22.7	26.2	24.8	23.5	26.7	25.3
		almeno una volta l'anno	33.1	27.4	29.8	33.3	28.1	30.3
		no, mai	21.1	15.5	17.8	21.4	16.2	18.4
	sovrappeso	almeno una volta a settimana	21.4	26	23.3	21.8	24.6	23
		qualche volta al mese	23.8	25.1	24.3	23.6	26.6	24.8
		almeno una volta l'anno	33.2	28	31.1	33.1	28.6	31.2
		no, mai	19.3	17.9	18.7	19.4	17.8	18.8
	obesi	almeno una volta a settimana	22.4	24.9	23.6	21.3	25.6	23.4
		qualche volta al mese	22.6	23.8	23.2	24.5	24.6	24.6
		almeno una volta l'anno	32.5	28.6	30.6	33.4	26.7	30.2
		no, mai	19.7	19.6	19.7	18.6	20.9	19.7

Dati estratti il 08 lug 2020 05:54 UTC (GMT) da I.Stat

Figure 11.1 Quantitative statistics is the frequency of weight control in 2016 and 2017

hand, mass media are promoting the traditional view of food of Italian culture and, on the other side, they promote nutrition and beauty standards that are not in line with the culinary tradition. People must orient themselves and find a "truth" between these suggestions that are in contrast.

Media are influenced by Italian politics, and I find that Jones, an English journalist who has lived in Italy for several years, has a very interesting vision of how Italian politics, the media, and collective imagination have changed in the last twenty years. I also used his book, *Il cuore oscuro dell'Italia* (Jones, 2003), to try to better show this context. We can see the importance of the female body in advertising related to sales of women's beauty products, such as creams to fight cellulite or to eliminate body fat (or even machines to lose weight).

Another noteworthy feature of Italian television is the fact that Berlusconi, a well-known figure in Italian politics, owns three national TV channels. The Italian media are therefore closely linked to this figure, who has dominated Italian politics since the 1990s. Jones (2003) shows that in 1983, Berlusconi bought Italia1, one year after Rete4: two Italian national television channels who rose at a time when private television in its entirety was unified by Berlusconi under the name of Mediaset. In 1990, he already owned 24.7% of market television advertising and he now owns 60%. On these channels, nothing other than football matches, rich men, and undressed women are shown. Jones defines this situation as a "cultural implosion" (2003, 180).

Berlusconi has lowered the standards of Italian television and, therefore, of Italian popular culture in general. He encouraged the construction of an imaginary link to the values transmitted by television and to superficial aspects and beauty. This man has not only influenced the Italian politics of recent years but he has, through his political and economic power, promoted a lifestyle and a set of values that Jones defines "*berlusconismo*" (is to say "Berlusconism").

In the text "The female body between science and guilt: The story of cellulite", Ghigi (2004) explains the role of French magazines in the construction of the concept of cellulite. It shows how two French magazines, "*Votre Beauté*" and "*Marie Claire*" have helped to show cellulite as a disease. In fact, these are two newspapers funded by pharmaceutical companies that manufacture anti-cellulite cosmetic products.

A similar situation is discernible amongst body tips from nutritionists and media advice about weight loss. If we start reading Italian newspapers, it seems that losing weight and reaching your "ideal weight" through dieting is natural and healthy, so working on your own body through strict rules is encouraged as something that can take our body to a condition of "normality". News articles thus push people to decide to seek help from a food specialist, since they are always mentioned in these articles for the sake of confirming what the author tells us from a scientific point of view.

It's thus clear that the information and the images transmitted by the television on one side and the advice given in newspapers on the other leads individuals to seek help to succeed in losing weight. We can therefore analyze the media, associating them with "rumours", which are discursive amplifications of the stereotype.

The media are political instruments that operate by following and reproducing the structures of power and control in the society in which they are produced.

In addition, the media are the main tool for the population to access the "truth". They are very powerful instruments that absorb the culture in which they are produced and, at the same time, reproduce it. There is a very strong discourse in the media around bodies—perfect, idealized bodies—related to weight loss. In addition to such discourse, there are always images—which represent a huge disclosure of information—that represent bodies as they are thought to be "perfect", and to which one thinks she must conform. Advertisements, movies, TV shows, newspapers, video clips—all have the same stereotypes of beauty, so it's really hard for the public to criticize what they see and feel, trying to distance themselves from these stereotypes in order to see the situation in its complexity. What the media produce is the fact of observing each other in a hostile way; they produce a human "panopticon" (Foucault, 1975) (Bourgois & Scheper-Hughes, 2003). Women look at each other by judging and analyzing each other; women are observed by men; people relate with each other in a violent and intrusive way.

Therefore, media increase the stereotypes of beauty and people reproduce them through their judging looks. The legitimacy of the media leads people to trust the information received by them. The media narrative is received by the people and even absorbed, becoming a part of the individual imagination; subsequently, the information is spread thanks to individuals. The consequence is the increase and reproduction of stereotypes (Das, Kleinman, & Lock, 1997). Moreover, the justification of people's views derives from science and medicine, in which people trust because they are believed to be objective and certain.

Information helps people to make sense of the world and build their own individual imaginations, connected to the collective imagination of the context in which they live. It is only in a society in which popular culture drives individuals to choose to lose weight and work on their own body that a lean and toned person can be an example of beauty; in other times—or in other contexts where there is no possibility of eating a lot and having the certainty of food—one will rather see beauty in different body types, such as curvy or fat bodies. People are therefore led to seek the help of a specialist, convinced by the media of the necessity of this aid.

Violence

During the interviews, I could observe a strong normative process reproduced and legitimized by nutrition experts, especially during the first visits, where the specialists took measurements of the patients' bodies.

> The first time I went, the doctor took all the measurements, she weighed me and did the pinch test.

… tells M., a 24-year-old girl who went to see a nutrition expert for a digestion-related issue, when I asked her about the experience of her first appointment.

> L., a 26-year-old girl who began a therapy path with a nutrition expert, explains to me that she went the first time because of an allergic reaction to the skin called "eczema":

> She weighed me and she took all the measurements: arms, torso, thighs, and for a short period I also used a small device to see how much effort I made during the day. To see if the diet worked.

…she explains when I ask her about her first session. Therefore, I ask her if the final goal of the course was to lose weight, and she replies no, that the fact of losing weight was a consequence of the diet that the nutritionist had given her. So, as I carry out the interviews and talk to people, I realize that the main motivation for going to a nutrition expert was not losing weight in the first place, but the approach during the meetings and the advice of the specialist made the loss of weight a secondary objective, when it was not even a primary one, to be able to fit what is generally identified as "normality".

When anyone asked for diets to lower cholesterol or to eliminate toxins from the body, the first thing the specialist did during my observation was to weigh the patient. Accurate body-related data were the basis for working on any request from the patient. To legitimize their work on the body, specialists also rely on the BMI (i.e. "Body Mass Index") and it is through the data relative to the BMI that patients understand whether they lay within the boundaries of "normality".

Basing one's analysis on numbers, taken as certain and real by specialists inasmuch as scientists, sometimes prevents them from listening to people and understanding their real needs. The BMI can help on some occasions, but it's about numbers, and people are more than that.

This reductive and deterministic interpretation of BMI also leads to a focus on weight loss as an end in itself, based on the assumption that this will improve health outcomes, rather than a focus on healthful eating and exercise patterns (Scrinis, 2013, 89).

Scrinis shows us that the deterministic interpretation of BMI pushes people to focus on the weight itself, assuming that weight shows us the individual's level of health, instead of focusing on a healthy and balanced diet and without focusing on the whole individual, which is much more complex and vast than the hard sciences show.

Experts often give patients a goal to reach, in terms of BMI and weight, even when the patient's need is far from a weight loss.

I realized that the normativity that I witnessed through my observations and that I heard about during the interviews is a form of violence. Violence can never be understood solely in terms of its physicality alone. Violence also includes assaults on the personhood, dignity, sense of worth, or value of the victim (Bourgois & Scheper-Hughes, 2003).

People feel obliged to completely remove food and not enjoy sociability. Once, for example, a patient, having learned that she had lost 1.2 kg, decided to ask the nutritionist if she could eat a pizza for her birthday dinner. The answer is clear:

> No, carbohydrates in the evening are turned into fat, it's biological. You have to go out without eating pizza!.

Sad, the patient told him that she thought he was going to let her eat pizza, maybe with a fast on the next day, but the specialist did not change his mind about this decision, relying on the science of nutrition. Another person I met (M.) tells me, before starting the interview, that she just received a message from her nutritionist and she tells me she is very stressed about meeting her soon.

Another woman tells me that she is available to get me into the office during the visit, but, laughing, she tells me that she will surely cry. Removing many ingredients causes people to make decisions that they then regret, as S. tells me (a 55-year-old woman who, in order to lose weight, started smoking again after she had stopped for ten years).

As Bourgois and Scheper-Hughes explain in the introduction to *Violence in War and Peace: An Anthology* (2003), it must be argued that often violent actions are socially authorized, encouraged, and seen as a moral right.

The violence I'm talking about is symbolic violence.

> Symbolic violence: soft, insensitive, invisible violence for its very victims, practiced essentially through purely symbolic means [...]. This extraordinarily ordinary social relation thus offers a privileged opportunity to grasp the logic of domination exercised in the name of a symbolic principle known and recognized by both the dominant and the dominated [...].
>
> *(Bourdieu, 1998, p. 12)*

The symbolic violence of which I speak is a violence sometimes imperceptible because it is too close to us and, above all, it is highly normalized and accepted. During my observations,

I was able to see that patients, even if they are under pressure and violence, are trying to make the doctor happy with the results. The relationship of domination is clear and obvious, and people are so "under his control" (C.) that they deprive themselves of moments of sociability and food to please him.

When I talk with M., a 24-year-old woman, with J., a 26-year-old woman, and with L., a 26-year-old man, who go to other specialists (less rigid and less strict), the three, at different times and without a specific question about the argument, tell me that these nutritionists sometimes left them too free to choose, without imposing anything and perhaps needing someone more rigid.

I see very well the logic of the symbolic violence, which makes it so that the dominated are accomplices to the dominant, so that, in turn, the patients ask the physicians to be more violent in order for them to be able to reach a goal often imposed on them by the dominant ones. Violence on patients is a violence that becomes "incorporated": people's bodies are changed because of this violence and it is through these bodies that we can understand that the doctors are acting in depth on the individual.

Foucault (1975) explains that the bodies of people are completely mixed in with politics and the power dynamics of the society in which they live. Power operates on bodies by modifying them and, therefore, it is necessary to understand that bodies can be studied not only as stable physical supports, but as entities that change according to different circumstances.

The microcosm, i.e. the physical body, can symbolically show the problems of the macrocosm, the social body. The study of people's bodies and the history of beauty stereotypes can clearly make us better understand the power dynamics that surround us—dynamics in which we find gender issues and problems related to access to knowledge and education.

I think that this discourse on violence should be rationalised as a discourse about gender violence because most people who decide to intervene on their bodies to change them are women. The science of nutrition and the act of imposing weight loss is linked to the ever-present view of women's bodies that aims at controlling and manipulating (Ghigi, 2004).

These doctors reproduce a violent normative discourse and modify bodies relying on cultural scientificity.

> *[The] male order is also inscribed in the body through tacit injunctions that are involved in the routines of the division of labour or collective or private rituals [...].*
>
> *(Bourdieu, 1998, p. 41)*

The masculine order that Bourdieu speaks about is inscribed in these bodies, judged, weighed, measured, modified by rigid regimes which do not take into account the person as a whole. The symbolic violence of which I speak is a violence upon which the science of modern Western nutrition lays its foundations.

To conclude, according to my observations and interviews, nutrition experts contribute to increasing discomfort with our own bodies and place themselves in a situation of domination and violent non-listening towards patients. The data that can be found about this argument are not vast and we should work to create statistics that can show, through quantitative data, that there are dangerous conditions for patients of nutritionists. This criticism of the science of nutrition does not aim at demonstrating its uselessness; on the contrary, I think that it would be very important to lead the nutrition experts to reflect on these topics, so that they can have, and therefore give, important anthropological tools to the patients. In addition to prescribing a diet, I argue that they should listen to patients and give them the opportunity to better understand the context in which their body is located as well as which structures of power. They should help to delegitimize gender violence that affects bodies and stereotypes of beauty with which women think they must comply. In any case, it is fundamental to understand and emphasize that the body's ability to represent social values does not prevent its ability to create new ones. The body reflects the social constructs and the social context in which it lives, but it also has the power to evolve them. We will focus on this power in the next paragraph.

Agency

After talking about the ways in which people are forced into following a diet, one must also understand that in sessions between the specialist and the patient, negotiation and re-appropriation processes on the part of patients were observed. Attending the office of the nutritionist, I witnessed several cases in which patients negotiated their diet, and sometimes there were occasions when the patients managed to obtain that for which they were bargaining. In addition, I was able to recognize resistance techniques to the diet and the doctor, which were very interesting to study. During the interviews, in addition, I realized that the prohibitions of the nutritionist were not always respected and that there was a strong agentivity on behalf of the patients and an appropriation of the injunctions.

Finally, we must reflect on the fact that starting a therapy is a choice, however conditioned by the political and social powers.

As mentioned above, it was during the direct observations that I became aware of the negotiation mechanism between the specialist and the patient. During the meeting, the specialist gave advice that patients sometimes listened without saying anything, but there were cases where a great opening on the specialist's part towards the proposals of the patients could be observed.

When I conducted the observations, Easter was approaching and a lot of people were talking about Easter weekend with their doctor. In Italy, during the days around Easter, people do not work, schools are closed, many families go on vacation and, on Sunday and Monday, the family gathers for rich lunches and dinners, based on traditional regional dishes.

A woman asked if she could eat a piadina—a bread made with pan with garnishes that is normally eaten on the shores of the Emilia-Romagna region—and the nutritionist approved. This conversation shows very well how diet is sometimes co-created between the specialist and the patient; I also find that it shows how we can work together to make the social and the dietary a dialog, trying to make it a common process of identification of nutrition strategies. Patients are able to have a higher level of power than the specialist and to impose their own needs and priorities. With the same patient, contrary to what happens with other people, the specialist asks (instead of imposing it) to insert in the therapy a day entirely based on bananas. The patient laughs and says that no, she does not want to eat only bananas, and the specialist replies: "Okay, whatever you want".

I realized that the imposition of diet practices was set aside especially with people who need therapy for medical reasons. It is, indeed, mostly needed with people who come to therapy for aesthetics-related reasons. With older people and people who have health problems related to nutrition, such as people considered obese, she was more permissive, she listened better, as if being rigid with others was more of a strategy aimed at leading them to continue the therapy.

I attended a meeting between the nutritionist and a girl with Downs Syndrome, who particularly impressed me because, unlike what I had seen at all the other meetings, it was the patient who made and proposed the diet. The specialist gave her advice about meals, which she hardly listened to, and the girl told the specialist what to write on her computer. In this case, the upheaval of power relations was unusual, and the girl actually represented the most powerful person in this relationship. It was she who had the knowledge needed to formulate her own diet and who also decided whether the advice of the specialist was good or bad. Indeed, without knowing exactly how her life was going, it was difficult for the specialist to be able to prescribe an appropriate diet. In the other cases, people were available to listen and follow some prescriptions, behaving differently than they do in the private sphere, without imposing too many views or decisions in the office, as they left the decisional power to the specialist.

I noticed that people were not following the advice of the specialist exactly. Sometimes, during the observations, the patients admitted to not having followed the diet for various reasons. For example, people admitted that it was difficult to combine diet and sociality together. During a meeting between the nutritionist and a couple, the patients said that they went to eat at a friends' house and that, on that occasion, they did not respect their diet. The man had eaten the food that their friends had prepared. The specialist had explained that it was not good to act that way, that it was necessary to take advantage of sociality while respecting the prescriptions. The man then answered: "But it is not polite, if the people cook and you do not eat".

Fournier (2012) explains very well how the practices prescribed by doctors such as a diet set by a nutrition specialist cannot be reduced to individual practices. Since the patient lives in a social world made up of other people to whom he is deeply connected, interactions between the patient and other members of the community must be taken into account.

One can easily understand how people cannot sometimes follow a diet because the diet is built without taking into account the real life of individuals, i.e. without taking into account relationships and moments where food is something that can unite people. Dietary advice is formulated in the closed session of the medical consultation and is primarily for an "atomized" individual who, once back in his daily life, will have to juggle between self-care and standards of sociability (Fournier, 2012).

So, patients listened attentively to the specialist during the appointment, but, after, they realized that the diet was impossible to respect in the daily life. There have been people, in addition, for whom food is also a form of comfort or an outlet, and for these people there are times when dieting particularly affects emotions. During the observation process, there was a patient who was talking to the nutritionist about a chocolate bunny that he had bought for Easter and, when the specialist told him that chocolate was a forbidden food, the answer of the patient was that he did not buy the rabbit as food, but he bought it to cheer him up.

A., a girl of seventeen, described her experience with a specialist when she was thirteen and she told me that, despite the fact that the doctor wanted to carry on, she and her mother had decided to stop. Since the choice to begin a therapy course is voluntary and not imposed—nor imposable—by doctors, specialists cannot do anything if patients decide not to continue. So we see very well how people implement their own ability to act, either during the course, because of the circumstances, or when they decide to stop the course. They listen to the specialist, but they also manage to listen to their own body and the emotional and social needs that keep them away from the specialist's office.

During the observations, I was able to observe that the patients were also implementing resistance techniques. That is to say, they expressed things that were absolutely contrary to the regime and to the specialist to see his reaction and to laugh together about the situation and the regime itself. A woman on her first return to the specialist's office began to talk about the fact that she made Tiramisù—a traditional Italian cake made of mascarpone cheese, cream, egg, coffee and cocoa—and showed the specialist several pictures of this cake.

Another woman, on her way back to the office, talks about the best bakeries in Bologna and about who had participated in a contest and offered cakes and pies, and she says that everyone is talking about this in the waiting room. While undressing to weigh herself, she tells she has eaten carbohydrates during a dinner, something absolutely forbidden by the nutritionist, because, as the specialist puts it: "Carbohydrates eaten after 1.30 pm become fat, it is biology". She also told me that it was a dinner between friends and her daughters and, therefore, a dinner between women and that eating carbohydrates that night made her happy.

People have the ability to act and decide what to eat, when, and in what quantity once they are no longer under the specialist's gaze, and so confessing to having "gone out of track" shows the weak power of the specialist to the specialist herself and changes the dynamics of power. People are able to play a role of resistance to injunctions and to rebuild a world of everyday values through social relations and nutrition itself; a nutrition setting that is seen as rigid, fixed, and full of rules indeed during a diet, but ultimately as a sphere of rebellion and creative power.

Conclusion

To conclude this chapter, I would first like to summarize what I have just said. I think I have explained how the Italian context is favourable to the situation I have just studied. The Italian political situation of recent years, through the media, has changed Italian popular culture by paying particular attention to aesthetics. A culture that is more and more interested in beauty, but that, at the same time, relies on science and medicine and which supports beauty stereotypes, which grow stronger day by day.

Through the observations I conducted in a specialist's office, I was able to make an analysis of the violence reproduced by nutrition experts, a violence sometimes imperceptible because, at times, it is requested by the clients themselves. Through normativity and prohibitions, people feel deprived of a significant part of their lives, which is related to food, but also to social bonds.

There is, however, a response to this privation; a response that comes directly from people and represents their agency.

At the same time, I offer a critique of the science of nutrition. To criticize this science does not mean that I think this it is, nor that it should be considered, useless. On the contrary, I find that in this historical moment it is fundamental to have affordable specialists whom people can address without running the risk to commence a diet without having knowledge about nutrition from a clinical point of view. Nevertheless, I also think that it would be fundamental to set up a different training course for these specialists. They are the first people that patients can trust in moments of weakness and moments of individual uncertainty—produced by a social crisis—about their own bodies. The figure of a person with such a social training, which can lead people to self-acceptance, is therefore needed in my own opinion.

Providing a diet to those who request it is normal, but it would be even more important to have the tools to talk to people about bodies as something in a specific political, social, and cultural context.

The science of nutrition is a science in which political, social, and gender forces operate; therefore, the violence that we see is a symbolic and structural construct, barely disencumberable from the society in which we live. This study thus aims at focusing both on an almost unexplored field of human sciences and, at the same time, showing how power dynamics are notable even in sciences that claim objectivity. With this new awareness I think that the work of specialists could be more effective and less violent on patients who ask for help. I also reckon it is time to address these issues because of their actuality and of the large portion of the Italian population affected by them. I therefore think, with this dissertation, that I can combine the strictness of socio-anthropological research with ethical commitment (Dei, 2005) to make anthropology a tool for helping people: a tool for patients—to better analyze the world in which we live, and a tool for doctors—to better explain the world in which we live.

References

Adams, C. (2016) *La politique sexuelle de la viande. Une théorie critique féministe végétarienne*, L'Age d'Homme, Lausanne.

Beneduce, R. (ed). (2008) *Violenza*, Meltemi, Roma.

Bordo, S. (1997) *Il peso del corpo*, Feltrinelli, Milano.

Bourdieu, P. (1998) *La domination masculine*, Éditions du Seuil, Paris.

Bourgois, P., & N. Scheper-Hughes. (2003) *Violence in War and Peace: An Anthology*, Wiley– Blackwell.

Counihan, C. (1999) *The anthropology of food and body. Gender, meaning and power*, Routledge, New York.

Das, V., A. Kleinman, & M. Lock (ed). (1997) *Social suffering*, University of California Press.

Dei, F. (ed). (2005) *Antropologia della violenza*, Meltemi editore, Roma.

Fischler, C., & E. Masson. (2008) *Manger. Français, Européens et Américains face à l'alimentation*, Odile Jacob, Paris.

Fischler, C. (1988) *Food, self and identity*, Social Science Information.

Foucault, M. (1975) *Surveiller et punir*, Gallimard, Paris.

Fournier, T. (2012) *Suivre ou s'écarter de la prescription diététique. Les effets du « manger ensemble » et du « vivre ensemble » chez des personnes hypercholestérolémiques en France*, Science Sociales et Santé, 30(2).

Fournier, T., J. Jarty, N. Lapeyre, & P. Touraille. (2015) *L'alimentation, arme du genre*, Association Francaise des Anthropologues, Journal des Anthropologues, 140–141.

Ghigi, R. (2004) *Le corps féminin entre science et culpabilisation. Autour d'une histoire de la cellulite*. Travail, Genre et Société, 12: 55–75.

Groleau, D., A. Young, & L. J. Kirmayer. (2006) *The McGill Illness Narrative Interview (MINI): an interview schedule to elicit meanings and modes of reasoning related to illness experience*, Transcultural Psychiatry, 43: 671–691.

Jones, T. (2003) *The dark heart of Italy*, Faber and Faber, London.

Leder, D. (1990) *The absent body*, The University of Chicago Press, London.

Merleau-Ponty, M. (1945) *Phénoménologie de la perception*, Gallimard, Paris.

Nadel, S. F. (1979) *Lineamenti di antropologia sociale*, Laterza & Figli, Bari.

Pizza, G. (2005) *Antropologia medica. Saperi, pratiche e politiche del corpo*, Carocci editore, Roma.

Quaranta, I. (2006) *Antropologia medica*, Raffaello Cortina Editore, Milano.

Régnier, F., & A. Masullo. (2009) *Obesité, gout et consommation. Intégration des normes d'alimentation et appartenance sociale*, Revue Française de Sociologie, 50: 747–773.

Scrinis, G. (2013) *Nutritionism. The science end politics of dietary advice*, Columbia University Press, New York.

12

THE CLINICIAN-PATIENT INTERACTION

Crossing the chasm of expectations

Gillie Gabay

Introduction

Clinician-patient interaction greatly influences patient trust in the clinician. The importance of the patient's trust in the clinician emerges from research findings indicating that high patient trust in the clinician improves patient-adherence to medication and to guidelines. A higher reported patient trust reduced readmissions in chronic illness and improved clinical outcomes and quality of life. There are, however, barriers to patient trust underlying the clinician-patient interaction. Barriers underlie gaps between patient expectations and the actual encounter with the clinician. Awareness of both clinicians and patients to gaps in their expectations from each other may enable them to overcome these gaps and use trust-building communication. The lack of patient-clinician communication compared to patient's expectations, whether they are clear or ambiguous, may impair the patient's trust in the clinician, despite the therapist's efforts to provide optimal care. In this chapter, I will introduce a dozen of examples of gaps in expectations of patients from clinicians and vice versa. These gaps affect the degree of patient trust, particularly in the absence of open communication about expectations, and the suggested recommendations demonstrate how to avoid deepening the gap between expectations and actual patient experience.

The medical institution distilled the power relations between the clinician and the patient, and therefore there is a distance between them. The standing table between them, the computer, the uniform, the white gown, or the green gown of surgeons signify this distance. The position of the clinician is higher than that of the patient. The clinician has the knowledge, capabilities, reputation, control, and access. In addition, the clinician-patient encounter usually occurs in the clinician's natural environment of the clinic or the hospital, where she feels comfortable with the patient. The patient is the clinician's partner in the struggle to fight a disease. How does formality versus informality promote this struggle? To what extent do cultural characteristics influence the expectations from the relationship? How may clinicians establish patient trust in the patient-clinician relationship? These and other questions are the focus of this chapter.

In the last decade, characteristics of the relationship between a therapist and a client in psychotherapy have been used to describe the clinician-patient relationship in medicine. The reason for adopting attributes from psychotherapy in medicine stems from meta-analyses that has shown that the quality of the therapist-client relationship has a marked effect on positive outcomes of therapy (Del Re, Flückiger, Horvath, Symonds, & Wampold, 2012; Flückiger, Del Re, Wampold, Symonds, & Horvath, 2012; Sharf, Primavera, & Diener, 2010). Characteristics that have contributed to successfully building a trusting relationship are: acceptance, empathy, concern, support, flexibility, honesty, confidence, human warmth, interest in the client, openness, and respect for the client. These characteristics built client trust in the clinician and enhanced the client's self-efficacy to assume responsibility for his or her well-being (Ackerman & Hilsenroth, 2003; Fife, Whiting, Bradford, & Davis, 2014). Based on these research findings, medicine aims to establish quality relationships between clinicians and patients to advance clinical outcomes.

Emphasizing the relationship itself between the clinician and the patient centers each one of the two parties and the relationship itself as a factor that influences the outcomes of the treatment (Thompson & McCabe, 2012). Meta-analyses that looks at whether coaching interventions strengthen the ability of clinicians to build a good relationship have found that coaching improved abilities of clinicians to focus on: treatment goals, mental well-being, coping, self-regulation, communication skills, meaningfulness, and attitudes towards patients (de Haan, Duckworth, Birch, & Jones, 2013; Hawkins & Shohet, 2012; Miller & Rollnick, 2012; Theeboom, Beersma, & van Vianen, 2014).

The patient depends on the knowledge, abilities, and skills of the clinician. The patient's suffering strengthens her dependence on the clinicians. Is the dependency unilateral? It is evident that the clinician also depends on the patient. The patient can provide accurate and comprehensive information about the specific symptoms of the disease in her body. For the accuracy of the diagnosis, the patient should feel comfortable to expose her weaknesses before the clinician and to discuss her physical limitations and characteristics of her natural environment. In cases where the clinician has bad news to share with the patient, dependence is strengthened, and clinician-patient trust is the key to better coping and managing the disease.

Therefore, the clinician-patient interdependence and effective communication between them may build patient trust.

Trust, central in any relationship, is at the core of the clinician-patient relationship (Gilson, 2003; Pearson & Raeke, 2000). Trust encompasses the patient's belief that, at the moment of truth, the clinician will meet expectations (Gabay, 2019a). The importance of trust in the clinician stems from research findings on a strong relationship between trust and patient adherence to treatment. Patient trust in the clinician has been associated with fewer readmissions, better long-term health, and better quality of life (Haskard, DiMatteo, & Heritage, 2009; Lee & Lin, 2009; Berry, Parish, Janakiraman, Ogburn-Russell, Couchman, Rayburn, & Grisel, 2008).

A longitudinal study of public trust in physicians across 29 countries found that public trust in physicians as a professional community is eroding over time. This finding suggests that there is much room for improvement in both patient trust in the clinician and in public trust in medical professionals (Blendon, Benson, & Hero, 2014). Known antecedents of trust in a clinician are: competency (technical ability, listening skills, reliability, honesty, and concern for patient well-being) and compassion and engaging in dialogue with the patient (Freburger, Callahan, Currey, & Anderson, 2003; Dalton, Bunton, Cykert, Corbie-Smith, Dilworth-Anderson, McGuire, Monroe, Walker, & Edwards, 2014; Hillen, Temna, van der Vloodt, de Haes, & Smets, 2013; Katon, Lin, Von Korff, Ciechanowski, Ludman, Young, Peterson, Rutter, McGregor, & McCulloch, 2010; O'Malley, Sheppard, Schwartz, & Mandelblatt, 2004; Piette, Heisler, Krein, & Kerr, 2005; Street, O'Malley, Cooper, & Haidet, 2008; Tarrant, Dixon-Woods, Colman, & Stokes, 2010).

Also, patients attributed higher trustworthiness to clinicians with high interpersonal abilities (Ganesan, Brown, Mariadoss, & Ho, 2010). In addition, the higher the clinicians' reputation, the higher was the patient's trust. Illness also affected trust. Moreover, the more severe or prolonged the patient's illness, the higher the trust. Furthermore, the duration of the relationship also affected trust. The longer the clinician-patient relationship, the higher was the trust.

As for demographics, the older the patient, the more secular, and the less educated, the higher was the patient's trust in the clinician. The demographic similarity between patient and clinician also contributed to trust. Finally, research showed that meeting patient's expectations enhanced the patient satisfaction with the clinician and raised the patient's trust in the clinician (Brown & Bussell, 2011; Phillips, Leventhal, & Leventhal, 2013). Clinicians whom patients perceived as having a poor bedside manner or as culturally incompetent lost trust in the patient (Fletcher, Furney, & Stern, 2007; Tarrant, Colman, & Stokes, 2008; Franks, Jerant, Fiscella, Shields, Tancredi, & Epstein, 2006). Another variable that was conducive to patient trust in the clinician, with a greater contribution than that of the above variables, is perceived control of patients.

Perceived control originates from social learning theory and moves on a continuum from external control to internal control. Patients with external locus of control attribute events and situations that occur in their world as the responsibility of external factors (luck, boss, weather, and so on). Patients with internal control view themselves as responsible and focus on action (Mearns, 2009). They seek relevant information about their situation, are more involved in decisions and take responsibility for improving their situation. Internal locus of control is an acquired mastery that can be modified (Hall, Dugan, Zheng, & Mishra, 2001).

Internal locus of control promotes healthy behaviors in patients, reduced health-damaging behaviors, and accelerated disease recovery. Heart patients with internal locus of control were released from intensive care and returned to work faster than were heart patients with external locus of control (Bergvik, Sørlie, & Wynn, 2012; Gabay, 2015, 2016; Lefcourt, 2014; Schwarzer, 2014). A retrospective study found that internal locus of control was a factor in reducing the number of readmissions in chronically ill patients (Gabay & Moskowitz, 2012). According to these findings, communication with the patient may enhance patient's perceived control by inspiring and assisting the patient to think of the resources in her environment, both internal and external, which she can use to improve her health (forums, mobile phone reminders for drug use) (Gabay, 2016; Gabay & Moskowitz, 2012; Gray-Stanley, Muramatsu, Heller, Hughes, Johnson, & Ramirez-Valles, 2010).

Locus on control has also made a difference for clinicians. Awareness of clinicians to the linkage between internal locus of control and improved clinical outcomes increased their willingness to adopt communication skills that enhance internal locus of control (Roseman, Osborn-Stafsnes, Amy, Boslaugh, & Slate-Miller, 2013; Zwack & Schweitzer, 2013). However, the basis for the clinician-patient interaction may be prone to barriers to trust, or dilemmas. A dilemma represents a situation in which there are two alternatives, equally good, from which one must choose. Unresolved dilemmas can direct the clinician's energy in ineffective directions, rather than direct it to creating value for patients.

A clear view of the alternatives to choose from may help establish trust-building communication. Many dilemmas lie beneath the surface and revolve around gaps between the patient's expectations from the relationship with the clinician. Lack of dialogue between the clinician and the patient about the patient's expectations, whether the expectations are clear or ambiguous, may impair trust, despite the clinician's efforts to provide optimal clinical care. Based on narrative interviews with twelve patients ages 35–81 upon their discharge from a lengthy hospitalization in acute care in an Israeli general public hospital, and a month thereafter, I identified a dozen gaps in expectations. The dilemmas are driven by gaps between the patient's expectations versus the patient's actual experience that, in the absence of an open communication about the expectations, may breach patient trust in a clinician. These gaps pose dilemmas for the medical professional and for the patient regarding their conduct. Next, I will present the dilemmas and propose the use of communication to overcome these barriers to trust and avoid deepening the chasm of gaps in expectations.

Dilemma 1: *Expectations of the chronically ill patient from the clinician versus the clinician's expectations from the chronically ill patient.*

> "This is my fourth hospitalization this year, instead of referring me straight to the ward, I have to wait for hours until the completion of the process in the emergency department, every time, it is exhausting."; "The resident recognized me, he knew who I was, but behaved as if it is my first time at the hospital."

The patient lacks medical training, but she has gained knowledge and experience with her illness. Due to the experience she has accumulated, she expects the clinician to acknowledge her experience and shorten the processes (Gabay, 2019a). The clinician expects the patient to monitor her body and report any change in important metrics. The clinician expects the patient to understand that the clinician must identify risks. Due to the need to detect risk, the clinician does not shorten processes for the patient, which may create discomfort and frustrate the patient, decreasing cooperation. If the clinician will not explain to the patient that in order to treat her, he or she must avoid preconceptions, and therefore cannot shorten processes, frustration may arise, breaching trust. If the clinician will not express acknowledgment of the patient's experience with her illness and the health system, the patient may lose confidence in the therapist.

Dilemma 2: *The professional knowledge of the clinician versus the authority of the patient.*

> "I knew it's not my Crohn's disease, I told them, but they kept wasting time on checkups for Crohn's;" "I am an educated patient and I know I can stop any procedure at any phase and they can legally do nothing. They can't touch me…. [Quiet] … What physicians say is not the Bible … they are shooting in the dark. Their knowledge is limited. Every physician has his or her own method but we know our bodies. We read about the disease and we know what's right for us. With me, I knew the antibiotics will cause a lot of side effects, they already damaged my memory with it in the last hospitalization, so I refused to take it and it caused much tension;" "I did not agree and they cannot make me … otherwise they would not ask me to sign … If they cannot do that without my signature, then the authority is mine."

Patients new to the disease feel fully dependent on their clinicians who may make decisions overlooking patient involvement. Although patients may lack information or familiarity with how the medical system works, some patients, despite lack of medical knowledge, exercise their right to make treatment decisions. Clinicians have a moral obligation to assure that patients have all the information they need and that they understand it, to enable them to make choices regarding treatment or no treatment.

The patient-clinician relationship, however, is unbalanced. Many clinicians believe they understand the patient's medical condition better than does the patient. Their purpose is to save lives or manage an acute condition, so they may exceed their authority and dictate the treatment to the patient. They feel uncomfortable when patients decide not to receive treatment, despite the patients' right to choose not to receive treatment. The clinician, who obtained a medical education and training that is geared towards action, has an internal conflict between the imperative to save the patient at all costs and the patient's right to autonomy. The poles are not flexible. However, blurring the boundaries between patient autonomy and the limits of medical authority can create ambiguity for both the practitioner and the patient that the clinician must clarify by exploring her attitude and communicating with patients to maintain trust (Gabay, 2019b).

Dilemma 3: *The patient's expectation of empathy versus the clinician's expectation of knowledge and professional conduct.*

> "The anesthesiologist was digging to find a vein and connect the tube, it was so painful, I was screaming my lungs out but he kept going and said nothing." At some point, my surgeon stepped in, heard me and scolded at him to immediately stop: "Why don't you do that when she is sedated?!"

The public's expectations for empathy from clinicians has become a daily, natural expectation that, while understandable from the patient's perspective, when viewed through the eyes of medical professional, it may not be a legitimate expectation. While the clinician may manage the patient's pain with empathy, the clinician may also find it difficult to express empathy. Empathy is an acquired professional skill that is not part of the formal training in the medical profession. The difficulty may be due, in part, to burnout in a chaotic, fast-paced, demanding work environment, with continuous exposure to trauma that creates numbness or lack of communication skills for complex situations. Professional care requires communication, listening, patience, understanding the patient's intentions and experience, not necessarily empathy. Is the lack of empathy a testament to a lack of professionalism? Studies show that the clinician's ability to be empathetic on the one hand and to accept his or her professional and personal boundaries on the other hand draws boundaries to empathy limiting burnout and building resilience among clinicians (Gabay, 2020; Rozenblum, Lisby, Hockey, Levtizion-Korach, Salzberg, Lipsitz, & Bates, 2011).

Patients, however, categorize their clinicians on two axes: the professional axis and the communication axis. There are four possible categories along these two axes: Professional but non-communicative clinician; A caring but unprofessional clinician; Not professional and not communicative clinician; and a professional, effectively communicating clinician. The pattern of communication does not necessarily indicate the clinician's level of professionalism, but the patient interprets a clinician who does not communicate well as someone who does not understand the human soul, and therefore, is less professional. After all, what is the quality of medicine if it lacks the mechanisms that encourage a clinician-patient dialogue? Thus, for the patient, the lack of empathy reflects the clinician's inhumanity or lack of professionalism, and therefore necessarily reduces trust.

Dilemma 4: *Good patient-clinician communication alleviates patient loneliness.*

> You lose yourself from day one. It hurts so much. My spirit is broken… [Quiet] … but I chose to alienate myself … I don't know why … I need it … maybe it's because when I shut my world from the outside I don't feel like a cripple … I don't know … I have a concealed hate towards anyone who can move their legs and no one can understand that but the doctors kept encouraging me, once I was out of the ICU, to invite my friends to visit but I was not ready to talk about books and movies as if everything is the same.

The sense of betrayal of the body, the anxiety and fear of the future, create self-alienation of patients resulting in a sense of loneliness even when the clinician communicates well. Interpersonal communication between the clinician and the patient may allow the clinician a glimpse into the patient's pain. The clinician does not know the pain. The clinician may only imagine the pain and the fear the patient experiences. Thinking she or he understands how it feels in the patient's shoes, entails the clinician's sin of pretension. The clinician may make an attempt to feel in the patient's shoes but she can do that only to a certain point. Loneliness stems from the loss of the patient's expectation that someone, including the clinician, will understand her. The loneliness is real, filled with fears, disappointments, perhaps with anxiety about the disease striking again. Sometimes, until the stable return to the routine the patient knew before the hospitalization, there will be loneliness. Compassionate communication regarding the patient's feeling lonely, without pretentions to know what the patient is feeling, will maintain trust (Gabay, 2019a).

Dilemma 5: *Active listening of the clinician to the patient, impacts patient extent of dramatization.*

> In the internal ward they treat you like meat, I kept saying things over and over but they kept at it. As if patients are their guinea pigs.

The more patients are under the impression that the clinician is not listening to them, their frustration grows, and aiming at getting the attention of the clinician, they attempt to impress the clinician by exaggerating and dramatizing the symptoms. The more drama the patient produces, the more the clinician holds on to facts. The more the clinician listens and develops a dialogue with the patient, the more patients will feel responsible to speak calmly and accurately, believing that the clinician will attend to her needs and meet them (Gabay, 2020). The patient will act knowing that the clinician will act by the best medical procedures and avoid exaggeration. Active listening will improve the quality of care because the clinician will receive refined information from the patient. Active listening will help build trust.

Dilemma 6. *Asking questions through the professional prism.*

> The doctor was the only one who cared and treated me as a person. He asked how it happened, asked about my children, what ages they were. He said since your children are so young and you may want to have more children, I recommend surgery to avoid future complications. The next day when he saw me he said nothing to me.

Asking the patient personal questions, the clinician may create an emotional attachment of the patient who may perceive the questions as personal and expressing special interest in her. The clinician may be perceived as hypocritical. One time, he is viewed as friendly to the patient, and another time he is viewed estranged. The versatility may violate trust. In order to produce a balanced view of the clinician in the eyes of the patient, the clinician must explain the reason for the questioning. The patient should also be trained—not just the clinician—to understand that if the clinician asks personal questions, they are important for medical decisions. Just as the clinician explains every medical procedure, it is advisable to explain the purpose of the questions to the patient as part of the process of making a medical decision.

Dilemma 7: *The clinician's routine and the patient's emergency.*

> I noticed that they are coming and going and talking about the surgery like a regular person would talk about their flower arrangement. Do they even see me? Do they know it's MY cancer?!

The clinician is at work, in his daily routine, at the hospital, while for most patients visiting the emergency room is a crisis, disconnected from daily routine. The clinician is almost fully alert, striving for zero errors. During surgery, the patient is under anesthesia and unaware of what is occurring in the operating room. The patient does not feel that the clinician is geared toward her. The patient is tense, scared, anxious, and self-assembled. The clinician, even if excited, struggles to exude calm and control. The clinician may, due to his daily routine, become numb, insensitive to the patient's unique condition, and fail to realize his mission.

Under these circumstances, the clinician and the patient may each experience a bad encounter that produces cynicism, doubt, rejection, judgment, anxiety, and resistance, and these feelings may breach trust. It is important that the clinician will be attentive to the patient's needs in the recovery phase in the hospital ward. If the patient feels the urgency of addressing his or her needs outside the operating room, she will view the value as high, and will feel that the clinician understands that she is in a state of emergency and will feel at the center, promoting trust (Gabay, 2019a, b).

Dilemma 8: *Timing of signing an informed consent form and ensuring the patient's well-being.*

> "You are laying there naked and awake feeling that you are losing everything. You are just ash, you are valueless. In those moments, nothing existed around me. I was alone again in the operating room. There is no past and no future. There is only a great grief of this moment, there is crying, excitement, fear, pressure. On the one hand, I was glad that I wasn't in the operating room but on the other hand I wanted to be a minute after the surgery ended. I was laying there for four hours next to the dining room, smelling the hospital cooking. I was laying in the entrance to the operating room, freezing. One nurse came and gave me a heated blanket. The anesthesiologist and the surgeon explained nothing. Then just before entering the operating room I was asked to sign an informed-consent form" (Interviewee 5); "No one told me what kind of pain I will have. I suffered terribly. I couldn't lay down, get up, I needed an adjustable bed, an adjustable chair. I suffered terrible suffering and did not prepare ahead."
>
> *(Gabay & Bokek-Cohen, 2019a, b)*

When a patient's signature is required in the informed-consent form, the traditional patient-clinician power relationship balances out. The patient may decide, without knowing the consequences of his decision. The clinician expects his or her reputation to determine the right choice, even if he lacks formal authority, which emphasizes informed-consent. In the Patient Rights Act, in many cases the patient is required to sign his/her consent for the invasive treatment minutes before his or her appointment. The clinician might mumble medicine, and everyone is waiting to take the patient to the operating room, which is inappropriate.

The last-minute signature is being asked of patients, despite the patient's right to decide on the procedure. Precisely when patients report being frightened, they are asked to sign an important form. It is precisely when the patient is mentally ready for surgery, calm, trusting his providers, that the patient has to deal with pressure, reducing his immunity. The patient should be allowed time to digest the information, even if he or she subsequently exercises his funda-mental right to forgo treatment, taking risks of worsening his medical condition, and not the risks of the invasive procedure (Gabay, 2019a; Gabay & Bokek-Cohen, 2019a, 2019b). Treating the signature as a last-minute ritual before surgery or procedure fails with confidence.

Dilemma 9: *Professionalism in the age of evolving knowledge.*

> The procedure was so traumatic. I was very ill. I weighed 47 Kilos instead of the normal weight of 70 kilos. I was in a bad situation looking for a second opinion. The doctor gave me an intensive steroid therapy. The right side of my body was paralyzed twice due to medications. I went to a neurologist who, instead of saying I don't know, gave me a medication for stroke prevention that should not be given to teens at all, it was negligent to give me a medication for adults. I dropped 15 kilos, I was not in

school, I was in bed with zero energy. It made me feel worse, I had a blood poisoning. I lost an entire school year.

Medical knowledge develops into sub-specialties. Few therapists know everything or have a whole view. Do clinicians feel comfortable admitting that they don't know? Is there legitimacy to say "I don't know" in medical school? Or "I know very little about this"? Does a clinician, a clinician who knows what she doesn't know, who emphasizes the limits of her knowledge and the depth of knowledge in her specific field of expertise, feel confident to refer a patient to where she may find answers? The clinician may get used to saying "I don't know," and the patient needs to understand that this statement indicates professionalism rather than lack thereof. That way the patient will remain calm will be if they meet a clinician who will say, "I don't know—I'll check".

Dilemma 10: *Empathy! General vs. Unique.*

> After several hours in acute-care, I needed something for the pain again. The physician said, "I understand that you are in great pain. Take your pain to a positive place, think Zen" ... So condescending! ... I was furious with him.

Waiting times, pain, the expectation for optimal care, all create high sensitivity in patients. Patients are affected by layers of thoughts, emotions, deliberation, and behaviors making the clinician-patient relationship complex. The clinician may combine professionalism with humanity. Professionalism is defined as empathy, compassion, accountability, integrity (Passi, Doug, Peile, & Johnson, 2010). Communication skills of clinicians must adapt to different situations. When the clinician does not know the patient, empathy must be general, not unique. Empathy is not compassion. Empathy is an attempt to understand how the clinician would feel if she were in the patient's shoes. The correct solution will come from the patient herself after she asks the clinician a series of questions specifying all options and she chooses which is right for her.

Dilemma 11: *Communication from "bottom" "up" versus circular communication.*

> The head of the Neurology Department wanted to know what was happening with me. He listened to me at length and then explained everything respectfully, at eye level. The relations I had with him were exceptional and greatly encouraged me. He and the nurse gave me a feeling that I would be OK. I felt in good hands.

Unlike any typical organization that has a rank, in the hospital the communication flows not only from "up" "down", i.e., from the clinician to the patient, but also from "down" "up", i.e., from the patient to the clinician. How do the clinician and patient perceive each other? Does the patient think he is a customer and is therefore always right about the service? The patient as a client wants his or her own, and at the same time is suffering, hurt. When a patient's dialogue with the clinician reflects the therapist's recognition that the patient knows his or her body and illness, the patient will see him as a highly knowledgeable and trusted partner. Dialogue is an integral part of diagnosis and preparation for surgery. Although the clinician knows a lot about the disease, the patient knows a lot about her body, what she is experiencing and to what environment she will return to after surgery (Gabay, Gere, Moskowitz, & Zemel, Forthcoming).

Understanding this balance is necessary for a clinician to assess the benefits of dialogue. No person is closer to himself than the patient, even if he does not express eloquence and clarity. The dialogue slows down the clinician in accomplishing the task, while also inspiring him to see the patient as a unique person, and not to just see the disease. This allows the patient to become a partner, to build a high level of trust and to be more successful in treatment.

Dilemma 12: *Transparency in clinician communication and patient weakness.*

> The Neurosurgeon came by to see me but didn't see me at all. He hardly spoke with me. When he turned to me he said: "You have excess fluid in your head that pressures your brain and explains your cognitive regression, loss of memory, and walking disorder. We will drill a hole in your head, insert a catheter, pull a tube from the brain down through your stomach and regulate the fluids to decrease the pressure in your brain." [silence]. I was scared to death. I felt intense cold throughout my body.

On the one hand there are benefits to telling the patient the truth, and on the other hand it is inappropriate to talk over the patient's head while they are awake. The patient is experiencing ego depletion and is emotionally charged, creating greater difficulty in containing his or her understanding of the clinician's discourse. How does the patient's best interest interact with the flow of communication between medical professionals on the team? If the patient is partially awake, a bush over his head reflects insensitivity to his feelings. The patient becomes an emotionless object (Gabay, 2019a, 2019b). Treating the body as a commodity may stem from the clinician's efficiency but jeopardizes patient well-being and fails to promote adherence and self-management of chronic illness.

In the name of efficiency, the patient may become an object. For the most part, the patient does not understand the discourse between clinicians and examines what happens next, through external factors. The patient may be concerned about the language of the clinician, who does not speak at eye level but has a peer discourse with a senior clinician or consultant. The patient sees the body language, the language of the medical jargon, and the social contract between clinicians. The clinician, as far as he was concerned, spoke a professional language appropriate for dialogues with colleagues but did so above the patient's bed, the patient raising concerns and anxiety when necessary.

In summary, my premise in this article is the belief in clinicians' ability to adopt more effective communication skills with patients. Although patients may understand the issue of their illness and health in general, namely health literacy, they expect clinicians, as a medical authority, to inspire them to take greater responsibility for their health. Encouraging patients to be active in communicating with their clinicians, will increase responsiveness and maintain patient trust in the clinician. Clinicians who are aware of dilemmas around gaps in expectations that may block clinician-patient trust will enable the clinician to choose alternatives to resolve the dilemmas. Awareness of patients to gaps in expectations will empower them to better comprehend the complexity of the situation (Helmes, Bowen, & Bengel, 2002; Leisen & Hyman, 2004). Comprehension and awareness of gaps underlying the clinician-patient interaction can be recalibrated at the time of treatment to build and maintain trust.

It is recommended to manage patient expectations regarding treatment, by explicit communication, as far as the clinician is able (Gabay, 2019b). Not only as a patient who can largely control her health but also as someone who actually takes responsibility for it. Collaborative communication of the clinician should focus on what the patient can do to improve the management of his illness. It focuses on the patient, not the illness. As part of the patient-centered care paradigm, the focus is to be on the patient. Health systems and policymakers are called upon to design training programs that aim at increasing awareness of clinicians regarding the effect of internal control on patient health promotion and on clinicians' readiness to adopt collaborative communication skills. Training that enriches the capacity to build patient trust in clinicians will contribute to the perceived quality of care among clinicians and will promote patients' health.

References

Ackerman, S. J., & M. J. Hilsenroth. (2003). A review of therapist characteristics and techniques positively impacting the therapeutic alliance. *Clinical Psychology Review, 23*(1), 1–33.

Berry, L. L., J. T. Parish, R. Janakiraman, L. Ogburn-Russell, G. R. Couchman, W. L. Rayburn, & J. Grisel. (2008). Patients' commitment to their primary physician and why it matters. *The Annals of Family Medicine, 6*(1), 6–13.

Bergvik, S., T. Sørlie, & R. Wynn. (2012). Coronary patients who returned to work had stronger internal locus of control beliefs than those who did not return to work. *British Journal of Health Psychology, 17*(3), 596–608.

Blendon, R. J., J. M. Benson, & J. O. Hero. (2014). Public trust in physicians—US medicine in international perspective. *New England Journal of Medicine, 371*(17), 1570–1572.

Brown, M. T., & J. K. Bussell. (2011, April). Medication adherence: WHO cares? *Mayo Clinic Proceedings 86*(4), 304–314.

Dalton, A. F., A. J. Bunton, S. Cykert, G. Corbie-Smith, P. Dilworth-Anderson, F. R. McGuire, M. H. Monroe, P. Walker, & L. J. Edwards. (2014). Patient characteristics associated with favorable perceptions of patient–provider communication in early-stage lung cancer treatment. *Journal of Health Communication, 19*(5), 532–544.

De Haan, E., A. Duckworth, D. Birch, & C. Jones. (2013). Executive coaching outcome research: The contribution of common factors such as relationship, personality match, and self-efficacy. *Consulting Psychology Journal: Practice and Research, 65*(1), 40.

Del Re, A. C., C. Flückiger, A. O. Horvath, D. Symonds, & B. E. Wampold. (2012). Therapist effects in the therapeutic alliance–outcome relationship: A restricted-maximum likelihood meta-analysis. *Clinical Psychology Review, 32*(7), 642–649.

Fife, S. T., J. B. Whiting, K. Bradford, & S. Davis. (2014). The therapeutic pyramid: A common factors synthesis of techniques, alliance, and way of being. *Journal of Marital and Family Therapy, 40*(1), 20–33.

Fletcher, K. E., S. L. Furney, & D. T. Stern. (2007). Patients speak: what's really important about bedside interactions with physician teams. *Teaching and Learning in Medicine, 19*(2), 120–127.

Flückiger, C., A. C. Del Re, B. E. Wampold, D. Symonds, & A. O. Horvath. (2012). How central is the alliance in psychotherapy? A multilevel longitudinal meta-analysis. *Journal of Counseling Psychology, 59*(1), 10.

Franks, P., A. F. Jerant, K. Fiscella, C. G. Shields, D. J. Tancredi, & R. M. Epstein. (2006). Studying physician effects on patient outcomes: physician interactional style and performance on quality of care indicators. *Social Science & Medicine, 62*(2), 422–432.

Freburger, J. K., L. F. Callahan, S. S. Currey, & L. A. Anderson. (2003). Use of the Trust in Physician Scale in patients with rheumatic disease: psychometric properties and correlates of trust in the rheumatologist. *Arthritis Care & Research: Official Journal of the American College of Rheumatology, 49*(1), 51–58.

Gabay, G. (2015). Perceived control over health, communication and patient–physician trust. *Patient Education and Counseling, 98*(12), 1550–1557.

Gabay, G. (2016). Exploring perceived control and self-rated health in re-admissions among younger adults: A retrospective study. *Patient Education and Counseling, 99*(5), 800–806.

Gabay, G. (2019a). Patient self-worth and communication barriers to Trust of Israeli Patients in acute-care physicians at public general hospitals. *Qualitative Health Research, 29*(13), 1954–1966.

Gabay, G. (2019b). A non-heroic cancer narrative: body deterioration, grief, disenfranchised grief, and growth. *OMEGA-Journal of Death and Dying*. doi.org/10.1177/0030222819852836.

Gabay, G. (2020). From the crisis in acute care to post-discharge resilience – The communication experience of Geriatric patients: A qualitative study. *Scandinavian Journal of Caring Sciences*.

Gabay, G., & H. R. Moskowitz. (2012). The algebra of health concerns: implications of consumer perception of health loss, illness and the breakdown of the health system on anxiety. *International Journal of Consumer Studies, 36*(6), 635–646.

Gabay, G. & Y. Bokek-Cohen. (2019a). What do patients want? Surgical informed-consent and patient-centered care – An augmented model of information disclosure. *Bioethics 34*(5), 467–477.

Gabay, G. & Y. Bokek-Cohen. (2019b). Infringement of the right to surgical informed consent: negligent disclosure and its impact on patient trust in surgeons at public general hospitals – the voice of the patient. *BMC Medical Ethics, 20*(1), 77.

Gabay, G., A. Gere, H. R. Moskowitz, & G. Zemel. (Forthcoming). Medical Professionalism at the Hospital. IGI.

Ganesan, S., S. P. Brown, B. J. Mariadoss, & H. Ho. (2010). Buffering and amplifying effects of relationship commitment in business-to-business relationships. *Journal of Marketing Research, 47*(2), 361–373.

Gilson, L. (2003). Trust and the development of health care as a social institution. *Social Science & Medicine, 56*(7), 1453–1468.

Gray-Stanley, J. A., N. Muramatsu, T. Heller, S. Hughes, T. P. Johnson, & J. Ramirez-Valles. (2010). Work stress and depression among direct support professionals: the role of work support and locus of control. *Journal of Intellectual Disability Research, 54*(8), 749–761.

Hall, M. A., E. Dugan, B. Zheng, & A. K. Mishra. (2001). Trust in physicians and medical institutions: what is it, can it be measured, and does it matter? *The Milbank Quarterly, 79*(4), 613–639.

Haskard, K. B., M. R. DiMatteo, & J. Heritage. (2009). Affective and instrumental communication in primary care interactions: predicting the satisfaction of nursing staff and patients. *Health Communication, 24*(1), 21–32.

Hawkins, P. & R. Shohet. (2012). *Supervision in the helping professions.* McGraw-Hill education (UK).

Helmes, A. W., D. J. Bowen, & J. Bengel. (2002). Patient preferences of decision-making in the context of genetic testing for breast cancer risk. *Genetics in Medicine, 4*(3), 150–157.

Hillen, M., S. el Temna, J. van der Vloodt, H. de Haes, & E. Smets. (2013). Trust of Turkish and Arabic ethnic minority patients in their Dutch oncologist. *Ned Tijdschr Geneeskd Netherlands, 157*(Suppl 16), 5881.

Katon, W. J., E. H. Lin, M. Von Korff, P. Ciechanowski, E.J. Ludman, B. Young, D. Peterson, C. M. Rutter, M. McGregor, & D. McCulloch. (2010). Collaborative care for patients with depression and chronic illnesses. *New England Journal of Medicine, 363*(27), 2611–2620.

Lee, Y. Y. & J.L. Lin. (2009). The effects of trust in physician on self-efficacy, adherence and diabetes outcomes. *Social Science & Medicine, 68*(6), 1060–1068.

Lefcourt, H. M. (Ed.). (2014). *Locus of control: Current trends in theory & research.* Psychology Press.

Leisen, B. & M. R. Hyman. (2004). Antecedents and consequences of trust in a service provider: The case of primary care physicians. *Journal of Business Research, 57*(9), 990–999.

Mearns, J., 2009. Social learning theory. In H. Reis & S. Sprecher (Eds.) *Encyclopedia of Human Relationships*, vol. 3, pp. 1537–1540. Thousand Oaks, CA: Sage.

Miller, W. R. & S. Rollnick. (2012). *Motivational interviewing: Helping people change.* Guilford Press.

O'Malley, A. S., V. B. Sheppard, M. Schwartz, & J. Mandelblatt. (2004). The role of trust in use of preventive services among low-income African-American women. *Preventive Medicine, 38*(6), 777–785.

Passi, V., M. Doug, J. T. Peile, & N. Johnson. (2010). Developing medical professionalism in future doctors: a systematic review. *International Journal of Medical Education, 1*, 19.

Pearson, S. D., & L.H. Raeke. (2000). Patients' trust in physicians: many theories, few measures, and little data. *Journal of General Internal Medicine, 15*(7), 509–513.

Phillips, A. L., H. Leventhal, & E. A. Leventhal. (2013). Assessing theoretical predictors of long-term medication adherence: Patients' treatment-related beliefs, experiential feedback and habit development. *Psychology & Health, 28*(10), 1135–1151.

Piette, J. D., M. Heisler, S. Krein, & E. A. Kerr. (2005). The role of patient-physician trust in moderating medication nonadherence due to cost pressures. *Archives of Internal Medicine, 165*(15), 1749–1755.

Roseman, D., J. Osborne-Stafsnes, C. H. Amy, S. Boslaugh, & K. Slate-Miller. (2013). Early lessons from four 'aligning forces for quality' communities bolster the case for patient-centered care. *Health Affairs, 32*(2), 232–241.

Rozenblum, R., M. Lisby, P. M. Hockey, O. Levtizion-Korach, C. A. Salzberg, S. Lipsitz, & D. W. Bates. (2011). Uncovering the blind spot of patient satisfaction: an international survey. *BMJ Quality and Safety, 20*(11), 959–965.

Schwarzer, R. (2014). *Self-efficacy: thought control of action.* Taylor & Francis.

Sharf, J., L. H. Primavera, & M. J. Diener. (2010). Dropout and therapeutic alliance: A meta- analysis of adult individual psychotherapy. *Psychotherapy: Theory, Research, Practice, Training, 47*(4), 637.

Street, R. L., K. J. O'Malley, L. A. Cooper, & P. Haidet. (2008). Understanding concordance in patient-physician relationships: personal and ethnic dimensions of shared identity. *The Annals of Family Medicine, 6*(3), 198–205.

Gillie Gabay

Tarrant, C., M. Dixon-Woods, A. M. Colman, & T. Stokes. (2010). Continuity and trust in primary care: a qualitative study informed by game theory. *The Annals of Family Medicine*, 8(5), 440–446.

Tarrant, C., A. M. Colman, & T. Stokes. (2008). Past experience, 'shadow of the future', and patient trust: a cross-sectional survey. *British Journal of General Practice*, 58(556), 780–783.

Theeboom, T., B. Beersma, & A. E. van Vianen. (2014). Does coaching work? A meta-analysis on the effects of coaching on individual level outcomes in an organizational context. *The Journal of Positive Psychology*, 9(1), 1–18.

Thompson, L., & R. McCabe. (2012). The effect of clinician-patient alliance and communication on treatment adherence in mental health care: a systematic review. *BMC Psychiatry*, 12(1), 87.

Zwack, J., & J. Schweitzer. (2013). If every fifth physician is affected by burnout, what about the other four? Resilience strategies of experienced physicians. *Academic Medicine*, 88(3), 382–389.

13
CONSTRUCTING ETHNOGRAPHIC DATA IN MEDICAL EDUCATION

Jonathan Tummons

Introduction: ethnography and medical education – a long association

There are so many versions of educational ethnography, and so many occasions when ethnography is erroneously equated with qualitative research more generally, that it can seem difficult to identify what an "ethnography of medical education" might actually consist of beyond the self-evident fact that it in some way pertains to the education of healthcare professionals. Even the commitment to longitudinal research that ethnography is perceived as demanding by those who are only casually acquainted with it, is challenged by the emergence of multiple models of shorter forms of ethnographic work. Likewise, the notion that ethnographic work is conducted by a sole researcher immersed in a physical location is disrupted by the emergence of methodologies that permit – require, even – teams of researchers who might, thanks to digital technologies, be working from different locations and might not even all be physically situated within the research site.

At the same time, if we accept the argument that the many different variants of qualitative research generally that are to be found in the research methods literature often in fact rest only on spurious differences – an issue that equally applies when considering variants of ethnography specifically – then any working definition of ethnography must be considered as contingent whilst still being sufficiently robust and workable (Hammersley, 2018). With that in mind, and drawing on well-established work in the field by Walford (2008), we can make sense of the ethnography of education in terms of seven key elements. First, educational ethnographies rest on a study of cultures. These might for example be the cultures of a medical school, of a ward, or of a waiting room. Second, it draws on multiple methods and modes of data. Participant observation has long been held as the main method by which ethnographies are done, but to this we will add the analysis of documents, texts, images, other literacy artefacts, interviews, as well as quantitative work when the research questions require the use of numerical data. Third, within an educational ethnography, the researcher is a participant and not a passive outsider, becoming engaged with the culture over time through prolonged time spent in the field and/or repeated visits over an extended period. Fourth, the ethnographer of education is the main research instrument and is always, necessarily, enrolled within the practice of the research. Therefore they are required to exercise awareness and reflexivity throughout, not in order to remove or otherwise negate the subjective point of view that will always inform their writing, but to be sensitive to what these subjectivities do and account for them. Fifth, ethnographies of education assume a commitment to representing and learning from the people being researched. How people talk about their work (in the broadest sense of the word), or how they understand and define their experiences, are essential aspects of the theory building of the researcher. Sixth, the theory-building that emerges from ethnography of education is to be understood as an itera-tive process, resting on cycles of theory work, empirical work, and engagement in the field. Theoretical frameworks should not be rigidly pre-conceived (they should respond to empirical data); nor should they be abandoned or abrogated (the theoretical "blank slate" of grounded theory is rejected here (Thomas & James, 2006)). And finally, ethnographies of education do not seek to be generalisable in the sense that a large-scale quantitative panel study claims to be generalisable. Rather, through the ever-deeper exploration of the single field or case being researched, theoretical generalisations can be established (Alasuutari, 1995).

In summary, ethnographies of medical education commit us as researchers to an immersive and invariably long-term study that rests primarily on participant observation and engage-ment with the material artefacts of the field whilst also drawing on other methods such as interviews or document analysis, that foregrounds the positionality of the researcher, and that has an explicit commitment to iterative theory building.

In this chapter I am going to explore the ways in which we can construct and then use concepts and methods relating to ethnographies of education that relate specifically to med-ical cultures, practices, and social phenomena. I will explore some of the different methods and methodological perspectives that are used by ethnographers of medical education through a consideration of some of the ways in which more recent forms of ethnography have mediated these practices. Finally, I shall conclude with a discussion of a recently completed three-year ethnography of distributed medical education in North America that serves to illustrate the key points that I raise within the discussion as a whole.

Methods for contemporary ethnographies of medical education

It is beyond the scope of a chapter such as this one to explore in depth the core methods that are used by ethnographers of medical education: there already exists a proliferation of articles and chapters that have discussed these (MacLeod, 2016; Reeves, Peller, Goldman, & Kitto, 2013). Rather, what I hope to show through the brief discussion of the core tenets of ethnography of education that follows are the ways in which these have been adjusted and stretched over time as a response to, for example, the emergence of new technologies, to new areas of research interest, or to new theoretical impulses.

Participant observation

Participant observation remains both the most widely-used and the most immediately recog-nisable method for the construction of data within ethnographic research, and has traditionally been informed by both practical as well as ethical concerns. For example, an ethnographer of medical education who is physically present within the research field might observe the treatment of a patient at a distance if appropriate and if relevant permissions have been obtained, but would be more able to participate more closely in other settings such as during a meal break (Atkinson & Pugsley, 2005). As ethnographers, we can also observe online as well as offline practices with equivalent veracity, and we can construct observational data entirely within and/ or from virtual spaces, or from either live-streamed or pre-recorded video. Whilst the extent to which our participation as observers can vary is a paradigmatic aspect of ethnography – the ways in which we establish ourselves either as "complete participants" or as "complete observers" are well-established in social research more generally – the *location* of the researcher in relation to the field has been rendered more complex by the emergence of online ethnographies. The field can now be blended and represented in and through digital as well as physical communities and spaces, such as in the study of Twitter use amongst medical students by Chretien, Tuck, Simon, Singh, and Kind (2015), who drew on *digital ethnography* in order to frame their research: they found that students used Twitter in a number of ways, predominantly to access resources and/or expertise relating to their studies. A rather different example can be found in Dyke's (2013) *blended ethnography* that explores the relationships between a community-based eating disorder prevention project in the North of England and online communities that valorise eating disorders, challenging the divide between empirical and virtual ethnographies through drawing equally on data constructed across both sites – the physical and the virtual.

Qualitative interviewing

Interviews continue to be a central feature of ethnographic research, invariably seen as subordinate to observation, although some methodologies do foreground or privilege the importance of interviewing as a way of understanding practice through the accounts of those people who are enfolded within it (in the case of *institutional ethnography*), or as ways of discursively constructing the fields of research through gaining information from those who travel within them (in the case of *multi-sited ethnography*). Andreassen, Christensen, & Møller (2020), in their exploration of *focused ethnography* within medical education research (one of a number of shorter forms of ethnography to have emerged in recent years), similarly argue that interviews take on an additional importance in order to compensate for the relatively short time spent by researchers in the field. More conventionally, the role played by interviews in supporting observation data within "traditional" empirical ethnographic research can be seen in the work conducted by Balmer, Master, Richards, Serwint, and Giardino (2010) in their study of the pedagogies of ward rounds within a general paediatric unit, resting on a combined data set of 143 hours of observation and 39 semi-structured interviews – a substantial body of qualitative data. At the same time, the increased use of online interviewing is becoming common within *virtual ethnographies*, and notwithstanding the critiques of "remote" interviews – that they lack immediacy and intimacy, that being face-to-face allows for better rapport, that gesture and body language are lost – the capacity to interview someone in a different country and in a different time zone is clearly of value for many researchers. As network connections become more stable, the fidelity of audio and video recording is rarely a barrier to the construction of robust data. Alternatively, email or online forum texts can be used where the asynchronous nature of such exchanges might allow for differing patterns of participation: a good example can be seen in the research by Crompvoets (2010) into the discursive construction of professionalism amongst International Medical Graduates in Australia, which rested entirely on online discussion within a framework positioned as *cyber ethnography*.

The analysis of documents, texts, and artefacts

One of the ways in which ethnographers can construct their understandings of the cultural practices that are of interest to them is through the systematic exploration of the material artefacts or objects of the field – the tools and equipment that people use, the stuff that decorates the walls within institutional spaces, or the documents that regulate the everyday work done within the research site. The use of photography, video, or audio in ethnography is, of course, not at all new – but current digital technologies have made it relatively straightforward for the ethnographer to gather, store, and share increasingly large numbers of images, sounds, and films. At the same time, the increasing sophistication of specialist software for qualitative data analysis allows for the systematic management of increasingly large and sophisticated multi-modal data sets (Tummons, 2014). It is easier than ever to record the artefacts and tools of the field, either to use as *visual data* in their own right or to reinforce other forms of data construction – for example through the use of elicitation techniques in qualitative interviewing. Research into feedback practices in medical education by Urquhart, Ker, and Rees (2018) provides an example of the ways in which the capacity to capture the material practices of students alongside interview data generates more meaningful and robust research data. In their research, Urquhart et al. analysed video footage of assessment and feedback episodes involving students within a range of both simulated and workplace settings. To provide a single example: the capacity of the researchers to watch and re-watch students receiving feedback whilst working with a prosthetic arm affords them the capability to associate particular moments of feedback with particular physical actions, as well as being able to explore non-verbal communication – an example of a body of rich data that would be simply impossible to capture without digital technology.

Quantitative data

Ethnographies of education are invariably categorized as qualitative in nature: indeed, the association of "ethnography" with "qualitative research" is so unthinkingly adhered to that the contribution and potential of numerical data that was once a common feature of ethnography of education has now been lost sight of (Walford, 2020). The "paradigm wars" that can be seen as informing more-or-less conflicting discourses relating to social research more broadly can also be seen at work within medical education research (Hodges, 2005), including, although not restricted to, the (to many people entirely spurious) "qualitative versus quantitative" methods debate. And yet it is self-evidently the case that many research questions require the researcher – whether styled as an ethnographer or not – to ask, "how many times", "how much of", or "in what number of ways" phenomena are seen or discussed. This is not to say that ethnographies of medical education need to rely on complex statistical operations: the use of numerical data can be relatively modest – for example, the numerical data constructed through counting particular types of interaction or exchange between people through a series of systematic observations within a workplace setting – whilst still generating meaningful insights and can be driven by simply pragmatic responses to the questions that the researcher is seeking to answer. For example, in her retrospective discussion of an ethnography of hospital waiting lists, Pope (2005) discusses the use of numerical data collected by the hospital at which the research took place alongside the qualitative data that is more stereotypically associated with ethnography. Such usage of qualitative as well as quantitative data speaks to the broader discourse of *mixed methods* research, although other commentators have argued that the mixed methods approach continues to perpetuate spurious divisions between different modes of data.

Methodologies for contemporary ethnographies of education

Changes and challenges to ethnographies of medical education are not restricted to matters of method, however: methodological standpoints are also in a state of flux, responding to the same theoretical shifts or technological developments that inform current and recent discussions of method. Once again, an exploration of these could easily fill a chapter – or indeed a book – by itself. Here, I shall focus on just two issues that pertain directly to the current discussion.

Standpoint

Research methodology textbooks and handbooks are replete with reflexive debates concerning the ethnographer's relationship to the field. But alongside well-established issues such as the scope or degree of the ethnographer's participation in the field (as already referred to), we can now add developments that derive from both technological advances as well as from methodological advances. These need not be discrete factors: the same technological developments that have allowed for the emergence of virtual or cyber ethnographies of research sites that are entirely situated online also allow for the easy sharing of large qualitative data sets across distributed research teams (as I shall discuss below). But it would be a mistake to assume that the development of new forms of ethnography of medical education rested primarily, or even partially, on technological as distinct from methodological innovation. The relative decline of the primacy of the individual researcher is not necessarily linked to the expansion of the digital. One relatively recent innovation can be seen in the emergence of *duoethnography*, which – as the name suggests – rests on an explicit commitment to a shared dialogue of meaning-making between the two researchers, and is clearly and critically explicated in a study by Docherty-Skippen and Beattie (2018) into emerging forms of professionalism amongst medical residents. A qualitatively different relationship between two researchers underpins the research by Harris and Rethans (2018) into the role of creativity in teaching physical examination skills, with one author occupying the recognisable role of the participant observer who is new to the research site, and the other occupying the role of insider researcher which in turn afforded a gatekeeper function. *Autoethnography* provides a further radical departure from "traditional" anthropological models of ethnographic research. Focusing on personal narrative and an incitement to change, autoethnography has been used extensively in health sciences research, in particular by service users seeking a vehicle for self-advocacy, and has more recently begun to be used by healthcare professionals and researchers (Farrell, Bourgeois-Law, Regehr, & Ajjawi, 2015).

Ethics and confidentiality

A pre-contractual basis of mutual trust is the ethical touchstone of any ethnography of education, a process through which the participants understand with clarity and transparency what the research is about and what they are being asked to agree to – to being observed, to being interviewed, to being photographed, and so on. At the same time, participants also need to be aware of the obligations placed on the researcher by this ethical contract – that the researcher will treat them respectfully, and will represent them fairly and truthfully, (eschewing for now postmodernist discussions as to what constitutes "a truthful account"). Nonetheless, such well-established tenets require modification in the light of the discussion thus far. For example, if we are observing an online community, we are always physically invisible, and not necessarily visible in a virtual sense, either because we are "lurking" or because we have chosen to adopt particular online identities. It is likewise a straightforward process for our respondents to disguise all or some of their identities online. How we present ourselves within such environments is a fundamental aspect of our ethical warrant, if we are to ensure that the consent of our respondents is informed. Ethical concerns also extend to how we construct and analyse our data. For example, the multi-modal texts that people generate within forums or on blogs are not passive, static collections of words and images; rather, they are the utterances of people in a space where talk has to be written down: as such, they should be treated as speech generated by people, not as texts waiting to be collected and analysed, and should only be used once consent has been obtained. Can we legitimately watch and read what goes on within online communities without having received informed consent from all of the users of the community? Is a blog post a private communication or a public document? Questions such as these demand a heightened reflexivity on the part of researchers.

Medical education in a digital age: moving beyond single-site anthropological ethnographies of education

Up to this point, what I hope to have shown – necessarily briefly – are some of the ways in which ethnographies of education (medical or otherwise) have developed in recent years. With this as our backdrop, I now turn to a more detailed methodological discussion, focused on *Medical Education in a Digital Age*. This research project (originally titled *Higher Education In a Digital Economy*, but as a research team we soon adopted the title that I have reproduced above) was a three-year ethnography of medical education in North America, funded by the Social Sciences and Humanities Research Council of Canada (SSHRC). The fieldwork for the project was conducted from 2012 to 2015. The broad aims of the project were to explore issues at one university in Canada surrounding the implementation, dating back to September 2010, of a new medical education curriculum distributed across two campuses. This new distributed medical education (DME) curriculum was designed explicitly to rest on information and communication technologies (ICTs). The need to establish *comparability of provision* in terms of both educational experiences and assessment methods across the two sites (referred to from now as Main and Satellite in order to maintain anonymity) was driven by an external professional framework established by the accrediting organisations, the Liaison Committee on Medical Education (LCME) for North America, as well as the Committee on Accreditation of Canadian Medical Schools (CACMS): wider North American accreditation allows graduates to access opportunities for postgraduate training and residency across all of North America.

In 2010, the already-established medical education programme at Main Campus was redesigned and extended to include a new site – Satellite – situated 400 kilometres away in a neighbouring province. Main Campus is (perhaps unsurprisingly, bearing in mind the nomenclature used here) larger and busier than Satellite Campus. The size of the student cohort for the medical programme at Main Campus is almost three times that of Satellite. Approximately eighty students enroll at Main each year, whereas the typical student cohort at Satellite numbers thirty. The new curriculum was designed to rest on information and communication technologies (ICTs) from the ground up, the application of technology (digital video, digital learning platforms, e-learning devices and the like) functioning as a means to enact synchronously the DME curriculum across the two campuses, with the establishment of a videoconferencing system at the centre of this technological framework. Through this infrastructure, the two campuses are linked so that for the undergraduate students, during their first two years of study (that is to say, before they take up their clerkships at the beginning of their third year of study in, for example, emergency medicine, paediatrics, or psychiatry), the curriculum is shared, distributed through the ICT network. That is to say, students at both campuses follow the same curriculum and attend the same lectures and other plenary activities, linked via the videoconferencing system. Two groups of students share not only the same lecture space but also the same lecturer, who addresses one group in person and the other via the videoconferencing system, although other elements of the course such as small-group sessions or laboratory-based sessions are delivered separately.

At both of the sites, large lecture theatres, smaller seminar rooms and even student lounges have been equipped with videoconferencing systems. Irrespective of size, all of these teaching spaces are equipped with an array of monitors that allow not only for the display of media-rich teaching materials (the curriculum is delivered on a paperless basis), but also for staff and students at one campus to see and to hear their counterparts at the other, during lectures, seminars, laboratory sessions and panel meetings. State-of-the-art camera and microphone systems within all of the teaching rooms allow for the synchronous teaching by one member of faculty staff across both sites, for question-and-answer sessions that students at both sites can take part in, and for the recording of lectures and seminars for future revision and reference. Press-button systems allow students to activate the microphones in front of them (in every teaching room there is a button and a microphone at every seat) so that their counterparts at the other campus can hear their questions. At the same time, the cameras in each room focus on the student body and transmit their image to large screens at both sites. Teaching materials are collected and for-matted in advance of each lecture or seminar by a specialist team of Audio-Visual staff who are generally responsible for the technological infrastructure – ICTs, cameras, microphones and so forth – that the curriculum rests on. These specialist teams work out of control booths (one at each site) from where they orchestrate the technologies that are in use during lectures, seminars, and other meetings. It is at Main Campus that the bulk of "real world" teaching takes place, with students at Satellite participating via the videoconferencing system: it is relatively uncommon for teaching to take place at Satellite and be transmitted to Main.

The key theoretical and empirical findings of our research project have been published else-where and I do not propose to rehearse them here (Kits, Angus, MacLeod, & Tummons, 2019; MacLeod, Kits, Whelan, Fournier, Wilson, Power, Mann, Tummons, & Brown, 2015; MacLeod, Kits, Mann, Tummons, & Whelan, 2016; MacLeod, Cameron, Kits, & Tummons, 2019; Tummons, Fournier, & Kits, 2015; Tummons, Fournier, Kits, & MacLeod, 2016, 2018). Rather, I shall focus on a number of methodological issues that emerged throughout our research, that resonate with the earlier discussion of method and methodology. But in order to contextualise this discussion, an awareness of the scope of the project is needed. Four different methods for constructing data were employed, all characteristic of ethnography. The first data set derived from observations (n=108), which were conducted in lecture rooms, seminar rooms, staff meeting rooms, and technicians' control rooms, and were carried out between January and November 2013. The second data set was constructed through semi-structured interviews (n=31), which were conducted with academic staff, administrative staff, technical/audio-visual staff, and students, and were carried out between July and December 2014 (staff interviews (n=16), lasting between 50 and 60 minutes), and February and April 2015 (student interviews (n=15), lasting between 26 and 56 minutes). The third was derived from textual analysis: documents (n=60) relating to curriculum design and implementation, professional accreditation, institutional policy, and technical design and implementation, were analysed between January and December 2013. The fourth and final data set was visual: photographs (n=136) of teaching rooms, administra-tive offices and audio-visual booths at both campuses were taken between January 2013 and January 2014.

Some of the issues that faced us, as researchers, were simply pragmatic, although these invari-ably hinted at or led to more profound problems. Consider, for example, the role of ICTs in enabling our research team to work. It was necessary for ICTs to be employed in order to allow us to do our work as an integral element of the ethnography. The geographical distances between the two campuses mirrored the distances between individual members of the research team: most of us were in North America, but some of us were in the United Kingdom. As has been seen in other ethnographies, problems can and do emerge relating to the time needed to learn how to use technology, the reliability of different ICTs, how to respond when tech-nology breaks down, and so forth. Our research team responded to a number of such matters. Many of these were almost prosaic: how do we mute our microphones when we are talking live and sharing PowerPoint slides using the GoToMeeting web conferencing tool? Should we use N-Vivo or Atlas-Ti – two excellent but somewhat different qualitative data analysis software (QDAS) programmes – to store, organise, and code our increasingly rich and unwieldy data, and how long will our chosen software take to learn to use? In the end, we went with Atlas-Ti, which provided us with powerful tools for analysis and also sharing of our multi-modal data sets, our coding structures, our memos, and our research notes, across all members of the research team. Given that the project members spanned eight different time zones, how could we ensure that we chose appropriate on-line meeting times? Questions such as these seem of course straightforward to anticipate with hindsight. That is to say, it is a simple task to imagine questions such as these arising amongst or being anticipated by a team of researchers. But the lived experience of a research project often belies the idealised plan.

In addition to the kinds of problems listed above relating to technical and practical work, the doing of the research work within and through a technologically mediated environment led to questions that might be seen as being more profound, certainly less procedural and certainly more philosophical – the kinds of issues that I considered in the earlier parts of this chapter. For example, the mediation of identity through ICTs raises considerable epistemological and ontological concerns. The production of discourse in an online space that is physically apart from the body is one such concern, necessarily resulting in a diminished space for paralanguage (facial expression, gesture and movement) within communication that necessarily impedes particular forms of communication and of meaning making. The rendering permanent of discourses that would, outside an environment mediated by ICTs, be temporary, is another. The knowledge that what one says is also being recorded and can be scrutinised by people who did not take part in the original (on-line) conversation can lead to changes in how one talks and, thus, to changes in how one presents and engages as a social being – a process that can be more or less deliberate.

If identity constituted one problematic element, then field constituted another. How were we to make sense of the site that we researched? Our field encompassed not only two geographically distant campuses but also a more nebulous online space and place, mediated by technology. At the same time, different members of the research team had differential relationships to these spaces, in terms of not only geographical proximity (or lack thereof), but also organisational and hence, arguably, cultural proximity as well: some of the team were insider-researchers; others very much outsiders. Issues of location and access were thus rendered complex in our research: the insider knowledge that allowed some of our research team quickly to negotiate routes to gatekeepers and key informants was tempered by the need – as for any researcher of their own workplace – to prevent damage to their organisation, and to prevent harm to their colleagues or vulnerable others. At the same time, this same insider knowledge provided significant insights when analysing data – insights that the outsider members of the team would otherwise not have been able to draw on.

Conclusion: there's more than one kind of ethnography

The *Medical Education in a Digital Age* project was funded for three years (the data collection phase), but it took six more years for the last of our findings to be peer-reviewed and published. During the course of our work, we shifted our methodological stance, and embraced a somewhat different theoretical framework to the one that formed our initial discussions. Our research generated a considerably rich body of multi-modal data, gathered over a protracted period of time. The data was analysed by a transatlantic research team and we were able to share our data and our analyses using specialist qualitative data analysis software, which in turn informed our discussions of research quality and warrant. Our research quite conspicuously challenged several of the tenets of "traditional" anthropological models of ethnography of education: we were a team of researchers, geographically separated, and variously engaged in the different processes of data construction, data analysis, and writing; our research spanned two physical locations but also included a consideration of online spaces; some of us were insider-researchers, others (myself included) were novices within this field; some of us were physically present in the field, observing practices, taking photographs, and conducting interviews, and others of us were only digitally present, watching video, scrutinising online documents, and reading transcripts. As a research team, our practices were certainly heterogeneous, and yet we were all clearly engaged in the same ethnography, albeit ethnography that defied a simplistic labelling, consisting as it did of virtual, multi-sited, and institutional elements.

Medical Education in a Digital Age contrasts strongly in several ways with the examples of ethnographies that I have cited in this chapter – and yet speaks to the same debates of method and methodology. All of the works that I have cited in this chapter constitute ethnographic research, irrespective of the time spent in the field, the number of people enrolled in the research team, or the relationship of the researcher(s) to the site where the research was conducted. Simply put, ethnographic research can involve two or more years of work for a single researcher (Atkinson & Pugsley, 2005) or it can require just eight months and involve a research team (Balmer et al., 2010). It can rest on the well-established methods of participant observation, the taking of field notes, and qualitative interviewing (Pope, 2005) or it can draw on multi-modal data sets that are managed and coded using specialist software packages (Urquhart et al., 2018). It can be conducted through access to an online space by an ethnographer who will never meet their respondents "in real life" (Crompvoets, 2010), or it can be constructed entirely through the subjective perspectives of the researcher, locating themselves at the centre of the ethnographic process (Gross, 2012). Simply put, the ethnography of education defies a simplistic formulation, but can nonetheless be understood as being able to be operationalised in a number of different, nonetheless commensurate, modes.

My argument, therefore, is that we need to have conversations about method that are at times abstruse. I acknowledge that these conversations do not provide straightforward answers: indeed, they raise more questions in turn. Instead, we position these conversations as part of a turn in ethnographic research more generally that seeks to promote greater reflexivity amongst ethnographers whilst at the same time avoiding overshadowing the empirical work that our ethnography rests on. And we need to be sensitive to the fact that ethnography moves on and will continue to do so. And yet, while we are busy subscribing to yet more methodological frameworks that might be accused of resting on only slight epistemological or ontological differences, we argue that these slight – not cavalier – differences are important in allowing our peers to locate the work that we are doing within the broader field of ethnography. At the same time, we also argue that these slight differences are just that: slight. Ethnography has always been changing and adapting, and it will continue to do so. We have much in common with the broad field of ethnography and ethnographic research more widely, and if we can be less self-conscious in our methods, we can put methodological debates in their place as part of an ethnography that is not defined in terms of being virtual, multi-sited, or rapid, but in terms that are shared across all of these ethnographic variations, all agreeing on the centrality of a commitment to immersion, to rich and exquisite description, and to a profound understanding of the cultural practices that are being explored.

References

Alasuutari, P. (1995). *Researching Culture: qualitative method and cultural studies.* London: Sage.

Andreassen, P., M. Christensen, & J. Møller. (2020). Focused ethnography as an approach in medical education research. *Medical Education* 54(4): 296–302.

Atkinson, P., & L. Pugsley. (2005). Making sense of ethnography and medical education. *Medical Education* 39(2): 228–234.

Balmer, D., C. Master, B. Richards, J. Serwint, & A. Giardino. (2010). An ethnographic study of attending rounds in general paediatrics. *Medical Education* 44(11): 1105–1116.

Chretien, K., M. Tuck, M. Simon, L. Singh, & T. Kind. (2015). A digital ethnography of medical students who use Twitter for professional development. *Journal of General Internal Medicine* 30(11): 1673–1680.

Crompvoets, S. (2010). Using online qualitative research methods in medical education. *International Journal of Multiple Research Approaches* 4(3): 206–213.

Docherty-Skippen, S., & K. Beattie. (2018). Duoethnography as a dialogic and collaborative form of curriculum inquiry for resident professionalism and self-care education. *Canadian Medical Education Journal* 9(3): 76–82.

Dyke, S. (2013). Utilising a blended ethnographic approach to explore the online and offline lives of pro-ana community members. *Ethnography and Education* 8(2): 146–161.

Farrell, L., G. Bourgeois-Law, G. Regehr, & R. Ajjawi. (2015). Autoethnography: introducing 'I' into medical education research. *Medical Education* 49(10): 974–982.

Gross, S. (2012). Biomedicine inside out: an ethnography of brain surgery. *Sociology of Health and Illness* 34(8): 1170–1183.

Hammersley, M. (2018). What is ethnography? Can it survive? Should it? *Ethnography and Education* 13(1): 1–17.

Harris, A., & J.-J. Rethans. (2018). Expressive instructions: ethnographic insights into the creativity and improvisation entailed in teaching physical skills to medical students. *Perspectives in Medical Education* 7(4): 232–238.

Hodges, B. (2005). The many and conflicting histories of medical education in Canada and the USA: an introduction to the paradigm wars. *Medical Education* 39(6): 613–621.

Kits, O., C. Angus, A. MacLeod, & J. Tummons. (2019). Progressive research collaborations and the limits of soft power. *Perspectives on Medical Education* 8(1): 28–32.

MacLeod, A. (2016). Understanding the culture of Graduate Medical Education: the benefits of ethnographic research. *Journal of Graduate Medical Education* 8(2): 142–144.

Macleod, A., O. Kits, E. Whelan, C. Fournier, K. Wilson, G. Power, K. Mann, J. Tummons, & A. Brown. (2015). Sociomateriality: a theoretical framework for studying distributed medical education. *Academic Medicine* 90(11): 1451–1456.

MacLeod, A., O. Kits, K. Mann, J. Tummons, & K. Wilson. (2016). The invisible work of distributed medical education: exploring the contributions of audiovisual professionals, administrative professionals and faculty teachers. *Advances in Health Sciences Education* 22: 623–638.

MacLeod, A., P. Cameron, O. Kits, & J. Tummons. (2019). Technologies of exposure: videoconferenced distributed medical education as a sociomaterial practice. *Academic Medicine* 94(3): 412–418.

Pope, C. (2005). Conducting ethnography in medical settings. *Medical Education* 39(12): 1180–1187.

Reeves, S., J. Peller, J. Goldman, & S. Kitto. (2013). Ethnography in qualitative educational research: AMEE Guide No. 80. *Medical Teacher* 35(8): 1365–1379.

Thomas, G. & D. James. (2006). Reinventing grounded theory: some questions about theory, ground and discovery. *British Educational Research Journal* 32(6) 767–795.

Tummons, J. (2014). Using Software for Qualitative Data Analysis: Research outside paradigmatic boundaries. In Hand, M. and Hillyard, S. (eds.) *Big Data? Qualitative Approaches to Digital Research.* Bingley: Emerald. 155–177.

Tummons, J., A. MacLeod, & O. Kits. (2015). Ethnographies across virtual and physical spaces: a reflexive commentary on a live Canadian/UK ethnography of distributed medical education. *Ethnography and Education* 10(1): 107–120.

Tummons, J., C. Fournier, O. Kits, & A. Macleod. (2016). Teaching without a blackboard and chalk: conflicting attitudes towards using ICTs in higher education teaching and learning. *Higher Education Research and Development* 35(4): 829–840.

Tummons, J., C. Fournier, O. Kits, & A. Macleod. (2018). Using technology to accomplish comparability of provision in distributed medical education in Canada: an actor–network theory ethnography. *Studies in Higher Education* 43(11): 1912–1922.

Urquhart, L.M., J.S. Ker, & C.E. Rees. (2018). Exploring the influence of context on feedback at medical school: a video-ethnography study. *Advances in Health Sciences Education* 23(1): 159–186.

Walford, G. (2020). Ethnography is not qualitative. *Ethnography and Education* 15(1): 122–135.

Walford, G. (ed.) (2008). *How to do Educational Ethnography*. Tufnell Press.

PART V

Visual/sensory ethnography

14

VISUAL ETHNOGRAPHY IN HEALTH AND HEALTHCARE

Concepts, steps, and good practices

Laura Lorenz and Bettina Kolb

Introduction

As with ethnography for the study of any phenomena, visual ethnography in health and healthcare involves placing one's self (as researcher) into the perspective (the "shoes") of the individuals or group being studied. The research process encourages empathy for people and their lived experience with health, illness, and healthcare, and recognises that reality (truth) is relative and different perspectives can co-exist. Ethnography requires researchers to reflect on their assumptions and life experiences and how these can influence study findings (Bloor & Wood, 2006). Visual ethnography in health and healthcare results in coproduction of knowledge as researchers, participants, and audiences talk about the visuals and what they mean (Pink, 2001).

Visual ethnography originated over 100 years ago, when photography was first used to illustrate observational findings. Initially, photos were perceived as "truth", or objective fact for "scientific documentation" of cultural and physical difference (Pink, 2001). In the mid-1900s anthropologists Gregory Bateson and Margaret Mead used photography to generate theory (Harper, 2003). For the past 50 years or more, visual ethnography has experienced a sea-change as ethnographers have put responsibility for documenting experience through visual methods (still cameras, video cameras, drawings, collage) into the hands of people whose experiences are the subject of study (Collier, 1957; Ewald, 2002; Wang, 1999). The perspectives of patients, communities, and clinicians on health, illness, and the delivery of health services are all rich areas for study using visual ethnography.

Visual ethnography in health and healthcare involves a range of methods, from photography (Wang, Burris, & Ping 1996) and video (Carroll, Iedema, & Kerridge, 2008), to drawings, and graphic facilitation (North, Sieberhagen, Leonard, Bonaconsa, & Coetzee, 2019). Words are integral companions to the visuals as participants assign meaning to their visuals in interviews, (Lorenz, 2011; Wang et al., 1996), focus group discussions (Bayer, Alburqueque, & Our Word Through Our Eyes Program, 2014; Gullón et al., 2019), and caption-writing (Wang, 1999). The meanings assigned by participants inform analysis (Pink, 2001) and, we argue, should be paired with participant-generated visuals throughout their research lives.

Visual ethnography can be useful for a range of purposes: to understand participants' lived experience with illness and health (Bayer et al., 2014; Gullón et al., 2019; Healey et al., 2011; Lorenz, 2011; Wang et al., 1996); with the organisation and delivery of healthcare (Carroll et al., 2008; North et al., 2019); and with the experience of nature and health impacts of climate change (Healey et al., 2011; Mattouk & Talhouk, 2017). Benefits of visual ethnography include back and forth conversations among participants and researchers (Harper, 2003; Lorenz & Kolb, 2009; North et al., 2019), with policymakers and decisionmakers (Carroll et al., 2008; North et al., 2019; Wang et al., 1996), and with community members (Bayer et al., 2014; Lorenz & Kolb, 2009; Wang et al., 1996). Visual methods can stimulate holistic accounts of healthcare practice (North et al., 2019), bring out tacit knowledge (North et al., 2019; Carroll et al., 2008), and help to make visible reasoning and values (North et al., 2019; Healey et al., 2011). Their use can establish shared understandings (North et al., 2019) and shared experiences (Cremers, Gerrets, & Grobusch, 2016), generate trust (Carroll et al., 2008; North et al., 2019), and foster empathy (Lorenz, 2011; Wang et al., 1996).

Another benefit of visual ethnography is also a risk. Visuals affect both emotion and cognition, which together influence learning, behaviour, and perception (Damasio, 1994). The brain stores information, retrieves it, reasons, and makes decisions using visual images (Damasio, 1994). Ethnographers using visual methods must reflect on the ways in which their knowledge and experiences – the information stored in their brain – influence what they see and how they interpret it (Lorenz, 2011).

Our focus in this chapter is on the use of *participatory* visual ethnography in health and healthcare, or methods that place responsibility for visual documentation into the hands of people who are often the subjects of research. We will now define some key concepts in participatory visual ethnography in health from our perspective.

Key concepts in visual ethnography in health and healthcare: A model

Based on the literature and our own work, we propose a model of key concepts to support the design and implementation of a visual ethnography in health and healthcare (see Figure 14.1). Our model shows a process that is empathic, trustful, participatory, interdisciplinary, and reflexive, and results in coproduction of knowledge.

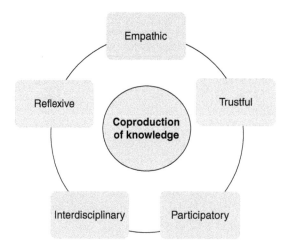

Figure 14.1 Key concepts for visual ethnography in health and healthcare

Empathic. Ethnography studies people in their everyday settings in order to "think oneself into the perspective" of the people being studied (Bloor & Wood, 2006, p. 70). Visual ethnography in health seeks to understand participants' experiences with health, illness, and healthcare. Seeing through participants' eyes requires hearing what they have to say about their visuals – why they created them and what they mean (Harrison, 2002; Harper, 2003; Pink, 2001; Wang, 1999). An empathic process involves honouring experiences that "diverge from established 'truth'" (Riessman, 2008, p. 186).

Trustful. Social distance between researchers and participants can result in a power imbalance and lack of trust (Bloor & Wood, 2006). Visual methods "are a powerful tool with which to establish trust and openness" (North et al., 2019, p. 13). Viewing research as a partnership is crucial to visual ethnography in health, and relies on what Carroll, Iedema, and Kerridge (2008) have termed "trustful entanglement" (p. 389). Transparency in documenting the research process contributes to findings that audiences will view as trustful (Riessman, 2008). And finally, trustful refers to ethics; participants trust that their data will be kept private and confidential. Researchers in turn trust that participants will adhere to ethical guidelines, for example asking permission before taking someone's photo.

Participatory. A participatory approach to visual ethnography in health positions participants – patients, community members, clinicians – as experts of their own lives (Rose, 2016). Ideally, participants are involved in all study aspects, from helping to determine the topic or questions to creating visuals, interpreting them, and reaching audiences (Wang & Burris, 1997). A participatory approach is inherently flexible (Bloor & Wood, 2006); research plans may have to be revised as participants express their needs and preferences, for example what photographs to take (Pink, 2001).

Interdisciplinary. Photographs and other visuals can help to bridge the discipline gap between researchers and participants and bring out their tacit knowledge (Kolb & Lorenz, 2014). The visuals encourage a participant to speak (Bloor & Wood, 2006). The research conversation prompts interdisciplinary learning and generates common understanding of issues, context, and solutions (Kolb & Lorenz, 2014). Visual ethnography can help children, persons with low socioeconomic status, and people living with disabilities to contribute to research in a thoughtful way (Lorenz & Kolb, 2009).

Reflexive. Reflexivity is "a critical feature of visual research" and deepens understanding (Mitchell, 2011, p. 5). Researchers may have multiple identities and perspectives (Rose, 2016), which inevitably influence "ethnographic knowledge, interpretation, and representation" (Pink, 2001, p. 23). Participants also practice reflexivity as they reflect on what they want to photograph and "develop critical awareness of visual representations" (Gubrium & Harper, 2013, p. 35). Transparency about reflexivity contributes to trustworthiness of research findings (Riessman, 2008).

Coproduction of knowledge. Applying the concepts described above leads to coproduction of knowledge. Visual ethnography involves co-construction of data (Harrison, 2002; North et al., 2019) and avoids knowledge extraction (Pink, 2001). Instead the focus is on coproduction (Pink, 2001). Discussing research visuals is an opportunity for dialogue and sharing of expertise, thus prompting mutual learning and creation of new, common knowledge (Kolb & Lorenz, 2014). Viewing audiences contribute to coproduction of knowledge as well (Pink, 2001; Cremers et al., 2016), as they translate study findings to policy, programming, and services (Lorenz & Kolb, 2009).

It is important to note that the boundaries between concepts in Figure 14.1 are arbitrary. They intersect and overlap in practice. For example, an interdisciplinary process relies on a trustful environment in which researchers and participants work together on multiple tasks.

A key aspect of visual ethnography that underlies all the concepts described above is ethics. An empathic process that is ethical means learning about participants' strengths as well as problems. A trustful process that is ethical involves providing opportunities for people to make informed decisions about participating. A participatory ethical process engages participants in learning about being a visual ethnographer and protecting individuals and communities from harm. An ethical interdisciplinary process supports meaningful communication across disciplines. Being reflexive about the emotions that participant data can evoke is also an ethical imperative. We will now illustrate use of the model as we examine two photos from a paper we co-authored (Lorenz & Kolb, 2009).

Using the model to examine two research photographs and their implications

Writing this chapter prompted us to return to a paper about our experiences with participatory visual methods to explore health topics in Morocco and the United States (Lorenz & Kolb, 2009). Sarah Pink (2001) and others have modelled revisiting visual ethnography data over time to gain new insights (Lorenz, 2011). Our starting point is one photo from each study. For each photo we describe the study research purpose and context before describing the photo in detail – an important analysis task (Rose, 2016) – and exploring ways in which the photo and related research process illustrate the concepts in our model (Figure 14.1).

Morocco. The first example is a photo interview study focused on the Sefarin *hammam* in Fez, Morocco. The hammam is a traditional "Turkish" bath where residents go for washing, religious ceremonies and drinking water, and it supports health care and hygiene. The Fez component was part of a larger study of hammam in five countries funded by the European Union and the Austrian Ministry for Research, to develop interdisciplinary strategies to envision and plan for the future of hammam buildings and their neighbourhoods.

In Figure 14.2 we see a waterway with trash and debris piled up in a cement channel and embedded in the shallow flowing water like rocks in a river. Some of the trash is enclosed in plastic bags, some is not. The water and debris take up two-thirds of the photo's landscape. In the top third of the photo, graffiti marks the channel wall that runs from left to right. A platform anchors the top of the photo and shows this area to be a channel for flowing water.

Empathic: The study involved local residents in taking photos and talking about them, to incorporate their viewpoint into future scenarios for the hammam. Using visual methods opened up an unexpected view as participants took photos in and from places where outsiders (foreigners, women) could not have entered. Without this picture researchers and the community would not have discussed health and hygiene related to water supplies outside the hammam.

Trustful: The study took place in a context where it can be uncomfortable for citizens to appear to criticise the government. Trust in the local partner organisation, which worked closely with local residents to support restoration and renovation of the *medina* (market), helped participants to feel that participation would be safe. The project's planned discussion and dissemination efforts, including public meetings and presentations, also created a contract of trust between residents and foreign scientists.

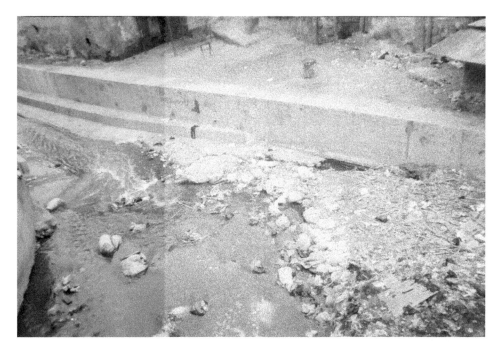

Figure 14.2 Polluted waterway. "All those who love their town don't want to see it in this condition, by the way the photo is very significant" – Participant, HAMMAM Case Study, Fez, Morocco, 2006.

Participatory: Participants were free to take any photos they chose, and to select which among them to discuss with a researcher. As shown in Figure 14.2, the participant changed the focus of her photo-taking and discussion away from the hammam to a polluted river outside the medina neighbourhood. Participation continued in community-wide events where the photos and captions were reviewed and discussed, and solutions suggested.

Interdisciplinary: The community meetings brought residents, policymakers, architects, urban planners, and social scientists together to view and discuss the photos, captions, and future scenarios. The photos became a common language for discussants with different disciplinary expertise and lived experience to share their perspectives.

Reflexive: Participants reflected on problems and strengths in their neighbourhood during photo-taking and the photo interview. For Figure 14.2, the participant was careful not to assign blame when pointing out the problem of the polluted river. Participation required subtle reflection on the local context and what would be safe and effective at motivating action to address something of importance to the resident.

Coproduction of knowledge: With Figure 14.2, a participant directed the researchers' gaze to a problem that challenged the study's narrow focus on the hammam. With her photo, the photographer expanded the project's lens to capture a health issue outside the hammam itself yet pertinent from her perspective to planning for health and urban renewal in her neighbourhood.

United States. Our second example used photovoice in a study of lived experience with acquired brain injury (ABI) (or any injury to the brain after birth) in a city in the north-eastern

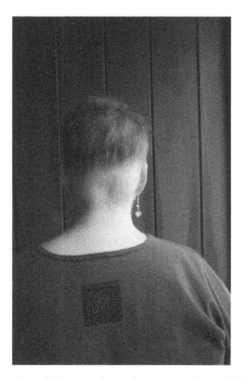

Figure 14.3   New depth of acceptance. "In my 17th year of recovery, I am no longer shamed by lack of hair and scar. It represents a new freedom, pride in what I have overcome" – Participant, Framingham Photovoice Study, 2006.

U.S. At the time (2006), most published research on ABI focused on measuring the impact of brain injury on function. There were few studies exploring the impact on people's lives, a topic relevant to patient-centred care, a quality of care issue. Participants were recruited from a brain injury support group. The study received funding from a state agency and the Brain injury Association of Massachusetts (BIAMA).

In Figure 14.3, we see a woman from behind. Her head and body comprise two-thirds of the frame. The focus of attention is the back of her head where the lack of hair shows a scar and fills the centre of the image. Short dark hair covers her head above the scar. Light enters the frame from the right, highlights her right ear and earring, and casts a shadow on the left side of the frame. The photo subject gave the camera to her mother to take the photo.

Empathic: With brain injury, self-stigma and stigma from others can inhibit quality of life and opportunities for healing (McLellan, Bishop, & McKinlay, 2010). Behavioural and communication problems after brain injury can cause community members to mistake it for mental illness (McLellan et al., 2010). Study participants wanted to increase awareness of brain injury in the community and in healthcare, and foster empathy for people living with it. In the photo we see the "patient" through her mother's eyes; family members are often integral to the care of their loved ones with brain injury.

Trustful: Participants awarded the researcher "guest" insider status because she had a brother with a brain injury and was friends with a group member. Further, the group's facilitator and the researcher worked closely together on study planning. These factors meant that participants felt trust in the researcher and research process.

Participatory: The Figure 14.3 photographer was responsible for changing the study topic from living with traumatic brain injury (TBI), caused by a blow or jolt to the head, to living with acquired brain injury (ABI), which includes brain injury from stroke, brain tumour, and infectious disease. Throughout the project her participation was intentional: when she noticed that few people had photographed strategies that support their healing, she took multiple photos showing her own strategies (such as doing word puzzles and games) and wrote captions for them. When writing her captions, she thought audiences would not want to read anything long, so she reworked her captions until they were like *haiku* – short and meaningful.

Interdisciplinary: The researcher brought questions to the study that asked about participants' recovery from brain injury. Participants protested the word "recovery" because in their minds it stigmatised them since they were unlikely to recover their former function or work. They asked to use the word "healing" instead. In her caption, the participant contests the word recovery as a short-term prospect and goal as she writes about being in her 17th year of recovery.

Reflexive: The participant who took this photo was reflexive about her life before and after injury. She took photos that helped her to discuss strengths and losses. The Figure 14.3 photo and caption prompted intense reflection and discussion in the group. Members saw her as a hero for losing her sense of shame about brain injury during the project.

Coproduction of knowledge: Participants were integrally involved in all aspects including the final exhibit. Figure 14.3, for which a mother and her daughter with a brain injury collaborated to produce the photo, is one example of the coproduction of knowledge that took place.

Visual ethnography in health and healthcare in practice

We have selected eight studies as examples of visual ethnography in practice (see Table 14.1). Each study was conducted in a different region of the world: Africa, the Arctic, Asia, Australia, Europe, the Middle East, North America, and South America. Each has a different sample and different purposes. The selected examples illustrate the use of four visual ethnography methods: photo-elicitation (Lorenz, 2011); photovoice (Bayer et al., 2014; Gullón et al., 2019; Healey et al., 2011; Mattouk & Talhouk, 2017; Wang et al., 1996); video ethnographic filming (Carroll et al., 2008); and graphic facilitation (North et al., 2019). Our examples are united by the use of participatory methods in visual ethnographies of health, illness, and the organisation and delivery of healthcare.

Table 14.1 illustrates the wide ranging use of visual ethnography in health and healthcare around the globe. Participants have included adolescents, adult community residents, medical staff, and patients. Topics include factors affecting participants' health, well-being and sexuality; community perceptions of environmental factors associated with physical activity; and ways that climate change is affecting health. The studies have helped to illuminate health and development needs of rural village women; understand lived experience with traumatic brain injury; develop culturally appropriate best practices for nursing care; and improve clinical communication within a hospital. They have a common intent: to have an action impact. We will return to these eight studies as exemplars for the steps of visual ethnography in health and healthcare.

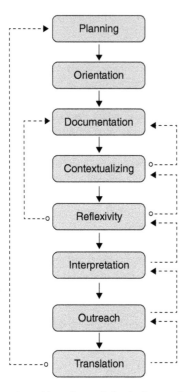

Figure 14.4   Steps of visual ethnography in health and healthcare

Visual ethnography in health and healthcare: Steps

We propose that visual ethnography in health and healthcare involves eight steps: Planning, Orientation, Documentation, Contextualizing, Reflexivity, Interpretation, Outreach, and Translation (see Figure 14.4). These steps draw on the work of Caroline C. Wang (1999) and our own research and practice (Lorenz & Kolb, 2009; Kolb & Lorenz, 2014; Kolb & Lorenz, 2020 *forthcoming*). In describing the steps, we provide "exemplars in practice" from the studies in Table 14.1.

Figure 14.4 shows the steps for planning and conducting a visual ethnography in health and healthcare. As noted by the dotted lines and arrows, some steps may be repeated multiple times. For example, participants may document their perspectives using visuals (photos, video, art) and contextualize them multiple times. Similarly, researcher reflexivity on personal life experiences that may influence findings can prompt a return to interpretation.

Step 1, *Planning*, includes deciding on the health topic of study, gaining entry into the study setting and seeking support from stakeholders (e.g., community elders or elected officials). At this stage you will determine how you will protect the privacy and confidentiality of participants, keep them and their communities or workplaces safe from harm, and obtain ethics approval, if needed. From a practical standpoint, Step 1 involves determining where and how often to meet, what cameras to use, and how to recruit participants. Carroll et al. (2008) is an example of planning. Before starting video filming at the study site (a hospital ICU), researchers conducted participant observation and interviews with ICU staff. Following two days of observation and interviews, staff agreed to have video-filming begin. A great deal of planning – creation of the filming protocol and intensive participant observation, notetaking, and interviews – preceded

Table 14.1 Participatory visual ethnography in health and healthcare: Examples from eight regions

Author/Year/Journal	Location	Focus	Population	Visual Methods	Notes/Implications
Bayer, Alburqueque & Participants/ 2014/ *Health Promotion Practice*	Peru	Factors affecting participants' health, well-being and sexuality; educate program planners, policymakers and community members	12 adolescents (aged 12–16 years) living in urban neighbourhoods	Collection: Photovoice Analysis: Participants described their photos using SHOWeD; sorted selected photos by themes; refined selections, captions and grouping for an exhibit	Provided insight into unique adolescent perspectives that others would not traditionally have access to or would not seek access to
Carroll, Iedema & Kerridge/ 2008/ *Qualitative Health Research*	Australia	Structure of clinical communication within a hospital ICU; development of interventions to improve practice in hospital ward rounds, daily planning meetings, and general interactions	Experienced and junior medical staff, nursing staff, and social workers working in a hospital	Collection: Video-ethnographic filming Analysis: Video-reflexive sessions were structured around specific questions prompting discussion of ICU practice complexity and implications for junior staff	Researchers and clinicians worked in partnership and made visible and discussable clinicians' tacit knowledge; resulted in restructured ward round and planning meetings to increase patient care time
Gullón et al./ 2019/ *International Journal of Environmental Research and Public Health*	Spain	Community perceptions of urban built, social, and political/economic factors associated with physical activity; develop policy recommendations	24 adults (12 men, 12 women) in two socioeconomically different districts of Madrid	Collection: Photovoice Analysis: Participants coded photo themes; researchers moved between data and theory and classified policy recommendations using the "ANGELO" framework	Changed perspective on relationships among researchers, citizens, and policymakers; generated changes to increase physical activity and improve population health
Healey et al./ 2011/ ARCTIC	Canada (Arctic)	Community perspectives on ways climate change is affecting the health of northern peoples	6 volunteers from *Nunaqut (Inuit)* communities and 2 graduate students	Collection: Photovoice Analysis: Group members collaborated to select a message for their photos, grouped them by theme, and created a model of relationships among themes	Participants and researches adhered to the Inuit principle of *Inuuqatigiittiarniq*, or working in an environment of respect and appreciation for one another

(continued)

Table 14.1 Cont.

Author/Year/Journal	Location	Focus	Population	Visual Methods	Notes/Implications
Lorenz/2011/ *Health (London)*	USA	Revisit photos, conversation and analysis from a study of patients' perspectives on lived experience with health and illness (traumatic brain injury or TBI)	1 adult with TBI accessing outpatient rehabilitation services	<u>Collection</u>: Photo-elicitation <u>Analysis</u>: Narrative analysis methods (thematic, structural, dialogic, and visual analysis) by researcher; member check	Patient photos focus the conversation, create collaborative understandings, and help researchers to practice empathy and learn *about* and *with* patients
Mattouk & Talhouk/2017/ *PLoS ONE*	Lebanon	Perceptions among rural youth of harmony with nature	77 young people (aged 7–16) living in 5 rural villages in north, central and south Lebanon	<u>Collection</u>: Photovoice <u>Analysis</u>: Thematic analysis of photographs and text (separately and together) by researchers	Presents youth as key agents of change for nature conservation; knowledge gained has influenced design of nature conservation activities
North, Sieberhagen, Leonard et al./2019/ *International Journal of Qualitative Methods*	South Africa	Afrocentric nursing practices related to engaging with families while their children are hospitalised in the ICU	Nurses providing care for children in an ICU	<u>Collection</u>: Graphic facilitation, sociograms, and photo-elicitation <u>Analysis</u>: Thematic analysis of interview and focus group transcripts by researchers, cross-case analysis afterwards by researchers, and member checks	Use of visual methods made visible the implicit (a.k.a. tacit) practices and values by nurses in both settings, as well as nurses' culturally specific caring practices with family members in both settings; findings used to develop culturally-specific protocols
Wang, Burris, & Ping/1996/ *Social Science & Medicine*	China	Empower rural women to record and reflect on their lives, especially their health needs, and educate policymakers	52 village women in rural Yunnan Province, China	<u>Collection</u>: Photo novella (photovoice) <u>Analysis</u>: Participants selected significant and favourite photos for exhibit and described them for researchers	Promoted outsiders' empathy (as opposed to paternalism, condescension or idealism) for village women; led to policy changes to address needs they identified

Abbreviations: ANGELO framework = Analysis Grid for Environments Linked to Obesity; ICU = Intensive Care Unit; SHOWeD = What do we SEE here; What is really HAPPENING here; How does it relate to OUR lives; Why does this situation EXIST; What can we DO about it the visual ethnography component. This level of planning engendered trust among researchers and the people whose interactions would be filmed.

In Step 2, *Orientation*, you begin to work with participants. They may help to decide on the study topic and questions. They learn about ethical issues: how to stay safe, and ways to protect the safety and confidentiality of others. Healey et al. (2011) is an example of orientation. Prior to data collection, participants and researchers developed an ethics checklist to guide their project (Qaugiartiit/Arctic Health Research Network, 2008). Participants agreed to work in an environment of respect and appreciation for each other, an *Inuit* principle. The participatory process used to develop ethics principles fostered community and participant trust, and, we suggest, improved interdisciplinary collaboration.

In Step 3, *Documentation*, participants document their perspectives using visual methods. For this step, a researcher may provide the photos, but in our work and the exemplars in Table 14.1, participants have visually documented their realities. Mattouk and Talhouk (2017) provides an example of documentation. The authors recruited 77 young people (aged 7–16 years) from 5 villages in Lebanon to document their understanding of and relationship with nature. At each site researchers facilitated two days of workshops; one to introduce the project and topic and practice taking photographs, and a second to discuss 3 photos and captions from each participant. The one-week documentation time-frame allowed researchers to engage a substantial number of young people in documenting their perspectives and provided trustworthy data to inform country-wide environmental education efforts.

Step 4, *Contextualizing*, involves participants in decoding or interpreting study visuals (Kolb, 2008). In interviews and discussion groups, participants describe the visuals in the context of their lives and experiences. They may write captions, on their own or in collaboration with others. Steps 3 and 4 may be repeated several times. North et al. (2019) is an example of contextualizing. For this study 48 South African paediatric nurses, with 3 working languages (English, Afrikaans, and isiZulu) contextualized their day-to-day interactions with parents of hospitalised children. While nurses described the timing, purpose and, location of nurse-family interactions, researchers drew a visual pathway of care that was posted on the wall of the nurses' staff room and amended throughout the project. The graphic became a shared visual reference of tacit and explicit knowledge that prompted continued discussion. The visualisations fostered a sense that researchers were listening and are an example of coproduction of knowledge.

Step 5, *Reflexivity*, demands rigorous self-reflection by researchers on life experiences that may influence how the data are seen and interpreted. Keeping a journal can support self-reflection and insight. During study implementation, participants may do emotional sharing, and writing in a journal can help researchers to explore the emotional impact of participants' stories. Lorenz (2011) is an example of reflexivity. The photos by the participant living with a brain injury generated emotional empathy in the researcher for the frustration and confusion in his life. In a return to this "case" years later, the author realised that she had ignored the participant's strengths – patience and persistence. And further, she realized her focus was likely influenced by strong feelings about their common work history in international development, when efforts to improve lives could mean being complicit in policies that contributed to harm. Being reflexive about emotions that emerge during the research process can foster trust in the findings.

Step 6, *Interpretation*, means digging deeper into the data to understand their meaning and implications. Often participants take part in interpretation, for example by grouping their photos into themes. When researchers do not involve participants in interpretation, a member check can support accuracy and credibility of findings. Bayer et al. (2014) is an example of involving participants in multiple aspects of interpretation. Thirteen participants (aged 12–16 years) in Lima, Peru first participated in interpretation by writing descriptions for their photographs using a structured approach (SHOWeD) (Wang, 1999). Second, they discussed their photos and descriptions with the group and received feedback. Third they reviewed all photos and captions, sorted them by message and theme, and chose some to represent each message and some for inclusion in a "photo story". Interpretation also involved developing the exhibit content and layout. For this study, interpretation was highly participatory.

Step 7, *Outreach*, involves communicating study findings to outside audiences to support the study's action purposes (if there are any). Outreach can include an exhibit, a website, booklets, reports, conference presentations, and graphic narratives or other arts-based "products" such as skits, songs, or poetry. Outreach provides opportunities to learn from outside audiences and identify ways to apply study learning. Wang, Burris, and Ping (1996) is an example of outreach. Sixty-two village women from two Yunnan Province counties in China participated in a pioneering "photo novella" project, later called photovoice. One outreach activity was a slide presentation for Provincial and County Guidance groups, which included "some of the most powerful policymakers in the province" (Wang et al., 1996, p. 1396). A second was an exhibit in the provincial capital attended by high-level Yunnan policymakers, 3,500 local residents, and 30 journalists. Inviting journalists was intended to capitalise on the media's influence on public and policymaker conversations. The project purposefully created empathy for village women's daily life struggles and strengths.

Step 8, *Translation*, involves translating visual ethnography findings to health policy, programming, and practice. This step can lead to peer-review publications, training manuals, policy advocacy, and professional development workshops. It requires a return to stakeholders identified in Step 1, to understand their perspectives. Gullón et al. (2019) is an example of translation. Twelve men and twelve women in two districts of Madrid, Spain used cameras to explore environmental factors affecting their physical activity and grouped their photos into 61 categories. Researchers transformed the categories into 14 themes and used the ANGELO framework (Analysis Grid for Environments Linked to Obesity) to generate 34 policy recommendations to support increased physical activity. The participatory translation process resulted in coproduction of knowledge by researchers and participants.

How you design and implement the eight steps of visual ethnography in health and healthcare described above is up to you. We are not creating a recipe to follow exactly. The steps are guidelines for planning and implementing your visual ethnography in health and healthcare, and the cited studies provide examples to inform decision-making for your study.

Conclusion

In this chapter we have mined the research literature to find and describe examples of the range of settings, participants, and methods used around the world for visual ethnography in health and healthcare. We provided a model to help you make choices that support key concepts of a model of visual ethnography in health and healthcare: empathic, trustful, participatory, interdisciplinary, and reflexive. We described eight process steps and cited an exemplar study to inform choices for each step: Planning, Orientation, Documentation, Reflexivity, Interpretation, Outreach, and Translation. In conclusion, we encourage you to adapt the model and steps to your context as you design and implement your own visual ethnographies in health and healthcare.

References

Bayer, A. M., M. Alburqueque, & Our World Through Our Eyes Program. (2014). Our world through our eyes: Adolescents use photovoice to speak their mind on adolescent health, well-being, and sexuality in Lima, Peru. *Health Promotion Practice, 15*(5), 723–731. doi:10.1177/1524839914530400

Bloor, M., & F. Wood. (2006). *Keywords in qualitative methods: A vocabulary of research concepts*. London: Sage Publications.

Carroll, K., R. Iedema, & R. Kerridge. (2008). Reshaping ICU ward round practices using video-reflexive ethnography. *Qualitative Health Research, 18*(3), 380–390. doi:10.1177/1049732307313430

Collier Jr, J. (1957). Photography in anthropology: A report on two experiments. *American Anthropologist, 59*(5), 843–859. doi:10.1525/aa.1957.59.5.02a00100

Cremers, A. L., R. Gerrets, & M. P. Grobusch. (2016). Visual ethnography: Bridging anthropology and public health. *Practicing Anthropology, 38*(4), 7–11. doi:10.17730/0888-4552.38.4.7

Damasio, A. (1994). *Descartes' error: Emotion, reason, and the human brain*. London: Penguin Books.

Ewald, W. (2002). *I wanna take me a picture*. Boston: Beacon Press.

Gubrium, A., & K. Harper. (2013). *Participatory visual and digital methods*. Walnut Creek: Left Coast Press.

Gullón, P., J. Díez, P. Conde, C. Ramos, V. Márquez, H. Badland, … M. Franco. (2019). Using photovoice to examine physical activity in the urban context and generate policy recommendations: The Heart Healthy Hoods study. *International Journal of Environmental Research and Public Health, 16*(5), 749. doi:10.3390/ijerph16050749

Harper, D. (2003). Framing photographic ethnography: A case study. *Ethnography, 4*(2), 241–266. doi:10.1177/14661381030042005

Harrison, B. (2002). Seeing health and illness worlds – Using visual methodologies in a sociology of health and illness: A methodological review. *Sociology of Health & Illness, 25*(6), 856–872. doi:10.1111/1467-9566.00322

Healey, G. K., K. M. Magner, R. Ritter, R. Kamookak, A. Aningmiuq, B. Issaluk, & P. Moffit. (2011). Community perspectives on the impact of climate change on health in Nunavit, Canada. *Arctic, 84*(1), 89–97. doi:10.14430/arctic4082

Kolb, B. (2008). Involving, sharing, analysing – potential of the participatory photo interview. *Forum: Qualitative Social Research, 9*(3). doi:10.17169/fqs-9.3.1155.

Kolb, B. & L. S. Lorenz. (2014). Let's see: Participatory visual methods in practice. In C. Fogel, E. Quinlan, & A. Quinlan (Eds.), *Imaginative inquiry: Innovative approaches to interdisciplinary research* (pp. 79–92). Palo Alto: Academica Press.

Kolb, B., & L. S. Lorenz. (2020 forthcoming). Photo interview and photovoice: Engaging research participants, empowering voice, and generating knowledge for change. In P. Bernhardt, R. Breckner, K. Liebhard, & M. Pohn-Lauggas (Eds.), *Visual analysis from socio-scientific perspectives*. Berlin: De Gruyter.

Leon-Quijano, C. (2017). Visual ethnography: Tools, archives and research methods. *Visual Ethnography, 6*(1), 7–17. doi:10.12835/ve2017.1-0073

Lorenz, L. S. (2011). A way into empathy: a 'case' of photo-elicitation in illness research. *Health (London), 15*(3), 259–275. doi:10.1177/1363459310397976

Lorenz, L. S., & B. Kolb. (2009). Involving the public through participatory visual research methods. *Health Expect, 12*(3), 262–274. doi:10.1111/j.1369-7625.2009.00560.x

Mattouk, M., & S. N. Talhouk. (2017). A content analysis of nature photographs taken by Lebanese rural youth. *PloS One, 12*(5), e0177079–e0177079. doi:10.1371/journal.pone.0177079

McLellan, T., A. Bishop, & A. McKinlay. (2010). Community attitudes toward individuals with traumatic brain injury. *Journal of the International Neuropsychological Society, 16*(4), 705–710. doi:10.1017/S1355617710000524

Mitchell, C. (2011). *Doing visual research*. London: Sage Publications Ltd.

North, N., S. Sieberhagen, A. Leonard, C. Bonaconsa, & M. Coetzee. (2019). Making children's nursing practices visible: Using visual and participatory techniques to describe family involvement in the care of hospitalized children in Southern African settings. *International Journal of Qualitative Methods, 18*, 1–18. doi:10.1177/1609-406919849324

Pink, S. (2001). *Doing visual ethnography: Images, media and representation in research*. London, Thousand Oaks, and New Delhi: Sage Publications.

Qaugiartiit/Arctic Health Research Network. (2008). Reviewer health research ethics checklist (draft). library.vlt.is/89/1/Ethics%20Review%20Checklist%20-%20draft%20-%20March%202008.pdf

Riessman, C. K. (2008). *Narrative methods for the human sciences*. Los Angeles: Sage Publications.

Rose, G. (2016). *Visual methodologies: An introduction to researching with visual materials – 4th Edition*. London: Sage Publications Ltd.

Wang, C. C. (1999). Photovoice: A participatory action research strategy applied to women's health. *Journal of Women's Health, 8*(2), 185–192. doi:10.1089/jwh.1999.8.185

Wang, C. C., & M. A. Burris. (1997). Photovoice: Concept, methodology, and use for participatory needs assessment. *Health Education & Behavior, 24*(3), 369–387. doi:10.1177/109019819702400309

Wang, C. C., M. A. Burris, & X. Y. Ping. (1996). Chinese village women as visual anthropologists: A participatory approach to reaching policymakers. *Social Science & Medicine, 42*(10), 1391–1400. doi: 10.1016/0277-9536(95)00287-1

PART VI

Auto/ethnography

15

INSTITUTION(ALIZATION), BUREAUCRACY, AND WELL-BEING?

An organizational ethnography of perinatal care within the National Health Service

Tom Vine

Introduction

The NHS is a highly politicised creation. The political left has long regarded it as principal pillar of a socially-conscious ideology. To the extent that it is now an integrant part of British tradition, those at the more conservative end of the political spectrum regard it with a sense of pride, too. However, the NHS has frequently been the subject of bitter critique in terms of its resourcing, provision, and specific purpose. Such critique is routinely invoked to win political points. Equally, spin doctors are often charged with developing campaigns to convince the public that opposition parties are not sufficiently committed to the NHS. For example, at the time of publication there was a frenzy of reports in the British media of Prime Minister Boris Johnson's alleged negotiations with US President Donald Trump to "sell off" the NHS to the Americans. In all probability these allegations were untrue. They do, however, illustrate the public's preoccupation with the NHS.

The point of this chapter is not so much to defend the NHS against the specific criticism with which it is routinely charged, but to bring to the fore the unseen and intangible aspects of its role. This necessitates a shift in mindset; it is not that the NHS needs to be run "more efficiently" as the prevalent counternarrative would have it, but that its institutional character and influences must be properly acknowledged if we are to reflect more meaningfully on the experiences it affords. I urge readers to consider both the hospital and the NHS as anthropological phenomena, rather than socially inert brokers of clinical expertise. To this end, in a (post-) industrial world, hospitals – and organizations more generally – have, to some degree at least, assumed the role of wider kin or provincial community. Organizations are not simply economic expediencies but are principal brokers of shared experience, identity, and existential security.

Reflecting on the ethnographic data presented, I challenge the negative perception of the NHS by suggesting that well-being (of newborn, family, and the wider community) is realised, not just through clinical expertise, midwifery, and caregiving but through the institutional characteristics inherent to health provision within the NHS. Rather than regard the NHS – and hospitals generally – as a necessary "institutional evil", it is through the very dynamics of the institutional culture they represent that a sense of health and well-being is routinely realised.

Institutions and institutionalization

On the very first page of *Modern Organizations* (1964), the eminent sociologist Amitai Etzioni penned the following:

> Our society is an organizational society. We are born in organizations, educated by organizations, and most of us spend much of our lives working for organizations. We spend much of our leisure time paying, playing, and praying in organizations. Most of us will die in an organization, and when the time comes for burial, the largest organization of them all – the state – must grant official permission.

As an organization theorist and ethnographer I recognise, perhaps more so than most, that organizations have become an integral part of our human geography. But what of *institutions*? In some respects the words organization and institution are synonymous; they refer to common underlying anthropological phenomena. But while the word organization is typically used positively, the same is not always true in respect of institution. This chapter deploys the latter label, in part in a bid to better understand – and challenge – its negative reputation but also because the derivative concept of institutionalization is relevant, too. It is worth stressing that the institution that tops and tails life (in terms of birth and death) for most of us in the industrialised world is the hospital; and in the UK, this is typically an NHS-affiliated hospital.

The words "institution" and "institutionalization" are routinely invoked negatively. Indictment comes from both the political left (consider, for example, the Left's preference for rehabilitation in place of incarceration as a means of addressing crime) and the political right (just try searching "NHS" on *The Daily Mail* website!). The bulk of the academic literature takes a comparable position. The scholarly attitude towards institutions – as distinct from organizations – has been molded by a critical discourse in which Goffman's (1961) "total institutions" and Foucault's (1973) prisons and psychiatric hospitals have become ingrained in the scholarly psyche as representative examples, so much so that Burrell (1988, 1997) suggests that the dark forces of institutionalization are latent in *all* organizations.

Institutions, we routinely tell ourselves, are inherently *dys*functional. But to what degree does this attitude resonate with formal definitions? The Oxford English Dictionary lists three definitions of institutionalization:

1. The action of establishing something as a convention or norm in an organization or culture.
2. The state of being placed or kept in a residential institution.
3. Harmful effects such as apathy and loss of independence arising from spending a long time in an institution.

While the second and particularly the third definition allude to the concept's negative characteristics (which Goffman, Foucault and Burrell all invoke), the first – and *primary* – definition is perfunctory. Indeed, in this primary sense, institutionalization innocuously describes the manner in which we assume the characteristics of an organization – how we are *enculturated*. And this, of course, is an intrinsic aspect of our social and organizational lives. While I have no desire to fall prey to accusations of misplaced concreteness, it is I think fair to say that we almost always think of institutions and institutionalization in terms of the subsidiary definitions, ignoring the functional – perhaps even positive – aspects conveyed in this primary definition. By way of illustration, think about how the word is assimilated in popular parlance. It tends to be used in very specific contexts. For example, it invokes the ideas of *being institutionalized*, or *institutional racism* or – simply – *bureaucracy*. Indeed, we tend either to assume that institutions have a totalising, oppressing, and alienating agenda or, for the less vociferous, that institutions both rely on and proliferate devitalising bureaucracy. Neither is empirically accurate, and yet such damnation persists. As recently as 2016, Graeber, for example, penned the following: "What the public, the workforce, the electorate, consumers, and the population all have in common is that they are brought into being by institutionalized frames of action that are inherently bureaucratic, and therefore, profoundly alienating. They are the instruments through which the human imagination is smashed and shattered" (Graeber, 2016, 99). Bureaucracies are by no means perfect. However, as we've noted of institutions more generally, it would be a mistake to overlook the fact that the conventional – and almost exclusively negative – perception of bureaucracy represents a convenient whipping boy irrespective of political hue. In *The Case for Bureaucracy,* Goodsell, for example, reflects on the fact that:

> Bureaucracy… is said to sap the economy, endanger democracy, suppress the individual and be capable of embodying evil. It is denounced on the right by market champions and public-choice theorists and on the left by Marxists, critical theorists, and postmodernists. One side of the political spectrum finds bureaucracy a convenient target because it represents taxes, regulations and big government, the other sees it as representing elitism, injustice to the underprivileged, and social control.
>
> *(Goodsell, 2004, 17)*

For Kallinikos (2006, 611), too: "The prevailing negative sentiment bureaucracy tends to evoke reflects a crooked… historical trajectory that has been engraved by a variety of socio-cultural conditions and forces that traverse the entire ideological and political spectrum of modern society". The overwhelmingly negative narrative associated with bureaucracy is attributable to at least two erroneous social inclinations, as Vine (2021) has noted. The first of these is our tendency to conflate bureaucracy's pathological extremes with its everyday reality. The second is the perennial misrepresentation of bureaucracy in the arts, specifically in dystopian literature and cinema (everything from Kafka's *The Trial* to Gilliam's *Brazil* have molded our attitudes towards bureaucracy). The problem here is that casting bureaucracy in this way ignores the existential value of institutions. As the celebrated theorist of bureaucracy Max Weber noted over a century ago, institutions provide a sense of routine, security, and predictability. To this end, a counter argument – that institutions may actually be *anti*-alienating – is beginning to gain traction. In recent years, a distinct cadre of scholars has presented data supporting this position: du Gay (1994, 2000, 2004, 2005, 2011), Goodsell (2003), Kallinikos (2003, 2004, 2006), and Styhre (2007) are foremost among their ranks. Interestingly, in many cases these scholars argue that it is actually *post*-bureaucratic endeavours that represent the greater concern in respect of alienation. Indeed, Vine (2018) reveals data that support precisely this: for the subjects of his research the wholesale movement away from the sense of existential identity and ontological security institutions provide was profoundly unsettling.

It is thus against this overwhelmingly negative perception of both institutions and bureaucracy that the NHS is compelled to continually defend and legitimise itself. Notwithstanding the defense outlined, I by no means wish to suggest that institutions are beyond reproach. Clearly not. I simply wish to suggest that a fresh approach to viewing the NHS-as-institution can be realised by viewing the institutional and bureaucratic aspects of the NHS not as necessary evils, but as important conditioning factors in and of themselves.

Method

I have presented a broad defense of the ethnographic method elsewhere (see Vine, Clark, Richards, & Weir 2018) and do not plan to rehearse this here. However, the ethnography presented in this chapter is rather different; it is an ethnography of convenience, an "opportunistic ethnography", if you will. My daughter, Sophie, was born in 2018 and in the run up to her birth I thought it would be interesting to experience and explore the event through the medium of ethnography. Now, I recognise entirely that this was to be a controversial decision. Would it be disrespectful to my wife? Would it be disrespectful to my new-born? Would it be disrespectful to my wider family? Would it be disrespectful to the hospital? I grappled with the ethics and found sanctuary in Briony Campbell's *The Dad Project* (2009). Through the medium of photography, Campbell documented her father's gradual demise from cancer. When her work was professionally exhibited, she commented that she too had debated whether or not to pursue the project. Ultimately, her father supported her in the decision to do it. Her work won numerous awards and is now a principal part of her father's legacy. Of course, while Campbell's work documented end-of-life hospital care, mine would focus on start-of-life.

My data is presented in the form of edited notes from a diary I kept at the time. True to the ethnographic spirit, I was careful to collect and convey as much detail as possible: in respect of people, processes, and physical environments. As an organization theorist, however, my primary focus was on recording, digesting and interpreting the *organizational dynamics* encountered. The entries in italics are repurposed directly from the diary I kept, and are presented in chronological order. The names of hospital personnel are pseudonymised throughout.

The story

Thursday 4th October 2018

Becky is 38 weeks pregnant. She didn't sleep at all last night and feels itchy all over. We ring the midwife and convey her symptoms. It transpires that she needs to go to hospital for blood tests. Upon arrival there is confusion with respect to the blood forms as by chance there is another Rebecca with a similar surname undergoing identical treatment. The confusion resolved, Becky's blood tests are completed. We're then introduced to a friendly midwife, Nikola, who records the baby's heartbeat and uterine contractions using a cardiotocography (CTG) machine. She suggests that Becky retains the CTG machine straps she's been issued for later tests. "We want to save our NHS money where we can!", she says in a Polish accent. Later, the blood test results confirm that Becky is suffering from cholestasis, a pregnancy-related liver condition. The paediatricians recommend induction because going full term can, apparently, increase the risk of stillbirth. We digest the news. Becky has wanted a natural birth all along. This is a significant deviation from "the plan". They want to admit her on Saturday.

Friday 5th October 2018

It's all happening so quickly. Becky's due date was originally the 15th October and we've assumed all along that since this is her first child, it will be late. We've had building works going on at home in readiness for the baby and the builders are yet to complete the job. The place is covered in dust. In effect, we now have 24 hours to prepare. The nesting begins. We spend the entire day cleaning the house and doing what we can to mitigate the dust. We keep reminding ourselves that our circumstances are not unusual; do any parents return from hospital to the perfect home? And what about the car? It's filthy. And we haven't yet fitted a baby seat. Apparently the hospital will not let you leave without a baby seat.

Saturday 6th October 2018

We're both exhausted. The house is still a little rough round the edges but the car is packed and we need to go. We arrive at the hospital just after 11am as instructed and head to ward F11. The Ward is opposite The Labour Suite, where Becky will eventually give birth. The Labour Suite is itself next to The Birthing Unit. Becky was hoping to give birth in The Birthing Unit, which unlike the Suite is geared towards natural birthing. Those plans have gone out of the window now.

We're welcomed by a very friendly nurse who shows us to Becky's bed. It's a bit like being at a hotel. Her bed is in a very spacious 6-patient bay. Becky has been given a bed by the window. There's a fully reclining chair alongside the bed – apparently for the "birthing partner". I feel a little uncomfortable saying "birthing partner". I recognise that it is deployed for reasons of inclusiveness (good), but can't help feeling it degrades the father's role somewhat (bad). I sit in the chair. It is permanently reclined which is a bit of a problem since I plan to be writing my ethnographic notes in this chair. Hmmm. I'm conscious about keeping notes – I haven't discussed doing so with Becky, let alone any of the hospital staff. I figure that Becky's got enough on her plate without worrying about what I'm up to. I don't mention it to hospital staff, as what is rather innocuous might suddenly raise concern and take on a life of its own. I figure I'm ok. Am I? Yes, this is fine. I think. We're left alone for about an hour to settle in.

Everything is spotlessly clean. There is an entertainment system for Becky to use, similar to those found on long-haul flights. There is a menu listing various options: internet access, TV, radio, films (including pay per view). There is even a power point for charging mobile phones – hospitals have clearly given up the battle trying to prevent patients and their families from using their phones. A woman comes past with a lunch menu. Shortly afterwards another midwife arrives. She takes various particulars, answers questions and reassures Becky. I don't discuss my feelings with Becky but it's at this very point that I begin to feel the warmth of the institution cradle me. It's a trite metaphor but it really does feel appropriate. A little later, while Becky is eating her lunch, I resume writing my diary in violation of my original intentions to only do so when she's sleeping. "What are you writing in your book?" Becky asks. I hesitate. "About hospital", I respond vaguely. "Ah, yes" she says, "That's how you process everything, isn't it?"

The nurses return to administer the first of two pessaries. I ask Claire whether much is likely to happen for a while. She replies, "No. To be honest, you ought to go home and get a good night's sleep". I leave as I hear Becky and Claire engage in the now familiar and ostensibly pointless – conversation about whether she's having a boy or a girl. "We don't know", Becky replies, "we want it to be a surprise". "Oooo" Claire says, "I wanted to know with my two. I couldn't bear the idea of getting lots of pink things, only to have a boy".

Sunday 7th October 2018

I wake at home about 9am. I make myself a coffee and phone Becky. She says she's feeling pretty good. We agree that I will continue with the domestic duties at our house before heading to the hospital for about 2pm. At about 11am, Becky calls and says she'd like me to come in earlier. She's in a fair bit of discomfort. This puts me in a quandary since the house is still not clean. I decide to whip out the Febreze and cut a few corners. I eventually arrive at the hospital for just after 1pm. Becky is experiencing contractions. She's determined to stay mobile and so we walk together to the hospital restaurant. She's breathless and it takes a while to complete the short walk. We're sure to return by 2pm, which is when they need her back. We count the intervals and duration of her contractions and I document the data in a notebook Becky has brought along. A midwife pops her head round at about 3pm to apologise for the delay – she says they're extremely busy. At about 3.30pm Becky begins to get frustrated. The drugs she's been administered are wearing off. "What's the point if they're not going to follow it up as scheduled?", she asks. "I'll have to start the whole process again!" She doesn't mention it but I get the feeling that she's worried about the effects of the delay on our baby. At 4.30pm, she's really distressed. I head to the nurses' station to convey our concerns to the midwives. They are frantically busy. While waiting for a nurse, I peruse the dozens of thank you cards that adorn the station. Without exception, the handwritten messages are glowing in their assessment of their experience on the ward. I eventually speak to the charge nurse. She apologises on behalf of her staff and explains that the delay is down to the fact that there have just been too many high risk patients that take priority.

We hear babies cry elsewhere on the ward – the sound of the "prize" at the end of the journey. My mind begins to wonder. It occurs to me that the sound of a baby crying is not dissimilar to that of an engine starting. Is that an appropriate analogy? The engine starting for the very first time as the car roles off the production line. Goddammit, why am thinking these thoughts? What use are they? Why can't I be useful?

And then – progress – well, at least for the woman in the bay opposite. Her waters break and she's transferred to The Labour Suite. Becky is the sole remaining patient in the bay. "I'll hopefully sleep better tonight", she says. Every cloud has a silver lining. The midwife walks through the door. "It sounds like you guys have been busy today", Becky says cheerfully. "It never rains… .", comes the response. "It's just horrible thinking how much the wait impacts on everybody… not everyone is as patient as you!" Patients have to be patient, I guess.

Heather comes by at about 6.30pm to do another inspection. She says Becky is a "9" and as a result they could technically break her waters now. "Hmmm", the midwife ponders, "I need to consult with my colleagues in The Labour Suite". Initially, we both assume that this is to seek relevant clinical advice. When she returns, however, it becomes apparent that it is really about operational capacity – without saying this in so many words. No matter. The penny has dropped. Health is like any other industry operating with scarce resources. The upshot is they can't fit Becky in right now. In a strange way, Becky is relieved.

At about 10pm, I head off to a local hotel where I've booked a room for the night. On my way out, I see one of my MBA students at the nurses' station. She too is heavily pregnant. It's a bit awkward. What's the protocol for this sort of interaction? I haven't the foggiest. "Good luck", I say.

Monday 8th October 2018

I text Becky at 7am, as planned. She calls me back a few minutes later to say they have transferred her to The Labour Suite and plan to break her waters shortly. I jump in the shower, check out of the hotel and head to the hospital. Upon arrival, I am greeted with the sight of my wife without underwear, waters broken. She's in a very chipper mood. Grinning, in fact. She's been transferred to her own room now. It feels very comfortable. Sunlight floods in through the skylight windows. It's rather beautiful.

We have been allocated another midwife, Toni and a midwifery student, Olivia. Becky and the two midwifes exchange pleasantries. Over the next couple of hours, we establish a wonderful rapport, trading jokes and anecdotes. As Becky's labour progresses, she shifts into her preferred position for giving birth: on all fours. The midwives busy themselves with various tasks, before positioning another cardiotocography machine adjacent to Becky's bed. They attach her CTG straps to Becky's bump. Silence. What the fuck? The reassuring sounds of the baby's heartbeat are absent.

[MY NOTES ARE INCIPHERABLE AT THIS POINT, FOR APPROXIMATELY HALF A PAGE]

They eventually find the heartbeat. I breathe an immense – and audible – sigh of relief. I study the midwives' faces. They maintain complete professionalism, but it is clear that this was a tense episode. As the heartbeat settles back into a steady rhythm, Toni explains to Becky that while she understands why it is that some women prefer to give birth on all fours, our baby's heart will probably find it easier to do its job in the conventional birthing position. Apparently the conventional position enables easier passage through the birth canal. She's right.

Our baby is born at just after 8pm. She pulls off my glasses at about 15 seconds into life, a trick she's repeated hundreds of times since. The experience is, of course, magical. Later on in the evening, I kiss my wife and new-born goodbye. On my way out of the ward, I notice a poster on the noticeboards: 'EPIC DAD: Restoring the Role of Fathers'. EPIC apparently stands for Encourager, Provider, Instructor and Carer. Wow. That's me now! And this poster is far from alone. The whole wall is plastered with notes of practical advice for new dads and advertisements for local self-help fatherhood groups. In my experience these sorts of notices (in GP Surgeries or Council offices, for example) normally target vulnerable sections of the community. As an educated white male, I'm unused to being targeted in this way. It feels strangely compelling.

Tuesday 9th October 2018

I text Becky at 7.50am and say I am on my way back to the hospital. I haven't slept very well; I was far too concerned about my new-born. I arrive at the hospital just after 9am. Becky hasn't slept well either, unsurprisingly. It is lovely to see them both. I kiss my daughter on the forehead as she sleeps in her crib. It feels unworldly. Becky is struggling with the feeding. Our baby appears to be too sleepy to feed but Becky is worried that the lack of sustenance is compounding the sleepiness: a vicious circle. A nurse called Matilda drops by and Becky explains the dilemma. Though young (early 20s) she's a no nonsense character. Matilda fetches a syringe and instructs Becky to express some colostrum. Matilda then dispenses the contents of the syringe directly into our baby's mouth. As she settles into my arms, we discuss baby names. We decide on Sophie. We both rather like the Ancient Greek etymology.

While Sophie sleeps, I listen to the conversations going on in the adjacent bays. Around one bed, the extended family has arrived and the customary conversation in respect of resemblance circulates. "I think I can see a bit of Robert in the baby's eyes…".. "Oh, I'm not sure, I think the baby looks more like Tristan's Dad". You get the idea. In another bay, a young couple trade insults and expletives. It is a stressful time that is bound to put tensions on already fragile relationships. Eventually, the Dad rings his own father and persuades him to collect them. "I'll pay you for the diesel money", he says down the phone. "It will probably be cheaper than the bus anyway". They apparently agree a rate and tensions begin to subside. A little later, a nurse – who I suspect was privy to this conversation too – drops by and suggests they stay another night in hospital. My suspicion is that this isn't strictly for clinical reasons, but to help ameliorate tensions. In another bay, a paediatrician addresses another new Dad, explaining that they are concerned about the baby's hips. "You'll receive details on an appointment in the post regarding an x-ray, scheduled for about 6 weeks from now. It is important that you keep the appointment". The Dad looks anxious. "Thing is", comes his response, "it really depends whether or not we can afford to get to the hospital.... we live an hour away and money is tight". The paediatrician empathises and reassures them that they will work out a way to minimise the financial impact.

Listening to these conversations brings home the reality of childrearing for low income families. And it feels particularly difficult to stomach given the fact that throughout this whole day, a professional photographer goes from bed to bed trying to persuade families to fork out for a photo shoot; she is representative of Bounty (a promotions company that provides new mothers with sample baby products; the infamous 'Bounty Pack'). She offers to take photos of your new-born with or without family and arrange prints in an array of sizes, mouse mats and keyrings. The conversation she has with the single mother to the bed next to us is especially revealing: "Would you like a professional photoshoot?" "To be honest", comes the response, "I have a photographer booked to take photos at home". "When is that booked for?", the photographer asks. "Well, that photographer said to call and book it as soon as I'm home and settled". "Well, the thing is", the Bounty photographer replies, "babies change so fast at this age that by the time you get photographed, your baby will have changed and you've lost the opportunity forever". At this point, the din of the hospital drowns out the conversation. Ultimately, I'm unsure whether the new mum succumbed to the pressures of the photographer. I really hope she didn't.

Discussion

The NHS is an institution designed principally to deliver clinical care on a national scale. But interpretation of the ethnographic data presented suggests it can be cast in other significant ways too: as *existentially-secure environment;* as *resource maximiser,* as *broker of community relations;* as *mediator between clinical orthodoxy and cultural contingency;* as *fractional matriarchy;* and as *validating institution.* Each is examined below.

NHS as existentially-secure environment: Bureaucracy is often assumed to be alienating; in practice, however, it is pivotal in realising a sense of security. On the face of it, an NHS hospital is considered to be secure purely in terms of physical security: swipe-card entry, video surveillance and personnel verification. But the sense of security it provides goes much deeper. The hospital perdures beyond the shift of any single member of staff. The concept of "the midwife" is a case in point. The midwife is rarely a single individual; technically it describes an office. Over the duration of Becky's pregnancy, we probably saw over a dozen midwives and yet, routinely referred to this as a distinct role: that of *the midwife.* More generally, the institution – bricks, mortar, and cultural entity – is a constant. It is for this reason, of course, that patients feel so wonderfully cosseted with. A cursory read of the thank you cards that are displayed round the nurses station – and indeed beyond – are testament to precisely this. Yes, the names of specific midwives are noted and individually thanked, but the central narrative presented in almost all of the cards I read is that the entire perinatal experience was expertly managed. In many cases this seems to come as a surprise. Of course, the birth of a child is a cause for celebration; but for many it is assumed that this is *in spite of* rather than *because of* the experience afforded by the hospital. The NHS hospital *is* a community; it serves as host to a complex organizational culture and it is a broker of identity. One is reminded of the film *Shawshank Redemption.* Upon release from prison after a life of incarceration Brooks hangs himself.

Far be it for me to suggest that hospitals are directly comparable to prisons (although as Foucault has famously observed, as institutions they are not dissimilar); the important point is that they serve as vital community and identity workspaces, a theoretical concept developed by Petriglieri and Petriglieri (2010). This is, I think, at least part of the reason the couple in one of the adjacent bays were so relieved when the paediatrician suggested that they stay another night.

NHS as resource-maximiser. I do not purport to suggest that my study represents a systematic evaluation of resource use within the NHS. Nonetheless, my training as a management academic has primed me to evaluate my various organizational experiences in terms of efficiency. To this end, I couldn't help but notice the specific manner in which discourses of resource preservation underpinned the perinatal experience. On the one hand it was clear to see how commercial pressures manifest themselves; the presence – and persistence – of the Bounty photographer was especially unnerving in this respect. But ultimately the Bounty episode represented a side of the operation that was peripheral to the perinatal experience. On the one hand, the presence of the photographer felt invasive; on the other – and notwithstanding the long-term game Bounty is playing in eliciting a sense of brand loyalty, the free products it supplies to new parents (some of whom are extremely cash-strapped) are appreciated. What was clear is that NHS money is being spent in areas that mattered; the various wards associated with perinatal care appeared to be extremely well staffed and the clinical care was excellent. In this respect, commercial considerations remained firmly subordinate to patient care. Resource preservation typically manifested itself in less evasive ways. A very clear example of this was Nikola's suggestion that Becky retain the CTG straps she was issued when we first arrived at the Hospital such that they could be used throughout the perinatal period. It felt especially pertinent that the advice was conveyed in a Polish accent. This was, I felt, a rather nice bringing together of international communities and their shared sense of the value and importance of the NHS, and particularly so in a multicultural climate muddied by the prospect of Brexit. More difficult to discern, however, was the fact that birth partners took on what I refer to in a forthcoming publication as "negotiated nursing". To this end, birthing partners are (a) afforded a sense of involvement, and (b) free up clinical staff to focus their energies on those patients who are either in need of more complex clinical attention and/or do not have familial support on hand. At one point I felt frustrated that I wasn't being useful, but upon later reflection I realised that my role as "birthing partner" was indeed more than to provide proverbial moral support: I regularly made Becky's bed and generally kept house. I brokered discussions between Becky and the clinicians at key moments, particularly when Becky was in a pain or felt anxious. I was even able to assist in terms of recording key medical information, such as Becky's contraction intervals. Now, the extent to which the involvement of family members in this way is a conscious aspect of the operational design isn't clear. My suspicion is that this is done intuitively and, as a practice is implicit rather than explicit. It has, in all likelihood, evolved naturally; the midwife's comment that "not everyone is as patient as you" is, I think, instructive in this sense. The hospital makes judicious decisions taking into consideration the support networks each patient has at their disposal. This approach represents a formidable challenge to the prevalent narrative that institutions and the bureaucracies they spawn are faceless, senseless, and de-individuating.

NHS as broker of community relations. One of the most remarkable aspects of the experience was the fact that it brought together people from very different walks of life. The interaction with families in adjacent bays both prior to and after the birth of our baby was illuminating. In my line of work as a university lecturer I rarely have an opportunity to interact with people from different social backgrounds. In an NHS hospital, you have no choice. Now, this all might sound delightfully patronising but it most definitely isn't intended to. While it certainly brings home the very different environments and networks of opportunity that babies are born into – even in a relatively affluent part of a developed nation – it was revealing to note how each of us seemed to appreciate and marvel at the hospital experience. We did not hear a single raised voice or complaint trained at the institution or its processes; it was, on the contrary, nothing but praise. And where we did witness tensions, these were inter-familial tensions with regards to personal finances, which the hospital did its very best to help ameliorate. Of course, and as the data show, the NHS is no utopia. The commercial pressures of the photography was, as noted, rather unsettling. But then, I have no doubt that such a measure would have been evaluated in utilitarian terms; the freebies offered to new parents (and the likely financial rewards attributed to the hospital itself) most likely outweighing the negatives associated with the commercial pressure heaped on patients.

Given the sense of community brokered by the institution, it is perhaps unsurprising that it delineates specific topics of conversation, too. One of the regular discursive tropes associated with both antenatal and perinatal experience is regarding the anticipated gender of the child. Initially, this was something I found vacuous and tiresome, even irritating. Eventually, however, I realised that it is not so much that people are genuinely interested in the sex of an unknown baby; rather this particular conversation serves as an anthropological medium. It is not just *something to talk about,* but it is a shared un/known which connects us and reveals something about one another. Becky's interaction with Claire was instructive in this sense. Claire commented that she wanted to know the gender of her second child in advance, because she couldn't bear the prospect of buying pink baby paraphernalia only to discover that she should have bought blue. Now, this sort of justification is unlikely to have had much traction with Becky, as a feminist. However, at the time rather than insincerely concurring or challenging the nurse in respect of gender politics, she rather shrewdly pointed out that where there's a sibling involved (which presumably there was in the case of Claire's second child), that sibling probably wants to know the sex in advance. Moreover, in the case of the clinician-patient dialogue, the conversation about prospective gender serves a second purpose: it has a cultural-therapeutic function. Patients appear to appreciate these exchanges of words precisely because they are *not* clinical; they alleviate anxiety.

It is, then, with these observations in mind that mothers-to-be and their birthing partners who are considering a home birth (or a birth in purportedly more natural environments) would do well to remember that the institution – the hospital – in our case the NHS, is not always an abstract representation of an oppressive patriarchal regime. To the extent that our experience is at least to some degree representative, parents who regard the only advantage of giving birth in a "clinical" environment is proximity to specialist care (should something not go according to plan), would do well to appreciate that the hospital is much more than a mediator of clinical expertise; it is a highly cultural – and enculturating – space. In a world in which ties of kinship and indigenous community have been displaced, it conveys a sense of community; it rekindles relations between different people's perceptions, hopes, and fears that we rarely have the opportunity to experience. For a brief period, at least, everything is taken care of for you; you are cocooned. It is, quite possibly, the closest most of us will get to a direct experience "of the state" at any point in our lives; it is also one of those rare occasions when the institution of family and the institution of the state are brought together.

NHS as mediator between clinical orthodoxy and cultural contingency. Given its clinical remit, it is to be expected that the NHS assumes a role of "safety expert", "educator" (as evidenced through the leaflets, posters and various online facilities) and "formal advisor". What is, perhaps, more noteworthy is that our experience suggests that the NHS is remarkably sensitive to cultural preferences. In the months leading up to the birth, Becky had undertaken extensive research regarding the childbirth process and had been persuaded that the convention of giving birth lying down on one's back was the result of a patriarchal healthcare discourse which puts control of the patient at the centre of its practice, often without realising it. As such, Becky had envisaged a birth on all fours, which is – apparently – more natural. Or, at least, this is the prevalent bourgeois narrative. Ultimately, Becky's birth plan reflected her desire to give birth on all fours. The midwives were acutely aware of this, and tried to accommodate it. They only intervened – and did so extremely sensitively – when it became clear that this preference may well have been restricting Sophie's passage through the birth canal. To this end, Becky's cultural preferences prevailed until the point at which their presence compromised our baby's safety.

The NHS as fractional matriarchy. It would be disingenuous, misleading, and rather patronising to suggest that NHS perinatal care is "run by women". What is clear, however, is that it might legitimately be cast as a fractional matriarchy: the perinatal institutional experience is one which, on the face of it at least, is mediated through a women-dominated environment. One of the diary entries from the 8th October reveals my own reflections on this at the time:

> Chitchat is something I've never quite got the hang of. This is, a woman-dominated environment. In fact, aside from birthing partners, there isn't a single male member of staff. Nurses, doctors, obstetricians, paediatricians, cleaners, housekeeping staff – all are women. As a result, a woman-centric culture dominates. The chitchat is most likely a technique the clinical staff use to help make patients feel at ease, but it feels natural rather than engineered. Are woman better at chitchat than men? Is it fair to ask these sorts of question?

Beyond observations in respect of conversational dynamics, it was also interesting to note that to some degree stereotypical gender relations appear to be reversed; women dominate the organizational environment while the posters on the wall are dedicated to male self-help groups and fathers-to-be camaraderie.

NHS as validating institution. The unborn baby is inscribed onto the bureaucratic apparatus long before the birth itself. We received the 28-page Pregnancy Notes booklet on our first midwifery appointment, which took place at our GP surgery. The midwife referred to this as "the bible", and it would – apparently – accompany us throughout Becky's pregnancy. Becky was instructed to bring it with her to each midwifery appointment and to any other medical meeting. In this day of electronic communication, the booklet felt rather reassuring. It was gradually filled in as Becky's pregnancy progressed and we completed the midwifery visit schedule. As I've argued elsewhere (see Vine, 2021), documentation or "paperwork" provides a sense of continuity; in this case continuity between hospital visits, different clinicians and other hospital stakeholders. To this end, it is an important bureaucratic artefact: hence "the bible". Upon arrival at the hospital, Becky was required to hand over this booklet. It later transpired that it wasn't to be returned to us. Interestingly, Becky revealed to me that this made her feel rather sad. In its place, however, we received a "My Personal Child Health Record" book, which has since become known as *Sophie's Red Book*. It serves a similar purpose, but focused this time on the infancy period.

The Pregnancy Notes and *Sophie's Red Book* are of course just two examples of how the NHS can be presented as a validating institution. More broadly, it is worth noting that everything is documented: from the meal choices for the mothers, the new born baby's feeding schedule, the decanted colostrum, the baby's weight, visiting hours, staff rosters. Perhaps most important of all, however, is the clipboard that graces the foot of the bed and "travels" with the patient as she moves around the hospital. These, of course, are the medical notes that provide the backbone of the clinical care; they frame it and co-construct its narrative.

Concluding thoughts

In my native field – organization theory – there is an ostensible distinction between "organization" (generally viewed positively) and "institution" (generally viewed negatively). As we have seen, however, this distinction is largely unfounded. Both refer to a common underlying anthropological phenomenon; a collective cultural entity. Institutionalization is rarely – if ever – paired with well-being. In fact, it is often assumed that institutionalization is more naturally paired with "*unwell-being*". As Graeber (2016) notes, institutions are "supposed to be alienating". The data imparted here challenges this portrayal.

It is not so much that we need to take more notice of positive – but often glib – comments about the NHS such as "those nurses work *so* hard", or "they're doing their best with very limited resources". Ultimately, comments such as these simply reinforce a perception that the NHS is a dysfunctional organization that subsists on the basis of goodwill. No, the provision of clinical expertise is just one aspect of healthcare. It is the institution that provides the experience; it is the institution that brokers the culture; it is the institution that affords a rare coming together of different walks of life, of different generations, of different ethnicities. In a secularized and increasingly commercialised existence, experiences such as this offer an invaluable glimpse of a shared purpose. Without wishing to discredit private providers of healthcare who doubtless do a terrific job, the services they offer are crafted in such a way that they afford the "customer" an array of choices in terms of healthcare plans, appointment times, and treatment options. In effect, they endeavour to provide their customers with a sense of control. But is such control necessarily desirable? One of the virtues of the NHS is that it necessitates the relinquishing of our control and this has a desirable existential effect: we feel cradled. To this end, we might feel vindicated in challenging the various adverse connotations of the word institutionalization. Such connotations include incarceration, racism, and – simply - bureaucracy. As an alternative to these negative quips, on occasion the lexicon affords instances of the term deployed in a more positive sense. For example, Brown's (2016) popular book *The Pub: A Cultural Institution*. The word here is understood in a desirable sense; the pub reflects a sense of community, tradition, and kinship. Pubs and hospitals are not dissimilar in these respects but – regrettably – this is rarely acknowledged in the case of the latter. As I pen these words (March 2020), the COVID-19 crisis is just unfolding. Calamitous as it is, one silver lining is that the crisis appears to have rekindled widespread respect and support for the NHS. Perhaps this represents a good opportunity for us to recognise the vitality of its institutional credentials.

And, finally; I wish to reflect on the nature of opportunistic ethnography. The ethnographic account delineated in this chapter can be described as opportunistic in at least two senses. First, it is opportunistic in that I was presented with a life experience and took the decision to interpret it through an academic lens; it wasn't formally arranged. Second, I recorded ethnographic notes both discreetly and only when time permitted (principally when my wife was sleeping and when my assistance – either emotional or physical – was not required). I thus "did ethnography" only when presented with opportunities to do so; I thus had very little control over the data collection schedule. On reflection, however, this experience of "opportunistic ethnography" wasn't altogether different to the more conventional – planned – ethnographies that I have undertaken in the past. Even when properly planned, and with solicited ethics approval, it is off-putting to scribble notes down while the action unfolds in front of you. (This is of course why ethnographers have a reputation for weak bladders; they must regularly scurry off to the toilet to write up their notes).

As this was opportunistic ethnography, there are two pertinent questions we are compelled to address. The first: is this *academic* research? Ethnographers – especially auto-ethnographers – are forced to routinely deflect vitriolic attack (see, for example, Delamont 2007), and I suspect that the notion of opportunistic ethnography will be especially troubling for such antagonists.

But I remain convinced not only that it is academic research, but that it offers insights which alternatives are unable to provide. While a more conventional, etic, positivist approach will have been able to report on broader trends about patient satisfaction, such approaches are unlikely to have yielded the sense of nuance and analytical depth presented here. It is hoped that this chapter has demonstrated to readers that our attitudes to both institutionalization and bureaucracy are somewhat skewed. The NHS – and hospitals more generally – are more than innocuous "providers"; they are cultural entities. In 2017, the British media reported on a man who had refused to leave his hospital bed for two years. Inevitably, the media were savage in their assessment of the circumstances; the man was labelled a "bed-blocker", pure and simple. Now, while his hospital residence clearly doesn't make financial sense, it does – I think – help illustrate the fact that hospitals are communities; they are agents of kin and are hence deeply social spaces. Women are, of course, welcome to give birth at home or elsewhere (my wife flirted with the idea of giving birth in a forest, for example) by way of "recreating" a "more natural" experience. But to what end? In one sense, these alternatives are indeed more natural; in another sense, however, they represent a wholesale rejection of community. We have, it seems, created a bourgeois discourse which tends to regard hospitals and the administration of clinical care as anti-community and anti-natural. This position lacks nuance; it is an over-simplification.

The second question: is this work *ethical*? As opportunistic ethnography, clearly the research could not involve advanced formal solicitation of ethical approval. Consequently, during the review process for this chapter, the editors suggested it might be best to frame the chapter not as research (since the orthodox academic research process necessitates formal ethical approval) but as "a reflective account". I'm perfectly content with this latter label but wish to stress that the distinction between "research" on the one hand and "reflective account" on the other is not necessarily instructive. On the face of it, a strict ethics approval process is desirable. However, there is a body of work that is beginning to challenge this assumption. For example, in their exploration of the ethical practices inherent to ethnography, Fine and Shulman (2009) note that non-disclosure of research intent (in the various forms of "faux-friendliness", "inverse-plagiarism" or "self-censorship", for example) are both inevitable and often ethically *desirable*. This is something that is echoed in Bochner and Ellis's (2016) work on ethical quandaries in autoethnography. Similar conclusions include research by Thomas, Hujala, Laulainen, and McMurray (2018) in respect of what they refer to as "wicked problems". More recently, Vine (2018) has theorised these tensions as "methodological paradoxes". Collectively, this emerging body of work reveals a greater degree of complexity in respect to research ethics than is routinely acknowledged by university ethics approval processes. This body of work raises at least three important points worth considering: (i) exercising respect and sensitivity to participants is, ironically, often only achieved by circumventing official ethics documentation and formal solicitation of approval; (ii) overly-authoritarian ethics approval processes are likely to yield more in the way of "under the radar" operations; and (iii) overly-rigid ethics approval processes significantly thwart intellectual creativity and innovation. I daresay many academics reading this book will have had first-hand experience of this final point.

As noted at the outset of this chapter, I grappled with the ethical ramifications of this research throughout the process, but ultimately found sanctuary in the work of Campbell (2009). Having been through the process myself, has my position changed? No. On the contrary there is a compelling argument to suggest that ethnographic work such as that presented is not only legitimate, but that as trained ethnographers we have an active *duty* to reflect on life events in this manner. After all, we have each had an extensive and privileged education and are trained to interpret social interactions in this way. Arguably, then, there is an obligation that we contribute to the ethnographic record wherever possible. As a colleague of mine once noted, if academic ethnographers reject these opportunities, journalists will embrace them instead. I have no desire to cast aspersions over the profession of journalism, but I dread to think what a rabid tabloid reporter might cook up in similar circumstances.

By way of summary reflection, then, my wife was right: ethnography *is* how I process things. Ostensibly, it is about academic research; in reality, it has become a way of life. Auto/ethnography is often charged by critics as self-indulgent. To some degree they are right. What is beyond dispute, however, is that it is cathartic.

References

Bochner, A. P. & Ellis, C. (2016) *Evocative Autoethnography: Writing Lives and Telling Stories*. New York: Routledge.

Burrell, G. (1988) 'Modernism, post modernism and organizational analysis 2: The contribution of Michel Foucault', *Organization Studies*, 9(2): 221–235.

Burrell, G. (1997) *Pandemonium: Towards a Retro-Organization Theory*, London: Sage.

Delamont, S. (2007, September 5–8) *Arguments against Autoethnography,* Paper presented at the British Educational Research Association Annual Conference, Institute of Education, University of London, pp. 1–7.

du Gay, P. (1994) 'Making up managers: bureaucracy, enterprise and the liberal art of separation', *British Journal of Sociology,* 45(4): 655–674.

du Gay, P. (2000) *In Praise of Bureaucracy : Weber, Organization, Ethics*, London: Sage.

du Gay, P. (2004) 'Against 'Enterprise' (but not against 'enterprise', for that would make no sense)', *Organization,* 11(1): 37–57.

du Gay, P. (ed.) (2005) *The Values of Bureaucracy*, Oxford: Oxford University Press.

du Gay, P. (2011) 'Chapter 1: 'Without regard to Persons': Problems of Involvement and Attachment in 'Post-Bureaucratic' Public Management'. In Clegg, S., Harris, M., and Höpfl, H. (Eds.) (2011) *Managing Modernity: Beyond Bureaucracy,* Oxford: Oxford University Press.

Etzioni, A. (1964) *Modern Organizations,* Englewood Cliffs, N.J.: Prentice-Hall.

Fine, G. A. & D. Schulman. (2009). 'Lies from the Field: Ethical Issues in Organizational Ethnography'. In S. Ybema, D. Yanow, H. Wels, & F. Kamsteeg (Eds.), *Organizational Ethnography: Studying the Complexities of Everyday Life* (pp. 177–195). London: Sage.

Foucault, M. (1973) *The Birth of the Clinic: an Archaeology of Medical Perception*. London: Tavistock.

Goffman, E. (1961). *Asylums: Essays on the Social Situation of Mental Patients and Other Inmates,* [1st ed.], Garden City, N.Y.: Anchor Books.

Goodsell, C. (2003) *The Case for Bureaucracy* (2004), Washington DC: CQ Press.

Graeber, D. (2016) *The Utopia of Rules: On Technology, Stupidity, and the Secret Joys of Bureaucracy,* London: Melville House.

Kallinikos, J. (2003). Work, human agency and organizational forms: An anatomy of fragmentation. *Organization Studies*, 24(4): 595–61.

Kallinikos, J (2004) 'The Social Foundations of the Bureaucratic Order', *Organization,* 11(1): 13–36.

Kallinikos, J (2006) 'The institution of bureaucracy: administration, pluralism, democracy: A review article', *Economy and Society,* 35(4): 611–627.

Petriglieri G., & J. Petriglieri. (2010) 'Identity workspaces: The case of business schools', *Academy of Management Learning & Education,* 9(1): 44–60.

Styhre, A. (2007) *The Innovative Bureaucracy: Bureaucracy in an age of fluidity,* London: Routledge.

Thomas, W., A. Hujala, S. Laulainen, & R. McMurray. (2018) *The Management of Wicked Problems in Health and Social Care,* London: Routledge.

The Economist. (2011) "Employment: Defending jobs". 2011-09-12. Accessed 7th December 2019.

Vine, T. (2018) 'Methodology: From Paradigms to Paradox'. In Vine, T., Clark, J., Richards, S., & Weir, D. (Eds.) (2018) *Ethnographic Research and Analysis: Anxiety, Identity and Self,* London: Palgrave Macmillan.

Vine, T. (2018) 'Home-grown Exoticism: Ethnographic Tales from a Scottish New Age Intentional Community'. In Vine, T., Clark, J., Richards, S., & Weir, D. (Eds.) (2018) *Ethnographic Research and Analysis: Anxiety, Identity and* Self, London: Palgrave Macmillan.

Vine, T. (2021) *Bureaucracy: A Key Idea for Business and Society,* London: Routledge.

Vine, T, J. Clark, S. Richards, & D. Weir. (Eds.) (2018) *Ethnographic Research and Analysis: Anxiety, Identity and* Self, London: Palgrave Macmillan.

16

CRITICAL AUTOETHNOGRAPHY AND MENTAL HEALTH RESEARCH

Stacy Holman Jones and Anne Harris

Introduction: A match made in heaven

Today I flew over the Midwest
filling out a questionnaire
on the emotional life of the brain
and personal capacity for resilience
against despair... .

...There are bridges
not built in me...
there are areas
that do not light up—

These lines from Bianca Stone's (2014, p. 11) *Reading a Science Article on the Airplane to JFK* capture the spirit of what creative and critical autoethnographic approaches can bring to mental health research. It is an approach that allows for critical interrogation of cultural structures that alienate, marginalise, and harm; it simultaneously provides a means for affective, evocative renderings of personal experience that go beyond the linear, logical, and representative. Thus, critical autoethnography is perfectly matched for the needs of mental health research, practice, and service provision.

Critical autoethnography is the study and critique of culture through the lens of the self. Autoethnography merges the practices of autobiography—writing about the self—and ethnography—the study of and writing about culture. Critical theory is concerned with understanding institutional, political, social and interpersonal power relations. In the context of autoethnography, this means understanding how our how experiences within cultures are enlarged and/or constrained by relations of power, oppression, and privilege (Holman Jones & Harris, 2018; Boylorn & Orbe, 2013). Thus, the "critical" in critical autoethnography[1] points to how we write about self and culture in dynamic and mutually animating relationship to critical theory.

Critical autoethnography offers health researchers creative ways to share and understand complex and dynamic selves, to engage in difficult conversations in ethical and meaningful ways, and to change how we relate in healthcare contexts, particularly in the area of mental health and wellness. Patricia Leavy (2015) writes that arts-based methods, including critical autoethnography, adapt the "tenets of the creative arts in order to address social research questions in holistic and engaged ways" (p. 4). They "connect us with those who are similar and dissimilar, open up new ways of seeing and experiencing, and illuminate that which otherwise remains in darkness" (Leavy, 2015, p. ix).

This is especially true for people with mental health diagnoses. In *Art Heals* (2004), Shawn McNiff points out that the arts have always been entangled with meaning-making and searching for the self in ways that recognize the complexity and multi-dimensionality of human experience, including psychological distress. Creative and narrative practices contribute significantly to mental health recovery in the areas of self-expression, self-discovery, and the rebuilding of identity that happens when people begin to see themselves as skilled and competent *artists* (Van Lith, Schofield, & Fenner, 2013, p. 13; Howells & Zelnik, 2009, p. 219).

Creative arts strategies have been found to be particularly effective for people who struggle with unstable identities and connections with others, and who are often overwhelmed with complex, often polarising emotions (Morgan, Knight, Bagwash, & Thompson, 2012, pp. 94–95). This fracturing of the self can significantly impact an ability to function in everyday life, to maintain relationships, to deal with stigma, and to achieve recovery (Kerr, Finlayson-Short, McCutcheon, Beard, & Chanen, 2015). One such diagnosis is borderline personality disorder, or BPD.

In this chapter, we explore what critical autoethnographic methods might offer mental health researchers, practitioners, and "people with lived experience"[2] of BPD. We'll do this by bringing the practice of critical autoethnography into conversation with research on arts-based approaches to mental health treatment and recovery. And, true to the commitments of critical autoethnography, we will bring our own stories of mental health diagnoses and stigma into this conversation with the hope that sharing these stories serves as a catalyst for understanding that leads to better ways of living.

BPD and critical autoethnography: Stripping back the insulation of shame

BPD is one of the most frequently diagnosed, yet most complex and misunderstood of all personality disorders (Chanen, Sharp, Hoffman et al., 2007). It is characterized by intense and highly changeable emotions, an unstable sense of self, impulsivity, and anti-social behaviours (NIMH 2020). As a result, people with BPD diagnoses often endure not only the burden of relational unintelligibility but also considerable societal stigma and significant levels of vilification from within health services (Veysey, 2014).

In addition, BPD is not only an under-researched area of mental health, it is—like autoethnography—a diagnosis and area of research frequently challenged along criteria of "validity," and "reliability," making both funding and effective care hard to come by (Miller, Muehlenkamp, & Jacobson, 2008). For many, particularly those who are "high-functioning," experiences of BPD are not noticeable or immediately recognisable to others, which throws the "validity" and "reliability" of diagnoses into question.[3] This can make it even harder for the sufferer, their families and healthcare providers to accept, or believe, that someone may have a personalty disorder. Approaches such as critical autoethnography, which help to link personal experience of the sufferers themselves with the current state of play in mental healthcare provision, can be vital to not only understanding but also improving the lived experience of people with mental health disorders (Donald, Duff, Broadbear, Rao, & Lawrence, 2017). This is because critical autoethnography brings together the concrete detail of the personal-in-community in ways that help us understand how stories animate and build affective understanding. Sophie Tamas, an autoethnographer who writes about trauma, mental health, and recovery, observes that

> Autoethnography is like stripping back the insulation of shame and fear and extending a bare-ish wire so that anyone can make a splice, can feel a current of connection, can imagine themselves into a particular body and place and time. This may seem risky but it's less draining than maintaining the illusion of safety… It's a method of attention, of calling myself to account as a practice of care and making-do and thinking-with some kind of community.
>
> *(2017, p. 110)*

For example, Sam Taylor et al.'s (2014) "Writing for Recovery" project illustrates how creative writing like autoethnography is an effective platform for people with long-term mental health conditions because it allows them to craft an individual identity, separate thought or emotion from the writer, and to observe experience from multiple perspectives (p. 5). They note that creative methods can help to "find the voice for newly emerging personal and communal identities beyond diagnoses, enabling the individual and shared re-storying of their past, current, and future experiences" (p. 9). Narrative techniques also offer opportunities to re-story the past while attending to the complex emotions and shifting identities present in any personal account of a life. For people seeking a form through which to tell and re-tell experiences of mental illness, treatment, and recovery, autoethnographic methods enable us to write voice, experience, and theory as "mutually entwined concerns" (Liggins, Kearns, & Adams, 2013, p. 105).

Telling selves: writing voice, experience and theory as mutually entwined concerns

And you have seen someone you love,
With a colossal
complex vehemence, die.
And it is pinned under glass
In perfect condition.

(Stone, 2014, p. 12)

For many people with borderline personality disorder (BPD), experiencing a "self" in relation to others is like riding the waves of the ocean: a constantly moving me who is more like a rise and fall, an encounter with the fleeting promise of a return to the collective "we" of the ocean. Critical autoethnography can help people with BPD diagnoses—indeed, all of us—embrace the difficulty of putting experience into words and make plain the impossibility of narrating a coherent sense of self in and through time (Harris 2014; Tamas 2018, 2013; Holman Jones 2011).

One technique for writing the complexity of self-other relations is to experiment with narrative voice, choosing a mode that reflects various selves and vantage points on experience (Adams & Holman Jones, 2018, pp. 148–150). For example, we can use first person voice to embody a "'confident I' who can proclaim itself and take ownership of the story on the page" (Faulkner & Squillante, 2016, p. 47), even when we don't share that same confidence. By writing in second-person voice—using "you"—we can immerse readers in an experience, showing them how they might feel in another person's shoes (Gutkind, 2008, p. 124). And third-person voice can create "a fitting psychic" distance from experience, allowing us to see things from a new, and sometimes safer, perspective (Wyatt, 2005, p. 814). In the following excerpt of autoethnographic text, Stacy experiments with 2nd person voice as she writes to a loved one lost to complications of anorexia; complications that years later she wonders whether could have been entangled with undiagnosed BPD.

> I knew you first in writings created for my audience—your careful and intricate synthesis of words we read in tandem, treasured course texts forever altered and refined: Annie Dillard's (2000) <u>For the Time Being</u>, Chela Mohanty's (2013) <u>Feminism Without Borders</u>, Wayne Koestembaum's (2001) <u>The Queen's Throat</u>, the whole of Butler, and Acker (1995), and Barthes (1986). Books I fell for in my chosen teacher's classrooms, now in ours. We layered our own speech, mark, and breath over and through these texts, inventing a language full of citation, reverence, remembrance.
>
> And then the stories—always the stories—impossible to accept, exhausting to write and to read: homeless after coming out, the Christian charity of your family a bludgeon; the desperate clutch at control[4] that starvation and compulsive exercising offered; the temporary oblivion of sugar and alcohol. Your brilliant spirit trapped in a weak and wrong body, agent and instrument of an inexhaustible violence.[5]
>
> Out of the chaos your voice called and questioned and I listened and said otherwise. In and through the crippling stories, others were born: unstinting efforts to mend the rift with family, taking their love in spoonfuls; cautious embrace of the curve and heft of flesh; resolute support of others wavering in and out of identity categories. And always, the relief at finding language to story the confusion, fear, and determination into being. At finding the words to tether mind to body and knowledge to desire[6] where they had come undone…
>
> Still, "desire is to lack what one has—and to give what one does not have."[7] This desire, this lack, this borrowed giving were our failure. We lost each other in language—words you could not say, names I could not claim, sentences we could not pry from our hands or loose from our hearts. Our stories became ransom notes, demanding to know what our connection might mean,[8] cataloguing debts we could not repay in text or deed. We wrote each other where we did not—could not—exist.[9] Until nothing was possible except the return of your poetry, my books, our shared history. Letter by letter, we dismantled the alphabet.
>
> *(Holman Jones & Adams, 2014, pp. 106–107)*

★★

While personal narrative makes room for telling stories in rich complexity and detail, experience doesn't always come in the form of a coherent story with a beginning, middle, and end, or even a story at all. In those moments, poetry can offer us a way to write silence, bodies, movement, and complex emotions. Tamas (2018) observes that writing prose allows her to create "a sense of being understood and appreciated" (p. 113), whereas she turns to poetry when she is "undecided, in motion" (2018, p. 113).

Poetry's line breaks and use of stanzas invites writers and readers *into* an experience by asking us to pay attention to rhythm, beat, and breath in equal measure to language. Poetry also asks us to consider how texts are both physical and visual representations that reflect and materialize our experiences, images, and bodies (Adams, Holman Jones, & Ellis, 2014, p. 75). The immersive, sensory-rich, mobile and open-ended nature of poetry is a helpful tool for people living with mental health diagnoses because it offers both a place to express difficult emotions while offering relief from the sense of isolation and othering that so often accompanies them (Bakare, 2009, p. 218).

Poetry also responds to critical autoethnography's call to braid together multiple voices/ perspectives, experiences, and emergent theoretics including affect theory, new materialist theory, and posthuman studies (Gale, 2018, Harris & Holman Jones, 2019, Wyatt, 2018, Wyatt, Harris, Hofsess, Holman Jones, & Murray, 2020). These theoretical frameworks ask us to write how emotions, events, and relationships come to be through tracing the electric current of sensory experience across the body or tracking experience as one would a weather system moving across a landscape. In the next excerpt, Stacy uses poetry as a tool for navigating the difficult emotional landscape of grief and regret that accompany any kind of loss and are perhaps felt more acutely when one loses a loved one to self-inflicted harm. She constructs a call and response poem *in memoria*, stitching together language drawn from personal letters and shared theoretical essays and books:

> *…I unfold all of your letters, trace each line, looking for you, wanting one more moment to gather*
> *and release a handful of your words… .*
> *She questions her name*
> *and the question is you:*
> *Will you continue?*
> *Will you provide?*
> *Could you recognize me?*
>
> *…Stuttering, faltering, shattered.*
> *What does it mean when I say*
> *You have touched me?*
> *To have failed, to have found*
> *what's missing in the wake of me?*
>
> *…In searching for what's missing*
> *in the wake of you. . . .*
> *I want to ask what it means*
> *to "apprehend your life and your death*
> *to give an account of its meaning,*
> *to acknowledge how your life/*
> *is bound to mine."[10]…*
>
> *My every word marked by your*
> *speech, moved by*
> *the flight of your thought.*
> *Each letter a monument undiscovered*
> *until now, until I turn, too late, to write*
> *to you. To dedicate my words,*
> *as they have been without source.*
>
> *…My fingers moving in memoria.*
> *Inscription and that which comes in a dream.*
> *Composing an altar to*
> *losing the alphabet.*
>
> *(Holman Jones & Adams, 2014, pp. 106–107)*

★★

Autoethnographic narrative and poetry offer us tools for writing selves, experiences, and relationships in all of their complexity and unfinishedness. The page is a space brimming with possibility, and we know that carefully crafted language is able to conjure the skin-tingling sense of atmospheres and the body-grip of emotions. When we extend our writing to include texts created for performance, we harness the power of critical performance autoethnography. Critical autoethnographers working in and through the method and lens of performance embrace, rather than erase, embodiment, viewing the body as the source of stories, movements, and speech that is created in the ethnographic exchange (Spry, 2016, p. 35). In the next section, we turn to critical performance autoethnography as a mode of research that focuses explicitly on embodiment, relationships, the affective and emotional in narratives of mental health challenges and does so with the aim of creating change.

Borderlines and belonging: embodying the change we seek

You know this. That the body lays down
while the mind bloats
on intellectual chaos.
And you have just eaten
a bag of cinnamon-flavored chips
and assessed that if you met
a wonderful new person
who ran from you in horror
you would fill their space
with calculated desolation.
(Stone, 2014, pp. 12–13)

The American Art Therapy Association affirms how performance-based approaches provide an "alternative means for communicating for those who cannot find the words to express anxiety, pain, or emotions" (qtd. in Morris, 2018). Performance also allows us to distance ourselves from painful and traumatic experience. For example, character-based work that depends not on mining personal experience but instead on embodying the story of another, can be particularly healing for individuals suffering from forms of mental illness that disrupt or impede a sense of coherent identity.

Catherine Goodwin, a drama therapist who works with people with BPD says that she finds "the distancing in dramatherapy to be essential in this work, enabling clients to openly express their feelings through the character or themes of the story or poem" (qtd in Morris, 2018), offering participants a reparative safe space where feelings and thoughts can be both heard and validated. It allows us to rehearse different ways of being in the world. As drama therapist John Casson puts it,

> in the theatre of our lives we can feel lost, forget our lines, lose a role, feel frozen, unable to move or change: we may need a prompt, a rehearsal for the next scene or to go back to a previous scene and sort it out. Acting can then enable us to move, to change.
>
> *(qtd. In Morris, 2018)*

Similarly, for scholars in the health disciplines, the "personal political body-to-body autoethnographic scholarship is moving us into a deeper epistemological desire" to work collaboratively with "a band of Others to begin and begin again" (Spry, 2016).

In addition to providing a space in which to distance ourselves from painful experience and to try—and safely fail—to rehearse new ways of being in the world, critical performance autoethnography creates "embodied and textual encounters between ourselves and those 'others' our cultures and beliefs have alienated and misunderstood" (Gingrich-Philbrook, 2013, p. 612). For people with BPD diagnoses, who are often those alienated and misunderstood "others," creating encounters in which they have a chance to speak with authority, mastery and, yes, with humour, about themselves and their experiences is a powerful tool. Such encounters allow us to directly address stigma and move us closer to acceptance and change. In the following excerpt from the verbatim play *All The Rage,* which Anne created from conversations with a BPD community in Melbourne, the character Mel rehearses a more confident persona called Brad, evoking identification through humour:

> (*Standup comedy club stage, mic and small table. 42 year old MEL walks to the mic with a buzzer in hand, enters to the soundtrack of "Borderline" by Madonna. Clears throat.*)
>
> MEL: Hello hello hello, my name is Brad. Like 'bad', but with an R'.
>
> (*no laughs*)
>
> MEL: You know that feeling when you sort of go, "It's a fucking new week starting, you know, and I'm just going to, oh fuck it, I'm going to open up a bottle of Scotch kind of thing." Know what I mean? How's everybody doing tonight? (*nothing*)
>
> Yeah? Well anyway. I get depressed on a Sunday. I don't know why. But I'm not here to talk about depression, I have a condition called borderline personality disorder, or BPD. It's all the rage. (*MEL pushes the buzzer which prompts a fake loud laugh track*)
>
> I've always known there's something wrong with me. My family's had depression my whole life, both my father and my mother's side. They're all bonkers – which came in handy when I was telling them about my BPD. At least they didn't pull the usual, "What the hell's borderline personality disorder? Just pull your fucking socks up" kind of thing. (*fake loud laugh track*). Yeah so anyway…
>
> I got pretty successful at a very young age, but by the time I was 32, I had a break-down, 32 and a half kind of thing, a breakdown. No idea what was going on. My doctor at the time said, "I really think you should go and see a psychiatrist, I think you've got something, you know, you're not getting better, you're getting worse." That was when I was about 37 or 38. I'm just trying to get the maths together.
>
> We did the questionnaire in the doctor's office and he said, "Well, for want of a better term - you're pretty fucked up, mate. You've got what we call borderline personality disorder," and he sort of ran through it all, shooting out questions: "Do you feel like this? Do you feel like that? "Do you ever go for drives and not remember how you got there?" Like, fuck, I do that all the time, you know?" I drive for eight hours and you wouldn't think through that eight hours kind of thing you'd just end up somewhere. I ended up in Sydney one time. So, I've been living with that now for about four or five years I'm going to be 42 in a month. Not that I believe in any of that birthday kind of crap. I don't know why people celebrate people's birthdays because it's not like I did anything, my mum and dad had sex and she squeezed me out. What did I do to be celebrated, you know what I mean? (*fake loud laugh track*).

In this excerpt, and the rest of the play, dark humour can be used to bridge differences between people with a mental health diagnosis, and those without. Through the very words of people with lived experience, we can challenge frightening and negative stereotypes about those with personality disorders, as well as allow us to laugh at ourselves. Despite persistent critiques of autoethnography as navel-gazing, it is a methodology that does just what Mel/Brad attempts above – offers a critique of a solitary and sometimes united self, and suggests the power of cultural and community belonging.

Critical autoethnography allows us to go beyond writing "self" in relation to "culture," writing multiple selves or "more-than-selves" and "beyond-cultures" in ways that help us move out of alienation and isolation and into a much-needed and desired space of belonging. In the next section, we consider how critical autoethnography might help generate a getting out of our "selves" and into spaces in which belonging and the messy, ambivalent negotiations of respect, family and culture are written and, possibly, revised.

Out of selves: critical autoethnography as ambivalent negotiation

Homi Bhabha (2001) identified the "ambivalent negotiations" (p. 55) of "third spaces," an interstitial place between cultures, identities and practices. In postcolonial literature, it is a place of hybridity in which the multiple and co-constitutive layers of individual-social-cultural work together in both messy and contingent ways (Bhabha 2004). Those with mental health diagnoses often find solace in telling stories of not known or not wanted families, childhoods, cultures; diasporas of might-have-beens.

Many, if not most people diagnosed with BPD receive those diagnoses in early adulthood. Anne was diagnosed after age 50, a phenomenon becoming more common. In these cases, the pattern of symptoms of BPD may first become evident in mid- to later life, or worsen during this time, and are often associated with the loss of a long-term, important relationship. While Anne can find examples of BPD traits and experiences in her early life, it was not until a series of losses in mid-life, particularly the discovery and rejection of her birth mother and the death of her adoptive mother, that BPD was diagnosed, a journey that took time, as well as letting go of any sense of authority about—in critical autoethnographic terms—self or culture.

Becoming willing to believe that acceptance might only come with the complete surrender of any sense of the self ("auto") is humbling and frightening and freeing, all at the same time. It is confusing. It is disorienting. It is a release from the shackles of the self, or whatever selves we come to believe we know. As both a personal and relational coming home, the work of multiplicity now moves us toward a new value of critical autoethnography, for getting *out of* self, and speaking back to cultures of oppression. In the following excerpt, Anne tells the story of finding a letter that foreshadowed the sequence of mid-life losses that led her to reconsider how longing and abandonment—family and not-family—shaped her ambivalent negotiations with BPD.

★★

We've recently moved to a new house and I'm unpacking a box of books. A white business-size envelope and old-fashioned artistic handwritten address popped out of one. The postmark is February 9, 1996. A letter from my birthmother, Dorothy. Outside of that letter, I've had no contact with her for over 20 years. Though I've been waiting for something to happen all my life.

> Dear Anne,
> You <u>want</u> to proceed and I don't.
> You refuse to <u>accept</u> my responses.
> Just because you <u>found</u> me doesn't mean you can have me.
> I do not want to be your <u>friend</u> nor do I want to be your <u>mother</u>.

I can only see the underlined words: want, accept, found, friend, mother. But I feel the loss of their surround. Her words, those five pages of handwritten text…were alive, and not only because something—anger, refusal, recrimination—had flowed out of it with such vivid animation. It was a threat to my life, as well as a way of life of belonging.

My adoptive mother, Anna Mae, died in 2007. She suffered with mental health problems for several years, on medication for depression, suicidal tendencies and at times hear voices (mostly the punitive, Catholic kind). She'd stopped eating, was blind from a stroke, and had survived a series of shock treatments her family had tricked her into consenting to. She endured most forms of degradation and loss a person can imagine. She did not go gently into that good night…

When I was younger, we were inseparable. She supported me in all my creative endeavours, sitting in the hard-backed chair in the corner of a friend's living room with her purse in her lap while we sang show tunes around the piano. The price for all of that connection was that I sometimes felt that my mother was devouring me, that I could never differentiate, never leave, never disappoint her, and I loved my mother, but I wanted my own life—queer and precarious and free…

While I was trying to escape Anna Mae's "devouring" motherlove, I wanted to find my birthmother with a clawing hunger. I dreamt in images, fleshbodies, my connection to hers like a virus, a mutation. I wondered what it would feel like to be held by the person from whose body I had come, what it would be like to look into a face like my own. I wondered, trespassed and invited loss as I wrote letter after letter to Dorothy…

(Holman Jones & Harris, 2019, pp. 42–45)

Judith Butler asks us to consider, "Whose stories do we read, and how important might the story be in telling a history"? (qtd. in Ahmed 2016, p. 492). Critical autoethnography can help those with BPD and their families to make the self and the interpersonal "third space" of the world more livable by embracing its multiplicities and challenges. Writing is a core part of this. For adoptees, and often for people with mental health diagnoses,

…the very term *autoethnography* presents a complication. *Ethno* is something we have often been decontextualized from (Holman Jones, 2005, 2011). *Auto* is what has been stolen from us. *Graphy* is how we stay alive… .Writing becomes inventing, not recording or evoking. This story-writing is a creative act, a political act, an act of survival.

(Harris, 2017, p. 25)

Through autoethnographic re/enactment of encounters we "enact the displacement and difference of our comings and goings; we make and remake home in the entanglement of here and there, now and then, strange and familiar" (Harris & Holman Jones, 2019, p. 64). The displacement becomes emplacement; rejection and misunderstanding become encounter. In this view, critical autoethnography becomes a powerful tool for choosing hope over cynicism, connection over alienation, despite the attendant risk and sometimes sorrow.

Conclusion: what can critical autoethnography bring to mental health futures?

And you want to be good.
And you want to be liked.
And you want to recover.

(Stone, 2014, p. 13)

We close by thinking speculatively of the reparative work that creative methods like critical autoethnography might bring to mental health research. Judith Butler (2015) argues that for a life to be livable—that is, for it to be a good life—we must strive for more than bodily survival (p. 209). If we are to live good lives, we must do so in meaningful relation with others (Harris & Holman Jones, 2019, p. 98). That critical autoethnography begins with the self—the "auto"—might suggest that such scholarship also ends with the "I" without considering the relational we. However, critical autoethnography is a deeply relational process; it is not a stage for a "single and unified subject [to] declare its will" (Butler, 2015, p. 156). Instead, critical autoethnography seeks to create a collective "we" by generating a conversation about how more of us can live *good* lives. Butler asks:

> What if we shift the question from "who do I want to be?" to the question, "what kind of life do I want to live with others?" It seems to me that then many of the questions you pose about happiness, but perhaps also about "the good life" – very ancient yet urgent philosophical questions – take shape in a new way. If the I who wants this name or seeks to live a certain kind of life is bound up with a "you" and a "they" then we are already involved in a social struggle when we ask how best any of us are to live.
>
> *(qtd. in Ahmed 2016, p. 491).*

What if critical autoethnography continues to push the question from "I" to the intra-action (Barad, 2007) of a series of emergent encounters experienced with others, asking first and foremost, Butler's "what kind of life do I want to live with others?" This question is at the centre of our life of multiplicities, and at the centre of the work we believe critical autoethnography can do.

Asking and answering this question by writing and performing critical autoethnography might approximate what Susan Best (2016) describes as "reparative aesthetics," work that "attenuates shame while also bringing to light difficult and disturbing issues," (p. 1) seeking "pleasure rather than the avoidance of shame, but … also signal[ing] the capacity to assimilate the consequences of destruction and violence" (p. 3). Reparative aesthetics draw on Eve Sedgwick's (2002) notion of reparative readings:

> Because the reader has room to realize that the future may be different from the present, it is also possible for her to entertain such profoundly painful, profoundly relieving, ethically crucial possibilities as that the past, in turn, could have happened differently from the way it actually did.
>
> *(p. 146)*

We hope this chapter and the excerpted texts suggest some ways of thinking about how critical autoethnographic scholarship can create a kind of reparative aesthetic in mental health research. Such works allow us the narrative, poetic, and embodied freedom necessary for co-creating affective, complex, and emotionally dynamic pictures of future-selves that do not remain stuck in—but do not disavow—painful pasts and presents. Mental health diagnoses can offer clarity to the "strangeness that seems to reside somewhere between the body and its object" (Ahmed 2016, p. 163) in ways that mental health service providers have yet to fully acknowledge. Critical autoethnography is a ready form for harnessing that clarity by shifting focus from the individual journey of, "who am I" to the relational encounter of, "what kind of life do we want to live with others?", a shift that can open significant possibilities for radical change within the mental health fields of practice and creative research.

Notes

1 We co-founded the Critical Autoethnography conference as a way of creating a small and therefore close community dedicated to making good on these unifying commitments. Our aim was to build communities of difference in the academy, supporting culturally—and onto-epistemologically—diverse autoethnographic practice (in particular from the global south), and exploring the critical potential of autoethnography as a theoretically-informed political project. Autoethnography is spreading rapidly in Australia as elsewhere, particularly amongst a rising tide of creative, practice-led, or arts-based postdoctoral degree structures. These artist-scholar-practitioners are turning more than ever to the potential of critical autoethnography to offer a rich arts-informed mode for weaving theory and practice in their culturally-embedded work and disciplines. But it also offers onto-epistemological possibilities for scholarship that emerge from diverse perspectives and knowledge-making practices and communities such as Australian Indigenous, New Zealand Maori, Tongan, and Samoan, among others, holding space for cultural and geopolitical diversity within the global critical autoethnography community. For more information, join our Facebook group Critical Autoethnography.

2 Some use the word "consumer" to describe persons with lived experience of mental health diagnoses and treatment. "People with lived experience" and "consumer" are equally inaccurate for representing those with experiences or diagnoses of mental illness; however they are the most common in wide usage at the time of writing.

3 The same holds true for questions about the rigor and veracity and of critical autoethnographic work, particularly in scholarly communities that hold objectivity and propositional logic as ideals.

4 Bordo, 1993, p. 59.

5 Butler, 2004a, p. 26: "The body implies mortality, vulnerability, agency: the skin and the flesh expose us to the gaze of others, but also to touch, and to violence, and bodies put us at risk of becoming the agency and instrument of all these as well."

6 hooks, 1994, pp. 198–199: "I asked students once… 'Do you think there is not enough love or care to go around? To answer… they had to think about …the way we try to separate mind from body." She notes that professors—and students—"must find again the place of eros within ourselves and together allow the mind and body to feel and know desire."

7 Barthes, 1986, p. 226.

8 Butler, 2004b.

9 Barthes, 1986, p. 52: "You wait for me where I do not want to go: you love me where I do not exist."

10 Butler, 2004b.

References

Acker, K. (1995) Seeing gender. *Critical Inquiry* 37(7), 78–86.

Adams, T.E., & S. Holman Jones. (2018) The art of autoethnography. In Leavy, P., (Ed.), *Handbook of arts-based research* (pp. 141–164). New York/London: Guilford.

Adams, T.E., S. Holman Jones, & C. Ellis. (Eds.) (2014) *Autoethnography*. London: Oxford University Press.

Ahmed, S. (2016). Interview with Judith Butler. *Sexualities*, 19(4): 482–492.

Bakare, M.O. (2009) Morbid and insight poetry: A glimpse at schizophrenia through the window of poetry. *Journal of Creativity in Mental Health*, 4: 217–224.

Barad, K. (2007) *Meeting the universe halfway: Quantum physics and the entanglement of matter and meaning.* Durham & London: Duke UP.

Barthes, R. (1986) *A lover's discourse: fragments.* New York: Hill and Wang

Beatson, J., S. Rao, & C. Watson. (2010) *Borderline personality disorder: towards effective treatment.* Australian Postgraduate Medicine: Vic.

Best, S. (2016) *Reparative aesthetics: witnessing in contemporary art photography.* London: Bloomsbury Press. Online edition: books.google.com.au/books?id=RZehDAAAQBAJ&source=gbs_navlinks_s

Bhabha, H. K. (2004) *The location of culture.* Abingdon: Routledge.

Bhabha, H. K. (2001) Unsatisfied: Notes on vernacular cosmopolitanism. In G. Castle (Ed.), *Postcolonial discourses: An anthology* (pp. 38–52). Malden, MA: Blackwell.

Bordo, S. (1993) *Unbearable weight: Feminism, western culture, and the body.* Berkeley: University of California Press.

Boylorn, R.M., & M.P. Orbe. (Eds.). (2013) *Critical autoethnography: Intersecting critical identities in everyday life.* Left Coast Press.

Butler, J. (2015) *Notes toward a performative theory of assembly.* Cambridge, MA: Harvard University Press.

Butler, J. (2004a) *Precarious life: The powers of mourning and violence.* London: Verso.

Butler, J. (2004b) Jacques Derrida. *London Review of Books,* 26: 32.

Butler, J. (2005) *Giving an account of oneself.* New York: Fordham University Press.

Chanen, A.M., & K.N. Thompson. (2016) Prescribing and borderline personality disorder. *Australian Prescriber,* 39(2): 49–53.

Chanen A.M., Sharp C., & P. Hoffman et al. (2007) Prevention and early intervention for borderline personality disorder. *Medical Journal of Australia,* 187(7): 18–21.

Dillard, A. (2000) *For the time being.* New York: Vintage.

Donald F., Duff C., Broadbear J., Rao S., & K. Lawrence. (2017) Consumer perspectives on personal recovery and borderline personality disorder. *The Journal of Mental Health Training, Education and Practice,* 12(6): 350–59.

Faulkner, S. L., & S. Squillante. (2016) *Writing the personal: Getting your stories onto the page.* Rotterdam, The Netherlands: Sense Publishers.

Gingrich-Philbrook, C. (2013) Evaluating (evaluations of) autoethnography. In Holman Jones, S., Adams, T.E., & Ellis, C., (Eds.), *The Handbook of autoethnography* (pp. 609–626). Walnut Creek, CA: Left Coast Press.

Gale, K. (2018) *Madness as methodology: Bringing concepts to life in contemporary theorising and methodology.* New York/London: Routledge.

Gutkind, L. (2008) *Keep it real: Everything you need to know about researching and writing creative nonfiction.* New York: W.W. Norton & Company.

Harris, A. (2017) An adoptee autoethnographic femifesta. *International Review of Qualitative Research,* 10(1): 24–28.

Harris, A. (2015) A kind of hush: Adoptee diasporas and the impossibility of home. In Chawla D., & Jones S.H. (Eds.), *Stories of home: Place, identity, and exile* (pp. 161–175). New York: Lexington Books.

Harris, A. (2014) Ghost-child. In Adams, T.E., & Wyatt, J. (Eds.), *On (writing) families: Autoethnographies of presence and absence, love and loss* (pp. 69–76). Rotterdam: Sense.

Harris, A., & S. Holman Jones. (2019) *The Queer life of things: Performance, affect and the more-than-human.* New York: Lexington/Rowman & Littlefield.

Holman Jones, S. (2016) Living bodies of thought: The "critical" in critical autoethnography. *Qualitative Inquiry,* 22(4): 228–237.

Holman Jones, S. (2011) Lost and found. *Text and Performance Quarterly,* 31: 322–341. doi: 10.1080/10462937.2011.602709

Holman Jones, S. (2005) Autoethnography: making the personal political. In Denzin N.K. & Lincoln Y.S. (Eds.), *The Sage handbook of qualitative research* (3rd ed., pp. 763–791). Thousand Oaks, CA: Sage.

Holman Jones, S., & T.E. Adams. (2014) Undoing the alphabet: a queer fugue on grief and forgiveness. *Cultural Studies ↔ Critical Methodologies,* 14(2): 102–110.

Holman Jones, S., & A. Harris. (2018) *Queering autoethnography.* New York: Routledge.

Hooks, B. (1994) *Teaching to transgress, education as the practice of freedom.* Routledge. New York.

Howells, V., & T. Zelnik. (2009) Making art: a qualitative study of personal and group transformation in a Community Arts Studio. *Psychiatric Rehabilitation Journal,* 32(3): 215–222.

Kerr, I.B., Finlayson-Short L., McCutcheon L.K., Beard H., & A.M. Chanen. (2015) The 'self' and borderline personality disorder: Conceptual and clinical considerations. *Psychopathology,* 48: 339–348.

Koestenbaum, W. (2001) *The queen's throat: Opera, homosexuality, and the mystery of desire.* New York: De Capo Press.

Kulkarni, J. (2017) Complex PTSD – a better description for borderline personality disorder? *Australasian Psychiatry,* 25(4): 333–35.

Leavy. P., (Ed.) (2019) Introduction to arts-based research. *Handbook of Arts-Based Research* (pp. 3–21). New York/London: Guilford Press.

Liggins, J., Kearns R.A., & P.J. Adams. (2013) Using autoethnography to reclaim the 'place of healing' in mental health care. *Social Science Medicine,* 91: 105–109.

McNiff, S. (2004) *Art heals: How creativity cures the soul.* Boston & London: Shambala.

Miller, A.L., Muehlenkamp J.J., & C.M. Jacobson. (2008) Fact or fiction: Diagnosing borderline personality disorder in adolescents. *Clinical Psychology Review,* 28(6): 969–981.

Mohanty, C. (2003) *Feminism without borders: Decolonizing theory, practicing solidarity.* Durham, NC: Duke University Press.

Morgan, L., Knight C., Bagwash J., & F. Thompson. (2012) Borderline Personality Disorder and role of art therapy: A discussion of its utility from the perspective of those with a lived experience. *International Journal of Art Therapy,* 17(3): 91–97.

Morris, N. (2018) *Dramatherapy for borderline personality disorder: Empowering and nurturing people through creativity.* New York/London: Routledge.

National Institute of Mental Health (NIMH). Borderline personality disorder. Online: www.nimh.nih.gov/health/topics/borderline-personality-disorder/index.shtml#part_145387

Sedgwick, E.K. (2002) Touching feeling: Affect, performativity, pedagogy. Durham, NC: Duke UP.

Stone, B. (2014) Reading a science article on the airplane to JFK. *Someone else's wedding vows* (pp. 11–13). Portland, OR: Octopus Books.

Tamas, S. (2018) Moving pieces. *Departures in Critical Qualitative Research,* 7(4): 113–122.

Tamas, S. (2017) The shadow manifesto. *International Review of Qualitative Research* 10(1): 110–113.

Spry, T. (2016) *Autoethnography and the other: Unsettling power through utopian performatives.* New York/London: Routledge. Online edition: books.google.com.au/books?id=YvvdCwAAQBAJ&printsec=frontcover&source=gbs_ge_summary_r&cad=0#v=onepage&q&f=false

Taylor, S., Leigh-Phippard H., & A. Grant. (2014) Writing for recovery: A practice development project for mental health service users, careers and survivors. *International Practice Development Journal* 4(1). Online: www.fons.org/Resources/Documents/Journal/Vol4No1/IPDJ_0401_05.pdf

Van Lith, T., Schofield, M., & P. Fenner. (2013) Identifying the evidence-base for art-based practices and their potential benefit for mental health recovery: A critical review. *Disability and Rehabilitation,* 35(16): 1–15.

Veysey, S. (2014) People with a borderline personality diagnosis describe discriminatory experiences. *Kōtuitui: New Zealand Journal of Social Sciences Online* 9(1): 20–35.

Wyatt, J. (2018) *Therapy, stand-up, and the gesture of writing towards creative-relational inquiry.* New York/London: Routledge.

Wyatt, J. (2005) A gentle going? An autoethnographic short story. *Qualitative Inquiry,* 11: 724–732.

Wyatt, J., Harris A., Hofsess, B., Holman Jones, S., & F. Murray. (2020) Material turbulence: Stillness, movement and the work of the lumen. *Liminalities: A Journal of Performance Studies* 16(1). Online: liminalities.net/16-1/lumen.pdf

PART VII

Observational methods in ethnographic research

17

ETHNOGRAPHERS IN SCRUBS

Ethnographic observation within healthcare

Melinda Rea-Holloway and Steve Hagelman

Introduction

It is 7 a.m. on a chilly Tuesday morning in Minneapolis, and we have just arrived at a large clinic where we will observe for the day. We are shadowing a family practice physician who has been caring for many of his patients for decades. He has a few patients already waiting and a full day ahead, so he gives us a quick tour of the exam rooms, his office, and the staging area where he spends most of his down time. He knows that we are there to learn about what it is like to manage patients who have diabetes, but he wants to know exactly *how* he can best assist us in accomplishing this task. He wants to understand what kinds of things we want to see and what types of conversations he should try to encourage with his patients. When we explain to him that he doesn't need to do anything special, that we just want to follow him, as he goes about his normal day, doing all of the tasks that he normally does, he raises an eyebrow, skeptically shrugs, and says that he hopes we will be able to get what we need.

The premise is simple: to really understand something, you should see it in action. If you want to understand what it is like to live with a specific illness, observe patients living with that illness. If you want to understand how physicians interact with their patients, watch them interacting. In practice, however, observational research is more nuanced and complex, and the literature available on observing in healthcare settings is scant. This chapter hopes to help fill that gap, outlining some of the techniques we find useful when doing fieldwork in hospitals, physician's offices, and in the homes of patients.

Healthcare observation contexts

We regularly do fieldwork in three different types of healthcare contexts and are often observing in a combination of them depending on the objectives of the research. They are (1) healthcare professionals (HCP)/patient interactions, (2) HCPs in the backstage, and (3) patients' daily lives at home.

HCP/patient interactions

Our pharmaceutical and medical device company clients are often interested in learning about HCP and patient interactions. It is our job to help them not only understand the nuts and bolts of these interactions, but the deeper social and cultural context surrounding these exchanges.

Specific project goals vary, but common observational foci for HCP/patient interactions might include:

- *Conflict and pain points.* We pay attention to those moments when the HCP and the patient disagree on a point or a plan of action. We try to isolate problem areas or topics where either participant struggles to communicate or to be heard. We focus on body language and note where, within the interaction, patients or HCPs seem to be tense or become more comfortable. We often see tension and conflict arise around the delicate balance that HCPs must try to achieve between providing ideal patient care and running a successful business. This sometimes causes conflict between the HCP and patient, between various HCPs, and between the HCP and the office staff. We pay attention to how dynamics change when fear, anger, annoyance, or frustration enters the room, and how conflict is revolved. We identify what seems to cause challenges and areas where interactions could improve. This might include trying to map out where things tend to break down or stall, or where the patient (or the HCP) seems to not get what they want or need.

- *Talking points and communication strategies.* We document how general norms of communication are practiced or are breached and how each interactant customizes their communication strategy for the other. One value in seeing HCPs taking care of multiple patients is that we get to observe the patterns and variations in their interactions. We pay attention to how they go about getting information from patients, how they explain key concepts to their patients and what prompts them to go off script. Understanding these habits and strategies helps clarify the assumptions, priorities, and overall philosophies HCPs have about their patients, the disease/illness, and its treatment. Sometimes there are important differences in how communication happens, depending on patient type or physician specialty. For example, during one of our projects observing the office visits of patients with diabetes we saw key differences in some of the assumptions that physicians made about their patients (and therefore how they communicated with them) based on whether they had type 1 or type 2 diabetes.

- *Power.* Power relations between physicians and patients have always been a key variable in the sociology of health and illness. We note how physicians (or patients) shape conversations and strategies that patients (or physicians) use to make themselves heard. Over the years we have found that different types of illnesses/diseases produce different types of HCP/patient power dynamics. The relative power position that each player assumes can greatly impact not only the content and direction of the in-office exchange, but also what might happen after the exchange. For example, patients who have rare disease diagnoses tend to occupy a more equitable power position with HCPs than those who have more common diagnoses. This is generally evident in the content and manner of the HCP/patient interaction but also in how roles and responsibilities tend to be assumed outside of the doctor's office. In addition, different types of HCPs arrive at the exchange with different power positions and this can render a materially different experience. We once spent several months observing HCPs insert central venous catheters and found that although the procedure was supposedly identical whether performed by a physician or a nurse, the HCP/patient exchange varied dramatically. Nurses tended to assume a role that was guided by medical knowledge and skill while also being sensitive and reactive to the patients' cues. Physicians on the other hand, tended to assert and reinforce their role as the expert, virtually ignoring patient input.

- *Identity and emotional content.* Sadness, fear, shame, anger, frustration, resentment, guilt, trust, love, and empathy are all frequently on display in HCP/patient interactions, and these emotions help the ethnographer better understand where and how a particular disease or illness fits into theoretical models of health and wellness, patienthood, and the sick role. In the aforementioned project on diabetes, we found that some type 2 patients tried to miti-gate some of the guilt and shame they felt about the condition by proactively outing some of their non-adherent behavior. Depending on the physician, this could serve to ground the interaction in blame and guilt or in compassion and encouragement.
- *Other players in the interactions.* We often imagine HCP/patient interactions happening in a vacuum with two people, the patient and the HCP, going about their business without out-side influence. Yet there are a variety of other players whose influence must be taken into account. Patients' loved ones, other HCPs, and staff members are often weighing in, pro-viding information and support.
- *Decision-making.* A key objective of most of our healthcare work is to develop a clear understanding of how HCPs make treatment decisions. We pay careful attention to the data points HCPs consider and how the conversation and the physical examination help the HCP diagnose their patient and decide on a plan of action.

HCPs in the backstage

Observing what HCPs do behind the scenes, outside of their interactions with patients is a second common focus area of healthcare observation. Getting a feel for these backstage moments helps the ethnographer not only understand the context surrounding the patient visit, but it also helps them understand the influences and challenges that impact an HCP's daily work.

Each healthcare space has its own unique culture with its own personalized norms, ideas, habits, and ethos. A first step in conducting fieldwork in any space is to try to get a sense of the overall culture of the place and how this culture impacts HCP behavior and patient experience. Observation is ideal here, because it gives the ethnographer an opportunity to watch, listen, and record a variety of types of data that might help to bring the culture of the space to life. We always recommend (if possible) spending some time getting a feel for the space before digging too deeply into anything else. Here are a couple of key "away from the patient" contexts we pay attention to:

- *Pre- and post-visit care and administrative work.* HCPs face some of their thorniest challenges during indirect patient care, and they can get almost catastrophically behind with this type of work. HCPs often struggle with, among other things, navigating health insurance pre-authorizations, trying to stay on top of required documentation, and tracking down test results or old medical records. Observing this backstage work is a must to get a more realistic understanding of an HCP's workflow because a simple description of it during an interview can be misleading. For example, a nurse once told us that she had one task to do (schedule a procedure for a patient) before she could to go lunch. It ended up taking her forty-five minutes and four phone calls to accomplish this seemingly simple task.
- *The division of labor.* Within each hospital, clinic, or office there are a number of HCPs, each playing a valuable role in providing patient care. We try to understand how jobs are conceptualized and how various HCPs assume roles and responsibilities. It is always helpful to try to understand what types of jobs are attached to each player and which jobs

tend to float between HCPs. This can vary a lot. When we were observing HCPs who provided flu vaccines to their patients, we found that it was hard to predict who within the practice was responsible for ordering and managing the vaccine supply within the office. In some practices, it was the physician/owner. In other practices it was a nurse or an office manager.

- *Material culture and tools.* Examining how HCPs arrange their space and use their tools can help round out an understanding of work habits, the culture of the place, and how they see their particular jobs. Observing HCPs who inserted central venous catheters (CVCs), we found that although they all used similar kits, the first thing that many tended to do when opening the kit was personalize it in some way. Some would add an item, others would remove items, but each would try to make it their own. This observation went a long way in helping us to understand not only the process of CVC insertion, but also how each HCP conceptualized their role in it—actively engaged in customizing the procedure rather than simply following prescribed steps. Observation is often a better approach than interviews for understanding material culture because the use of objects and space is so routinized that people may not be able to accurately describe it.

Patients' daily lives at home

The day-to-day context of how patients live with a specific medical condition or carry out specific health behaviors is a third and final common focus area of healthcare observation. We typically try to understand the ways in which health status impacts (1) daily life/routines/quality of life, (2) material culture and tools, (3) identity, (4) relationships, and (5) emotions.

- *Daily life/routines/quality of life.* Interviewing patients is important, but often it is the observation of daily habits that reveals how a particular medical condition impacts his or her life or how patients struggle with symptoms or treatment regimens. So, no matter what medical condition our participants have, we always begin with a deep dive into their daily habits and routines. We look for ways in which the medical condition alters their schedules and how they go about accomplishing mundane things. Some medical conditions tend to disrupt routines and rituals more than others.
- *Material culture and tools.* In most of our healthcare studies, patients rely on a variety of medications, medical devices, and other tools to help them treat their condition. They also often rely on non-medical tools to help them with comfort care, identity/impression management, and maintaining a feeling of control. Identifying these tools can help us not only understand the general roles that health and illness play in daily life, but also how a specific medical condition alters a patient's environment. When we studied patients with chronic pain, for example, we found that they had an assortment of items in their living rooms or kitchens that we don't typically see there (TENS machines, yoga mats, acupressure balls, ointments, patches, etc.). When we studied patients with a pulmonary disease that makes movement exhausting, we found that they often altered their living space to minimize walking, confining furniture and daily necessities to a small area of their house. We have found that items signifying some conditions are worn like a badge of honor (pink ribbons), while items signifying other conditions can be stigmatizing (insulin pens, oxygen tanks, etc.).
- *Identity and relationships.* Being diagnosed with a medical condition, whether acute or chronic, usually impacts the way that people see themselves and their place in the world. It can wreak havoc on feelings of independence and can fundamentally change not only perceptions of

self, but their actual statuses. Having a serious medical condition also impacts relationships, and it is important to get a clear understanding of how the condition effects the delegation of roles and responsibilities within the household as well as the quality and tone of personal exchanges. A few years ago, when we studied women with metastatic cancer, we found that the condition often caused serious relationship conflicts and, in some cases, dramatically changed relationship dynamics.

- *Emotions.* Being diagnosed with a serious medical condition almost always results in strong and powerful emotional responses and these tend to change over time. We try to get a sense of participants' emotional journeys and identify any key factors that signal points of transition or make it better or worse. In some of the more serious chronic conditions we have studied, we have found that patients who had figured out a way to take a more active role in their treatment tended to feel better about themselves and their health.

Planning for fieldwork

Developing a research plan

The first steps in any research project is identifying what you are trying to understand, who will help you understand it, and how you will find them. Once the basic scope of the research is in place, we develop a field guide that outlines our research objectives and helps direct both interview and observational data collection. We typically collect both in a fluid and dynamic way. There isn't a clear-cut boundary where we stop observing and start asking questions or vice versa, but we always try to begin with some observation. This allows the ethnographer to get a feel for the language used, how players move through the space, and where participants seem to struggle. This helps provide better context for framing questions.

Throughout the research process we use the field guide to help focus what we pay attention to, but there are always interesting, unexpected things going on beyond what it outlines. The key to good observational research is to create a field guide that focuses data collection enough to ensure that research objectives are met, while at the same time remaining open and flexible. Spradley (1980) offers a starting point via some general observational questions that can serve as a start for a field guide:

1. What people are here?
2. What are they doing?
3. What is the place like?
4. What are the events that take place here?
5. How are social situations clustered in space?
6. How do actors play different roles in different places?

These are all very open and exploratory, the sorts of questions you'd ask if you found yourself on a strange planet (besides, of course, "which way back to Earth?"). If you're entering your fieldwork just "wanting to learn" then these questions will provide you with something to latch on to. As you get to know the environment more, then it will be natural to tackle more specific topics. Here are some additional questions, useful for doing fieldwork in healthcare spaces:

1. What is delegation of responsibility and division of labor like?
2. How does change happen within the practice?

3. How are interactions/treatment around X disease/illness different than interactions/treatment around other diseases/illnesses?
4. How do HCPs and patients define/understand X? And how do understandings differ?
5. How do HCPs and patients learn about X?
6. What sort of language/words are used to explain and talk about X?
7. How do HCPs make treatment decisions?
8. What types of challenges do they face?
9. What kinds of ideas, values, and beliefs are evident in the space?
10. Which tools are used most frequently?

If you still need some direction on what to observe, sometimes it can help to look for things to count or draw. We once did a project for a fast food chain where most of our data was observational—hanging out in the restaurants for hours on end without our beloved video cameras. Some of our observations were watching people interact with each other and the space, but we also counted a lot. We timed how long it took people to eat their meals and how this varied by group composition. We took pictures each hour of different parts of the restaurant and compared customer counts throughout the day. You need to be creative and flexible to make the most out of an observational setting, and sometimes it makes sense to count and tally. For healthcare observations, you might consider counting how many minutes it takes HCPs to do various activities. It might be interesting to measure how much time they spend with their patients, identifying the factors that can extend or abbreviate these interactions. If you're using video, you can always time events later.

We have also used counting in the past to understand the process of how people brush their teeth. We used the video we had collected to time the different steps of brushing (like prepping the toothbrush, the actual brushing, and rinsing). Not only were we able to find cross-cultural differences in brushing time and brushing sequences, breaking down the act forced us to look at toothbrushing from an intense, exacting perspective. Counting and timing can not only be useful in its own right but can force you to look at your observational data in a different way, taking into consideration factors that might account for or help explain observed differences.

Drawing can also be a useful tool when observing a setting. Maps, for one, can be invaluable. Mike Youngblood, in his 2017 presentation about observational research at EPIC (an industry conference), suggested mapping out a space and then making multiple copies of the map to document the range of uses of the space. If you're in the backstage of a doctor's office, for example, you might have a page devoted to each healthcare provider you're observing and draw out each of their pathways, getting to know how different staff members use the space differently. It can also be useful to map out HCP and patient movements in exam rooms to understand how physical proximity may play a role in their interactions.

Planning the logistics

Building extra time into the timeline. Plan to spend more time in the field than you think you need. For one, developing rapport is challenging when observing someone at work, and it can take a while for HCPs to get comfortable to your presence. More time also allows you to see HCPs working in a wider variety of situations, with different staff members, different patients, and at different parts of the day, which all can help give you a better, more comprehensive understanding of what's going on at the practice.

You also may need additional fieldwork time if you are observing interactions that are not very common. Once a client wanted us to observe nurses interacting with patients with a rare condition called Pulmonary Arterial Hypertension (PAH). PAH patients generally make up a small part of the HCPs' practices, and nurses may see only a few of these patients on any given day. Other times it may be impossible to know how many of a given type of patient will be seen at a given practice on any given day. For example, if you are trying to observe how gunshot wounds are treated, it may be very difficult to predict when a patient with a gunshot wound might arrive at any given emergency room. Having a flexible timeline can be a lifesaver in circumstances like these, allowing the ethnographer some wiggle room to spend time in the practice or hospital waiting for targeted patients or contexts.

Preparing physically and emotionally.

Doing healthcare research can be physically draining and surprisingly difficult if you are not used to it. Wear comfortable shoes because you will be on your feet all day and eat a big breakfast because you might not get a chance to eat once you're there. There also may be physical demands you can't plan for. When doing our CVC fieldwork in the radiology department, we had to wear heavy lead aprons while trying to position our cameras over our heads to capture a delicate procedure without getting in anyone's way.

Healthcare research can also be emotionally taxing as you sit in on life and death conversations or meet people facing devasting challenges. It can be hard for the ethnographer, especially if you have a long field period, to observe so many people struggling with their health. You must also be prepared to have difficult conversations with patients, even if you are only there to observe. One time when we stepped in to get consent from a cancer patient to observe a procedure she was about to undergo, she quickly signed the consent, but then grabbed our hands and began to tell us how afraid she was of dying.

Heath care fieldwork can also include discussions of embarrassing symptoms or require patients to partially undress. Ethnographers need to be able to read sensitive situations and react appropriately, which can mean excusing ourselves from the room, diverting our eyes or cameras, or transcending the discomfort. This can happen at any moment in the field, because you never know what a patient visit will hold. Nor will you know what the patient will consider "sensitive," but as a general rule, we have found that most patients, if they understand what we are doing and why we are doing it, are pretty comfortable having us sit in, even during sensitive moments. The patient role and the setting itself, the exam room, also might make people more comfortable than they would otherwise be showing and talking about their bodies. Still, occasionally some patients are *not* comfortable, and given the power dynamics of the patient/HCP relationship, the ethnographer has to be alert and sensitive to the possibility that a patient might feel obligated to consent to our presence when they would rather not. Body language often cues us into their discomfort and we typically excuse ourselves from the room.

Consideration and protection of personal health information

The protection of personal health information is always one of our top concerns when conducting healthcare research. HIPAA is a set of rules and regulations in the United States designed to protect patient privacy and we have to abide by those rules. Other countries have similar privacy laws, and it is important to familiarize yourself with local regulations. The HCPs may also have certain steps they want you to take regarding their patients' health information. Your organization or client may have certain requirements, too. Some key safeguards are:

- Have clear, comprehensive informed consent statements that outline what information is being collected and how it is going to be used.
- Make sure patients know that they do not have to consent and that declining to participate will not impact their care.
- Only collect patient information when necessary.
- Don't collect information from someone who hasn't given consent, and if this happens accidentally, have a planned procedure for dealing with it. This sounds easy, but patient information is everywhere in clinics and hospitals (in charts pulled up on monitors, in conversations between HCPs, in patients who walk in front of video cameras, etc.).
- Establish and document security measures for digital and physical data.

The use of video cameras requires special care in healthcare research. With a pen and paper, ethnographers can avoid writing down names, physical descriptions, and anything else that would need to be protected under HIPAA, but a video camera doesn't allow for the same selective data collection. Having the ability to record our fieldwork has greatly improved our accuracy, our ability to capture detail, and has enriched our analytical process, but its use does require additional vigilance.

The fieldwork

Once you've done all of your pre-work: recruiting and prepping your participants (see separate chapter), developing a field guide or research plan, prepping emotionally and physically for the work, and getting familiar with privacy laws, it is time to get in there and do some observational research. The most important thing here, besides taking decent notes and/or video, is to be *human*! Fieldwork (especially healthcare fieldwork) requires the ethnographer to be alert and sensitive to the cues of their participants. We have seen some ethnographers make the mistake of assuming they need to be more clinical during healthcare research, but we have found that participants are more comfortable and more willing to share when we engage in a more informal and conversational manner.

Sometimes participants or their family members can initially be suspicious and building rapport can be challenging, but it is essential in making participants comfortable enough to show you their authentic experiences. It can help to communicate with your participants frequently before the fieldwork begins so they have a better understanding of the process, your motives, and you as a person. Once you are actually in the field, it is useful to reiterate your goals and process, stressing that *they* are the expert and you're just there to learn from them. This helps put the participant in a position of control and can make the entire situation a little less intimidating and a lot more authentic.

Doing research in context also helps. People are much more comfortable spending time with a stranger on their own turf. Once we did a study on restless legs syndrome, a condition where a tickling or twitching in the legs causes discomfort, only relieved by moving them. Since symptoms tend to flare up at night, we were on call, often going to their homes around bedtime. These late-night visits could have been awkward for participants, but we stressed that their experiences were so valuable that we wanted to visit them, on call, at any hour. For a condition where patients' symptoms are often downplayed and even ridiculed by their friends and family, us just being there, sensitive to their situation, helped to alleviate suspicion and discomfort.

In addition to just showing the participant that you really care, it helps to:

- *Be yourself.* You might need to be a notch friendlier or more sociable than usual, but you should still be yourself. People will see right through you if you're disingenuous.
- *Dress appropriately.* Business casual works for observing HCPs, but if you're in patients' homes, you need to dress down.
- *Offer a hand when needed.* As an observer you don't want to interfere with the very thing you're trying to observe, but there will be times when lending a hand, besides being a nice thing to do, helps build rapport. We often find ourselves helping with the groceries, being their sous chefs, or handing them a tool.
- *Talk about things they're interested in.* People tend to really enjoy talking about themselves, their family, and their things. Noting a kid's picture, an interesting piece of art on the wall, or a motorcycle in the driveway can all make for good ice breakers.

Building rapport can be more challenging when you're observing someone at work. Where small talk might be fine for rapport building in other settings, when your participant is trying to get things done, it can be an annoying nuisance. What can you do then? It is always important to make sure that you frame your presence in the right way. This is often done before you arrive at the clinic or hospital, but you will inevitably encounter people who didn't know you were coming or don't understand why you are there. Making sure that participants know that you are not there to judge or grade them, but rather to learn from them is key to making HCPs comfortable with your presence.

Active engagement is another good strategy for building rapport during workplace observation. Showing authentic interest in them and what they are doing will go a long way in making them feel comfortable. Again, stress their expertise (and your lack thereof) and show interest in the things they show you. If verbal engagement in the situation would be too intrusive, use nonverbal cues and body language to show that you're paying attention and are engaged in the process.

Avoiding disruption of normal processes

For non-participant observation there's an old notion that the observer should be a fly on the wall, not impacting the environment, just simply watching. Of course, that's never really possible. Limiting your impact on the situation, however, is attainable by balancing being involved enough so that people are comfortable with your presence while staying out of the way enough where business can go on (almost) as usual.

We've found that there are a few things you can do to keep out of the way of a practice's normal operations and workflow. Rule number one is to only ask questions during the HCP's downtime (if they have any!). Even then it is important to ask if they would mind a question or two. Some HCPs can keep up their work and talk to you at the same time. Others stop dead in their tracks when they answer your questions. You need to take extra care with these latter participants and just be conscious about how much your questions are impeding their work.

The ethnographer also needs to be aware of their physical presence. Exam rooms are typically small, and we find it best to get the HCP's input on where we should stand. Usually we look for a spot where the HCP can easily enter and leave the room as well as have physical access to their patient. Essentially, we want to stay out of the way. You also may need to position yourself in an angle where you capture the HCP on video but not the patient in cases where you want to avoid filming them. Typically, you will be in just a few exam rooms with a given HCP, so it doesn't take long to get in a routine.

Outside of the exam room, the ethnographer needs to avoid frequently traveled pathways—again staying out of the way. If you're standing in a high traffic area, it won't take long to realize it. Choose a new spot. If you're videotaping, you also might position yourself where you can avoid collecting patient data unnecessarily. You should avoid pointing your camera at an angle where it captures patients in the background or where it captures a computer screen that is displaying patient data. This also means turning your camera off in hallways or waiting rooms when you can.

Observing complex, segmented spaces

There is a lot going on in healthcare settings and healthcare providers always seem to be on the move. Although it is easy to settle in and shadow a single HCP, sometimes it makes more sense to bounce around and selectively follow multiple healthcare providers throughout the day. If you are interested in seeing interactions around a certain condition, your "sample" is composed of those targeted interactions, not the HCPs. As such, you need to be with whoever might be engaging in those interactions at any given time (as long as it is amenable to them!). Observing multiple HCPs at a single practice can also provide deeper insights into the workings of the practice, the different roles and responsibilities that different actors play, and how different HCPs might approach their work and their interactions with patients differently. An individual is rarely the unit of analysis for our healthcare studies.

Logistics of dealing with and managing "others." One of the biggest differences in doing field-work in a clinic or a hospital rather than in-home visits is the number of people you'll meet. Even if you are shadowing a single HCP they'll interact with other HCPs and patients who might not directly be a part of your research. You might meet upwards of twenty or more patients on a given day (and their family members) so you'll spend a lot of your time explaining yourself and gaining consent. We have found it valuable to have a second person in the field whose main job is to hang out in the waiting room telling patients about the research, letting them know what to expect, and getting consent forms signed ahead of time.

You will also need to explain yourself to non-participating patients and staff who are curious about what you're up to. If you're not collecting any of their data, this can be as simple as saying, "I'm doing research." That might be all you have time for, but it is important that everyone feels comfortable with you there.

Conclusions

Healthcare environments require that ethnographers remain flexible and ready to adapt at any moment in the field. You can use the same approach to observation and rapport building and get vastly different results at different practices. One practice might treat you like a huge nuisance where in another they might enjoy the experience and hate to see you leave. There are lots of different factors like the personalities of the HCPs, how busy they are, the kinds of patients they have on a given day, whether their bosses told them you were coming, and simply what kind of a mood they are in on the day you show up.

You have to expect the unexpected. Expect to run into challenging personalities. Expect to run into emergency situations and general chaos. Expect that some practices won't let you access everything or everyone you'd like to. Everywhere is different, but it is this unexpectedness that should reassure you that you are capturing real life. Real life isn't always black and white. It can be crazy, and it can go off script. The insights from ethnography are equally as surprising and dynamic, and that's what makes this work so worthwhile.

References

Spradley, J. P. (1980). *Participant Observation*. Belmont, CA: Wadsworth Publishing Company.

18

ETHNOGRAPHIC INVESTIGATIONS OF A DIAGNOSTIC IMAGING DEPARTMENT

Ruth Strudwick

Introduction

The doctoral study summarised in this chapter explores the workplace and professional culture in a Diagnostic Imaging Department (DID). The primary focus of the study was on the profession of diagnostic radiography, looking at how diagnostic radiographers work and interact with one another, with other professionals, and with their patients. This study was carried out in one DID in an NHS hospital in the East of England. The professional culture was studied using ethnography. Participant observation was carried out over a four-month period in the DID by me as the lead researcher. I took on the role of observer as participant during the observation period (Gold, 1958). The four-month observation was followed by semi-structured interviews with a purposive sample of ten staff working in the DID to explore some of the issues uncovered by the observation in further detail. Thematic analysis was used to analyse the data from the observations and interviews (Fetterman, 1989). The objectives of the study were: to describe the culture in a DID and highlight the current workplace cultural issues that face diagnostic radiographers, to explore how people learn to become a diagnostic radiographer and how they become professionally socialised, and to observe and describe how radiographers communicate and interact within the DID.

There has been very little written about the professional culture within the profession of diagnostic radiography or about radiographers and how they work and interact. Consequently, the work of diagnostic radiographers is not widely understood, and their work has not been examined in depth.

Diagnostic radiographers mainly work in acute healthcare settings with most diagnostic radiographers employed in the United Kingdom (UK) by the National Health Service (NHS), working in acute NHS hospital trusts. Diagnostic radiographers are responsible for producing diagnostic images of the human body using different imaging modalities and technologies. They mainly work in uni-professional teams of radiographers within the DID. Diagnostic radiographers interact with and work alongside other healthcare professionals and NHS employees within the DID including; nurses, support staff, porters, domestic staff, clerical workers, and secretaries. Diagnostic radiographers also carry out imaging examinations in other parts of the hospital, such as wards – accident and emergency (A&E) – and operating theatres. In these situations, they work singlehanded within a multidisciplinary team, alongside other healthcare professionals (Radiography Careers, 2008). Radiographers interact with different patients of all ages, abilities and disabilities. The human interactions are the variables within their work, and this is often an unseen aspect of the radiographer's role.

Radiography became a graduate profession in the early 1990s. Much of the research in radiography has been and still is quantitative, as the profession is perceived to be science and technology driven. However, qualitative research within radiography is increasing as we begin to understand how radiographers work (Adams & Smith, 2003; Ng & White, 2005).

Ethnography is useful as a methodology in investigating the professional culture of the diagnostic radiography and starting to uncover some of the hitherto hidden aspects of the profession. Ethnographic research can seek to highlight the norms, values, and beliefs of a professional group, and also provide a description of the group, its cultural artefacts, hierarchies, and group structure (O'Reilly, 2005). Hafslund, Clare, Graverholt, and Nortvedt (2008) commented that the practice of diagnostic radiography is largely reliant on tradition and the way things have always been done.

It is important, at the outset of this chapter for me to outline my position as a researcher. It is acknowledged that in qualitative research, it is the researcher that is the research instrument, and not the methods used (Richardson & St. Pierre, 2005). I am a diagnostic radiographer with 24 years' experience. I worked as a diagnostic radiographer in practice for eight years, then I moved into higher education and I am currently an associate professor at a university in the East of England. I have had close involvement with many diagnostic radiographers working in hospitals associated with the university. These are the hospitals where the student radiographers that I teach go for their practice placements, which account for 60% of their training course. The hospital where this study was undertaken is one of these placement hospitals.

My perspective is therefore not one of a detached, objective researcher. I am familiar with the working practices of diagnostic radiographers as I am one! I also know how the department functions on a daily basis. I am also familiar with current issues within the profession of radiography, both in clinical practice and in education. As the subject lead for radiography at the university, I have contact with many of the diagnostic radiographers in the region due to the student radiographers having practice placements at these hospitals. I therefore knew many of the participants before I started this research. Those I did not know personally knew who I was because of my role in the university.

The issue of role and identity was an important consideration for me as I explored how I fitted into the research field and what my influences were on the research setting and the data collection. All researchers are to some degree connected to, or a part of their research setting, particularly in a qualitative study (Aull-Davis, 2008). This was even more pertinent as I was studying my own profession. During the observation, as I became more accepted within the group, the radiographers asked my opinion about their work and discussed their practice with me. It was at times like this that I had to consider the role I was playing (as a researcher), remember why I was there in the DID and decide just how much I should participate in the conversations that occurred between staff members. This made me consider my own role and identity. I knew that I was present as a researcher and not as a radiographer, therefore I wanted to gain information from the participants, but it was difficult to know just how much to ask, how much to be a participant, and whether I should simply observe or be part of conversations. The participants were obviously aware of who I was, as well as my current role and job title and the fact that I was there as a researcher. Before the research commenced, I spoke to all of the staff about my study at their staff meeting and handed out my participant information sheets and consent forms. Therefore, all of the radiographers were aware of why I was present in the DID at the start of the study. However, seeking and giving consent is complex, particularly with participant observation. Participants may change their mind during the course of the study, or they may not fully understand the nature of the research (Sin, 2005). Participants formed their own opinions about me and about my research. They may also have considered my position and whether they thought I could be impartial. It may also have been that because of my known position as a radiography educator that they chose not to disclose their true thoughts and feelings and may have been more reserved. Oakley (1981) suggests that the ethnographic researcher needs to "be friendly but not too friendly" (p. 33). Rapport with the participants is required in order for them to disclose information, but some detachment is required in order to see the research participants as sources of information and to discover new information.

My previous experience as a practitioner and my current role as an educator had the potential to influence the study (Aull-Davis, 2008). Because of my professional experience I have a good understanding of radiography, the role of the diagnostic radiographer, the terminology used, and the "cast of characters" (Roberts, 2007). Therefore, I was able to make judgements about the things I was observing based on my previous experiences as a diagnostic radiographer. I believe that this gave me an advantage over a non-radiographer studying the professional culture as the participants did not need to provide lengthy explanations to me about what they were doing and why (Aull-Davis, 2008). However, I am also aware that I entered into the study with some pre-conceived ideas which, although I was aware of them, will have subconsciously influenced the way I conducted my observations, interviews and the data analysis. Aull-Davis (2008) suggests that because of their personal history and closeness to the subject being studied, ethnographers "help to construct the observations that become their data" (p. 5). I was studying my own profession, and so it was difficult to grapple with some of the less than ideal findings, for example when observing poor communication between radiographers and patients. I developed a rapport with my participants and so it was then difficult not to suppress some of the findings and present a more subjective viewpoint to find in favour of my profession and the participants (Becker, 1967). Oakley (1981) suggests that in order to be effective, the relationship between researcher and participant should be non-hierarchical and that the researcher needs to invest of themselves, and to give of themselves in order to receive information. This allows for the development of rapport between the researcher and participant but could lead to further subjectivity and bias.

Methods

In order to study the culture, two research methods were selected; 1) observation within the DID to identify issues, and 2) interviews with staff members from the DID to further explore the issues highlighted by the observations. The research was carried out in one DID in a medium sized acute NHS teaching hospital by one researcher over a period of seven months. The purpose of the research was not to seek generalisable results but to gain understanding and meanings about the culture in which diagnostic radiographers work (Creswell, 2007).

The whole approach was inductive, in that theories were built and tested throughout the study. Findings were explored as the study progressed with the analysis beginning almost as soon as the data were collected.

Observation

The study commenced with a one-week period of observation within the DID for me to gain an understanding of the way in which the DID functioned. At the beginning of the observation I started with an initial mapping of the DID (Hodgson, 2002). O'Reilly (2005) suggests that a plan or description of the field (in this case the DID) assists in description of the culture.

Observation involves sound, movement, touch, and smell. Edvardsson and Street (2007) argue for a "sensate field researcher" (p. 25) who is able to "accurately document and reflect on the use of sensate material" (p. 30).

After the initial one-week observation I continued regular observations in the department. The observations for this study were undertaken for one day per week, and the day of the week was altered as well as the time of day in order to observe the DID in its natural state. After a few days in the DID it became apparent that the main viewing area was the "hub" of the DID. I spent more time observing there than in any other place within the DID. I took on the role of "observer as participant" from the four researcher roles in observation outlined by Gold (1958). I considered being a participant observer, the advantages of working as a radiographer and also carrying out the research would mean that I would really be a part of the team with my own patients and my own work to discuss. However, I discounted this idea as I felt that if I was working as a radiographer I may miss out on interactions between staff as I could be alone in an X-ray room, imaging patients.

Two members of staff did not consent to be observed so I had to ensure that I did not observe them. This was done by consulting with the work rotation in the DID to see where they were working.

During the period of observation, I took field notes in a small notebook. I used these field notes to record my observations and my own thoughts and feelings. Allan (2006) says that the researcher's thoughts and feelings are also important data. Often when I wasn't observing in one particular area I would still find out about events in other areas of the DID as staff members would discuss what had been going on during breaks and lunchtimes in the staff room.

It was difficult at first to adjust to being in the department but not working there. As a practitioner I had a feeling of guilt about not having a clinical role and being able to assist the radiographers. This was particularly true when the department was busy. Rudge (1995) highlights this tension and talks about the ethics of assisting in the practice area when your role there is to be a researcher and to observe. Johnson (1995) suggests that healthcare professionals as researchers will feel torn between the needs of the patients and the researcher role.

In studies of this nature the "Halo effect" often occurs (Asch, 1946) where participants being observed want to be seen in a favourable light. Other writers describe the "Hawthorne effect" (Vehmas, 1997; Bowling, 2004) where participants are aware of being observed and alter their behaviour. Some of the radiographers engaged me in the team, and spoke to me frequently, whereas others were quite happy to ignore me. However, after a week of my period of observation many of the staff members included me in the team and admitted to forgetting why I was actually there. This reinforced my understanding that over a period of time the researcher will begin to fade into the background and participants will behave as they would if the researcher were not present (Ellen, 1984; Bowling, 2004). It is, however, important to acknowledge that it is not possible to be completely overt; people may forget that the researcher is present and it is not always easy to explain fully the nature of the research (O'Reilly, 2005). It is difficult to balance the need to be open and honest with the need to fit in and become unobtrusive.

My decision to wear a uniform helped me to integrate into the department. However, this prompted thoughts about how I felt to be wearing a uniform and yet not being involved in the care and imaging of patients. As professionals, the wearing of a uniform is a powerful statement and it helps us to take on our professional role and persona. I struggled with the fact that I was dressed as a radiographer but was not "being" a radiographer. This is referred to by Cudmore and Sondermeyer (2007) as "being there but not being there". It has been argued that without true immersion in the culture the researcher cannot provide an authentic account (Allen, 2004). Therefore I spent the whole of each day of the observation with staff, including eating lunch and taking tea breaks in the staff room. This helped me to become integrated into the team and recognised as a part of the staff group. Chesney (2001) describes the veils of research and how the actual researcher (the person) can be hidden. She advocates being open, honest, and up front – not hiding the real you.

Another challenge was being able to fit in, in order to cause as little disruption as possible (Bonner & Tolhurst, 2002). I intended to become a familiar part of the work setting within the DID in order that staff members continued to work as normal. Coffey (1999) encourages carving out a space to be, a location that allows for observation but does not intrude on events. To this end I selected places to stand that were as unobtrusive as possible. This often involved standing in a corner in the viewing area or behind the lead glass screen of an X-ray room where I could see what was going on but I wasn't in the way of the radiographers and did not interrupt their work flow.

I continued with the observations until I felt that I had reached data saturation, a point when no new information is generated (Creswell, 2007).

Interviews

Interviews were used following the observations to explore issues further. I was able to interview a cross-section of staff from the DID. Ten interviews were carried out with key informants, these were identified during the observations (see Table 18.1). This was a purposive sample (Bowling, 2004).

The interviews were semi-structured and explored further the issues highlighted by the observations (Johnson, 1995; Coffey, 1999). The interviews were carried out over a period of one month. This was two months after the observation had finished, which gave me some time to reflect on the observations before carrying out the interviews. This was useful as I was able to carefully consider my interview questions and schedule.

The questions used during the interviews were open and exploratory. These questions were based on the themes extracted from the observations and also explored further some of issues uncovered by the literature review. The interviews were recorded onto a digital recording device and transcribed verbatim. The data produced were contextualised and I began to look at issues and events from the insider's or emic perspective (Fetterman, 1989).

Data and data analysis

The act of capturing data may shape what is said and in turn influence how it is analysed (Miles & Huberman, 1994). Data analysis is the process of systematically searching, arranging, and making sense of the data (Creswell, 2007). The data gathered from observations and interviews were analysed to look for common themes or patterns of behaviour and actions (Fetterman, 1989). During data analysis, the original research question and subsequent questions were revisited to look for answers. It is important to acknowledge that data analysis is not a distinct phase of the research process; rather data collection and analysis are simultaneous and

Table 18.1 The key informants chosen for the interviews

Research number	Gender	Role and Grade	Length of time worked at Anytown
DR1	Female	Band 5 radiographer, works in general department	7 months
DR4	Female	Band 6 radiographer, works in general department	2.5 years qualified and 3 years as a student
IA4 (imaging assistant 4)	Female	Band 3 imaging assistant, works in general department	19 years
Manager	Male	Band 8A. Manager of DID	26 years
SenDR2	Female	Band 7 advanced practitioner, fluoroscopy	7.5 years
SenDR7	Male	Band 6 radiographer, works in general department	4.5 years
SenDR12	Female	Band 6 radiographer, works in general department	15 years
Stud2 (student 2)	Female	3rd year student	2.5 years as student
SuptDR1	Female	Band 7 radiographer, responsible for main department	11 years
Supt DR4	Female	Band 7 radiographer, acting CT superintendent	7.5 years

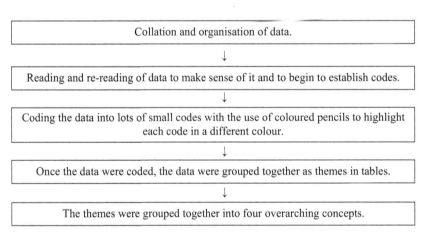

Figure 18.1 Data analysis flowchart

continuous processes (Bryman & Burgess, 1994). The collection and analysis of data are closely linked and each shapes the other in an iterative process.

Once the process of data ordering was complete, it allowed for the data, in coded form, to be grouped together under overarching concepts. I decided on four overarching concepts. Overarching concepts are used to group together similar codes to provide more order and structure to the data. Some of the themes were relatively easy to group together, whereas others were not. There were also several themes that had links between them, and bridged the overarching concepts. The flow chart below (Figure 18.1) illustrates the stages of data analysis that were followed:

Table 18.2 The overarching concepts and themes.

Relationships with patients	Relationships with colleagues
Involvement with patients	*Use of dark humour*
Task focussed interactions	Team working and communication between
Time pressures and waiting times	Diagnostic radiographers
Avoiding confrontation	Interprofessional relationships
Categorising patients	Diagnostic radiographer – radiologist relationships
	Discussion and story telling
	Role modelling
Structure and environment	*Characterising the role of the Diagnostic radiographer*
Blame culture	*Visible product*
Structure, organisation, routine – the way things are done	Diagnostic radiographers' views about research, Continuing Professional Development and
Workflow	evidence-based practice
Behaviour in different areas	Extended role and barriers
	Dealing with radiation

The four overarching concepts and the themes are shown in the Table 18.2 below, with the overarching concepts shown in bold text. When looking at the data, four more meaningful themes emerged and these are referred to as key themes. These four key themes were more prominent in the data and, following discussion with my supervisor, who acted as a member checker, it was felt that these were familiar anecdotally through experience and deserved more in depth analysis. These four key themes appeared more frequently throughout the study, from both the observations and the interviews. The four key themes demonstrated new knowledge about the culture within the DID and were not found to be discussed in depth in the literature. The four key themes were; involvement with patients, use of dark humour, blame culture and visible product. The four key themes are shown in italics in Table 18.2.

Conclusion

The DID is a task-focused, target-driven environment where throughput of patients is important. It is time-pressured, and efficiency is paramount. This working environment influences the way in which radiographers behave and interact with their patients and colleagues. Diagnostic radiographers behave in a very task-focused manner which to some observers may appear to be uncaring. They like to take control of the patient interaction and concentrate on the task of producing diagnostic images.

There are many barriers to extended role and the relationship between the diagnostic radiographers and the radiologists is a contributing factor. In the past, the diagnostic radiography profession has been dominated by the medical profession and some of this remains within the DID. The radiologists have a certain amount of control over opportunities for extended role within their own DID.

New staff members or students come into the culture with new ideas and suggestions and these tend to be prevented from being implemented as they do not conform to ideas that are acceptable. This therefore maintains the cultural status quo. The DID is a closed community, which makes interprofessional working and liaison between professions difficult. The use of ionising radiation by radiographers as part of their role and the confusion this can cause to other professionals can also put a strain on interprofessional collaboration. Diagnostic radiographers can use their knowledge of ionising radiation as power.

Diagnostic radiographers interact with equipment and computers and this is an important part of the job. Diagnostic radiographers are one of the only professional groups that have a visible product (an image) as a result of their interaction with the patient. This visible product is there for all time as a record of the interaction between the radiographer and the patient. Radiographers can therefore be very defensive of the images they produce. This can also result in radiographers putting more emphasis on the image production than on the care of the patient.

There is a system of work within the DID, and a way things are done. There is expected and acceptable behaviour. Diagnostic radiographers tend to conform to the acceptable pattern of behaviour as this contributes to the smooth running of the service within the DID. This expected behaviour is passed on through role modelling and by radiographers to students as they learn to become radiographers and copy the behaviour of others. Radiographers share their knowledge with one another and spend a lot of the time informally teaching their colleagues. Discussion about the job and storytelling are integral to the culture within the DID. Radiographers learn how to behave in different areas of the DID by observing and copying the behaviour of others. Students talk about emulating others and how they observe and copy what they perceive to be good behaviour and how they decide not to copy what they deem to be less acceptable behaviour.

Diagnostic radiographers communicate with patients in a task-focused manner. They make a rapid assessment of their patients, categorising and depersonalising them in order to deal with them. In categorising their patients, radiographers can make decisions about how the patient might behave and how much time might be needed for the examination. They use their previous experiences and expertise to make decisions and judgments about their patients. Diagnostic radiographers do not like to become involved with patients on an emotional level; they exercise professional detachment and do this for self-preservation. They try to avoid a display of emotion and try to avoid emotional engagement. It appears that it is not acceptable for a radiographer to become upset in front of patients or relatives. Radiographers learn their patient care from one another, and this is very much like an apprenticeship model which results in little change in practice. Like many professionals working with the public, diagnostic radiographers use dark humour as a coping strategy. Dark humour is used to diffuse a potentially upsetting situation and also to check that a colleague is okay. It is rare to see radiographers discussing an upsetting situation without the use of humour.

The team working between the radiographers in the DID can appear choreographed as they become used to working together and taking on different roles within the team. The diagnostic radiographer quickly adjusts to this team approach to tackling the workload. Discussion with colleagues is an important part of the culture in the DID, and radiographers often discuss their work with one another as they are carrying it out. Diagnostic radiographers exhibit different behaviours in different parts of the DID; there are front areas where they interact with patients and the public, taking on a professional appearance, and then there are back areas which are much more informal, where radiographers behave in a more relaxed manner.

What does this tell us about the culture in the DID?

Symbolic interactionism can be used to explain how diagnostic radiographers learn to behave and become socialised into the culture of the DID. This takes place as each radiographer comes to understand the behaviour and intention of the acts of others around them, and then guides their own behaviours to fit in to this culture (Manis & Meltzer, 1978). Socialisation into the workplace, often termed occupational socialisation involves the internalising of norms, beliefs, and values in order to "become" a diagnostic radiographer. This is done through situated learning (copying and learning the acceptable behaviours), observing others, and interacting with others (Atkinson & Housley, 2003). The diagnostic radiographer produces a social performance which is based on a cultural script which has been learnt from others (Madison, 2005). The culture in the DID is based on learnt behaviour. The culture is governed by the diagnostic radiographers and they have control over the culture. They decide on the acceptable behaviours, norms, beliefs, and values and how things should be done.

Like many work-based cultures, the culture within a DID is fixed and rigid. It does not change easily. Any changes take time and are not always well-received. The old way of working, the way that things have always been done, perpetuates through learnt behaviour and through conformity to expected behaviours. Pediani and Walsh (2000) warn that any change in practice takes time and needs to be simple, understandable, and made relevant to those involved. The implications of this are that any change or development takes time and meets resistance.

References

Adams, J., & T. Smith. (2003) Qualitative methods in radiography research: a proposed framework. Radiography, 9(3): 193–199.

Allan, H.T. (2006) Using participant observation to immerse oneself in the field: The relevance and importance of ethnography for illuminating the role of emotions in nursing practice. Journal of Research in Nursing, 11: 397–407.

Allen, D. (2004) Ethnomethodological insights into insider-outsider relationships in nursing ethnographies of healthcare settings. Nursing Inquiry, 11(1): 14–24.

Asch, S.E. (1946) Forming impressions of personality. Journal of Abnormal and Social Psychology, 41: 258–290.

Atkinson, P., & W. Housley. (2003) Interactionism. London: Sage.

Aull-Davis, C. (2008) Reflexive Ethnography, a guide to researching selves and others, 2nd Ed. London: Routledge.

Becker, H.S. (1967) Whose side are we on? Social Problems, 14(3): 239–247.

Bonner, A., & G. Tolhurst. (2002) Insider-outsider perspectives of participant observation. Nurse Researcher 9(4): 7–19.

Bowling, A. (2nd Ed) (2004) Research methods in health – investigating health and health services. Maidenhead: Open University Press.

Bryman, A., & R.G. Burgess. (Eds) (1994) Analyzing Qualitative Data. London: Routledge.

Chesney, M. (2001) Dilemma of self in the method. Qualitative Health Research, 11: 127–135.

Coffey, A. (1999) The ethnographic self. London: Sage.

Creswell, J.W. (2007) Qualitative Inquiry and Research Design – Choosing among five approaches, 2nd Ed. London: Sage.

Cudmore, H., & J. Sondermeyer. (2007) Through the looking glass: being a critical ethnographer in a familiar nursing context. Nurse Researcher, 14(3): 25–35.

Edvardsson, D., & A. Street. (2007) Sense or no-sense: The nurse as embodied ethnographer. International Journal of Nursing Practice, 13: 24–32.

Ellen, R. F. (ed.) (1984) Ethnographic Research. A guide to general conduct, New York: Academic Press.

Fetterman, D.J. (1989) Ethnography – Step by Step. California: Sage.

Gold, R.L. (1958) Roles in Sociological fieldwork. Social Forces, 36: 217–223.

Hafslund, B., J. Clare, B. Graverholt, & M.W. Nortvedt. (2008) Evidence-based radiography. Radiography, 14: 343–348. doi: 10.1016/ j.radi.2008.01.003.

Hodgson, I. (2002) Engaging with cultures – Reflections on entering the ethnographic field. Nurse Researcher, 9(1): 41–51.

Johnson, M. (1995) Coping with data in an ethnographic study. Nurse Researcher, 3(2): 22–33.

Madison, D.S. (2005) Critical Ethnography: Method, Ethics and Performance. London: Sage Publications.

Manis, J.G., & B.N. Meltzer. (1978) Symbolic Interaction – A Reader in Social Psychology. Boston: Allyn and Bacon Inc.

Miles, M.B., & A.M. Huberman. (1994) Qualitative Data Analysis: An Expanded Sourcebook. London: Sage.

Ng, C.K.C., & P. White. (2005) Qualitative research design and approaches in radiography. Radiography, 11(3): 217–225.

Oakley, A. (1981) Interviewing women: a contradiction in terms, in Roberts H Doing Feminist Research. London: Routledge.

O'Reilly, K. (2005) Ethnographic Methods. London: Routledge.

Pediani, R., & M. Walsh. (2000) Changing practice: Are memes the answer? Nursing Standard, 14(24): 36–40.

Radiography Careers. (2008) www.radiographycareers.co.uk accessed 18 January 2008.

Richardson, L., & E.A. St. Pierre. (2005) Writing – A Method of Enquiry. In Denzin N. K. and Lincoln Y. S. (Eds.) The Sage Handbook of Qualitative Research, 3rd Ed. Thousand Oaks: Sage.

Roberts, D. (2007) Ethnography and staying in your own nest. Nurse Researcher, 14(3): 15–24.

Rudge, T. (1995) Response: Insider ethnography: researching nursing from within. Nursing Inquiry, 2: 58.

Sin, C.H. (2005) Seeking Informed Consent: Reflections on Research Practice. Sociology, 39(20): 277–294.

Vehmas, T. (1997) Hawthorne effect: shortening of fluoroscopy times during radiation measurement studies. British Journal of Radiology, 70(838): 1053–1055.

19

THE ALIVE! PROJECT

Understanding the intersection between faith and soul food using ethnographic methods

Deirdre Guthrie and Elizabeth Lynch

Now let me hear you say that [CBPR]!! CBPR—Community based participatory research. Now, your silence means what the heck is that?!...[I]t means that the research is community-based and not research institution-based. You follow what I'm saying? And also means that it is community-led! And not just academic research institution-led. For the most part, historically, we've probably experienced research as being somebody else's experiment ON us. ...This particular style of grant recognizes that the community has many of its own answers. And that has to be done in partnership with research. ...We're not bringing a program to the congregations about health disparities. The congregations are building a program. You catch the difference?

(Ragland, undated).

With these words, the Reverend Alan Ragland emphasized the importance of the community taking the lead in health research. According to the Centers for Disease Control and Prevention (2014), Black Americans are more likely than White Americans to die of cancer and heart disease, more likely to suffer from diabetes and asthma, and less likely to receive preventive care and screening. At Rush University's Department of Preventive Medicine, researchers recognize that the growing Black–White disparity in cardiopulmonary diseases is partly due to a greater prevalence of nutrient-poor diet and sedentary lifestyle among Blacks than among Whites. It is also due, however, to environmental factors such as education, income, geography, and access to healthcare. In addition, the higher morbidity seen among Black Americans is linked to the structural violence of racism that manifests as a stress burden, which may erode health in a process one research team calls "weathering" (Geronimus, Hicken, Keene, & Bound, 2006). However, the impact of discrimination is complicated by factors such as a person's coping style, economic situation, and gender.

Health behavior interventions have the potential to reduce this health disparity, and can benefit from the "thick description" approach drawn from anthropology to help explain human behavior (Krumeich et al., 2001). This article uses the term "health program" instead of "intervention" to emphasize the study's collaborative and participatory design. This outcome is due, in large part, to a lack of cultural tailoring to and a sense of mistrust by African Americans of the medical research process. Thus, Rush University's Department of Preventive Medicine set out to collaborate between academics and clinicians at Rush University Medical Center and church leaders from five African American churches to help congregations and their communities build healthier lifestyle behaviors in order to reduce the higher rate of health disparities found in the African American community. In addition to the author's independent role of medical anthropologist, Rush's interdisciplinary research design team included clinical psychologists, theologians, and public health researchers.

In recognition of the challenges mentioned above, and with the belief that the researcher has a responsibility to the group being studied, Rush researchers located the ALIVE! program within the Black Church in the Greater Chicago area and advocated for a holistic and trans-lational research approach based on the tenets of community-based participatory research (CBPR) methods (Israel, Schulz, Parker, & Becker, 1998).

CBPR is a collaborative approach to research that equitably involves community members and researchers in all aspects of the research process. The eight principles of CBPR defined by Israel and partners dictate that the study influence the development, implementation, and dis-semination of health disparity research for meaningful and sustainable change as follows:

1. The "community" in CBPR must reflect a specific unit of identity.
2. The "research" in CBPR must explicitly recognize and seek to support or extend social structures or social processes that contribute to the ability of community members to work together to improve health.
3. A collaborative partnership must be stressed during all phases of the research.
4. The academic–community team must integrate knowledge and action for the mutual benefit of all partners.
5. The research must address health from a broader perspective, encompassing not only phys-ical, mental, and social well-being but also the social, economic, cultural, and political factors that perpetuate social inequalities.
6. CBPR must be iterative and flexible.
7. Partnerships must address health from an ecological and positive perspective rather than a focus on pathological behaviors or circumstances.
8. Partnerships must plan for and disseminate findings to all partners.

The potential for success of what became known as the ALIVE! project was heightened because it was initiated from within the African American church. Following a forum hosted by Rush University Medical Center Reverend Alan Ragland of Third Baptist Church of Chicago approached the presenters to ask how pastors could obtain support in their efforts to improve their own health behavior before "teaching and preaching" to their congregations. Following this, five pastors and Rush researchers met for a six-month period of structured self-care support, during which time the researchers noticed that clergy used scripture to think about their health behaviors and to support each other's healing.

In addition, the centrality of the church in the lives of African Americans raised the possi-bility that this church-based, codesigned health program could break down the barrier of mis-trust between medical researchers and laypersons, be culturally tailored to meet congregants' needs, and accomplish wide reach and sustainability. In cities such as Chicago; Atlanta, Georgia; Baltimore, Maryland; Dallas, Texas; and Oakland, California, churches have become key sites for health education, screening, and testing for African Americans. Community residents encourage their neighbors to get regular checkups, organize exercise groups, and teach one another how to cook with healthy ingredients. In the process, pastors have emerged as key allies in these public health efforts. In fact, successful collaborations among medical professionals, academics, and congregants go back at least 25 years to Wholistic Health Centers and the Health and Human Services Project of the General Baptist State Convention of North Carolina (Tubesing, Holinger, Westberg, & Lichter, 1977).

Because the role of the church is significant in forming identity ("Inevitably a church teaches its members either directly or indirectly how to deal with aggression, anger, pride, sexuality, competition, social relations, child rearing, and marital relations" (Taylor & Chatters, 1991)), it is a key site at which to study how participants come to identify or disidentify with internal and external resources that support healthy behaviors to achieve "coherence," a global life orientation or way of viewing life as structured and meaningful (Antonovsky, 1979).

Methods

Anthropologist Paul Farmer, MD, posits that the principle of "accompaniment," drawn from liberation theology, is central to the success of public health interventions. Farmer (2013) writes:

> The power of this simple idea came to me in contemplating patients facing both poverty and chronic disease. They missed appointments, didn't fill prescriptions, didn't "comply" with our counsel. …But when we began working with community health workers to take care to patients, the outcomes we all sought were much more likely to happen. Instead of asking "why don't patients comply with our treatments?" we began to ask, "How can we accompany our patients on the road to cure or wellness or a life with less suffering due to disease?"

Accompaniment on the ALIVE! project meant establishing credibility through prolonged engagement (scope), persistent observation (depth), and member checking (Lincoln & Guba, 1985). Rush staff consistently attended church services to show a dedicated presence and build long-lasting relationships that would eventually allow for a detailed, "thick description" accounting of field experience (see here for a listing of ALIVE staff and church partners: http://thealiveproject.org/about-us/personnel/). Researchers did so to test the external validity of the research claims and eventually to see if these claims were transferable to other places, times, people, or situations. Elizabeth Lynch, PhD, the project's principal investigator (PI), commented on the uniqueness of the approach in medical research:

> At every level we have done things differently as a result of working with the pastor and community. We spent much more time focusing on "relationships" without trying to collect data. You don't really ever hear relationship building being such an integral part of research but we spent about a year just getting to know people.

Relationship building for this project included a range of activities, from holding retreats at religious centers for pastors, lay leaders, and each church's advisory board, to conducting a commemoration ceremony following the needs assessment (from here on, NA), to using creative ways of engaging people to think about their relationships to mind, body, and spirit to develop an *ethnographic* approach. Both qualitative and quantitative methods HAVE their place in public health projects. While qualitative data provide rich contextual background, quantitative data can strengthen both internal validity (whether ethnographers' interpretation of data jibes with that of data sharers) and external validity (the generalizability and representativeness) of the data.

The Rush research team initiated its NA by collecting background data through textual analysis on church materials such as websites and church calendars. This step gave researchers

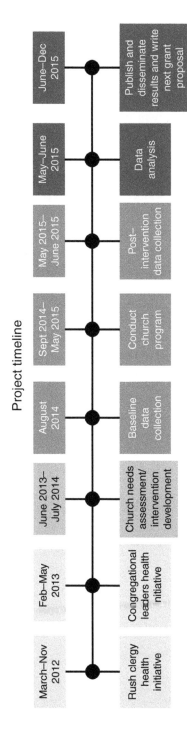

Figure 19.1 Project timeline

a sense of the organizational culture and structure of each church and its demographics and helped them assess community capacity and resource inventory. Researchers conducted "windshield tours" to see if churches were located in food deserts or near community gardens or whether the areas discouraged or supported physical activity. Then, through pastor recommendation, the team identified church leaders with informal qualitative methods skills as well as an interest in supporting wellness, who later became advisory board members and inside ethnographers (lay experts).

This article highlights three qualitative methods used during an NA for the ALIVE! wellness program that helped secure buy-in from research participants and provided explanations of how African American church members view wellness and faith. These three strategies are the pairing of insider (lay expert) and outsider (professionally trained) ethnographers to conduct interviews and analyze data; participant observation; and "going beyond the focus group" to use prompts, such as scripture readings and film screenings, to elicit authentic engagement. These features were chosen because they democratize the research process by building trust-based and long-term relationships, developing lay leadership, and emphasizing lay knowledge, thereby securing collaboration in this community.

Inside/outside ethnographers

An essential piece of the research design was the training of cultural brokers composed of insider/outsider teams. Insiders are lay experts who know and understand the contexts in which cultural narratives arise and the unstated messages in those narratives. In the case of this project, they "talk church" fluently and help researchers translate key terms, expressions of beliefs, rituals, identities, and behaviors of the African American Church-going culture. Yet they are also able to step outside of that discourse to translate local meanings (cultural, spiritual, and emotional). Insider ethnographers also have preexisting relationships with church networks in which trust may already be established.

Outsider ethnographers enhanced the project through their formally trained skills in ethnographic methods and their distance from church culture and perspective outside of church politics, which allowed them to ask naïve questions and trouble cultural assumptions.

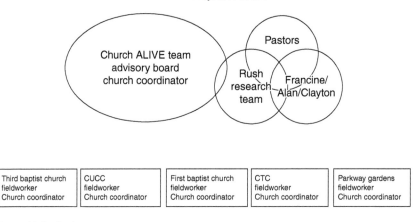

Figure 19.2 Project structure

Insider/outsider teams were involved in all aspects of the health research process: conducting participant observation, forming research questions, observing church events and sermons, conducting interviews, surveying congregants, facilitating community dialogues, and analyzing data. All of the ethnographers underwent training, which consisted of an afternoon of methods training prior to placement, assigned reading, practice interviews and participant observation, weekly individual feedback on their transcribed data and reflections, and three team meetings by phone during which strategies were shared and findings discussed by the group

A job description was sent to each church pastor to identify candidates with lay skills to conduct interviews, take notes, and help facilitate dialogues 10 to 15 hours a week for $10 per hour. In addition to serving as a cooperative learning and training vehicle for fieldworkers, our entire team, which eventually consisted of the church advisory board leaders, spiritual leaders and pastors, Rush researchers, and fieldworkers, came to a deepened understanding of the data. It also served a secondary purpose: to glean additional insight on the research process itself.

The ALIVE! team as a whole consisted of the following participants:

1. AB leaders, who are insiders with their own expert knowledge and insights, to help identify faith-based resources and use them in community-designed projects and health/wellness ministries
2. Spiritual leaders, including pastors, who model and encourage healthy behavior (through sermons, self-practice, programs, etc.), including Rev. Francine Stark, who offers methodological tools that promote self-awareness and self-care using *lectio divina* (divine reading, discussed in detail later)
3. Rush researchers, who were experts on collecting, analyzing, and measuring data into transferable and replicable research with funding resources
4. Fieldworkers, who serve as liaisons and build bridges between these groups and interests and who document and provide useful data on church culture

Fieldworkers spent two weeks training on fieldwork methods with assignments that involved practicing participant observation (PO), field note taking, and coding themes. They then began working on the project five to 10 hours a week, during which time they were expected to attend at least one church meeting, document their observations and reflections (the first stage of data analysis), and send the documentation to the research team for review and feedback once a week. Constructive critiques focused on discussing how to thicken "thin" descriptions of church observations and identifying missed opportunities to follow up on responses during interviews. Also emphasized was the strength of each person's unique positional perspective, which ranged from being able to share emotional testimony as a person of faith to having insights into living with chronic disease. Through this iterative process of data collection and analysis, the team began to identify patterns, gaps, silences, contradictions, and emotional moments in interview scripts and during Bible studies and sermons. Also garnered was information relating to the three project themes: 1) what makes one feel more "ALIVE!," 2) identifying resistance or barriers to feeling more ALIVE! and strategies to confront them, and 3) connecting faith to communal wellness. Eventually, the team was able to generate and refine research questions and provide the background context from which to interpret and understand why the health project was needed, what particular needs it filled, and the challenges and potential of the project, which the team then presented to the Advisory Board members and the Rush researchers.

Participant observation

For purposes of comparison, ethnographers attended two different levels of church activities: sermons (pastoral) and smaller educational program meetings (Bible studies). Participant observation (PO), which involves both prolonged engagement and persistent observation, is substantiated by the belief that what people do often matters more than what they say in terms of revealing the embodiment of culture. Prolonged engagement meant allotting enough time in the appropriate field setting—church Bible studies and sermons—to understand the cultural phenomena and dynamic being explored: the intersection of faith and healing. And in order to create conditions for the co-construction of meaning, we needed to lay the groundwork for rapport and trust, facilitated by the pastors' support of the project.

Drawing from Lincoln and Guba (1985), the observer should be in attendance long enough to:

- become oriented to the situation so that the contextual and structural factors (shaping the culture of faith and wellness) are appreciated and understood,
- be able to detect and account for distortions that might be in the data (e.g., researcher begins to blend in; respondents feel comfortable disclosing information beyond their organization's "mission statement" or that "tows the party-line"),
- rise above his or her own preconceptions,
- build trust, and
- create a detailed accounting or thick description of the patterns of cultural and social relationships—in the ALIVE! context, those that surround faith, food, and health.

PO during the NA itself consisted of Rush researchers attending church sermons and Bible studies in the spirit of accompaniment and to facilitate trust-based relationships among congregants, observe church dynamics in practice, begin to learn and translate the discourse of "talking church," and deepen understanding of the context and environment in which church members worshipped. For example, the embodied, visceral experience of participating in a call-and-response sermon in which prayer, preaching, singing, saxophone or organ playing, and testimony were layered into a seamless, multidimensional worship experience, provided a unique environment in which to study spiritual practice within African American aesthetics because "participation" overtook "observation" on a physiological level.

Ethnographers documented the turnout at these meetings and noted the characteristics of participants (age, gender, etc.), the theme and purpose of the meeting, its structure and leadership, evidence of church politics, what the most "exciting" or "tense" moment was at the meeting, and if any "surprises" occurred. They were asked to look for church communication patterns and dynamics that might inform a model for being "alive," including the style of the pastor (use of storytelling, humor, political anecdotes, song, etc.), emotional moments that particularly resonated or inspired the congregation, and attitudes or metaphors expressed along the mind – body or faith – wellness continuum. Other observations related to the NA could be noted at the ethnographers' discretion, and a space on the observation form was designated for reflections on and reactions to what had just occurred.

Throughout the needs assessment, this kind of PO helped generate more informed research themes to guide the formation of interview scripts and complicated baseline data obtained through other means (survey, interview, focus groups). More specifically, it allowed Rush researchers to view the vital role of pastors as role models and authority figures with the power to interpret and translate scripture into guidelines for daily life practice; to recognize that the site of Bible study meetings might be a forum in which to convey the integration of mind, body, and health; and to acknowledge active engagement and aerobic activity in the pew as an expression of "being alive."

Beyond the focus group: Prompting real engagement on food and spirit

Throughout the interactive process with congregational members and leaders of the NA, two specific types of community dialogue sessions seemed to elicit the most spirited and authentic response on healthy eating and spirit. The first was the use of *lectio divina* with lay leaders, which, according to Rev. Francine Stark, is a phenomenological process of personal reflection on scripture that originated in the monasteries of the Christian church. It is a process by which the reader cultivates the ability to listen deeply, to hear the "still, small voice of God" (1 Kings 19:12):

> No eye has seen, no ear has heard, no mind has conceived what God has prepared for those who love him, but God has revealed it to us by His Spirit. The Spirit searches all things, even the deep things of God. For who among men knows the thoughts of a man except the man's spirit within him?

Origen, a third-century A.D. scholar and Christian theologian from Alexandria, taught that the reading of scripture could help move people beyond elementary thoughts and discover the higher wisdom hidden in the Word of God. Rev. Stark explains that today the practice has been adapted to contemporary congregations for use in spiritual retreat and transformation. Participants are frequently encouraged to keep journals of their reflections as a way of crystalizing their thoughts, deeper understandings, and discernment about their relationship with God. She breaks down the process into five parts:

1. *Lectio*—Reading the Word
2. *Meditatio*—Pondering the "Living Word"
3. *Oratio*—Praying the Word
4. *Contemplatio*—Resting in the Word
5. *Operatio*—Living the Word

According to Rev. Francine Stark, a co-investigator on the ALIVE! project, "When pastors talked about change, scripture was used time and again as the lead-in to deeper, more reflective discussions about health and their need and right to claim it for themselves. As the team talked about this observation, we realized that the same use of scriptures that support deeper understanding and shared reflection for the pastors could be used to support congregational members in their discernment about their health concerns and commitments." *Lectio Divina,* or Divine Reading, would emerge as an effective practice used with church members during advisory board meetings to prompt their thinking about integrating spiritual and physical health.

The second vehicle for authentic engagement was the screening of the documentary *Soul Food Junkies,* which seemed to provide entry into otherwise difficult topics around food. The reason may be that its director, Byron Hurt, is an African American man who wanted to explore the relationship between soul food and health in the African American community following the premature death of his father, who loved soul food. The themes resonated with the congregants and generated a dynamic dialogue on topics that were not being raised in medical researcher-led venues, such as the powerful role of African American women in nourishing communities and the undeniable reality of health disparities, which Hurt called "soul sickness" as he documented the impact of diabetes, high blood pressure, and colon and pancreatic cancer on African Americans.

Lay leaders who, prompted by scripture, had been meditating and reflecting on their own life experiences with food, exercise, stressors, disparities, and health and wellness now became even more powerful cultural brokers, as they led dialogues following the church screenings of the film. They were able to both affirm and celebrate family food traditions as well as examine unhealthy behaviors and practices that had the potential to hurt family members and community well-being. In turn, researchers benefited by observing these dynamics during lay leader training and community dialogues, and gained a more sophisticated understanding of health stressors and facilitators among congregants. These conversations also included other perspectives from those who did not participate in more formal exchanges (interviews, focus groups, surveys).

Issues of internal validity

After each observation, interview, or group discussion, each fieldworker reflected on what he or she had observed, the environment, and the overall tone of the interview, effectively "thin-slicing" what church members were saying and doing around wellness and health. In this way, the team began to identify patterns, gaps, silences, contradictions, and emotional moments, providing the background context from which to interpret and understand what wellness needs existed among the church members. Reflexive analysis also helped reveal and address researcher bias, thus increasing the credibility of the findings.

In their reflections, the ethnographers considered how the teaching of scripture might inform congregants' health practices, how the communal experience of Bible study served to connect and inspire congregants to healthier behaviors, and whether Bible study taught a transcending of the body over an integration of bodily needs with spirit and, further, how an emphasis on bodily transcendence might inform health decisions or behavior. They also considered in what ways congregants or church leaders talked about the body and wellness that differed from a clinical public health perspective (e.g., use of words like "sacrifice" as a positive offering to God or discussion of spiritual food as nourishment).

Each time the data were gathered and coded by fieldworkers and Rush researchers to note the translational gaps, regular meetings were held to "member check" and update the rest of the team. Continuous feedback from church members helped in evaluating the appropriateness of the research questions and presented the opportunity to revise or amend the emerging health program design. The aim of this (or any) dialogical hermeneutic method built around such ongoing dialogue and negotiation with coparticipants is to achieve "validity" when the investigator's description matches the group's understanding of the problem or needs to be assessed.

For example, on the topic of clashing discourses, it became clear that community members were open to hearing objective measures of assessing health, but many did not consider language that referred to "an epidemic of obesity" as value free, instead conflating it with (White) body image preferences. Another example of such language was African Americans' negative association of "health food" as "White people's food" that lacked "soul" (flavor, passion). Also noted was an emerging pattern of a stated preference for health to be supported collectively, on the level of the congregation as a whole, rather than restricted to individualized self-care strategies.

What follows is an example of the updates in which emerging themes were shared with members of the advisory board for review and feedback as part of the commitment to member checking:

> Good morning. We've been attending Bible studies and sermons and interviewing your pastors and members of your congregation. We've received a lot of helpful information about how people view wellness, particularly in spiritual terms (one church

member defined it as "having faith in the face of adversity") and the challenges to staying well. At Rush, public health researchers define wellness in more physical terms, such as healthy eating and life-sustaining physical activity. In this project we seek to integrate our definitions of wellness—the physical, mental, and spiritual—to achieve a vibrant holistic sense of well-being. We've heard that people see their churches as having a tremendous role to play in the health of their congregations. The church is described as a "hospital, a safe place, where people go to heal and hear the truth" and that it's full of tremendous social support among fellow believers "who will hold us accountable and encourage us." That "we come to church when we are sick, whether spiritually, physically, mentally, for the word of God is health and life to all who find it." And, in terms of a key component of our project, *nutrition* and wellness, we've heard a lot about the cultural and emotional attachments to food. We screened the film *Soul Food Junkies* and discussed how our favorite dishes can be cooked in ways and with ingredients that support our health and wellness. We are listening … and today we'd like to talk with you more about where to go from here… .

Results

Our methodology informed the assessment by identifying thick descriptions that contextualized needs among church members in the following ways:

- The foundation for wellness is spiritual faith experienced in interaction with community.
- Faith and wellness are defined not in terms of self-help but in interaction with others.
- Soul food is a representation of love.
- Divine reading of scripture (*lectio divina*) with wellness themes helps integrate mind, body, and spirit.
- The pastor's service as a role model ties the concept of faith and wellness to the community.
- Racism persists as a collective reality and stressor.

Each description is discussed in detail, with a concluding paragraph for each explaining the implication for need based on that description.

Wellness as faith experienced with community

Perhaps the most important finding was that wellness in the community studied was defined in psychosocial and spiritual terms and that its experience is deeply phenomenological and embodied as an expression of spirit. One collective summary definition that followed a community dialogue was that "wellness is how one attains or maintains a peaceful and positive mindset, even in the midst of stress, in order to have a positive impact upon one's community and the next generation." Church members therefore emphasized a need and desire to feel mentally "balanced" and at peace in order to clear a "space for prayer" as well as make healthier choices pertaining to food and physical activity. "If you have an even keel," explained one church member, "you don't allow unimportant things to stress you out; everything else falls in place. Being health conscious means you do some type of exercise and eat healthy, be conscious, and at least don't overdo it. But mental [health] is most important."

Another respondent said she felt that the inability to find this space "weakened her immune system" and increased her chance of making unhealthy choices. To be "alive" meant "to have a clear, free mind, regardless of what was going on around you." Such harmony was sought in the churches, which were compared to "spiritual hospitals" where one sought inspiration through trying times by believing in God and the social support of the congregation, again pointing to its significance as a communal and health resource. Faith was described in terms of putting one's trust in God and letting "Thy will be done." For some, this faith was critical to resilience: "Without the church I wouldn't have had that fortitude... .God brought me this far; he's still there, taking care of me." So, to varying degrees, faith also involved "letting go, and letting God," which indicated that people differed in how much control they felt they ultimately had on their life circumstances, including health outcomes. As one church member stated, "You can be emotionally broken down ... and when you get down ... you need God to make you well." Or as another remarked, "I think if you have faith and are able to pray that you have a chance of healing and being cured more quickly." One woman who worked in a neighborhood hospital emergency department commented, "My God, all my years in the hospital ... you see everything... babies born you don't think will make it... then you see who's in charge... .[It's] important to be still and know 'He is.'"

Another congregant recalled being anointed with oil by her pastor before a high-risk surgery:

> My own experience has led me to believe that faith is the greater healer. I have been told a couple of times ... that I would be paralyzed because of the health conditions that I have. I have prayed. ... [My life] has changed drastically but I can still walk. ... I've learned to adjust, but all that's through faith ... God is not going to allow [paralysis] to happen. You need your faith.

One church leader who counseled congregants advised them against practicing "blind faith": "I believe that God is involved in all things, but I also believe there is a place for science. It's finding balance. ...So when people approach me and they say, 'I don't need a therapist' or 'I don't need my Prozac or Albuterol,' I explain that God helped man create that. ... And when that doesn't work I show them my pills."

Implications for need: A successful wellness program must integrate physical health with mental and spiritual health, respecting that the latter is viewed as the foundational priority.

Faith and wellness defined by interactions

Faith as an expression of spiritual wellness was seen as communal and linked with a duty toward sharing and spreading the word through one's personal story or testimony. One pastor reminded congregants, "Life is full of trials; being a Xtian [Christian] doesn't mean you stop bearing crosses. People will disappoint you. You will disappoint yourself. But stay focused on what God has called you to do. Stay faithful. Go tell it!" One church member related, "When you are an active participant [in your faith], you are not focused on you, you are focused on other things. Like other people... when you give of yourself, blessings come. I was grounded in that."

An insider ethnographer and former marine described his "calling" to God in visceral and emotional terms. He said the presence of God was so clearly channeled through his preacher on the day he walked into church that his leg began to shake and he found himself spontaneously uttering the sermon even though he was unfamiliar with the words. As he described the importance of this moment, how it marked the beginning of his becoming "truly accountable" in his life and deeply devoted to this particular pastor, his voice cracked and his eyes welled up in tears. When he spoke at meetings with Rush researchers, other attendees noted feeling an emotional charge in the room because every utterance was a shared experiential testimony, evoking and this openness evoked an engaged response with his interview respondents.

Implications for need: A successful wellness program needs to be framed as a collective effort that incorporates congregational interaction as support. Furthermore, "testimonies," the act of sharing how one was called to God in front of a community that bears witness, can be analyzed to explore whether such callings inspired positive changes in health practices.

Soul food as love

The sharing and offering of soul food is a deeply symbolic practice that expresses cultural pride, generosity, and love. At the same time, a lack of information on how to eat nutrient-rich food prepared in healthful ways is acknowledged as a challenge, as is access to affordable, fresh produce. The deep personal meanings of celebration and abundance that accompany food sharing among loved ones is best expressed by our interview respondents as "fellowship." It is present in every Sunday dinner, holiday festivity, and church potluck, although older church members complained that it is threatened by today's "fast-food generation." One pastor described the strong fellowship tied to food as "resource sharing": "Food not only builds relations and stronger fellowship, food is an equalizer between family, friends, and even strangers." A church member noted, "I think it's just reflective of the whole Southern mentality [that] we don't have much money but we do have food, and what we do have we can share. More is always better." With regard to abundance, the tradition of serving large portions of rich, "tasty" (often high in salt or fat) food is a matter of pride, particularly for those church members who remember growing up in a setting of deprivation and hardship. Congregants prioritize preparing certain dishes that their fellow church members consider delicious and pleasing to the eye over dishes considered "healthy."

As one respondent notes, "Food is comforting, which makes us feel good and gives us good memories. New, healthier foods won't have warm fuzzy feelings, just obliga-tion." That is, food that has strong emotional associations that make up one's identity are much more engaging than food that church members do not identify with and may even consider White people's food. This disidentification points to the challenge of helping church members create a positive identification with healthy eating behaviors, activities, and practices. Other attitudes expressed around food described the associations of Black people and soul food:

> [P]eople get defensive… and we have many cultural issues in the Black community around what we eat and how it's fixed and what it means, and it even gets tied to what it means to eat Black, being Black… [E]ating healthy is a White thing. Yes, some people will say eating healthy is Black people trying to be White, uppity, too good to eat some pig's feet!

For pastors who struggled to maintain healthy eating habits amidst the church socials featuring a bounty of fried chicken, candied yams, and sweet potato pie, the effort to adjust church menus to reflect more healthful food choices was difficult. But they understood what was happening when they were handed plate after plate of steaming, tantalizing-smelling food. One pastor, who had diabetes, recognized the love behind the offerings, even as she had to reject the food for her health:

> It's their caring, it's their love, it's the way that they love me, it's the way Black folks have shown their love through the generations. Somebody dies, you bring food; somebody is sick, you bring food. Whatever is going on, you bring food, and food makes it better.

Another pastor asked his congregation to consider, "If Jesus was coming to supper, what would you feed him? A Big Mac, fries, and a Coke? Or real food?"

Congregants were encouraged by the discussion that followed the prompt at the end of the *Soul Food Junkies* film, which describes ways to cook soul food that are healthful while embracing the importance of community traditions. Ethnographers documented the ideas circulating throughout the churches:

> I've heard individuals express interest in learning how to cook from their elders, creating a church community garden to teach children about growing produce, and starting a church cookbook using recipes from elders with modifications to make traditional recipes healthier.

Ethnographers discovered that older adults, many of whom had been raised in rural areas, were a resource of "untapped knowledge potential" for sharing positive health behaviors, including a history of gardening. Many saw the "younger generation" as having lost these healthier habits. Most elders perceive a tremendous difference in the ways "kids" live today and perceived their own childhood as healthier. Reasons included more physical activity, more chores, time spent outdoors, and less access to processed or fast food:

> We've gotten to the point where we've become microwave people. That's why we've got to depend on stores and government regulations to make sure that we have food that is healthy before we throw it in the microwave and we cook it to death or we boil all the nutrients out of it. … A lot of people, they don't like to eat vegetables that are supposedly "al dente." You wanna cook it until it's wilted, has no life whatsoever.
>
> When I was in school, sometimes I would get up and do work before school, and get dressed, have to walk to catch the bus. … And these children today, they're not motivated… .[W]e ate food that we raised on the farm, and now all they want is a burger. A nugget. A chicken nugget… .They don't want this pot of greens or vegetables, no type of vegetables. They may skip that. And then, they smoke… . It's a lot different.

The study's ethnographers learned that a majority of congregants they spoke to were open to and interested in participating in a wellness program that focused on healthful eating, had many ideas to offer within their church, and were aware of a lot of confusion around what foods were "healthy" and nutrient rich. As one outsider ethnographer noted,

> I've heard from individuals who switched from serving soda to serving juice or punch or lemonade, I've heard about ice cream and other desserts being called "low-calorie" foods (in comparison to things with icing), and I've heard of cakes being mentioned in lists of "healthy" content. It seems that many people are simply not clear on nutritional content.

At the same time, many healthy habits were already in place. "Lots of people mentioned cooking with smoked turkey instead of pork and baking things instead of frying them," one ethnographer noted. Many churches were already practicing healthy rituals that could be expanded or drawn on, such as the "Daniel Fast" with its five components—food, fitness, focus, faith, and friends—which are incorporated through sermons, readings, journaling, mobile apps, and a cookbook that could be expanded or drawn on. During the fast, congregants are invited to consider what temptations they struggle with and how faith, friends, and focus could help them resist such temptations. Over the holidays, LaDawne Jenkins, Project Director on the research team and a pastor's wife, urged congregants to be mindful of their eating and keep a food diary. "[T]hink about how the food is making you feel. ... Are you stuffed, are you full, are you feeling still hungry because you didn't get enough? Just observe the whole setting."

Implications for need: The screening of *Soul Food Junkie,* the practice of existing Bible-based rituals such as the Daniel Fast, the keeping of food diaries, and the sharing of healthful recipes and food practices by older adults can be tools for a successful wellness program. These steps emphasize the importance of community and celebrate food as expressions of generosity, pride, and love in a way that avoids death language (Gunderson & Pray, 2009) and allows church members to begin to engage in self-inquiry around their own food practices.

Divine readings with wellness themes

During sermons and Bible study meetings, some scripture referred to the "fleshly" body in negative terms associated with sin and death. Noting this association, researchers sought to know how congregants perceived the physical body and health in this light. For example, the following passage was read and interpreted during a Bible Study:

> For we know that the Law is spiritual; but I am of flesh, sold into bondage to sin... .
> For I joyfully concur with the law of God in the inner man, but I see a different law
> in the members of my body, waging war against the law of my mind, and making me
> a prisoner of the law of sin which is in my members. Wretched man that I am! Who
> will set me free from the body of this death? Thanks be to God through Jesus Christ
> our Lord! So then, on the one hand I myself with my mind am serving the law of God,
> but on the other, with my flesh the law of sin.
>
> *(Romans 7:14–25)*

The pastor then turned to his congregation to render his interpretation:

> Since Adam and Eve we have this proclivity to sin. (Reads) "Wretched man that I am!
> Who will set me free from the body of this death." If we yield to flesh, we serve sin... .
> When we forgive we release ourselves. Praying in stressful situations puts us in that
> spiritual mode... .God is spirit and we need to see the difference between physical
> and spiritual... .Jesus shows his humanity. He breaks down in private prayer and pleads
> tearfully "the spirit is willing but the flesh is weak. Father, take this from me, spare
> me.'"...So I ask you, are we spiritual beings having an earthly experience, or earth
> beings having a spiritual experience?

As an emphasis on and identification with the spirit over the physical body became clear, the research team considered how to support mental and physical health alongside spiritual faith to create what Rev. Stark called "a holy trinity" of wellness. Rev. Stark elaborates:

> It was decided that vegetables would be the focus of the project and that there would be at least 12 classes for the church participants around eating habits, recipes, nutrition, and behaviors. The use of scriptures as a means of understanding why it is important to develop disciplines around healthier eating and exercising seemed to evolve as the congregational members claimed what they learned from their *lectio divina* practice. It was further decided, therefore, that a Bible study curriculum would also be necessary for the participants to be well grounded in their reflections about why eating vegetables was important and also as a means of helping them to overcome barriers to their better health behaviors.

At monthly meetings, at least four church leaders from each church gathered to contribute to the ALIVE! project and began to use *lectio divina* at those meetings. According to Stark:

> The response was phenomenal! This was a time for their personal spiritual development and a way by which they could share thoughts and feelings about getting to healthier places within their own lives. They all used the same short scripture…there was a time for personal reflection and journaling, and then they met in small groups to share their specific insights.

Church leaders (AB members and ethnographers) stated that the *lectio divina* process allowed them to access their own deeper truths around what they needed to bring more health into their lives and give them voice. According to Rev. Stark, as time progressed, they seemed more open to offer suggestions and to state very clearly what they felt would and would not work within their congregations. Lay leaders suggested nine themes inspired by scripture that Rev. Stark used as a baseline to develop her monthly Bible study curriculum around healthful eating and practice:

1. Made in the image of God
2. Commitment
3. Planning and structure
4. Health and stewardship of food
5. Support and accountability
6. Overcoming obstacles and stress
7. The importance of being and mindfulness
8. Our brothers' and sisters' keepers
9. Being a voice for the voiceless

Implications for need: Lectio divina allows successful implementation of the wellness program by serving as a catalyst for participants to deepen their engagement in the program and by facilitating integration of mind, body, and spirit.

Pastor as role model

The role of the pastor in the African American church is unique, historical, and powerful. In interviews and focus groups, Rush researchers learned that the pastor's engagement in adopting a healthy lifestyle through participation in the wellness program was viewed as the most important factor in changing congregational health. As one congregant noted,

> It's good to start with churches. Historically in our community, that's been where people felt credibility. If my pastor said that we should protest, vote, get education, then that's what we should do.

One of the inside ethnographers told of being on a mission to Africa to try (unsuccessfully) to educate a village against drinking unsafe well water:

> But once the word spread that the chief was no longer drinking the well water…suddenly most of the villagers stopped drinking the well water too. What we had been trying to accomplish in five months, the chief accomplished in a matter of days. Maybe there is a correlation here in this story to faith and health and wellness? Or the power of our leaders and where change must come from in order to affect people's lives?

The pastors who participated in this program charismatically engaged their congregations through the sharing of topical and political events, song, humor, and personal anecdotes relevant to the African American community. Congregants commended their pastors for being "passionate," "knowledgeable," and "interactive" and for "connecting scripture to real life." Their pastors were credited with making church "a safe place" in which members could openly "show their love and support for one another." One congregant said, "Our pastor is a church mother, so we all have the faith that she has already been where we are going and we are interested in her acquired wisdom." She added, upon reflecting on the distrust among church members with the medical community, that doctors might benefit from modeling some aspects of the pastor–congregant relationship. "Perhaps patients are so far removed from the medical community because the doctors are removed from those that they treat." Through observing these interpersonal communication dynamics, the team began to understand how each pastor might incorporate wellness content into his or her teachings.

One challenge pastors faced as a direct result of their popularity and important role in church life was the threat of burnout. One pastor related to me that the joke about the Baptist Church was that the pastor "dies in his church," unlike with other churches. These pastors acknowledged that the support of their congregations in working toward and maintaining certain wellness goals was critical to their own successful health outcomes, as well as to the church as a whole. As discussed earlier, the pastors were the ones who had initiated a self-care program with the guidance of Rush researchers and had then decided to try to expand the benefits they experienced to their congregations.

Implications for need: The pastor is a powerful role model whose personal health must be supported by the congregation. Likewise, pastors who model and teach wellness practices and behavior to their congregations from the pulpit and thereby enhance the likelihood of the wellness program's success.

Racism as collective reality

One factor that was conspicuously absent, for the most part, from interviews and focus group discussions was the impact of racism on the health and well-being of congregants. However, through PO at church services, the existence of racism on an institutional level was commonly and explicitly referenced, often by connecting current events to biblical themes. For example, during a sermon one pastor described the context in which a guilty murderer was freed while Jesus was kept in custody, and then paused to say to his congregation, "Isn't it interesting that the Zimmerman trial is still going on after two years?" (George Zimmerman is known for shooting an unarmed African American high school student in Florida and was acquitted in 2013 of second-degree murder.) In another biblical example, the pastor described how Jesus challenged a high priest and then referenced forced confessions and police brutality. Another pastor observed during a Bible study how "Jesus was political and wouldn't back down even from the most powerful," leading to a heated discussion around the day's U.S. Supreme Court decision to dismantle a key provision of the Voting Rights Act, one of the pillars of the Civil Rights Movement (Justice Clarence Thomas, an African American, was instrumental in bringing the Court to this conclusion):

> The USA is in a sad state to vote down this act. And Clarence Thomas, he benefited from affirmative action and then betrays his own community! Well, I suppose nothing has changed. Guess what? I woke up this morning and I am still Black!

The film *Soul Food Junkie* makes the case that aspects of the national food system are organized as a "class apartheid." It tracks a food history originating from slave survival gardens to Jim Crow laws that barred African Americans from restaurants to the Black Panthers breakfast programs. As with discussion of the Supreme Court decision to void part of the Voting Rights Act, some commentary following the film's screenings centered on racism as a barrier to well-being and a source of resistance to outside "intervention." One church member plainly stated, "I can't stand it when people tell me what to eat." Another congregant remarked, "Those same foods, fried chicken, chittlins, and pig's feet, brought Negroes through slavery and Jim Crow, so they must have some nutritional value because they kept us alive and strong long enough to do the master's work."

Implications for need: Institutionalized racism might not be openly discussed with White outside researchers but is openly acknowledged among congregational members at church events. Racism is likely a contributing factor challenging physical, mental, and spiritual health but proved difficult to assess. For a wellness program to be successful, it must find a way to address issues of structural violence that endanger health by either limiting access to resources or causing stress-induced "weathering."

In conclusion, applying ethnographic methods to this NA resulted in the research team's understanding of important elements about church and African American culture that would influence the wellness program design: how congregants defined the intersection between faith and health (that faith is foundational and communally imagined); that food is deeply personal and signifies abundance and generosity; that *lectio divina* is useful as a method to engage participants and help integrate the mind, body, and spirit; and that pastor investment in and modeling of the wellness project is vital to its success. This study also found that racism is still a stressor that impacts the community but in ways that are yet undefined in terms of how it affects personal health and wellness.

Discussion

As much work in the critical anthropology of development has documented, the conceptual ideal of accompaniment within translational CBPR research is often undermined by tensions around power sharing, incompatible timelines, clashing discourses, and the need to balance community stakeholder interests with the demands of scientific criteria that rely on objective measures (Wallerstein & Duran, 2010). What is considered "scientific integrity" can be understood as "either conceptually or logistically flexible" by professional investigators or as based more on "trust, accountability, and overall benefit to the community" by community investigators (Diaz, Johnson, & Arcury, 2015).

The NA methodology described in this article was successful in that it allowed the health program design to be coproduced by the congregation. Two central factors contributing to the successful collaboration were (1) choosing the site of the church, already considered by congregants to be a kind of spiritual hospital, to launch the health program and (2) securing the endorsement of pastors. As one researcher stated, "Understanding where 'authority' comes from in the church community was enhanced by partnership with the pastors at every level. For example, at critical points we had Rev. Ragland on a video explaining why it was important to be healthy—in scriptural terms. And Rev. Stark developed our Bible study curriculum to show that, as one participant said, 'God cares what I eat.'" The fact that the program was initiated by Rev. Alan Ragland, who invited other pastors and Advisory Board members with high levels of experience and education to the project was also instrumental to helping achieve clearer lines of communication around research goals and processes and to navigating what one researcher called "the often vast cultural divide between academia and the community."

Still, many challenges were encountered in conducting this research. On the quantitative medical research end, some professionals questioned the utility and "scientific rigor" of using PO prior to beginning the needs assessment. But ultimately a majority of the Rush researchers on the team argued that an understanding of the beliefs, values, and needs of the people within the church was required before attempting to gather the quantitative data needed to measure, replicate, and operationalize health behaviors within a wellness program.

Medical researchers on the team described how CBPR methods informed the NA as follows.

Benefits

1. Recruitment of participants two months. For a typical study, recruiting more than 200 people would take two years or so. In the church setting we chose, all the potential participants were in one place and the pastors helped accelerate recruitment.
2. The methods led to understanding that the church's assets—strong faith in the community and commitment to using the Bible (and the pastor's interpretation of it)—are central guides to life and allow members to cope with extraordinary life challenges.
3. In CBPR, as researchers identify discrepancies in findings, it presents a learning opportunity to strengthen relationships and clarify communication.
4. Researchers and community members were perceived as being on equal footing, which contributed to much more open communication and sharing of ideas.
5. This study design allowed for improved cultural tailoring of the health program to be most appealing and effective for the congregations.
6. As a result of the study, more people in the community could potentially benefit from the services offered by the program, and the attention to building relationships with the community made it clear that this is a priority for the researchers as well.
7. The methods used allowed the team to realize that the church is the original version of behavioral "intervention," a finding that was eye-opening. The learned people—pastors, elders, Bible study teachers—inserted context around the sacred word—scripture—in a setting that provided shared experience, accountability, and social support, all elements known to increase the chance for sustained behavior change.

Challenges

1. Community members who helped with recruitment (and participants) may not fully understand the risk of dropout and the problems that causes later such as biased outcomes.
2. There may be distinct motivations for academic versus community partners and it takes a lot of trust on both sides to engage in a project together without fully understanding the perspective of the other. Trust issues are critical on *both* sides, the academic partner also can have a lot at stake in the relationship/project.
3. Academic language does not always translate to communities with the same meaning, so this causes some translational challenges. Example: use of the word "intervention."
4. Lots of cooks in the kitchen makes it slow going.
5. The academic medical center is still largely entrenched with hierarchies of expertise. Acknowledging the value of lay knowledge in research may take time and can go against institutional norms..
6. Offering a standard randomized controlled trial (RCT) may not be acceptable to the communities we work with, as one group doesn't get the target intervention, and this feels unfair. However, this poses challenges to many within the scientific community who feel this compromises the study's scientific rigor. Perhaps most significantly, CBPR differs from controlled trials in that the subjective experience of participants is acknowledged and the reflexivity of both researchers and participants is viewed as "evidence" worth documenting. The challenge is to be creative in developing methods that allow for all participants to potentially benefit.

Church member feedback

This section discusses feedback from church members related to their experience serving on the Rush ethnographer team. Individuals cited different challenges, many of which related to their comfort level in the ethnographer role but some reflecting a concern about the medical institutional commitment to the process. When asked why they thought their pastors had recommended them to Rush researchers for the position, many thought it was their interest in nutrition and health. Others cited their communication and "people" skills. One young woman experienced doubt about her ability to perform well in the role, "but you don't tell the pastor 'no' so I said 'fine' and came [on the team]."

When asked about their experience interviewing their fellow congregational members, the church members' responses varied in accordance with the way they felt their personalities fit with the role of ethnographer. One ethnographer who was working on her master's degree in divinity understood the importance of translating cultural meanings and had faced such translational challenges during a mission to Zaire (the aforementioned mission trip during which she and her colleagues were trying to convince local villagers to stop drinking well water). Another described herself as an "introvert" who said recruiting interview respondents helped her "get out of her shell." Initially, she had not felt qualified to analyze the data "because I don't have a degree," but she learned to recognize the value of her perspective "because my summary reflections showed really interesting patterns within my community."

As ethnographers began to feel more comfortable with the research process, they began to own their role as true collaborators, translating interview protocols using language that was more conversational and accessible and using their own examples to clarify concepts in the interview scripts that were confusing to participants.

When asked about what they could have done differently, they talked about asking more follow-up questions, pointing out where they had received feedback on their transcripts in those areas. But they also learned to develop their own reflexivity and "trust my own intuition," not "push" respondents, and "stay present to notice what's not being said." Some noticed that the tone of the interviews shifted once the tape recorder was turned on and respondents felt "afraid who was going to get this information." Others felt resistance from cooks in the churches who seemed wary of being judged and protective of their position in the church. Another ethnographer was surprised to discover the mind-set of some of her fellow congregants who were "honest about not changing their behavior until a negative diagnosis forced them to." Yet another was equally surprised to discover how much knowledge already existed among her fellow church members, especially the elders.

Because the community tends to have an action-oriented agenda rather than a research-oriented one (Israel et al., 1998), at times the NA process felt abstract to congregational members. Lay leaders and inside ethnographers sometimes pushed for something concrete to offer church members early in the process. When asked if taking the time to talk to congregants during the NA helped them establish a sense of ownership in the project and enhance their engagement, views were mixed. One ethnographer said, "Not really. It's hard to motivate people to change if they don't want to change or wait until crisis to consider changing." Another mused, "I think it made people think about their health in a deeper way, like 'how can I practice some of these healthy habits?'…but people did struggle to relate faith with the body." And another one reflected, "I don't know yet…my take was, after we spoke they went on with their lives…people talk about having Rush people [medical researchers] come over, but ultimately we have to keep it going ourselves."

All ethnographers agreed that it was much easier to recruit participants and explain the needs assessment directly following some form of institutional partnership support. "In the first few months it was hard to get people to commit to an interview because they didn't know what I was doing," explained one ethnographer. Publicity was needed to "generate excitement" and "establish legitimacy," and it eventually took many forms, from the creation of a brochure to a public announcement from their pastor to the commencement ceremony, which officially anointed the participants into the ALIVE! program in a formal ritual. As more congregants became aware of the project and partnership with the medical center, they became more willing to talk with the ethnographers.

At the end of the NA, ethnographers were asked how their training in ethnographic methods could be improved. It was agreed that ideally, an expert ethnographer (with formal training) would have been assigned to partner with each lay ethnographer at each of the five churches. The one graduate student who had been hired for this purpose to "float" among the five churches was not enough.

Our outside ethnographer felt that the insider/outsider concept was a good one because, on her end, "people take time to explain things they might not with members of the congregation. 'Here in the black community we do X, Y, or Z…or we have a history of not trusting doctors because of X, Y, or Z." But she agreed that the teams would have benefited from a stable 1:1 insider/outsider ratio at each church.

We were allotted three months for PO, which is quite a long time for a public health intervention but is considered short by anthropological fieldwork method standards. Trained as an anthropologist, our outsider ethnographer felt the squeeze. "I would've liked more time to establish trust and build and sustain relationships. As an outsider 'floating' among all the churches, I felt I had to scramble each week to find interviewees." However, despite these constraints, she agreed with the other ethnographers that she had gathered data that were valuable to the NA. As for whether the NA established congregational investment in the project, she commented, "I think that will depend on whether or not they see their suggestions built into the health program: cooking lessons, cookbooks, community gardens… ."

In sum, CBPR methods were successful in eliciting the necessary thick description to contextualize and articulate the needs among congregants and enable coproduction of an effective public health program design. The findings did inform the design in integral ways. Ethnographers learned how congregants view their health and bodies, why Black church members might be resistant to public health interventions around food, what method could help integrate faith and body and help participants identify their spiritual selves with healthy lifestyle behaviors (*lectio divina*), and what would legitimize the program (pastor endorsement and active involvement as well as medical expertise on behavioral change and wellness). Lay ethnographers were indispensable in helping interpret data gathered at all stages of the NA and translate meanings around the intersection of health and faith for members of their community.

Limitations and future research

In terms of logistics, the insider/outsider team was challenged by a deficit of insider ethnographers compared to outsiders (the ratio being 2:5) and would have benefited from a 1:1 ratio with more time allotted for intra-team discussion to analyze findings and PO. The importance of PO in contributing to the needs assessment was evident in the findings around racism, which were commonplace in sermons but did not surface in interviews with Rush staff. Because the impact of race on health was conspicuously absent from interviews and focus groups, its impact on health disparities remains inconclusive and is a limitation of the study. At the same time, it is a testament to the legitimacy of incorporating ethnographic methods such as PO into public health needs assessments.

In contrast to most public health methodologies, a predetermined structure for developing methods to control variables in the ethnographic approach is problematic. Existing scientific, methodological, or theoretical knowledge about cultural systems must be open to discovery. Whitehead (2005) calls fieldwork in this vein an "iterative process of learning episodes" that is highly flexible and creative. But this is also what makes fieldwork and ethnography so problematic for researchers and funders, whose stance toward the research problem is more positivist in its epistemological and ontological framing.

Ultimately, the structures of funding agencies and research guidelines reduce thick descriptions and context into measurable and replicable outcomes, in this case, the measurable goal of increasing fruit and vegetable intake. But the health program also included psychosocial elements informed by the NA: Pastors linked their Christian beliefs/values and care for the body to their testimony about their own personal health journey. Bible study curriculums contained mechanisms for connecting mind, spirit, and body as a "holy trinity" of health. The mechanism of change thereby sought to align personal Christian values with health behavior in a supportive and educational setting. In this way, the public health program was much more tailored to the needs of the community and allied with CBPR ideals than most, but the fact that racism was not addressed in the design, even when it was documented as a community concern in sermons, and in discussions following the screening of *Soul Food Junkies,* points to persistent challenges to incorporating ethnographic methods into public health projects in meaningful ways.

How researchers from various disciplines define the nature of what is being studied and how best to understand it affects the collective research much more than the methods employed (qualitative/quantitative) do. Therefore, understanding the researchers' different epistemological orientations is critical. Is the program containing practical and evidence-based, high quality biomedical expertise meant to change behavior toward eating more vegetables, or can it be redirected to not so much intervene as *accompany* participants in their self-directed journey toward wellness? If the latter is a goal (which it is under the philosophy of CBPR), first researchers must understand why the identification with certain beliefs and practices around food is so deeply personal and communal, prompting church members to proclaim, "food is love."

The public health scientist's motivation to measure and replicate is driven by the important and pressing need to solve public health problems and support a healthier society. But, if pressured by funding deadlines or the necessity to offer something concrete beyond theorizing or descriptive testimony, we fail to understand the cultural practice or process at hand, and, in our haste to measure it, we do our work and our research participants a disservice. The NA to the ALIVE! project incorporating insider/outsider ethnographers, PO, and dialogue sessions that went beyond the focus group is an important corrective to existing public health protocol and an important step toward understanding the complex historical context and relationship between health disparities and food and faith cultures.

Acknowledgements

Special thanks to "insider ethnographers" Jasmine, Marvis, BJ, Virginia, Ray, and Aubry. We acknowledge the Pastors and members of Third Baptist Church of Chicago, Covenant United Church of Christ, First Baptist Church of Park Forest, Faith Community Church, and Parkway Gardens Christian Church, and especially the church coordinators and church leaders who served on the ALIVE Church Leaders Advisory Board. This work was supported by the Institute of Minority Health and Health Disparities of the National Institutes of Health [R24MD007994 to EBL]. The content is solely the responsibility of the authors and does not necessarily represent the official views of the National Institutes of Health.

References

Antonovsky, A. (1979). *Health, stress, and coping.* San Francisco, CA: Jossey-Bass.

Centers for Disease Control and Prevention. (2014, December 31). LCWK1. Deaths, percent of total deaths, and death rates for the 15 leading causes of death in 5-year age groups, by race and sex: United States, 2013. Retrieved from http://www.cdc.gov/nchs/data/dvs/LCWK1_2013.pdf

Diaz, A. E. K., C. R. S. Johnson, & T. A. Arcury. (2015). Perceptions that influence the maintenance of scientific integrity in community-based participatory research. *Health Education & Behavior 42*(3), 393–401.

Farmer, P. (2013, December 23). How liberation theology can inform public health. *Partners in Health.* Retrieved from www.pih.org/blog/dr.-paul-farmer-how-liberation-theology-can-inform-public-health

Geertz, C. (1973). *The interpretation of cultures: Selected essays.* New York, NY: Basic Books.

Geronimus, A. T., M. Hicken, D. Keene, & J. Bound. (2006). "Weathering" and age patterns of allostatic load scores among Blacks and Whites in the United States. *American Journal of Public Health, 96*(5), 826–833.

Gunderson, G., & L. M. Pray. (2009). *Leading causes of life: Five fundamentals to change the way you live your life.* Nashville, TN: Abingdon Press.

Israel, B. A., A. J. Schulz, E. A. Parker, & A. B. Becker. (1998). Review of community-based research: Assessing partnership approaches to improve public health. *Annual Review of Public Health, 19,* 173–202.

Krumeich, A., W. Weijts, P. Reddy, & A. Meijer-Weitz. (2001, April). The benefits of anthropological approaches for health promotion research and practice. *Health Education Research*, 16(2), 121–130. https://doi.org/10.1093/her/6.2.121.

Lincoln, Y. S., & E. G. Guba. (1985). *Naturalistic inquiry.* Newbury Park, CA: Sage.

Lynch, E., E. Emery-Tiburcio, S. Dugan, F. S. White, C. Thomason, L. D. Jenkins, C. Feit, E. Avery-Mamer, Y. Wang, L. Mack, & A. Ragland. (2019). Results of ALIVE: A faith-based pilot intervention to improve diet among African American church members. *Progress in Community Health Partnerships: Research, Education, and Action*, 13(1), 19–30. (Article) Johns Hopkins University Press.

Taylor, R., & L. Chatters. (1991). Religious life. In J. S. Jackson (Ed.), *Life in Black America* (pp. 105–123). Newbury Park, CA: Sage.

Tubesing, D. A., P.C. Holinger, G.E. Westberg, & E.A. Lichter. (1977). The Wholistic Health Center Project: An action-research model for providing preventive whole-person health care at the primary level. *Medical Care, 15*(3), 217–227.

Wallerstein, N., & B. Duran. (2010). Community-based participatory research contributions to intervention research: The intersection of science and practice to improve health equity. *American Journal of Public Health, 100*(Suppl. 1), S40–S46.

Whitehead, T. L. (2005). Basic Classical Ethnographic Methods, CEHC Working Papers, TL Whitehead Associates. http://tonywhitehead.squarespace.com/tools-products/

PART VIII

Note-taking and writing up

20

FIELDNOTES IN ETHNOGRAPHIC RESEARCH

Ruth Strudwick

Introduction

Field notes are qualitative notes created by the researcher during qualitative fieldwork. They can be used during observation, interviews, and focus groups. Initially, field notes were places where researchers could record their own private thoughts and ideas regarding their research interviews and observations (Phillippi & Lauderdale, 2018). Often in healthcare research, these field notes were not considered to be robust data and were therefore not included in the data analysis and remained private (Ottenberg, 1990). However, it is now recognised that field notes can be considered data which can be analysed and interpreted. Field notes are used to enhance data and provide a rich context for data analysis (Creswell, 2006). Field notes aid in providing thick and rich descriptions of the research setting and the context (Phillippi & Lauderdale, 2018).

During this chapter we will focus on the use of field notes during observation. Field notes in this context are used to note the behaviours, activities, and events that occur whilst the researcher is observing the participants. The notes are intended to be read as evidence that gives meaning and aids in the understanding of the culture, social situation or phenomenon being studied. Field notes allow the researcher to access the subject and record what they observe in an unobtrusive manner. They may constitute the whole data set collected for a research study, for example when observation is the only method used, or they may contribute to the data and be used alongside other data, for example from surveys, interviews, or focus groups (Schwandt, 2015). Gall, Borg, and Gall (1996) advise that field notes do not just need to be words, rather sketches and diagrams can also be part of the notes.

Ethnographic research involves observation of the participants within their natural setting. Marshall and Rossman (1989) define this observation as "the systematic description of events, behaviours, and artefacts in the social setting chosen for study" (p. 79). Observation allows the researcher to describe the situations through field notes to provide a "written photograph" of the situation under study (Erlandson, Harris, Skipper, & Allen, 1993).

So, it seems that writing field notes is relatively simple and straightforward; you go to your research site, observe what is happening, and then write it down. However, what should the researcher be writing down? There is very little guidance in the literature, there appears to be an assumption made that researchers will know what they need to record. However, decisions made at the start of the observation will have an impact on the final research report and there could be a lack of recording of useful information (Wolfinger, 2002). Research texts say that the researcher should take field notes, but there is very little emphasis on what should be recorded in these notes. Wolfinger (2002) suggests that when in the field, ethnographers need to continually ask questions and decide what to write about. They need to think about what they are noticing, what they are focusing their attention on, what they decide is important, and how much detail to record. Ethnography places a lot of discretion at the hands of the researcher – they are the research instrument and the research is iterative and inductive, i.e. the researcher's experiences in the field will guide the direction of the study. The researcher can therefore identify what they think to be important, interesting, and worthy of being noted down.

Merriam (1998) suggests that the researcher needs to focus on what the purpose of the research is in order to determine what they should observe. However, she also says that where to focus and when to stop cannot be determined ahead of time.

There are, of course, some practical considerations. It is best practice to write notes during the observation as things happen so that they remain fresh in the memory – many authors suggest that this is the best approach (Lofland & Lofland, 1984; Berg, 1989; Goffman, 1989). However, in some settings it may not be possible to note things down at the time and an observer taking notes might distract participants or cause the observer to miss important aspects of events (Muswazi & Nhamo, 2013). The notes taken in the field could be seen to be preliminary findings, which can then be built upon and completed more fully after the event. Therefore the researcher needs to consider how to write their notes in the setting and give themselves time to review these notes after the period of observation. Hammersley and Atkinson (1991) suggest that the focus of an ethnographic study will narrow over time. This means that the researcher will reduce the detail in the information recorded. This is a natural response as the researcher becomes more familiar with the setting and behaviours. This also needs to be considered as there may be information that is missed as a consequence. The information recorded by the researcher may also be influenced by the perceived audience, and they may be reserved about what to include and how to record the information (Emerson, Fretz, & Shaw, 1995). The researcher also needs to consider if they are happy for participants to read their notes or if they want to keep them private; this will obviously have an effect on what is recorded.

Prior to field note collection the researcher will need to plan their approach. They need to plan where will they locate themselves, how long they will be observing for, and how they will record their notes. Observation and note-taking can be tiring, and it is important to remain focused on the task at hand.

Notes will include both descriptive and reflective data. The descriptive information will largely be factual, e.g. date, time, location, setting, actions, behaviours, and conversations observed. The reflective information will include thoughts, feelings, ideas, questions, and concerns that you have as a researcher during the period of observation.

Spradley (1980, p. 78) provides a list of things to consider:

- Space: the physical place/places
- Actor: the people involved
- Activity: a set of related acts that people do
- Object: the physical things that are present
- Act: single actions that people do
- Event: a set of related activities that people carry out
- Time: the sequencing that takes place over time
- Goal: the things people are trying to accomplish
- Feeling: the emotions felt and expressed

Other authors provide useful tips for the researcher. Taylor and Brogdan (1984) suggest that the observer should be unobtrusive in clothing and actions, become familiar with the setting beforehand, keep the observation time short at first to maintain concentration, and be honest with the participants about what they are doing. Merriam (1998) adds that the researcher should pay attention by shifting from a "wide" to a "narrow" angle, focusing on the whole group and then individuals. He also suggests looking out for key words or phrases.

Field notes should also be ordered chronologically – this ensures that notes are taken in the order that they occur.

Advantages and disadvantages of field notes

As we are all aware, participant observation allows the researcher to see the "backstage culture"; if they are recorded well, then field notes can provide a unique insight and a detailed description of the setting. If this is the case, field notes will provide rich data which can be analysed (Muswazi & Nhamo, 2013). The field notes can assist the researcher in their interpretation of the observational data and can also lead to the development of future research questions and ideas. Field notes can be valuable in recalling events at a later date and providing information for other researchers or for constructing questions for follow-up interviews or focus groups.

One major disadvantage of taking field notes is that they are recorded by one observer and are thus subject to the researcher's memory of events (Canfield, 2011), and possibly, the conscious or unconscious bias of the observer. It is best therefore to record field notes at the time or immediately after leaving the site to avoid forgetting important details. The data recorded by the researcher will be based on their own individual interest and what they consider to be important. It may be, therefore, that some things are missed or not recorded by the researcher.

The recording of field notes may prevent participants from giving information when the researcher is present or modifying their behaviour. These changes in behaviour are termed the "Halo" and the "Hawthorne" effects (Asch, 1946; Vehmas, 1997; Bowling, 2004).

In some settings, whilst the researcher is taking notes, they may miss something or cause a distraction to the participants which could result in them altering their behaviour. Note-taking can also interrupt the communication between the researcher and the participants.

Credibility, trustworthiness, and authenticity should always be considered, just like with any other qualitative data collection method. It is important that the researcher introduces themselves in their writing in order to ensure their credibility to their readers. The reader will always be asking "is this account of events believable?" Therefore the researcher needs to ensure that sufficient detail is provided in the field notes to ensure that their account of events is credible, trustworthy, and authentic. Descriptive information as well as facts will need to be included in order to provide that "written photograph" of the situation under study that Erlandson et al., (1993) encourages and which was discussed earlier in this chapter.

Application to my own study

In my own ethnographic study of the culture in a diagnostic imaging department, I carried out participant observation for four months and during that time I took field notes in a small notebook. I used these field notes to record my observations and also my own thoughts and feelings about what was going on. Allan (2006) suggests that the researcher's thoughts and feelings are also important data. In my notes I clearly differentiated between my actual observations and my thoughts on those observations. I felt that it was important to record how I felt about what I had observed. When I typed the observations up afterwards I used italics to represent my feelings.

I recorded actions, interactions, what people said, how they behaved, what was happening, and what I saw. Along with this I recorded the location in which these events occurred and the context.

The field notes that I took were personal to me and I chose what to record (Coffey, 1999). This involved my decisions about what was significant (Agar, 1980; Anspach & Mizrachi, 2006). Abbott and Sapsford (1997) state that the interpretations, values, and interests of the researcher are a central part of the research. My ideas obviously directed where I observed and what I observed. It may be that I could have missed some elements of the culture and events that occurred. Although often when I wasn't observing in one particular area, I would still find out about events in other areas of the department as staff members would discuss what had been going on during breaks and lunchtimes in the staff room.

It was decided, in discussion with the manager of the department, that I should wear a radiographer's uniform for the duration of the observation. It was felt that this would be less intimidating for both staff and patients and I would fade into the background more easily. Coffey (1999) says that the researcher should have an acceptable appearance, which includes dress, demeanour, and speech. Hammersley and Atkinson (1991) agree, suggesting that the personal appearance and impression created by the researcher can influence data collection.

I chose the locations from which to observe after my initial survey of the imaging department, during which I tried to determine the main areas of the department where interactions between staff took place and areas which would provide me with useful and meaningful data. I was able to observe a cross section of the staff working in the imaging department, on different days of the week, at different times of the day, and in different locations. I wanted to build a picture of the whole department and how it worked.

During the period of observation I learnt my own style. When I started I found it difficult to decide what to record and how to record it. I developed a note form with my own abbreviations which I typed up as soon as I reached home when the work was still fresh in my mind. I used the drive home to reflect on my day and did a lot of thinking in the car. I was keen to formally record the data as soon as possible after the event to reduce the chances of inaccuracy.

Summary

Field notes are a useful data collection method to use with participant observation. The researcher needs to carefully consider how they will record information and decide on the data to be recorded. Field notes need to be credible, trustworthy, and authentic. They can be used to recall events, assist in data analysis, and help to frame future research questions. If used well, field notes can be key in uncovering the hidden aspects of the culture being studied.

References

Abbott, P. & R. Sapsford. (Eds.) (1997) Research into Practice – A Reader. OU Press, Buckingham.

Agar, M.H. (1980) The Professional Stranger – An Informal Introduction to Ethnography. Academic Press, London.

Allan, H.T. (2006) Using participant observation to immerse oneself in the field: The relevance and importance of ethnography for illuminating the role of emotions in nursing practice. Journal of Research in Nursing 11: 397–407.

Anspach, R.R. & N. Mizrachi. (2006) The field worker's fields: ethics, ethnography and medical sociology. Sociology of Health and Illness 28(6): 713–731.

Asch, S.E. (1946) Forming impressions of personality. Journal of Abnormal and Social Psychology 41: 258–290.

Berg, B.L. (1989) Qualitative Research Methods for the Social Sciences. Allyn and Bacon, Needham Heights, MS.

Bowling, A. (2nd Ed.) (2004) Research Methods in Health – Investigating Health and Health Services. Open University Press, Maidenhead.

Canfield, M. (2011) Field Notes on Science & Nature. Harvard University Press.

Coffey, A. (1999) The Ethnographic Self. Sage, London.

Creswell, J.W. (2006) Qualitative Inquiry and Research Design – Choosing Among Five Approaches, (2nd Ed.). Sage, London.

Emerson, R.M., R.I. Fretz, & L.L. Shaw. (1995) Writing Ethnographic Fieldnotes. University of Chicago Press, Chicago.

Erlandson, D.A., E.L. Harris, B.L. Skipper, & S.D. Allen. (1993) Doing Naturalistic Inquiry: A Guide to Methods. Sage, Newbury Park, Canada.

Gall, M.D., W.R. Borg, & J.P. Gall. (1996) Educational Research: An Introduction, (6th Ed.). Longman, White Plains, NY.

Goffman, E. (1989) On Fieldwork. Journal of Contemporary Ethnography, 18: 123–32.

Hammersley, M. & P. Atkinson. (1991) Ethnographic Principles in Practice. Routledge, London.

Lofland, J. & L. Lofland. (1984) Analyzing Social Settings (2nd Ed.). Wadsworth, Belmont, CA.

Marshall, C. & G.B. Rossman. (1989) Designing Qualitative Research. Sage, Newbury Park, CA.

Merriam, S.B. (1998) Qualitative Research and Case Study Applications in Education. Jossey-Bass Publishers, San Francisco.

Muswazi, M.T. & E. Nhamo. (2013) Note taking: A lesson for Novice Qualitative Researchers. Journal of Research and Method in Education, 2(3): 13–17.

Ottenberg, S. (1990) Thirty years of fieldnotes: Changing relationships to the text. In Sanjek R (Ed.) Fieldnotes: The Makings of an Anthropology (pp. 139–160). Cornell University Press, Ithaca, NY.

Phillippi, J. & J. Lauderdale. (2018) A Guide to Field Notes for Qualitative Research: Context and Conversation. Qualitative Health Research, 28(3): 381–388.

Schwandt, T.A. (2015) The SAGE Dictionary or Qualitative Inquiry, (4th Ed.). Sage, Thousand Oaks, CA.

Spradley, J.P. (1980) Participant Observation. Holt, Reinhart & Winston, New York.

Taylor, S. & R. Brogdan. (1984) Introduction to Qualitative Research: The Search for Meanings, (2nd Ed.). John Wiley, New York.

Vehmas, T. (1997) Hawthorne effect: shortening of fluoroscopy times during radiation measurement studies. British Journal of Radiology, 70(838): 1053–1055.

Wolfinger, N.H. (2002) On writing fieldnotes: collection strategies and background expectancies. Qualitative Research, 2(1): 85–95.

21

WRITING AND REPRESENTATION

Michael Klingenberg

Introduction: Laboratory to fact

This chapter is a discussion on the transformation of observation into text. In order to make a number of methodological points about writing and representation in ethnography, I will employ analytical concepts from Actor-Network-Theory, which helped me make sense of the world during my doctoral studies. I will begin by briefly outlining these concepts and their operationalisation in the field of nursing selection which my thesis was concerned with.

Actor-Network-Theory (or ANT), first developed by Latour (1999b) proposes that differences and equivalences between actors do not precede but are a result of interactions between such actors (Latour, 2005). In their seminal study, Latour and Woolgar (1986) demonstrate how scientific facts are not based on discovery, but are brought into being through a series of translations, that is, actions that allow entities to change shape and location and yet be taken for the same, to represent each other. Translations constitute specific summaries, emphasising and deemphasising parts and thereby orientating attention to specific concerns (Berg, 1997). Through translations, connections are forged which, in theory at least, could have been different. Whether such connections are successful depends on the characteristics of the actors involved. This includes theoretical assumptions about how research should be performed, or how science should be done. Law (2004) evocatively termed this backdrop for conceptualising the world "hinterland".

Hinterlands determine practice through specific training but can also be found in inscription devices, the techniques and apparatuses that help make the inaccessible accessible. These inscription devices perform translation in a framed and framing way. They come with their own possibilities and limitations on capturing what is "out there"; they already contain a specific idea of what can be described or "found". Through translations, the world is scaled up and down in order to make it accessible, in order to say something about a moment in time that can then be extended to again represent the world. In a laboratory, a substance which may or may not exist, invisible to the human eye, can, through centrifuges and computers, become graphs; graphs become numbers; numbers become published papers; and papers, if persuasive enough to be accepted as *evidence*, become proof that the substance does in fact exist "out there" in the world. The work that brought the substance about has disappeared from record and thereby from view (Latour & Woolgar, 1986).

In my doctoral work, I ethnographically engaged with selection for undergraduate nursing degrees in the UK. This selection is often positioned as the comparison of two points in time: selection method and outcome (see HEE, 2014 for an outline of this specific argument). My thesis claimed that if nursing selection is understood as practice, attributes such as personal values become the product of local interactions during selection events, rather than traits inherent to applicants. Through interactions of selection materials (such as interview forms) and translation and orientation of applicant speech by selectors into words on notepads and later into scores, selector work is successively removed, and action becomes solely associated with an applicant.

In this chapter I would like to make a similar point about writing ethnographically. Sketching out a trajectory from observation to published text, writing here will be interrogated as a practice. Concepts from ANT will help to illuminate this trajectory: technologies of translation force the observed world and ethnographic texts into particular shapes and particular messages about the world. This process is facilitated by personal, socio-theoretical, and methodological hinterlands. Such hinterlands, for example, play a substantial part in how journal articles on healthcare ethnographies can be written. The final section will argue that ethnographic texts, when written in the way outlined here, constitute scientific work in that they do not represent observation but enact the world. A text is all there is.

Throughout this chapter I will make reference to my own doctoral work and the resulting thesis (Klingenberg, 2018) as well as a published paper based on this work (Klingenberg & Pelletier, 2019). I will begin by discussing processes that turn participants' actions into observations and such observations into records.

Translations: the fleeting made durable

It is often said that ethnographers are protective of fieldnotes, not wanting to share undigested ideas (Emerson, Fretz, & Shaw, 1995; Van Maanen, 2011); I am doing it here to discuss how the world (selection in nursing somewhere in the UK, somewhere in time) becomes translated into specific records of that world, which in turn become, through further translations, a text, in this case a doctoral thesis.

> The first candidate I see is Pratibha. Pratibha, wearing a pink jacket and a smart black outfit, stands outside the booth and breathes in deeply. When Pratibha walks in, she introduces herself to the selector; the selector doesn't mention her name. The selector is Sara; her clipboard is down, and you can see the photo for the next question.
>
> Sara asks the question and Pratibha says something which I can't remember, then mentions the 6C's and tries (by using her fingers, which she points at with other fingers) to remember all of them. When Pratibha talks (often using her hands, while Sara's hands are crossed), what is most apparent to me, or interesting, is that she talks about nursing using the terms "we" and "our" as in: we have to do this, and it is our job. Pratibha isn't a nurse.
>
> When Pratibha becomes quiet, Sara asks "would you like me to repeat the question". Pratibha says yes and keeps talking; she starts talking about herself but quickly changes to hypothetical examples; no examples from experience are talked about. Pratibha sometimes uses the term "them" when referring to patients, as in: "a good nurse makes them feel like a person". Sara looks at Pratibha throughout and smiles. I can't see Sara writing. At some point, probably when Pratibha stops talking again, Sara asks: "is there anything else you want to add?". Pratibha starts talking about her job

then. She works in a care home, where she sees good and bad practice. Sara circled a 2 ("identifies a strength, but no objective data") for the station and the word "acceptable". Sara has not written anything other than that. (A few days later I will have the chance to talk to Sara about how she marked one applicant. She will tell me that she never writes, only if somebody fails a station. I have seen her in the past; I think she once showed me how she goes through the grid to justify judgement.)

(Fieldnotes)

Not all selectors wrote things down. Selectors, where they did not write, either gave as a reason: the fact that they needed to pay attention or that they only wrote when an applicant was to be rejected. As this judgment can only be made after some time during the interview, transcriptions in these cases constituted further reductions: in only transporting the reasons for rejection, everything that could be understood as a counterargument disappeared from record. Writing therefore is a selective action and for Latour and Woolgar (1986) it is precisely this selective recording, this emphasising of what is made important through translation and made unimportant through omission that orders actions into one narrative where other narratives are possible.

(Thesis)

Above I juxtapose two extracts: one from fieldnotes taken at one site of observation (a university), the other from my doctoral thesis. In my notes I make reference to an applicant first talking about herself and then giving what I termed "hypothetical" examples of healthcare. My hunch had been that applicants might talk about nursing utilising specific registers and that selectors might use specific categories of selection (formally or informally) based on such talk. This hunch took my attention to places where it otherwise might not have travelled. The idea of specific registers, however, did not make it into the thesis.

One reason for this can be found in the context in which the study took place and the materials employed to make observations last. I had not asked for ethical approval to audio-record selection interviews or for permission to formally interview individual applicants. Doing so would have made the study unfeasible within the allocated timeframe. I tried to write during interviews as quickly as I could, but, not being able to write shorthand, I could never write enough to produce sufficient data to honestly make the point outlined above. In the end I gave up. Writing on notepads and digitally recording transported words differently and fieldnotes became different to what they might have been. Moreover, writing things on paper allowed me to check what had (just) been written (glancing over a page triggered a thought that, when dictating, may not have occurred to me). When dictating, an attempt at recall often preoccupied me to the extent of obscuring a new thought, which may have been interesting and differently directed my ideas about the field.

Here, the impact of interactions of the human and material world is made visible. Watching and listening cannot hold events beyond the very moment they occur. Such events need to be translated and inscribed to become (more) durable, with inscription devices framing the shape of what is translated (Latour & Woolgar, 1986).

Fieldnotes do not constitute "raw" but "partially cooked" data (Madden, 2017, p. 141). What can and will be said about the field is already inscribed in these notes (Geertz, 1973) and further translations are necessary to turn fieldnotes into ethnographic texts. Atkinson (2015) suggests that processes of translating fieldnotes into empirical content are guided by considerations of economy and cogency, with economy referring, for example, to available space and cogency to the persuasive appeal of an account. In order to achieve economy and cogency, Atkinson proposes rhetorical and narrative techniques such as metaphors or synecdoche (stand-ins, meant to make the field more accessible through evocative description) and emic or etic categories (either those discussed as employed by participants or those proposed by the ethnographer) which collectively seek to explain parts of the field as social world. In my thesis, I created, for example, the metaphor of *heroic talk*, in itself an etic category, which positioned applicants as somehow better than professional nurses. These are not, however, purely narrative devices making field and analysis thereof more accessible, but constitute summaries in the sense that they allow parts of the world to be emphasised and other parts to drift in the background (Berg, 1997). Importantly, such summaries position the analysis, the translation, and the making accessible of data as a function of the ethnographer. As Madden (2017, pp. 141–142) puts it: "Making meaning from data is a rewarding process, and the ethnographer is responsible for it". It is interesting that both Atkinson and Madden, although emphasising the predominant role of the ethnographer in making meaning, seem reluctant to permit substantial autobiographical content in ethnographic texts.

Yet, the way an ethnographer is translated into written text produces specific accounts. What may be termed *autobiographical content* is constituted by the ethnographer writing about themselves in relation to conducting the research, interacting with the field and an acknowledgement of the ideas that have influenced various stages of the ethnographic work, from conception to writing up. This process is often termed "reflexivity". Atkinson (2019) discusses reflexivity as an important aspect of ethnographic work in that ethnographies always constitute the social world they aim to represent. More often, however, ideas of reflexivity appear to refer to the impact of the researcher on the field. Madden (2017, p. 23) for example writes that "reflexivity is not really about 'you, the ethnographer'; it's still about 'them, the participants'. The point of getting to know 'you, the ethnographer' better, getting to know the way you influence your research is to create a more reliable portrait, argument, or theory about 'them, the participants'". Madden seems to argue that writing about one's own influences in the ethnographic process allows the reader to access participants more directly, to somehow remove the ethnographer influence and see a "truer" picture of the field. Understanding reflexivity this way allows for a notion of ethnography in which the work of the ethnographer can (at least partially) be made visible through writing, and through this visibility somehow become removed from an overall account (for example, in the split between being "self-aware" and "researcher self-aware" discussed by Greene, 2014, p. 9). The field becomes purer, akin to a notion of reality rather than a co-constructed account of interactions. Although the problem of representing the real is acknowledged in most ethnographic texts (see Atkinson, 2015, 2019), a wealth of such texts, especially those that are published in journals as research papers, seem to constitute what van Maanen (2011) termed "realistic tales": accounts in which the ethnographer appears as the mostly neutral recorder of a real world. My thesis and subsequently published journal article fall squarely into this category.

Sixty thousand words of fieldnotes from one site of observation which contained the field note excerpt above, made reference to "I" or "me" about 2,500 times. The thesis chapter that included the quote above referred explicitly to me only 84 times, but more importantly in almost all instances as a passive recipient of action. I had written myself as an immutable mobile (Latour, 1990), with action seemingly passing through me, unchanged and not changing me.

One reason for this might be found in the notion of strangemaking when translating fieldnotes into argument (Atkinson, 2015). Strangemaking might be understood as a form of writing oneself "clear" (O'Connell, 2017). To perform what Atkinson (2015, p. 155 original emphasis) labels *ethnographic abduction*, to provide meaningful analytical accounts, the ethnographer has to move away from pure description, taking a step back to compare local instances with ideas, patterns, theoretical concepts. But it might be precisely this move of writing an immediate experience or fieldnotes into an unfamiliar version that provides the writing with the notion of a realistic representation (whether this is desired by the ethnographer or not, whether declarations affecting the opposite are made or not). Reflexive accounts here constitute selective summaries (Berg, 1997), creating a narrative that appears to aim at full (or near full) representation of the observed.

In the case of my research I made my own world strange to myself by reading theory, writing with theory and, importantly, by consistently translating my own writing until it felt like I wrote with someone else's notes. I wrote notes about my notes and notes about those notes, creating summaries and different summaries until what I wrote did not look like notes anymore but an analytical account of selection in nursing. In a way I had written myself (at least in part) out of an ethnography of which I was clearly a part *in order to write ethnographically*. I had somehow got lost in translation. Later, through a discussion of reflexivity in the methodology chapter of my thesis and (later still) in about 15 lines in a journal article, I translated a version of myself back in.

The process of reflexivity as purifying accounts of social worlds by emphasising particular ideas and actions of researchers is accelerated through the separation of autobiographical sections from sections that present empirical content and analysis. It is much rarer that the same influences are specifically written into accounts of the field and analyses thereof. Van Maanen (2011) argues that such "confessional tales" are often published as separate papers, and my reflections on writing here might constitute precisely such a confession.

So far I have discussed translations from the world to text and to text again. Such translations do not operate in a vacuum. In the next section I will focus more specifically on the function of theory in the production of ethnographic texts.

Hinterlands: contingent accounts

Hinterlands are the assumptions on which doing ethnography and translating the field into a final text are based. Such assumptions may be translated into the notion of theory, which informs understanding of ethnography and thereby produces specific ways of writing ethnographic accounts. They also help to understand interactions and data in specific ways, thereby framing data collection and analysis.

Classic healthcare studies have been written with various social theories (for example Boundary Work in Allen, 2001; Symbolic Interactionalism in Becker, Geer, Hughes, & Strauss, 1961; ANT in Mol, 2002; Habitus formation in Sinclair, 1997) as well as current research (for example Logics of Care in Lehn-Christiansen & Holen, 2019; Discourse Analysis in Moreau & Rudge, 2019; Street-Level Bureaucracy in Oute & Bjerge, 2019). These theories permit and possibly compel ethnographers to look at social fields in specific ways, forging an organisation of observation and representation of the observed: for example Foucauldian discourse analysis will emphasise text and power relationships enacted within (Foucault, 1972), where ANT will make the ethnographer look beyond interactions between humans and include the material world in their observations and writing. Any of these theories might reject being used as a framework. Yet being aware of a theory already produces particular interactions between ethnographers and the field. For example, a Foucauldian approach would ask to collect and analyse data differently, focusing on how certain positions become available and unavailable in the performance of texts. ANT was not proposed as a framework by Latour (2005) and not "implemented" as such by me in the sense that I didn't set out to interrogate selection by employing concepts from ANT; I didn't look for instances of translations or hinterlands, but instead used these concepts to make sense of the data generated. However, knowing about ANT already framed some of the things that could be said about the field of selecting for nursing degrees and in fact permitted me to order and make sense of data in the first place (Atkinson, 2015).

Theory allows the legitimisation of statements that otherwise might not easily be made ("reaching theoretical saturation" may sound more convincing than having run out of time or become bored with hearing the same things over and over again). Theory helps to make sense of, and determines, actions, with the notion of strangemaking discussed above a good illustration of this function. Through juxtaposition with data, theory, in a fashion, makes ethnographic accounts generalisable (Atkinson, 2015), and theory supplies shorthand with which to transport ideas across time and space, as demonstrated in the introduction to this chapter and in the following example.

In my thesis, the main argument of the literature review revolved around the fact that claims made in the psychology literature on selection are based on the assumption that values are, to some extent, static entities which can be externalised and measured, and that the tools for measuring such entities, if used expertly and correctly, will work independently of the context in which they are used. For some time, I struggled to order the literature and my ideas into a coherent argument. At the same time, my supervisor suggested a particular examiner and advised me to read a number of papers they had published. It was in reading these papers that I encountered the concept of "affordances" (Oliver, 2005), helping me to make sense of the literature reviewed. In this instance, part of my supervisor's hinterland (knowledge of people and their academic output) had been translated through adaptation of concepts into the structure and main argument of my literature review. In turn, my literature review had taken these concepts outside of a specific context (learning technologies, Oliver, 2016) and inserted them into a new field, that of selection in nursing.

A choice of theory therefore might not be straightforwardly methodological. I had come to doctoral studies from a positivist background. However, assumptions about the world I had were challenged when I was introduced to ideas of psychoanalysis as an analytical framework. Whilst participating in a reading group, I engaged with a number of poststructuralist ideas including ANT, which did not inevitably make ANT the theoretical framework for my theses. Nevertheless, a seed had been planted where earlier it might have fallen on barren ground.

These examples emphasise the contingency of social theory in the production of ethnographic texts. However, hinterlands operate beyond theoretical frameworks.

Hinterlands, as well as translating sociological ideas into ethnographic work, can be constituted by theories about ethnography and ethnographic writing itself. Madden (2017, pp. 158–159), for example, sees ethnography as a systematic approach which should be reflected in the way ethnographic writing is structured: stating and explaining an interest, describing the world as observed, analysing and interpreting, and, finally, justifying the decision to undertake ethnographic work by way of "resolution or conclusion". For Atkinson (2015), good ethnographic writing is constituted in the integration of theory with empirical data; for others, good ethnographic writing is constituted in the way marginalised actors are given voice without being voiced (Skeggs, 2007). And although few authors describe their methodological contemplations as instructive (for example Atkinson 2019), ideas about the value and function of ethnography will find their way from writing about ethnography into writing ethnography (and, like this chapter, back into writing about ethnography). Whether ethnography is written about as neutral (Conroy, 2017) or political (Zuiderent, 2002); as novel and cutting edge (Atkinson, 2015); as a form of social science constituting an amalgamate of the subjective and measurable world (Madden, 2017); or as social criticism (Clough, 2001); whether the function of ethnography is seen as empowering participants (Heyl, 2007) or to undermine common-place assumptions (Atkinson, 2015); whether by showing the complexity of routine work, the routinised character of supposedly complex interactions, or the highlighting of issues of conflict and power (Smith, 2007): whatever the story about ethnography, it has the potential to influence ethnographic writing, persuading to adapt or reject. This is not to say that such versions of ethnography are contradictory or incommensurable, however: they constitute different ideas about ethnography directing the writing in specific ways.

One approach to legitimise texts as ethnographic or *something else* might be the way the empirical, autobiographical, and theoretical are integrated, emphasised, and deemphasised. An overemphasis of the empirical might be seen to lack the analytical depth required to constitute an ethnography (Atkinson, 2015; Madden, 2017). Overemphasis of theory might produce a text that is not recognisable as an account of social interactions but a philosophical treatise of abstract concepts. A lack of autobiographical account might lead to accusations of poor practice or lack of transparency, but will also potentially transform the text into something akin to an objective account or "realist tale" (Van Maanen, 2011). Overemphasising the autobiographical may be seen as paying lip-service to conventions that are not based in methodological considerations, or as a transgression of ethnographic etiquette which requires the interest to be based in the world of the social actors and not in that of the researcher (Atkinson 2015).

Texts may be written for specific audiences and formats (Van Maanen, 2011). These audiences come with their own hinterlands, often translated as rules or guidelines for acceptance or publication. Doctoral dissertations may require different compositions of the three components discussed above to a journal article or journalistic work. (The preceding statement was left deliberately vague; it is not meant to instruct.)

This work is not only the effect of conscious decisions or intent. Although some audiences might be anticipated, it is impossible to know about them, their hinterlands, their assumptions. An example might be found in the responses to drafts of the paper which was based on my doctoral work (Klingenberg & Pelletier, 2019). This paper had been written with a particular style in mind, "with theory", as in the thesis excerpt above. A summary of observations, intertwined with analytical concepts, served to make a theoretical point about the field. Although interested, one reviewer rejected it as ethnography: it didn't have an ethnographic "feel". For this reviewer, the paper did not contain enough instances of empirical content (interview excerpts and vignettes) and not enough instances of autobiography (here the visibility of the author in the field); for another reviewer the paper lacked cogency, a clear justification and explanation of theoretical concepts and their relationship to the data presented. My point here is not to challenge the ideas of reviewers but to demonstrate how hinterlands are imported into texts and how they work to shape texts differently. Persuasion, although orientated and orientation work, is not pure agency but, again, the outcome of interactions. Ideas (based possibly on experience, education, ideological leanings, see Atkinson 2015) meet and need to be negotiated, producing a different text. Such negotiation is not always played out as direct interaction: whether a text is experienced as saying something meaningful or interesting or is seen to constitute ethnography, good or bad, an author may never know.

Not all of the ideas discussed above are reflected in my doctoral thesis (even less so in the subsequent publication). Where a reflexive account in the thesis may have emphasised some hinterlands, in the published paper choices on theoretical frameworks and analytical concepts were written as purely methodological, based on interrogation of theory and field. No word about reading groups, potential buttering up of examiners, no word about the late addition of theory that forced me to rewrite some of the analysis. Including such accounts never occurred to me. Having written with ideas on how to produce ethnographic texts, having been immersed in texts that seemed to produce accounts of observation of, rather than interaction with, the field, I wrote what, to me, constituted (and I hoped to be received as) good ethnographic texts. Hinterlands had become style and style method.

Of course, there are other ways of writing ethnographies, for example postmodern (Lather, 2007), feminist (Skeggs, 2007), experimental (Mienczakowski, 2007), or more overtly auto-biographical, as autoethnography (Reed-Danahay, 2007). These texts operate with different hinterlands, emphasise different elements and may be hailing different audiences (Park, Pelletier, & Klingenberg, 2014). Such forms of writing, however, seem to be rare in ethnography-based articles in healthcare-related journals, specifically those written by authors with a healthcare background. This might be explained to some extent by how ethnography is positioned in healthcare. Through the discourse of "evidence-based-practice", ethnography is placed in the same context as positivist research (Messac, Ciccarone, Draine, & Bourgois, 2013). Often it is written *about* as different from prevailing positivist research, making important contributions based on methodological and philosophical differences (see for example Charmaz & Olesen, 1997; Conroy, 2017; Lambert, Glacken, & McCarron, 2011; Pope, 2005; Reeves, Peller, Goldman, & Kitto, 2013; Savage, 2006). The hinterland of evidence-based-practice requires certain justifications for methodologies and textual conventions based not necessarily on particular socio-theoretical assumptions about the field but on ideas of outcome and neutrality. Assumptions about the need to evidence academic work (and worth) by way of largely journal-based publications, and the way the quality of these papers is measured (often using categories akin to measuring studies of effect), become translated into publications: in order to be valued as part of an evidence-based-practice canon, ethnographies in healthcare are often written in precisely the style of research that ethnography claims to be different from. Papers published in the BMJ (see for example Alderson, Russell, McLintock, Potrata, House, & Foy, 2014; or Swinglehurst, Greenhalgh, Russell, & Myall, 2011) are structured like papers based on trials with references to "outcome measures" and "results". Although these papers may constitute extreme cases, they serve to make a general point about ethnographic texts in healthcare-related journals: they are written as scientific texts, first stating the contingent nature of ethnography and then deleting contingencies from the text, most importantly the ethnographer who becomes a neutral observer of the world. Clough (1998) suggested more than 20 years ago that ethnography should relinquish the desire to be science and become social criticism. Healthcare ethnography as text becomes different practice then, but in the current context of healthcare, where ethnography is seen as important to describe the marginalisation of patients and workers, this may not only be impractical or professionally perilous but also apolitical. In order to become/stay relevant, ethnographic writing might have to continue to justify itself by borrowing textual conventions from positivist research; to oscillate between scientific style and non-positivist message.

Conclusion: world to word to world again

In this chapter I have attempted to demonstrate some of the processes that help translate observed events into written accounts. These processes constitute scientific work in the sense that the world is not simply observed but constituted in the process of recording (Latour & Woolgar, 1986). The vast world of healthcare in all its facets is reduced to selection events in three universities in the UK. These events in turn are limited through selective observation and this observation becomes fieldnotes. A multitude of interactions are summarised, for example, as metaphor or analytic category, thousands of words of fieldnotes become thousands of words of analytical writing which in turn become a thesis and then a published paper. Through adjusting of emphases, texts become more or less "neutral", more or less "real", more or less "ethnographic", more or less "permissible evidence". Through selective inscribing, through emphasising and deemphasising, scales become adjusted: the world is now small enough to be accessible (Latour, 1999a). Further translations help to make big again these accessible instances.

Through hinterlands such as social theory, local events can not only be compared to but *made the same* with events outside of the direct field of observation. But writing does more: through the processes of translation outlined above, a version of the world is being created. As all other versions are blocked from view, this version remains the only durable. This version, then, becomes, retrospectively, what was. Representation becomes the represented: word becomes world (Latour, 1999c), ethnography becomes scientific practice. This work serves to extend into the future, not only of the interrogated social world (nursing selection and how it is understood/researched may be framed by publish texts) but of ethnography *per se*. In writing ethnography in specific ways, blueprints, new hinterlands, are created: what is and can be said about and with ethnography is already inscribed in the way ethnography is written and therefore (to be) done. Writing ethnographic texts here constitutes present, past *and future*.

References

Alderson, S. L., A.M. Russell, K. McLintock, B. Potrata, A. House, & R. Foy. (2014). Incentivised case finding for depression in patients with chronic heart disease and diabetes in primary care: An ethnographic study. *BMJ Open, 4*(8), 1–9.

Allen, D. (2001). *The changing shape of nursing practice*. London: Routledge.

Atkinson, P. (2015). *For ethnography*. London: Sage.

Atkinson, P. (2019). *Writing ethnographically*. London: Sage.

Becker, H. S., B. Geer, E.C. Hughes, & A. Strauss. (1961). *Boys in white. Student culture in medical school*. Chicago; London: University of Chicago Press.

Berg, M. (1997). *Rationalizing medical work*. London: The MIT Press.

Charmaz, K. & V. Olesen. (1997). Ethnographic Research in Medical Sociology. *Sociological Methods & Research, 25*(4), 452–494.

Clough, P.T. (1998). The end(s) of ethnography: Now and then. *Qualitative Inquiry, 4*(1), 3–14.

Clough, P.T. (2001). On the relationship of the criticism of ethnographic writing and the cultural studies of science. *Cultural Studies - Critical Methodologies, 1*(2), 240–270.

Conroy, T. (2017). A beginner's guide to ethnographic observation in nursing research. *Nurse Researcher, 24*(4), 10–14.

Emerson, R., R. Fretz, & K. Shaw. (1995). *Writing field notes in ethnographic research*. Chicago; London: The University of Chicago Press.

Foucault, M. (1972). *The archaeology of knowledge*. Abingdon: Routledge.

Geertz, C. (1973). *The interpretation of cultures*. New York: Basic Books.

Greene, M. J. (2014). On the inside looking in: Methodological insights and challenges in conducting qualitative insider research. *The Qualitative Report, 19*(29), 1–13.

HEE. (2014). *Evaluation of Values Based Recruitment (VBR) in the NHS* (Vol. 2014). Vol. 2014. Retrieved from www.hee.nhs.uk/sites/default/files/documents/VBR literature review.pdf

Heyl, B. S. (2007). Ethnographic Interviewing. In P. Atkinson, A. Coffey, S. Delamont, J. Lofland, & L. Lofland (Eds.), *Handbook of Ethnography* (pp. 369–383). London: Sage.

Klingenberg, M. (2018). *Making a difference: selection in nursing*. University College London.

Klingenberg, M. & C. Pelletier. (2019). The practice of selecting for values in nursing. *Journal of Organizational Ethnography, 8*(3), 312–324.

Lambert, V., M. Glacken, & M. McCarron. (2011). Employing an ethnographic approach: Key characteristics. *Nurse Researcher, 19*(1), 17–23.

Lather, P. (2007). Postmodernism, Post-structuralism and Post(Critical) Ethnography: Of Ruins, Aporias and Angels. In P. Atkinson, A. Coffey, S. Delamont, J. Lofland, & L. Lofland (Eds.), *Handbook of Ethnography* (pp. 477–492). London: Sage.

Latour, B. (1990). Drawing things together. In M. Lynch & S. Woolgar (Eds.), *Representation in Scientific Practice* (pp. 19–68). Cambridge, Massachusetts: MIT Press.

Latour, B. (1999a). Give me a laboratory and I will raise the world. In M. Biagioli (Ed.), *The Science Studies Reader* (pp. 258–275). London: Routledge.

Latour, B. (1999b). On recalling ANT. In J. Law & J. Hassard (Eds.), *Actor Network Theory and After* (pp. 15–25). Oxford: Blackwell.

Latour, B. (1999c). *Pandora's hope: essays on the reality of science studies.* Cambridge: Harvard University Press.

Latour, B. (2005). *Reassembling the social: An introduction to actor-network-theory.* Oxford: University Press.

Latour, B. & S. Woolgar. (1986). *Laboratory life: the construction of scientific facts.* Princeton, NJ; Chichester: Princeton University Press.

Law, J. (2004). *After method: Mess in social science research.* Abingdon: Routledge.

Lehn-Christiansen, S. & M. Holen. (2019). Logics of care in clinical education. *Journal of Organizational Ethnography, 8*(3).

Madden, R. (2017). *Being ethnographic* (2nd ed.). London: Sage.

Messac, L., D. Ciccarone, J. Draine, & P. Bourgois. (2013). The good-enough science-and-politics of anthropological collaboration with evidence-based clinical research: Four ethnographic case studies. *Social Science and Medicine, 99,* 176–186.

Mienczakowski, J. (2007). Ethnodrama: Performed research-limitations and potential. In P. Atkinson, A. Coffey, S. Delamont, J. Lofland, & L. Lofland (Eds.), *Handbook of Ethnography* (pp. 468–476). London: Sage.

Mol, A. (2002). *The body multiple: Ontology in medical practice.* Durham and London: Duke University Press.

Moreau, J. T. & T. Rudge. (2019). How "care values" as discursive practices effect the ethics of a care-setting. *Journal of Organizational Ethnography, 8*(3), 298–311.

O'Connell, R. (2017). Ethnography. In J. Swain (Ed.), *Designing Research in Education. Concepts and Methods* (pp. 148–172). London: Sage.

Oliver, M. (2005). The problem with affordance. *E-Learning and Digital Media, 2*(4), 402–413.

Oliver, M. (2016). What is technology? In N. Rushby & D. W. Surry (Eds.), *The Wiley Handbook of Learning Technology.* Hoboken: John Wiley & Sons, Inc.

Oute, J., & B. Bjerge. (2019). Ethnographic reflections on access to care services. *Journal of Organizational Ethnography, 8*(3), 279–297.

Park, S., C. Pelletier, & M. Klingenberg. (2014). The missing self: competence, the person and Foucault. *Medical Education, 48*(8), 741–744.

Pope, C. (2005). Conducting ethnography in medical settings. *Medical Education, 39*(12), 1180–1187.

Reed-Danahay, D. (2007). Autobiography, Intimacy and Ethnography. In P. Atkinson, A. Coffey, S. Delamont, J. Lofland, & L. Lofland (Eds.), *Handbook of Ethnography* (pp. 407–425). London: Sage.

Reeves, S., J. Peller, J. Goldman, & S. Kitto. (2013). Ethnography in qualitative educational research: AMEE Guide No. 80. *Medical Teacher, 35*(8), e1365–e1379.

Savage, J. (2006). Ethnographic evidence. *Journal of Research in Nursing, 11*(5), 383–393.

Sinclair, S. (1997). *Making doctors: an institutional apprenticeship.* Oxford: Berg.

Skeggs, B. (2007). Feminist ethnography. In P. Atkinson, A. Coffey, S. Delamont, J. Lofland, & L. Lofland (Eds.), *Handbook of Ethnography* (pp. 426–442). London: Sage.

Smith, V. (2007). Ethnographies of work and the work of ethnographers. In P. Atkinson, A. Coffey, S. Delamont, J. Lofland, & L. Lofland (Eds.), *Handbook of Ethnography* (pp. 220–233). London: Sage.

Swinglehurst, D., T. Greenhalgh, J. Russell, & M. Myall. (2011). Receptionist input to quality and safety in repeat prescribing in UK general practice: Ethnographic case study. *BMJ (Online), 343*(7831), 983.

Van Maanen, J. (2011). *Tales of the field: on writing ethnography.* University of Chicago Press.

Zuiderent, T. (2002). Blurring the center: On the politics of ethnography. *Scandinavian Journal of Information Systems, 14*(2), 59–78.

PART IX

Journals and diaries

22

ETHNOGRAPHIC DIARIES AND JOURNALS

Principles, practices, and dilemmas

Graham Hall

Introduction

The activity of keeping a diary, that is, of maintaining a regular "personal life-record" of experiences, thoughts, beliefs, and feelings (W. Thomas & Znaniecki, 1918, p. 1832; also, Jones, 2000, p. 55), can be traced back almost 2,000 years. Since then, diary writing has become in many societies "a pervasive narrative form" (McDonough & McDonough, 1997, p.121) which is used for multiple purposes. For example, diaries might be kept to record facts or as a scientific record, to create a chronicle for posterity or as a memoire, to document artistic struggle or as a literary diary, or to bear witness or provide a personal testimony of suffering (Alaszewski, 2006). Diaries can also provide an important source of data for naturalistic and ethnographic research, giving "voice" to people other than researchers themselves (Plummer, 1983) by "tracking the contemporaneous flow of public and private events that are significant to the diarist" (ibid., p. 48).

Alaszewski (2006) points out that diaries are an often neglected source of data in comparison to surveys, interviews, focus groups, and so forth. That said, their use in health-related research can be traced back to the 1970s (e.g., Robinson's (1971) study of illness behaviour; Banks, Beresford, Morrell, Waller, and Watkins's (1975) research into the primary healthcare needs of a group of women). And more recently, diary studies within healthcare research have, for example, explored the lives of people with dementia (e.g., Bartlett, 2012) and their caregivers (e.g., Valimaki, Vehviläinen, & Pietila, 2007), those at risk of depression (e.g., Wichers, Myin-Germeys, Jacobs, Peeters, Kenis, Derom, Vlietinck Delespaul, & van Os, 2007), and those suffering from pain and fatigue (e.g., Broderick, Schwartz, Vikingstad, Pribbernow, Grossman, & Stone, 2008). Meanwhile, the health-related experiences of often marginalized or overlooked groups have also been uncovered through diary studies, for example, those living with HIV/AIDS (e.g., F. Thomas, 2007), older people (e.g., Jacelon & Imperio, 2005) and, indeed, younger people (e.g., Liao, Skelton, Dunton, & Bruening, 2016). Yet whilst the use of diaries in healthcare research is becoming more frequent, the literature surrounding this approach remains relatively scarce (Alaszewski, 2006; Worth, 2009). Consequently, this chapter aims to outline the principles which underpin ethnographic diary study design, the range of forms and formats that diary studies might take in practice, and the ways in which diary data might subsequently be approached and analyzed. As with any research methodology, implementing a diary study effectively is not without its challenges.

Diaries: initial understandings

Because of their origins and subsequent long history of being used as a social activity (see Introduction), diaries have an "everyday meaning" which reaches beyond their use as tools for research (Elliott, 1997, para. 4.2). Consequently, many researchers and research participants come to diary studies with their own thoughts and beliefs about what a research diary is or should be, and what keeping a diary involves (ibid.). Yet common to most (if not all!) understandings is that diaries are "self-report instruments used repeatedly to examine ongoing experiences" (Bolger, Davis, & Rafaeli, 2003, p. 580). Thus, their defining characteristics are:

- *regularity*: a sequence of regular timed and/or dated entries are made over time
- *personal*: diaries are maintained by identifiable individuals, who also control access to them
- *contemporaneous*: entries are made at or close to the time of experiences and events, rather than recalled a significant time later
- *a record*: diary entries record what the author considers relevant and important at that time, and might include activities, thoughts and feelings, interactions, and so forth (participation in a research study might require participants to focus on a particular aspect of their life or health experience, as we shall discuss later in the chapter).

(Alaszewski, 2006)

In the context of ethnographic healthcare research, therefore, diaries offer the opportunity to uncover and explore social, psychological, and physiological processes within everyday situations and in particular contexts (Bolger et al., 2003). They capture the "little experiences of everyday life that fill most of our working time and occupy the vast majority of our conscious attention" (Wheeler & Reis, 1991, p. 340, cited in Bolger et al., ibid.), and thus, as Bolger et al. continue, they enable researchers to discover and examine reported experiences in their natural and spontaneous context in a way that is not possible via other methods. Thus, as Myin-Germeys, Oorschot, Collip, Lataster, Delespaul, and van Os (2009, p. 1533) put it, they open "the black box of daily life". Additionally, by reducing the amount of time between an event and the recording or account of that experience, diaries significantly reduce the extent of recall error or bias compared to, for example, interviews (Alaszewski, 2006; Bartlett, 2012; Bolger et al., 2003; Verbrugge, 1980).

Diaries are therefore well-suited to ethnographic research, which looks at "uniquely situated realities" embedded within layers of context (Blommaert & Jie, 2010, p. 17). They can reveal the complexity of events and experiences by prioritizing participants' knowledge, understandings, and beliefs, and drawing on their "emic" perspectives (Davis, 1995) on events and contexts (i.e., participants' own "insider" understandings). Diaries give participants a degree of control and "voice" (Bartlett, 2012), whilst the ethnographic researcher's point of departure at the start of a study is the "ignorance of the knower" (Blommaert & Jie, 2010, p. 10), subsequently addressed by collecting and analyzing the diary data as the research progresses (Clayton & Thorne, 2000). Consequently, diary studies can provide researchers with a mechanism for unpacking what is often taken for granted in accounts of health, illness, and healthcare (Elliott, 1997).

Yet as most accounts of diary studies make clear, beyond this broad understanding of what diaries are and what diary-based approaches can offer, there are an array of possibilities in the design and implementation of diary research, whilst the analysis and interpretation of data also raises a series of potential dilemmas. As Janssens, Bos, Rosmalen, Wichers, and Riese (2018, p. 1) point out, there is "no golden standard for the optimal design of a diary study", as this depends on the aims and related research questions of the study. Diary-oriented researchers thus face a series of choices when designing their approach that will affect the quality, integrity and interpretability of the data (Polit & Hungler, 1993). Or, as Blommaert and Jie state with an explicit focus on ethnography, "the process of gathering and molding knowledge is part of that knowledge; knowledge construction *is* knowledge; the *process is the product*" (2010, p. 10, original emphasis).[1]

Developing the "solicited diary": key considerations for the ethnographic researcher

Research undertaken through diary studies almost always refers to accounts obtained via "solicited diaries", that is, those kept by participants at the researcher's request.[2] Although, as we have seen, these aim to "let people be heard on their own terms" (Bell, 1999, p. 266), solicited diaries are not private documents. They are maintained by participants with the researcher in mind, and in the knowledge that another person or people will read (or listen to, in the case of audio-diaries; see below) and interpret what is recorded (Elliott, 1997; Jacelon & Imperio, 2005). Although some of the more problematic implications of this knowledge can be minimized by developing clear guidelines, protocols and training for participants (see below), reported difficulties ranging from diarist embarrassment at what they are recording (e.g., Day and Thatcher, 2009), to the potentially fraught nature of providing an account of ill health for others (e.g., Elliott, 1997), to simply "pleasing the reader" (e.g., Davis, 1995). Clearly, therefore, the guidelines that researchers provide to participants and the diarists' knowledge that their accounts will be read means that solicited diaries must be viewed as co-constructed by the researcher and the diarist (Mackrill, 2008).

Participants, consent, and trust

As the discussion above outlines, therefore, ethnographic diary research is interested in the experiences, knowledge, and understandings of the research participants themselves. Although diarists may be a sample from a broader population, it is neither possible nor desirable to generalize to the wider population – although, of course, any insights that emerge may well have some relevance to, or prompt reflection about, other apparently similar contexts. Clearly, then, for an ethnographic diary study to be successful, participants need to be "on board" with the goals of the research and with its approach. Additionally, given that they are being asked to reveal something of themselves through their diary, that is, those aspects of their lives and thinking that researchers cannot otherwise access, diarists' belief and trust in the research team is central to the success or otherwise of any project.

Thus, there are a number of key issues for researchers to consider when recruiting diarists. These include making the purpose of the study and the reasons for an individual's recruitment clear, outlining how diaries will or should be maintained (see below), and also, importantly, establishing how trust between the researcher and participants might be developed (Alaszewski, 2006, p. 60). As Alaszewski (ibid.) summarizes:

- Is the researcher acceptable to the group?
- To what extent will the researcher's presence disrupt natural relations and activities?
- How can the researcher build up relationships and persuade members of the group to keep personal records of activities?

Consequently, gaining participants' informed consent is central to diary studies. This can be relatively unproblematic in many contexts. For example, patients contributing to Webster, Jowsey, Lu, Henning, Verstappen, Wearn, Reid, Merry, and Weller's (2019) exploration of experiences of hospital stay simply provided written informed consent. In contrast, however, Bartlett (2012) developed a form of "process consent" in her study of people with dementia, a context where ongoing consent was more difficult to establish. Following initial signed consent at the start of the project, participants were asked for further verbal consent at each stage of data collection and reminded that they could withdraw at any point (p. 1719). Furthermore, in contexts where literacy is limited or there are cultural or contextual reservations around signing documents, consent may need to be recorded orally in ways which are fully documented and, if possible, witnessed (Declaration of Helsinki, 2000).

Yet the willingness of participants to engage with the task of keeping a diary in ways which, for example, "go beyond" the superficial and reveal personal experiences and thoughts, takes a sustained period of time and effort (for more about the length of diary studies, see below), and dealing with potentially difficult health issues may require more than "just" informed consent. As noted, participants need to *trust* the researcher. For Bartlett's (2012) work with people with dementia, for example, trusting relationships were initially developed through a pre-diary interview by the researcher in the participants' own homes (i.e., a private, comfortable and safe space), in which diarists could ask any questions they might have about the study. In her investigation of the emotional well-being of people living with HIV/AIDS in Namibia, however, F. Thomas (2007) needed to navigate a range of socio-cultural norms about both the focus of the study (displaying and talking about emotions) and the nature of diary writing. As an evident outsider to the community who did not speak the preferred languages of the participants, trust was developed in conjunction with health workers who were already well-known to the diarists, and who continued to provide assistance and monitor the diary process throughout the study. In F. Thomas's research, as with most other ethnographic diary studies, agreement that the data would be anonymized and, in its raw form, read only by agreed members of the research team was central to the development of trust and the subsequent success of her project (see also, for example, Clayton & Thorne, 2000; Day & Thatcher, 2009; Freer, 1980; Kuntsche & Robert, 2009).

A structured or unstructured diary?

Although ethnographic research aims to minimize "the disruptions and distortions" of the research process on participants' experiences and understandings (Alaszewski, 2006, p. 78), just asking individuals to keep a diary is, for many, a change of behavior – as Alaszewski points out, keeping a diary is a minority habit (ibid.). Consequently, a key consideration is how to give diarists control over what they record, in order to enable them to follow and report on their own agenda within the constraints of a research study's own aims and objectives, or, as Mackrill puts it, "attaining relevant data without restricting the diarists writing flow unnecessarily" (p. 8). A tension in diary study design is, therefore, the extent to which diary entries should consist of participant-led "free text" or be structured around more explicit guidelines provided by the research team outlining what diarists should focus on.

An early study of women's health experiences, which initially asked participants simply to record their common health problems on a day-to-day basis, labelled the results of this unstructured approach as "disappointing" (Freer, 1980, p. 279). Meanwhile, Hall's (2008) initial guidelines for participants simply to record "anything you think was interesting" (p. 115) became more focused over time, at the request of the participants themselves, who felt lost in the array of possible topics they might document, and with the consequence that the data became more immediately relevant to his own research goals. Yet Webster et al.'s (2019) study of patients' hospital-stay experiences asked participants to complete an unstructured diary "in their own words, recording negative and positive experiences or anything else they considered noteworthy" (p. 1), whilst J. Thomas's (2015) investigation of the professional socialization of nursing students followed a similar approach. Key to the success of unstructured approaches such as these is the subsequent way in which data in analyzed, often through the identification of emergent, participant-driven themes and a grounded theory approach (for further discussion of data analysis, see below).

Undoubtedly, however, the majority of diary-based research provides participants with at least some guidelines to follow (Alaszewski, 2006; Mackrill, 2008), although, unsurprisingly, these can vary from study to study. Some studies might provide a combination of open and closed questions for diarists to reflect upon, whilst others may even give participants examples of the kinds of data researchers are hoping for (ibid.). Yet Alaszewski (2006) argues that researchers need to avoid instructions that are too prescriptive, as these will restrict diarists' freedom of expression, and their control and voice in the research. Consequently, ethnographic diaries are likely to be "open in structure and informal" (p. 78). In this respect, diary guidelines can be somewhat similar to interview guides, potentially creating a "dialogue" between diarists and researchers (Clayton & Thorne, 2000; Mackrill, 2008), especially when deployed alongside other research tools such as follow-up interviews (see below).

Recording diary entries

In any diary-based research, the precise design and format of the diaries that participants will keep will depend on the goals of that particular study, the kinds of data consequently required, and the expectations, abilities, and needs of the diarists themselves; every study is unique (Alaszewski, 2006). And, although paper and pen diaries are the most familiar approach in diary-based studies (Bolger et al., 2003; Worth, 2009), many researchers are now, as Bartlett (2012) puts it, "modifying and modernizing" diary research. Thus, while paper and pen diaries match the socially-constructed expectations of many research participants, new technologies, both offline (e.g., digital cameras and handheld audio- or video-recorders) and online (e.g., recording via SMS or online platforms) are increasingly deployed across a range of contexts.

In some cases, the decision to record data through non-paper and pen approaches might be taken for practical reasons. Kuntsche and Robert (2009), for example, asked their young adult participants to provide regular data about alcohol consumption via SMS for reasons of cost and because the young people concerned were familiar and comfortable with phone technology; consequently, retention rates in the study were maintained. Yet beyond dealing with practical constraints such as these, adopting new and innovative diary formats can allow more detailed and intimate access to participants' experiences. In Williamson, Leeming, Lyttle, and Johnson's (2015) exploration of new mothers' experiences of breastfeeding, audio diarists recorded whilst actually feeding their child. Worth's (2009) use of audio diaries with visually impaired teenagers "allowed the research to get closer" to the lives of the young people involved (para. 1), enabling them to express more clearly their identities through narrative-based reporting. Meanwhile, F. Thomas (2007) asked diarists in her study of people living with HIV/AIDS to keep a photographic record (i.e., via 'autophotography') of important people, objects, or places in their lives alongside their written diaries, arguing that this was inclusive and empowering for participants as it drew upon their own perceptual orientations, rather than on the knowledge frameworks of the researcher. Of course, given the range of possible ways of recording data, researchers can, where appropriate, offer participants a choice of format for keeping diaries in accordance with their own needs and preferences (e.g., Bartlett's (2012) research on people with dementia; Jacelon and Imperio's (2005) study of older adults). As Bartlett (2012) suggests, this may provide participants with a greater sense of control over the research process and allow them to draw more effectively on their own strengths in keeping their diaries. It is evident, therefore, that audio, video, and other non-traditional forms of diary recording are "much more than a simple change of format when literacy is a constraint" (Worth, 2009, para. 2.1); they offer researchers and participants new ways of making sense of health-related experiences.

Further key considerations in diary study design relate to their duration and how often participants need to update their diaries. Longer duration studies and diaries which are time-consuming to maintain – due to either the detail required or the regularity with which entries are kept – require more commitment and effort from participants. This has implications for diarists' retention or drop-out from the research as, in order to obtain high quality and regular data, diary studies require a level of participant dedication "rarely required in other types of research studies" (Bolger et al., 2003, p. 592–593). Reducing the length of the study or the amount of effort participants must expend in maintaining their diary is, of course, one way of addressing the problem, but this is likely to be at the expense of the depth of the data which is recorded. Therefore, although Jacelon and Imperio (2005) suggest that the optimal time for keeping a solicited diary is 1–2 weeks, the duration of diary-based research clearly, and once again unsurprisingly, depends on the aims of the particular study. For example, Worth's (2009) visually impaired teenagers maintained their audio diaries for 2 weeks whilst Bartlett's (2012) participants with dementia recorded their experiences for 1 month. In F. Thomas's (2007) study of people with HIV/AIDS, participants kept diaries for varying lengths of time (between 1 and 6 months) according to their own capabilities and the demands on their time. And in Webster et al.'s (2019) exploration of the hospital-stay experiences of patients, diaries were kept for the length of time participants were hospitalized.

Meanwhile, more structured approaches to diary design might require participants to record their experiences at either "interval-", "signal-", or "event-contingent" times (Bolger et al., 2003). Interval-contingent approaches require participants to update their diaries at regular, predetermined times throughout the study (e.g., Kuntsche & Robert (2009) asked participants to note and comment on their recent alcohol consumption at 9pm on Friday evenings for the duration of the project). Signal-contingent designs contact diarists through a messaging service (e.g., a phone call or SMS), to ask them to record their experiences at that time (e.g., Csikszentmihalyi, Larson, & Prescott (1977) contacted 25 teenagers at random times over the course of a week in order to explore their behavior traits in their own particular contexts). And event-contingent studies ask participants to report each time a specific event occurs (e.g., Williamson et al. (2015) asked first-time mothers to audio record their experiences of and feelings about breast-feeding during or shortly after feeding sessions over a week-long period). Clearly, however, many studies are organized in less structured ways, encouraging diarists to record the experiences which they consider to be relevant, as and when they occur (e.g., F. Thomas's (2007) study of people with HIV/AIDs in Namibia).

Maintaining participation

As we have seen, keeping a diary in any form places time and effort demands on diarists, and, while researchers will aim to reduce these demands, the risk of participants producing superficial or incomplete data or even dropping out remains, particularly in longer studies. Alongside clear guidelines (see above for the complexities of balancing researchers' wishes, needs, and structures with the freedom for participants to express what is important to themselves), Alaszewski (2006) suggests that initial face-to-face training may be useful, in which researchers can check instructions, answer queries, clarify how additional support will be given, and so forth. If diarists are confident from the outset in what they are doing and can see it meets the needs of the research, they are more likely to participate fully. Additionally, such face-to-face sessions can also develop trust between participants and researchers (see above), and both relationships with diarists and the quality and depth of the diary data they provide can benefit from in-study briefing meetings and/or by checking a sample diary entry early in the study (e.g., Bartlett, 2012; Hall, 2008; F. Thomas, 2007).

Furthermore, in much ethnographic research, diary approaches are pursued in conjunction with other methods of data collection which also provide opportunities for developing constructive researcher-participant relationships, identifying methodological difficulties, and exploring the quality of the data. In the diary-interview method (Zimmerman & Wieder, 1977), for example, diaries are maintained following an initial introductory interview, and subsequently collected and read by researchers as the basis for follow-up interviews that further explore the participants' reported experiences and perspectives. Interviews can be both during and at the end of the diary-keeping period, and the diary-interview method has been regularly deployed in healthcare research (e.g., in Bartlett's (2012) study of people with dementia, Elliott's (1997) investigation of the need and demand for primary healthcare, and Jacelon and Imperio's (2005) work with older adults).

A final consideration for many diary researchers is whether diarists should be paid or otherwise rewarded for their participation. While some projects might simply lack the resources to provide incentives for participants, a number of researchers argue that paying participants reinforces unequal power relationships (e.g., Ansell, 2001). Others, however, regard incentives as either a practical means of recruiting and maintaining the participation of diarists (e.g., Kuntsche & Robert's (2009) study of young Swiss adult's alcohol consumption) or consider a lack of incentives to be exploitative (e.g., F. Thomas's (2007) work with people with HIV/AIDS in Namibia). Yet as these two very different examples illustrate, context matters and will influence the way in which this issue is navigated. That said, the majority of published healthcare-related studies make no reference at all to participant rewards, and it seems reasonable to assume that many hope or believe that the act of keeping a diary and contributing to research will be rewarding enough in and of itself to encourage and maintain effective participation over time.

Analyzing diary data: possibilities and paradoxes

The analysis of ethnographic diary data aims to impose some order on what is often a large volume of information (Polit & Hungler, 1993) in order to identify "essential interpretations" of the research participants' context and experiences (Clayton & Thorne, 2000, p. 1516). A variety of analytical frameworks are open to researchers ranging from, for example, content analysis and grounded theory to conversational and narrative analysis[3], and, ultimately, the choice of approach will depend on the goals of the research and the researcher's understanding of the extent and nature of the data (Alaszewski, 2006). The majority of studies cited in this chapter, for example, thematize their findings following a content or grounded theory analysis (e.g., Bartlett, 2012; Day & Thatcher, 2009; F. Thomas, 2007; Webster et al., 2009), with fewer examples of narrative analysis (e.g., Worth, 2009).

Yet whatever approach is adopted, thinking through the processes underpinning collection and construction of the data reveals a number of issues which need to be addressed when analyzing and subsequently representing or summarizing the data (Richards, Ross, & Seedhouse,

2012). Thus, diary data analysis needs to be systematic and honest; it cannot be pursued in a mechanical or "by numbers" way – researchers need to recognize the difficulties inherent in understanding other people's reported perceptions (Burnard, 1991).

The role of the researcher

As the discussion throughout the chapter shows, the researcher's actions and decisions underpin and fundamentally shape the diary data and its analysis. In effect, "the researcher is the primary research instrument" (Richards et al., 2012, p. 33) in ethnographic diary research. As we have seen, the depth and relevance of the data to the aims of the study can depend to a substantial extent on the researcher-participant relationship, while decisions about the format of diaries and the level of guidance about what they should or might record all significantly affect the data.

Meanwhile, as ethnographic approaches require researchers to immerse themselves in the "lifeworld" of participants in order to explore and represent their insider perspectives, data analysis is necessarily interpretive, "an attempt to make sense of subjective representations of facts and events 'out there'" (Blommaert and Jie, 2010, p. 63). In other words, the researcher is inseparable from the analysis, and one researcher's interpretation of diary data may consequently differ from another's. To lessen or avoid the risk of particularly one-sided views, however, more than one researcher within a research team might analyze the data in order to reach shared understandings. Furthermore, researchers can check their interpretation and understanding of experiences and perceptions brought together within the data through a process of "respondent validation" with the diarists themselves (Richards et al., 2012). And, of course, researchers can triangulate their understandings of diary data with other data sources within a study (see, for example, the diary-interview approach, above).

The participants and the data

It is also important to reflect on the ways in which individual participants might contribute to a diary study's overall body of data, and what this means for the subsequent analysis. As noted earlier in the chapter, diary keeping is a social practice that varies across and within class and cultural groups, and researchers thus need to be aware of the possibilities of recruitment bias during participant selection (Williamson et al., 2015). Furthermore, participants in any study will probably vary in their attitudes towards and comfort with self-narration (ibid.), some warming to the task and being more predisposed to developing an identity as "a writer" than others (Elliott, 1997). Beyond the challenge of managing participant retention and avoiding drop-out (see above), therefore, individual diarists are likely to produce accounts of differing length, detail, and comprehensiveness. There will be differences in what they are willing and able to articulate, and certain phenomena may be consistently over- or under-reported, processes over which the researcher has no control (Breakwell, 2012). Diarists may also report events and experiences either when they happen, or record them at the end of each day (or at other times), with potential implications for recall and their levels of immediate emotional engagement with what they describe. Day and Thatcher (2009), for example, outline how, following particularly emotive diary entries, participants often clarified in later commentaries that they were no longer feeling that way (see also, Hall, 2008). Meanwhile, Fine (1993, p. 271, citing Douglas, 1976) raises the possibility that participants might, whether deliberately or not, "mislead, evade, lie, and put up fronts", and notes that researchers should be "suspicious" of the data they receive.

Meanwhile, it seems possible that the actual act of keeping a diary may cause participant "reactance" (Bolger et al, 2003), that is, it might change their experience or behavior in relation to the phenomenon being explored. Williamson et al. (2015) note how a diarist's continued commitment to breastfeeding was potentially linked to her participation in their study. Bolger et al. (2003), however, downplay the overall impact of reactance on the validity of diary data, arguing that any initial changes of behavior fade over time as participants become more used to the enterprise through a process of "habituation". Yet even if participant *behavior* does not change (or does not change much), there is clear evidence that the ways in which many participants in diary-based healthcare studies *think* about their experiences does change over the course of the research. Williamson et al. (2015) suggest that diarists may develop more complex understandings of the phenomena being explored, as, for example, documented by Elliott's (1997) investigation of participants' primary healthcare experiences in which diary entries changed in tone over the course of the study as participants became more reflective in writing about the topic. Alternatively, diarists' initial understandings might change during a study in order to fit in with the conceptualizations of the researchers (Williamson et al., 2015). Furthermore, keeping a diary might have therapeutic effect and outcomes for some participants, as they reflect on health and illness, and the emotional impacts this may have (Day & Thatcher, 2009; Williamson et al., 2015). Yet F. Thomas (2007) raises a particularly significant dilemma for researchers, not only in terms of analysis but with regard to research ethics more generally, suggesting that "the very process of diary keeping undoubtedly played a role in creating some of the emotions recorded" in her study of the emotional impact of HIV/AIDS on participants in Namibia (p. 79). Bartlett (2012) similarly observes some of her diarists with dementia becoming aware of, and frustrated with, their diminished reporting skills.[4]

Consequently, the "truths" that ethnographic diaries are attempting to uncover are multiple, contingent, and only ever partial (Williamson et al., 2015). Furthermore, practicalities such as particular participants' handwriting may limit researchers' access to the data in written diaries (Day & Thatcher, 2009), while Bartlett (2012) reported that some data were not usable in her study, as they were either too intimate or unrelated to her project focusing on living with dementia. Diary researchers, unlike interviewers, cannot spontaneously and immediately put diarists "back on track" (Mackrill, 2008).

Overall, therefore, ethnographic diary researchers are faced with the challenge of dealing with data which they may in some way "distrust", that is partial, and that may contradict itself over time and at times be irrelevant to the study's aims, in addition to data in which it is almost certain that some diarists' voices will appear more strongly and more articulately than others'. However, while Allport (1942, p. 96) worries that "few diaries turn out to be ideal", Mackrill (2008) argues that variation within and between data is not a weakness in comparison to methodologies that produce "similar data" – similar data does not straightforwardly equate to reliability when dealing with participants' insider understandings of their own experiences. Likewise, all accounts, even those purported to be "scientific" are "context-bound and speak to certain people, times, and circumstances" (Plummer, 1983, p. 14). What really matters in ethnographic research is that the data provides "as full a subjective view as possible" (ibid., p. 14) in order to gain a "detailed perspective on the world" (p. 20).

Key in any analysis of ethnographic diary data, therefore, is that it is clearly grounded in the original diary entries, that it should be dynamic and open to change during the analysis process, and that it should treat all data systematically thereby allowing for a full review of all the material (Jones, 2000). Furthermore, the exploration of data should clearly map findings to original diary entries, in order that the processes of data analysis and interpretation are transparent to others – the decisions within data collection and analysis, and their implications, should be made explicit to people other than the primary researcher or analyst (ibid.). Too often, however, these process are perhaps not explicit enough when the findings of diary-based research are disseminated.

Concluding comments

This chapter has mapped the key principles which underpin the design and implementation of diary studies in ethnographic healthcare research, illustrating the array of possible practices available to researchers seeking to develop solicited diary approaches, and highlighting a range of dilemmas which they might face in both diary design and the interpretation of diary data.

Essentially, diary studies facilitate the investigation of phenomena as they unfold over time via participants' own descriptions and understandings of events and experiences – information that is often hard to access by other means. By definition, therefore, diaries are "insider accounts" of participants' lives in relation (usually!) to the phenomenon being investigated. Ethnographic research studies are situated in specific contexts, and diaries can provide an effective means for finding out in detail about background settings and contextual influences. They offer researchers methodological and theoretical flexibility – as we have seen, many aspects of participants health and healthcare can be explored, and a wide range of frameworks can be deployed when analyzing diary data. And diaries can be used in conjunction with other research tools, most typically interviews, contributing to deeper understandings of healthcare issues and concerns via the process of careful data triangulation.

Furthermore, diaries provide research participants with a more evident sense of control within the research process. They are a "space" for diarists to reveal (or, perhaps, conceal!) their own perspectives, providing opportunities for freedom of expression that might be less evident to participants in, for example, interviews. Diarists might write about issues that researchers do not anticipate, and make connections between topics that researchers might not otherwise see (Mackrill, 2008). And, by enabling diarists to record events and experiences more immediately than other research tools, they go a significant way to addressing the difficulties around participant recall in research.

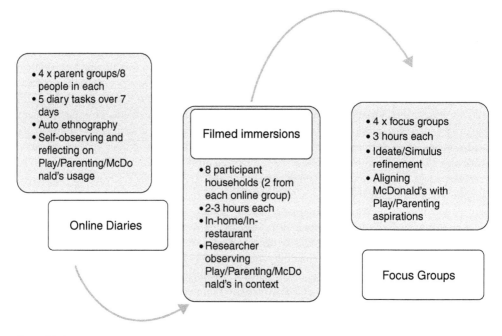

Figure 22.1

That said, the implementation of diary-based ethnographic research is not without its difficulties. Long-term diary studies can be costly to run, and avoiding bias in participant selection is challenging. Successful studies require significant diarist dedication and commitment; written diaries require participant literacy, whilst audio diaries are likely to require a degree of technological ability and familiarity. Participants in a project will contribute with differing degrees of openness and reflectivity, and issues surrounding forgetfulness and recall are never entirely absent. The ceding of some control of the research to participants through diary approaches thus has both advantages (see previous paragraph), but also carries risks in terms of the potential relevance of the data to the goal of the study. Researchers may try to lessen this risk by providing diarists with a clear focus and guidelines about what to record, which may also lessen some diarists' anxiety about whether they are engaging with a project "correctly". However, the extent to which diaries are or are not structured can potentially affect the richness of the data and lessen the extent to which diaries truly reflect diarists' priorities. Diary studies also raise a number of ethical issues. How might researchers respond to instances of distress recorded by participants? Might the act of keeping a diary actually cause some participants emotional harm, for example, by asking them to reflect on illness or trauma or reminding them of declining skills and abilities? In such instances, understandings of how "harm" impacts on individuals perhaps needs balancing with the potential long-term benefits of the research to the participant group as a whole (F. Thomas, 2007).

Despite these challenges, however, ethnographic diaries offer healthcare researchers an approach to undertaking research which is truly participatory. Contributing to a diary study can enrich diarists' lives, encouraging them to investigate and reflect on their own situations and contexts, and, to some extent, becoming co-researchers in the research project; and, as Mackrill (2008, p. 13) notes "the more curious diarists are about the research project, the better the data they are likely to produce". Ethnographic diary studies thus mediate the relationship between researchers and participants, making the 'whole person' visible (Bartlett, 2012).

Notes

1 Although the focus in this chapter is on the use of diaries for ethnographic research, it is important to note that diaries can be used to collect quantitative data for experimental and survey-based studies. For example, Parkin, Jacoby, McNamee, Miller, Thomas, and Bates's (2000) investigation into the impact of beta interferon therapy on patients with multiple sclerosis asked participants to record, via a numerical scale, their day-to-day experiences of a variety of dimensions of the illness over a period of 6 weeks, the subsequent statistical analysis looking at the cost effectiveness of the treatment for health service providers.

2 A notable exception is Jones's (2000) discussion of the value of an unsolicited diary in understanding the symptoms and treatment of a cancer sufferer, which the patient had kept unprompted, as their own "personal document" (p. 558). See also, Lester's (2004) edited collection of psychological studies.

3 Wide-ranging and nuanced discussions of these approaches can be found within the literature around research methods. Broadly speaking, however, in Content Analysis, the information in diaries is used to identify a reality external to the diary texts themselves, breaking them down into constituent parts and reassembling them into a pre-existing understanding of the world. Analysis is rooted in a grounded theory approach when it does not start with a clear idea of what these patterns will be, but themes and categorizations instead emerge during the researcher's interpretation of the data (Alaszewski, 2006, citing Charmaz, 2003). Meanwhile, Conversational Analysis engages in detailed textual analysis to explore how diarists represent and record social interaction, whilst Narrative Analysis focuses on how diarists structure their accounts, and the linguistic and discourse devices they use to represent their identities and intentions, that is, to "tell their stories" (Alaszewski, ibid.).

4 For F. Thomas (2007), this led to a reconsideration of what might be meant by "avoiding harm", what level of potential harm might be deemed (un)acceptable, and how to balance the cost to individuals against the potential longer-term benefits of the research to the researched group as a whole. Consequently, both she, and Day and Thatcher (2009) in their study of the relationship between stress and emotions for a group of athletes, worry about the researcher's inability to react appropriately to participants' emotions due to the time lag in accessing the data, their lack of training in counselling, and the need to "remain objective" when reading the raw data (Day and Thatcher, ibid., p. 256). For Fine (1993), however, notions of objectivity in ethnographic research are "an illusion" (p. 286); the world is always "known" from a perspective. Equally, Fine challenges the notion that ethnographers should necessarily be "kindly" towards participants (p. 270).

References

Alaszewski, A. (2006). *Using Diaries for Social Research*. London: Sage.

Allport, G. (1942). *The Use of Personal Documents in Psychological Science*. New York: Social Science Research Council.

Ansell, N. (2001). Producing knowledge about 'Third World women': the politics of fieldwork in a Zimbabwean school. *Ethics, Place & Environment*, 4(2), 1010–1016. doi: 10.1080/13668790123027

Banks, M., S. Beresford, D. Morrell, J. Waller, and C. Watkins. (1975). Factors influencing demand for primary medical care in women aged 20–44 years: a preliminary report. *International Journal of Epidemiology*, 4(3), 189–195.

Bartlett, R. (2012). Modifying the Diary Interview Method to research the lives of people with dementia. *Qualitative Health Research*, 22(12), 1717–1726. doi: 10.1177/1049732312462240

Bell, L. (1999). Public and private meaning in diaries: Researching families and childcare. In A. Bryman and R. Burgess (eds) *Qualitative Research*, vol. 2. London: Sage.

Blommaert, J. and D. Jie. (2010). *Ethnographic Fieldwork: A Beginner's Guide*. Bristol: Multilingual Matters.

Bolger, N., A. Davis, and E. Rafaeli. (2003). Diary Methods: Capturing life as it is lived. *Annual Review of Psychology*, 54(1), 579–616. doi: 10.1146/annurev.psych.54.101601.145030

Breakwell, G. (2012). Diary and narrative methods. In Breakwell, G., Smith, J., and Wright, D. (eds) *Research Methods in Psychology* (4th edition). London: Sage. pp. 392–410.

Broderick J., J. Schwartz, G. Vikingstad, M. Pribbernow, S. Grossman, and A. Stone. (2008). The accuracy of pain and fatigue items across different reporting periods. *Pain*, 139(1), 146–157. doi: 10.1016/j.pain.2008.03.024

Burnard, P. (1991). A method of analysing interview transcripts in qualitative research. *Nurse Education Today*, 11(6), 461–466. doi: 10.1016/0260-6917(91)90009-y

Charmaz, K. (2003). Grounded theory: objectivist and constructivist methods. In Denzin, N. and Lincoln, Y. (eds) *Handbook of Qualitative Research*. London: Sage.

Csikszentmihalyi, M., R. Larson, and S. Prescott. (1977). The ecology of adolescent activity and experience. *Journal of Youth and Adolescence*, 6(3), 281–294. doi: org/10.1007/BF02138940

Clayton, A-M. and T. Thorne. (2000). Diary data enhancing rigour: analysis framework and verification tool. *Journal of Advanced Nursing*, 32(6), 1514–1521.

Davis, K. (1995). Qualitative theory and methods in applied linguistics research. TESOL Quarterly, 62(2), 113–122. doi: 10.2307/3588070

Day, M. and J. Thatcher. (2009). "I'm really embarrassed that you're going to read this": reflections on using diaries in qualitative research. *Qualitative Research in Psychology*, 6(4), 249–259. doi: 10.1080/14780880802070583

Declaration of Helsinki (2000). *Bulletin of the World Health Organisation*, 79(4), 373–374.

Douglas, J. (1976). *Investigative Social Research*. Beverly Hills, CA: Sage.

Elliott, H. (1997). The Use of Diaries in Sociological Health Research. *Sociological Research Online*, 2(2). www.socresonline.org.uk/2/2/7.html

Freer, C. (1980). Health diaries: a method of collecting health information. *Journal of the Royal College of General Practitioners*, 30(214), 279–282.

Fine, G. (1993). Ten Lies of Ethnography: moral dilemmas of the research field. *Journal of Contemporary Ethnography*, 22(3), 267–294. doi: 10.1177/089124193022003001

Hall, G, (2008). An ethnographic diary study. *ELT Journal*, 62(2), 113–122. doi: 10.1093/elt/ccm088

Jacelon, C. and K. Imperio. (2005). Participant diaries as a source of data in research with older adults. *Qualitative Health Research*, 15(7), 991–997. doi: 10.1177/1049732305278603

Janssens, K., E. Bos, J. Rosmalen, M. Wichers, and H. Riese. (2018). A qualitative approach to guide choices for designing a diary study. *BMC Medical Research Methodology*, 18(140). doi: org/10.1186/s12874-018-0579-6

Jones, K. (2000). The unsolicited diary as a qualitative research tool for advanced research capacity in the field of health and illness. *Qualitative Health Research*, 10(4), 555–567.

Kearns, R. (1996). AIDS and medical geography: embracing the other? *Progress in Human Geography,* 20(1), 123–31. doi.org/10.1177/030913259602000109

Kuntsche, E. and B. Robert. (2009). Short Message Service (SMS) Technology in Alcohol Research – a feasibility study. *Alcohol and Alcoholism*, 44(4), 423–428. doi: 10.1093/alcalc/agp033

Lester, D. (ed.) (2004). *Katie's Diary: Unlocking the Mystery of Suicide*. Hove: Brunner-Routledge.

Liao, Y., K. Skelton, G. Dunton, and M. Bruening. (2016). A systematic review of methods and procedures used in ecological momentary assessments of diet and physical activity research in youth: an adapted STROBE checklist for reporting EMA studies (CREMAS). *Journal of Medical Internet Research*, 18(6): e151. doi: 10.2196/jmir.4954

Mackrill, T. (2008). Solicited diary studies of psychotherapy in qualitative research – pros and cons. *European Journal of Psychotherapy and Counselling,* 10(1), 5–18. doi: 10.1080/13642630701869243

McDonough, J. and S. McDonough. (1997). *Research Methods for English Language Teachers*. London: Arnold.

Myin-Germeys, I., M. Oorschot, D. Collip, J. Lataster, P. Delespaul, and J. van Os. (2009). Experience sampling research in psychopathology: opening the black box of daily life. *Psychological Medicine*, 39(9), 1533–1547. doi: 10.1017/S0033291708004947

Parkin, D., A. Jacoby, P. McNamee, P. Miller, S. Thomas, and D. Bates. (2000). Treatment of multiple sclerosis with interferon β: an appraisal of cost-effectiveness and quality of life. *Journal of Neurology, Neurosurgery and Psychiatry*, 68(2), 144–149. doi: org/10.1136/jnnp.68.2.144

Polit, D. and B. Hungler. (1993). *Essentials of Nursing Research. Methods, Appraisal and Utilisation,* 3rd ed. Philadelphia: J.B. Lippincott Company.

Plummer, K (1983). *Documents of Life 2: An Invitation to Critical Humanism*. London: Sage.

Richards, K., S. Ross, and P. Seedhouse. (2012). *Research Methods for Applied Linguistics Studies*. Abingdon: Routledge.

Robinson, D. (1971). *The Process of Becoming Ill*. London: Routledge and Kegan Paul.

Thomas, F. (2007). Eliciting emotions in HIV/AIDS research: a diary-based approach. *Area*, 39(1), 74–82.

Thomas, J. (2015). Using unstructured diaries for data collection. *Nurse Researcher*, 22(5), 25–29. **doi:** 10.7748/nr.22.5.25.e1322

Thomas, W. & F. Znaniecki. (1918–20). *The Polish Peasant in Europe and America* (5 volumes). Boston: Richard G. Badger, The Gorham Press.

Valimaki, T., K. Vehviläinen, and A. Pietila. (2007). Diaries as research data in a study on family caregivers of people with Alzheimer's disease: Methodological issues. *Journal of Advanced Nursing*, 59(1), 68–76. doi:10.1111/j.1365-2648.2007.04273

Verbrugge, L. (1980). Health Diaries. *Medical Care*, 18(1), 73–95. doi: 10.1097/00005650-198001000-00006

Webster, C., T. Jowsey, L-M. Lu, M. Henning, A. Verstappen, A. Wearn, P. Reid, A. Merry, and J. Weller. (2019). Capturing the experience of the hospital-stay journey from admission to discharge using diaries completed by patients in their own words: a qualitative study. *BMJ Open,* 9(e027258), 1–10. doi:10.1136/ bmjopen-2018-027258

Wheeler, L. and H. Reis. (1991). Self-recording of everyday life events: origins, types, and uses. *Journal of Personality,* 59(3), 339–354. doi.org/10.1111/j.1467-6494.1991.tb00252.x

Wichers, M., I. Myin-Germeys, N. Jacobs, F. Peeters, G. Kenis, C. Derom, R. Vlietinck, P. Delespaul, and J. van Os. (2007). Evidence that moment-to-moment variation in positive emotions buffer genetic risk for depression: a momentary assessment twin study. *Acta Psychiatrica Scandinavia*, 115(6), 451–457. doi: 10.1111/j.1600-0447.2006.00924.x

Williamson, I., D. Leeming, S. Lyttle, and S. Johnson. (2015). Evaluating the audio-diary method in qualitative research. *Qualitative Research Journal*, 15(1), 20–34. doi: 10.1108/QRJ-04-2014-0014

Worth, N. (2009). Making use of audio diaries in research with young people: Examining narrative, participation and audience. *Sociological Research Online,* 14(4): 9. doi:10.5153/sro.1967

Zimmerman, D. and D. Wieder. (1977). The diary-interview method. *Urban Life*, 5(4), 479–498.

PART X

Narrative analysis

23
NARRATIVE ETHNOGRAPHY
How to study stories in the context of their telling

Ditte Andersen

Introduction

As humans we make sense of the world through storytelling, and when we encounter disruptions in life caused by illnesses, accidents, or other significant impairments of our wellbeing, we can make our suffering meaningful and connect to others by sharing our stories. Disruptions spur storytelling for two immediate reasons. First, in an existential sense, disruptions derange our sense of selfhood and course in life. Focusing on disruptions caused by severe illness, Arthur Frank stated, "Stories have to *repair* the damage that illness has done to the ill person's sense of where she is in life, and where she may be going. Stories are a way of redrawing maps and finding new destinations." (Frank 1995, 53, emphasis in original). Second, on the more mundane side, storytelling is needed for practical reasons; "Stories of the illness have to be told to medical workers, health bureaucrats, employers and work associates, family and friends." (ibid.). People ask us – and we ask ourselves – what happened? What will happen in the time to come? What needs are to be cared for right now?

This chapter presents narrative ethnography as a methodology for researchers that want to study storytelling among the people whose wellbeing is disrupted by illness, injuries, or other calamities. The methodology may also be used by researchers that want to study the ways care workers, nurses, doctors, and other treatment providers use storytelling. The defining feature of narrative ethnography is that the methodology is tailored to study storytelling in context and thereby examine narrativity in its own right. The first step for narrative ethnographers is to go beyond an appreciation of stories as standalone creations, and to take the storying process into account. As Jaber Gubrium & James Holstein explain:

> The difference between sharing stories, on the one hand, and noticing, cataloguing, and analyzing the corpus of narratives for similarities and differences on the other, is a leap in imagination, highlighting narrativity as something separate and distinct from the stories themselves.
>
> *(Gubrium & Holstein, 2008, 241)*

The narrative ethnographer moves attention beyond the stories in themselves to the narrative practice of storytelling. Attention is often drawn to questions about power, inequality, and change as researchers reveal how storytelling rights are unevenly distributed in institutional setting, e.g. among patients, nurses and doctors in a hospital, or clients and professionals in therapy. Researchers may observe how some narrators sweepingly convince audiences of the claims they make and the morals of their story, while other people tell stories that appear incoherent, are silenced in the room, or disbelieved.

> Disadvantaged people are often less well trained in the requirements of telling an institutionally appropriate story, they are less likely to be seen as narratively competent, and their very experiences make them less able to tell the kind of story that is required.
>
> *(Polletta, Chen, Gardner, & Motes, 2011, 123)*

Narrative ethnographers may reveal how patients and professionals create narratives even before they are told in institutional settings such as a hospital or in therapy. In her pioneering work, Cheryl Mattingly showed how patients and professionals negotiate a configuration of time by creating a whole – a plot – out of a succession of events. The emplotment makes clinical actions meaningful by placing them within a larger therapeutic story. Mattingly makes clear how "[n]arrative plays a central role in clinical work not only as a retrospective account of past events but as a form healers and patients actively seek to impose upon clinical time" (Mattingly, 1994, 811). Patients and professionals use stories to navigate in the moment-to-moment interaction as well as to figure out a sensible direction to take during longer treatment courses. Hence, stories "have powerful consequences upon how the present is experienced and what future actions seem most reasonable, likely, or appropriate" (Mattingly, 2010, 52).

In the subsequent sections, I describe how narrative ethnographers can study various dimensions of stories and storytelling in general, and next I provide three specific examples of narrative ethnographic studies that orient towards 1) treatment recipients, 2) treatment providers, and 3) therapeutic frames of treatment.

Stories

Following Gubrium and Holstein (2009), I will present the distinction between "the whats" (the story content) and "the hows" (the storying process) as vital for narrative ethnography. This section turns attention to "the whats" and describes various strategies for researchers that want to analyze stories in ways that clarify how the stories are used and what the consequences are for tellers and audiences.

One strategy for researchers that want to forefront story content is to produce typologies, i.e. categorize and conceptualize narratives on the basis of differences and similarities. In *The Wounded Storyteller*, Frank proposes that severe illness spurs three types of narratives linked to plots of restitution, chaos, and quest. A narrative type, Frank explains, "is the most general storyline that can be recognized underlying the plot and tensions of particular stories" (Frank 1995, 75), and though we all tell unique stories, we compose these stories by "adapting and combining narrative types that cultures make available" (ibid.). The restitution plot outlines a storyline of health being disrupted and then restored, a chaos story has a non-plot stripped of narrative order and expectations, while the quest plot has the storyline of a journey where the ill person gains something such as new insights and a deeper sense of gratefulness through the experience.

Typologies provide useful overviews as long as researchers keep in mind that in real life people mix and combine narrative types. Researchers must avoid presenting typologies as over-simplified generalizations through a nuanced approach to the particularities of local storytelling. In the case of illness stories, a person may at one moment narrate a story drawing on the resti-tution plot and express an expectation of getting well again soon, yet in more bleak moments the same person may convey a feeling of chaos and express a lack of any sense of direction in life, and just a moment later describe the illness as a driver of personal growth. The benefit of typologies is that it enables narrative ethnographers to see patterns in storytelling and observe how stories are produced in various contexts. As Frank states "both institutions and individual listeners steer ill people toward certain narratives, and other narratives are simply not heard" (Frank, 1995, 77). The section on treatment recipients' recovery narratives exemplifies how narrative ethnography can uncover this.

Plots are one aspect of story content researchers can focus on; themes and the struc-ture of narratives are other. Catherine Riessman (2008) describes thematic analysis as the approach that orients to story content par excellence. She suggests that researchers pursuing this strategy keep stories "intact" "by theorizing from the case rather than from component themes (categories) across cases." (Riessman, 2008, p. 53). This means that a narrative eth-nographer wanting to produce a thematic analysis looks at a person's story as a whole and studies its meaning via the themes she opts to include. The overarching question is: what is the person's story about? In contrast, a structural analysis decomposes story into components to reveal the part played by various elements. "Like thematic analysis," Riessman notes, "structural approaches are concerned with content, but attention to narrative form adds insights beyond what can be learned from referential meanings alone" (Riessman, 2008, p. 77). The structural analysis looks at the distinct parts of the story and how they are assembled into a narrative. The overarching question is: how does the person organize her story? (Instructive examples of how to do thematic and structural analysis are accessible in Bengtsson & Andersen, 2020).

Narrative environment

Narrative ethnographers studying stories told by people who experience their lives being disrupted by illness, injuries and other calamities undermining their wellbeing often observe storytelling in contexts like treatment and therapy. The concept of "narrative environment" as presented by Gubrium and Holstein (2009) can be useful in a study of how specific contexts, such as a hospital unit, influence the form and content of narratives produced under their auspices.

The concept of narrative environment draws on insights produced by decades of research, producing insights into the institutional shaping of stories. In a review of this work, Francesca Polletta and colleagues distinguish between one line of scholarship that shows "that organizations do what they do in part through the stories they tell and elicit" (Polletta et al., 2011, 115). Healthcare workers share stories about how they manage difficult patients, solve puzzling problems, and deal with ethical dilemmas as a way to communicate relational and technical know-how as well as normative obligations. Stories are also ways for people to convey organizational schemas and logics of action that are subsequently enacted in the organizational routines. A second line of scholarship "has centered on the first-person stories that people in institutions – plaintiffs, petitioners, suspects, employees, students, members of therapeutic groups – are asked or required to tell" (ibid.). Patients, clients, and other participants in insti-tutional settings often encounter expectations to the content of stories. For example, in one narrative environment stories may be expected to include emotions, while emotions in another narrative environment undermine a story's proficiency.

Research demonstrates that people "usually end up conforming to the stories that are expected of them" (Polletta et al., 2011, 116). However, some participants do resist, and it is important to "preempt the notion that narrative environments determine the form and content of narratives" (Gubrium & Holstein 2009, 183). The narrative environment is a context that influences storytelling but it never dictates stories. The social, cultural, and organizational context provides storytellers with resources that can be used as creatively as the imagination and skills of the narrator allows.

Storytelling

In this section we turn to "the hows" of storytelling (Gubrium & Holstein, 2009) to highlight the interactive aspects of the storying process. By approaching storytelling as an interactional achievement, researchers can make clear how narrators collaborate and perhaps conflict over the meaning of experiences in the past and expectations of the future.

Crafting out stories that make sense of the blooming, buzzing confusion of the world is hard work, yet it is work we seldom notice as it is not done self-consciously. A narrative ethnographer has to open up this work for analysis, and one way to do this is through observing how stories unfold in social interaction and remaining alert to how conversational partners collaborate in the production of meaning (Gubrium & Holstein, 2009, 94). In this, we should not only notice how things people say contribute to the building of meaningful narratives but also consider how inactions (e.g. silence) discourage some narratives from ever emerging.

In narrative ethnography, the storyteller is approached as an active and situated agent. In terms of methodology, this means that the researcher orients to and documents the interactions and circumstances of narrative production. Storytelling is an interactional accomplishment when it is carried out in collaboration with people we communicate directly with but also in private moments when we try to make sense of things on our own. We use culturally shared resources such as language, concepts, genre repertoires, and narrative templates for sense-making. Sometimes audiences are present, at other times they are only imagined, but they are always part of our storytelling.

One way to forefront the storying process is to focus on the performative aspects of storytelling. Riessman summarizes the rationale behind dialogic and performance-oriented narrative research as follows:

> Stories don't fall from the sky (or emerge from the innermost "self"); they are composed and received in contexts – interactional, historical, institutional, and discursive – to name a few. Stories are social artifacts, telling us as much about society and culture as they do about a person or group. How do these contexts enter into storytelling? How is a story coproduced in a complex choreography – in spaces between teller and listener, speaker and setting, text and reader, and history and culture? Dialogic/performance analysis attempts to deal with these questions.
>
> *(Riessman, 2008, 105)*

Addressing questions like these often call for ethnographic methodologies or at least an ethnographic sensibility towards the "complex choreography" as Riessman terms it. Ethnographic fieldwork is not the only way to study stories in the context of their telling. However, as the enterprise requires methods that can capture empirical material of narrative practice in its contextual complexity, fieldwork may stand out as the obvious choice. In any case, the researcher somehow has to be on the scenes of story construction to observe how stories are shaped by the contingencies of communication (Gubrium & Holstein, 2008, 250). Of course, qualitative interviews are also scenes of storytelling (Holstein & Gubrium. 1995), and the three examples that follow shortly illustrate how both interviews and ethnographic fieldwork can be combined in different ways in narrative ethnography.

Narrative control

The concept of "narrative control" (Gubrium & Holstein, 2008) can be productively employed in narrative ethnographies studying stories in the context of illness, injuries, and other calamities undermining wellbeing. Gubrium and Holstein coined the concept to foreground the ways in which storytelling is mediated by interactional and institutional forms of control that reflexively enter into narrative accounts.

> Narrative ethnography opens to empirical inspection the social processes and circumstances through which narratives are constructed, promoted, and resisted. We can actually see and hear how those concerned actively call on or otherwise respond to the contexts, contingencies, and resources of narration to fashion their accounts. In other words, we can actually witness *narrative control* being exercised.
>
> *(Gubrium & Holstein, 2008, 256, emphasis in original)*

Narrative control should not be conceived of as completely constraining storytelling. Rather it is an underlying condition that is always present in one form or another. One form is interactional control that arises in the give-and-take of social interaction. Narrative ethnographers may observe how some storytellers take and are being granted a narrative space that allows them to string together multiple sentences into a story without derailing interruptions while other participants remain unsuccessful in claiming this space. Narrative control can also take institutional forms, e.g. by formalizing expectations to narrative formats. For example, in a context such as an Alcoholics Anonymous meeting participants are expected to present a personal story that fits with the larger 12-step narrative (Cain, 1991, Carr, 2011). Narrative control can take on many forms and must be observed by the narrative ethnographer in the context where it is exercised.

How to study storytelling in context: three examples

This section presents three examples of narrative ethnographic studies on storytelling in the context of treatment. The first study exemplifies a focus on treatment recipients' narratives, the second on treatment providers' narratives, and the third on therapy as a frame for storytelling. Each subsection clarifies the translation process from research question to methodological design and contributions of the narrative ethnographic study.

Example I: a study of recovery narratives

The first example (Andersen, 2015), focuses on young people in a Danish drug treatment program. Researchers have long demonstrated the importance of narratives in recovery processes where individuals need to make sense of a past extensive drug use and construct a future non-addict identity (e.g. McIntosh & McKeganey, 2000). However, it has not been studied much how recovery narratives actually develop in the everyday context of drug treatment. One reason for this shortage is the reliance of most studies on qualitative interviews, and while the researchers in these studies often recognize the importance of contexts, they have not analyzed how the drug treatment context shapes narratives moment-to-moment. Narrative ethnography has the potential to do this. In line with this, the research question addressed in this first example is: "How do recovery narratives develop moment-to-moment in a drug treatment context for young people".

In terms of research design, detailed ethnographic data is necessary to address this question. Data such as audiotaped treatment talk enables detailed study of interactional storytelling and in this study this kind of data proved to have much value. For example, a fine-grained analysis of a long and informal group session with four young women and a treatment provider showed how the young women gradually, encouraged by the treatment provider, changed their narratives of past drug use to include more shame. Previous research (e.g. Carr, 2011) already has demonstrated how drug treatment has a tradition of a gendered production of shame targeting young women, but narrative ethnography expands on this literature by demonstrating how this is actually produced moment-to-moment. Audio-recorded data is not the only way to do this kind of narrative ethnography, and the study also benefits from interviews and field notes. The important thing is that data needs to be thick and detailed enough to allow for an orientation to contexts and social interaction in the analysis.

The study shows how a local treatment context works as a narrative environment that shapes treatment recipients' narratives. The institutional settings examined in the study work in different ways. For example, the pleasures of drug use are tabooed in one of the treatment centers where the narrative environment favors stories that link extensive drug use to painful problems, while the young people in another treatment center were encouraged to include pleasurable aspects in their stories of past as well as present drug use. The demonstration of how a local narrative environment shapes stories contributes to the general understanding of interactive storytelling in encounters between professionals and clients in treatment settings. The narrative environment of any particular drug treatment matters because it shapes the stories participants tell; silencing some stories, encouraging others. Stories and narrative environments are locally unique. Contextualized storytelling is ubiquitous.

Example II: a study of treatment providers' use of storytelling

The second example (Andersen, 2014) shows how narrative ethnography can illuminate professional treatment providers' use of stories in their day-to-day work. Humans use storytelling to make sense of their experiences and orient themselves in the turmoil of everyday life. In the context of drug treatment, we know from previous research (e.g. Paik, 2006, Carr, 2011) that a persistent challenge for treatment providers is to figure out how best to work with clients that make claims the professionals consider inauthentic. The treatment provider needs to understand what is going on (is my client lying? is he or she delusional?) in order to figure out how to proceed. The research question in this study is "How do treatment providers use storytelling to make sense of what they experience and figure out how to proceed in their daily work".

The research design combines an ethnographic case study with an interview analysis. Encounters with puzzling problems and recalcitrant people in institutional settings stimulate storytelling as the professionals need to figure out what kind of problems they face and how to handle them (Polletta et al., 2011). Aware of this, a case with a young man pseudo-named Jerry was selected for the case study. The ethnographic fieldwork documented daily conflicts between Jerry and his treatment providers over a time period of several weeks. Jerry kept saying that being enrolled in drug treatment helped him and that he was doing better, while his treatment providers disagreed; they thought he was doing worse and was not benefitting from treatment. The narrative ethnography uncovered how the treatment providers tried out different stories to make sense of the situation, and the subsequent interview analysis found the same story templates in a broader population of treatment providers.

The narrative ethnography contributes with an identification of three distinct types of stories that treatment providers activate to make sense of client inauthenticity: (1) professionals routinely refer to what this study labels the story of institutional conformism, portraying institutionalized clients who have developed a habit of saying the "right" things rather than the "real" things, (2) in the somewhat taboo story of ulterior motives, clients are interpreted as making inauthentic claims because they want to obtain something externally from drug treatment (e.g., avoid prison or work training programs), and (3) the story of disorders explains inauthenticity as a result of pathology. The study illuminates how professionals assert narrative control through storytelling and how specific stories carry specific consequences and may ultimately contribute to the exclusion of some clients from treatment.

Example III: a study of treatment as a frame for storytelling

The third example (Andersen & Sandberg, 2019) demonstrates how a treatment setting works as a frame for storytelling. The specific treatment setting examined is a Danish anger management program. Previous research has critiqued conventional anger management programs for disregarding participants' values honoring masculine performances of being tough, risk-seeking, and capable of violence (Laursen & Laws, 2016). In contrast, the program in this study represents a liberal approach that endorses such values while still encouraging participants to reform their behavior and avoid causing anger-related harm. The research question of the study is "How does this program work as a frame for the participants storytelling and narrative presentations of past, present, and future selves?"

The research design is based on ethnographic fieldwork and extensive field notes from all sessions in a therapy course. A detailed narrative analysis shows how the program works as a frame that communicates certain expectations through subtle or not so subtle cues. For example, the walls of the therapy room exhibit a collection of photographs of angry, threatening men. The photographs work as visualizations of anger. All photographs portray men who are white, able-bodied, and strong-looking, while there are no pictures of, for example, angry women or children. This creates a link between anger and a certain type of masculinity. Further, their threatening postures link anger with the potential of physical aggression. Through this as well as many other cues, the therapeutic frame conveys an expectation that participants in this program value a kind of "hyper masculinity" (Bengtsson, 2016). The study shows how this is a classed and gendered frame that some participants align with while others do not. Thus, a participant that told stories countering the expectations of the program (for example, stories about how he feared rather than enjoyed fighting) spurred awkward silences and the participant became reluctant to share stories in the treatment sessions.

The study clarifies how a treatment program that seeks to accommodate a particular form of masculinity may unintentionally marginalize participants that "fail" to align with this. Treatment providers must have some kind of "imagined program participant" in mind when they prepare and organize therapy; they have to consider what kind of needs they are to accommodate and how to do this (cf. Henriksen, Andersen & Presser, 2019). However, this study calls for a meticulous reflexivity concerning how program expectations frame participants' storytelling and how storytelling opportunities are ensured for participants who counter these expectations.

Conclusion

Narrative ethnography is a methodology tailored to study stories in the context of their telling. For humans that encounter disruptions in life caused by, for example, illness, accidents, or other impairments of wellbeing, storytelling is an important way that we make our suffering meaningful and connect to others. Researchers that want to understand this and open the process of sense-making up for analysis may use narrative ethnography. Narrative ethnography is useful in investigations of what it is people do through storytelling, e.g. how treatment providers communicate logics of action through storytelling or how treatment recipients narrate a process of recovery, and it can be adapted to studies focusing on treatment recipients and treatment providers, as well as therapeutic frames.

References

Andersen, D. (2014). Storytelling in drug treatment: How professionals make sense of what they consider inauthentic client claims. *Contemporary Drug Problems, 41*(4), 491–506.

Andersen, D. (2015). Stories of change in drug treatment: a narrative analysis of 'whats' and 'hows' in institutional storytelling. *Sociology of Health & Illness, 37*(5), 668–682.

Andersen, D. & S. Sandberg. (2019). 'Of course you like to fight': Frames for storytelling in a liberal anger management programme. *Acta Sociologica, 62*(1), 96–109.

Bengtsson, T.T. (2016) Performing hyper-masculinity: Experiences with confined young offenders. *Men and Masculinities, 19*(4), 410–428.

Bengtsson, T. & D. Andersen. (2020): Narrative analysis: Thematic, structural and performative. In Järvinen, M., & Mik-Meyer, N. (Eds.). (2020). *Qualitative Analysis: Eight Approaches for the Social Sciences.* London: SAGE Publications Limited.

Cain, C. (1991). Personal stories: Identity acquisition and self-understanding in Alcoholics Anonymous. *Ethos, 19*(2), 210–253.

Carr, E.S. (2011) *Scripting Addiction: The Politics of Therapeutic Talk and American Sobriety.* Princeton, NJ: Princeton University Press.

Frank, A.W. (2013). *The Wounded Storyteller: Body, Illness, and Ethics.* University of Chicago Press.

Gubrium, J.F. & J.A. Holstein. (2008). Narrative ethnography. *Handbook of Emergent Methods,* Hesse-Biber, S & P. Leavy (eds). New York: The Guilford Press, pp. 241–264.

Gubrium, J.F. & J.A. Holstein. (2009). *Analyzing Narrative Reality.* London: Sage.

Henriksen, T.D., D. Andersen, & L. Presser. (2020). "Not a Real Prostitute": Narrative imagination, social policy, and care for men who sell sex. *Sexuality Research and Social Policy,* 17, 442–453.

Holstein, J.A. & J.F. Gubrium. (1995). *The Active Interview.* Thousand Oaks: Sage.

Laursen, J. & B. Laws. (2016) Honour and respect in Danish prisons: Contesting 'cognitive distortions' in cognitive-behavioral programmes. *Punishment & Society* 19(1), 74–95.

Mattingly, C. (1994). The concept of therapeutic 'employment'. *Social Science & Medicine, 38*(6), 811–822.

Mattingly, C. (2010). *The Paradox of Hope: Journeys through a Clinical Borderland.* Los Angeles: University of California Press.

McIntosh, J. & N. McKeganey. (2000). Addicts' narratives of recovery from drug use: constructing a non-addict identity. *Social Science & Medicine, 50*(10), 1501–1510.

Paik, L. (2006). Are you truly a recovering dope fiend? Local interpretive practices at a therapeutic community drug treatment program. *Symbolic Interaction, 29*(2), 213–234.

Polletta, F., P.C.B. Chen, B.G. Gardner, & A. Motes. (2011). The sociology of storytelling. *Annual Review of Sociology, 37,* 109–130.

Riessman, C.K. (2008). *Narrative Methods for the Human Sciences.* London: Sage.

24

IN THE QUEST OF RESILIENCE IN ELDER PATIENTS

Solutogenics

Gillie Gabay

Introduction

In 2035, estimates are that 50% of the population will be 65 and older with a life expectancy of 100 years and an expansion of chronic illness (Hall & Høy, 2012; Martin & Schoeni, 2014). When chronic illness becomes acute, patients are re-admitted to the hospital and suffer from psychological trauma (Fridh, Kenne Sarenmalm, Falk, Henoch, Öhlén, Ozanne, & Jakobsson Ung, 2015; Uhrenfeldt, Aagaard, Hall, Fegran, Ludvigsen, & Meyer, 2013). Researchers define resilience as a shift from focusing *on* the psychological trauma to focusing on coping *with* the trauma (Luthar, Cicchetti, & Becker, 2000; Maley et al., 2016; Manning, Carr, & Kail, 2016). In chronic illness, resilience of patients reduces readmissions, depression, and anxiety, and enhances engagement, adherence, determination to fight the disease, self-management of illness, quality of life, and recovery (Karatsoreos & McEwen, 2013; Maley et al., 2016).

Resilience is modifiable entailing the tolerance of uncertainty in health adversity (Karatsoreos & McEwen, 2013; Manning et al., 2016). Drivers of resilience are: self-efficacy, problem-solving, and emotional regulation (Aelbrecht, Rimondini, Bensing, Moretti, Willems, Mazzi, Deveugele et al., 2015; Trivedi et al., 2009; Trivedi, Bosworth, & Jackson, 2011). Studies on resilience of elders after discharge from hospitalizations are scarce. In this chapter, I explore the linkage between experiences of elders with clinicians while in acute-care and post-discharge resilience.

For the purpose of this chapter, I borrowed the Salutogenic theory of resilience (Antonovsky, 1991). The Salutogenic theory expands one's ability to transform one's world and therefore increases elders' ability to deal with medical adversity (Antonovsky, 1991; 1993; Mittelmark & Bauer, 2017; Mittelmark & Bull, 2013; Pelikan, 2017; Vinje & Ausland, 2015). As any empowering theory, the Salutogenic theory views people as able to control their health and well-being (Antonovsky, 1991; 1993; Mittelmark & Bauer, 2017).

An anchor of the Salutogenic framework is the sense of coherence (SOC) which encompasses three dimensions: comprehensibility, manageability, and meaningfulness. These three dimensions promote resilience. Antonovsky (1991; 1993) defined the dimension of comprehensibility as the patient's perception that her world is understandable and information is clear and structured. Antonovsky (1991; 1993) defined the dimension of manageability as the patient's perception that she has adequate resources to cope with health events. Manageability results in motivation to invest energy in effective coping. Antonovsky (1991; 1993) defined the dimension of meaningfulness as one's perception that it is worth it to cope with health challenges, as life is meaningful. This chapter seeks to close a gap in the state of the science exploring the resilience promotion of elders after being hospitalized in acute care. The research question is: Which conduct of clinicians had an impact on patients' trajectory from psychological trauma in acute-care to resilience after discharge?

The Study

Aims

While studies on communication with patients mainly focus on outpatient settings, studies on experiences of elders when communicating with clinicians in acute care and their effect on elders' well-being and resilience following discharge from the hospital are scarce and poorly understood (Hall & Høy, 2012; Jerofke, Weiss, & Yakusheva, 2014; Sürücü, Besen, Duman, & Erbil, 2018). This chapter seeks to identify communication pathways that activate elders' navigation from psychological trauma in acute-care to post-discharge resilience. This explorative study responds to calls of researchers to elucidate communication pathways that could improve elders' experiences in lengthy hospitalizations and promote their resilience following discharge (Atwal et al., 2007; Eggly, Albrecht, Kelly, Prigerson, Sheldon, & Studts, 2009; Hall & Høy, 2012).

Snowball sampling served to recruit participants. Interviews were audio-taped, transcribed verbatim, and translated from Hebrew to English. Two interviews were conducted with each participant. The first interview was held within the first two days post-discharge and the second a month thereafter, to capture the period of high-risk for negative outcomes, new acute conditions, readmission, disability, and morbidity (Manning et al., 2016; Rosenberg et al., 2015). Participants were six secular Israelis ages 68–81, recently discharged from a lengthy hospitalization in acute-care at a large medical center (1200–3200 beds) due to cancer, heart disease, and neurological disorders that put them in mortal danger. The information saturation method was applied to determine the sample size (Browne, Roseman, Shaller & Edgman-Levitan, 2010; Figueroa, Joynt, Zhou, Orav, & Jha, 2017). Qualitative narrative studies are interpretive, eliciting others' perspectives, and are the preferred strategy by qualitative researchers, including in medical education (Malterud, Siersma, & Guassora, 2016). To generate an unstructured narrative, the one general question that I asked was (Josselson, 2013): "How did you arrive at the hospital and what did you experience there?"

I analyzed each set of interviews separately searching for central themes upon discharge and a month following discharge. Communication of clinicians with patients occurred only during the hospitalization and not during recovery phase following discharge. Data analysis was thematic, guided by Aronson (1992). The analysis explored elders' experiences by dimensions of comprehensibility, manageability, and meaningfulness. I identified themes, i.e., units derived from patterns such as recurring meanings and feelings by bringing together elements of ideas or experiences, which often, when viewed alone are meaningless, but that make sense in a specific context. Themes emerged from the data through six analytical steps:

1. Reading and re-reading the interviews and listing patterns of experiences through direct quotes for each dimension
2. Identifying all data relating to the patterns already classified
3. Sorting all data according to the corresponding pattern

4. Combining and categorizing related patterns into sub-themes to obtain a comprehensive view of the emerging patterns
5. Piecing together themes in a meaningful way to form a comprehensive picture representing the interpretation of participants' collective experience in the hospitalization and post-discharge
6. Obtaining information allowing to make inferences regarding resilience based on the literature.

I present themes separately for participants' experiences during the hospitalization and for participants' experiences following discharge.

Findings

Hospitalization experience

Comprehensibility

a. Enhancing health literacy – two out of six clinicians encouraged participants to read about their disease and be more aware of their conditions, and assured that the participants understood the information:

> She (the nurse) referred me to a certain site in case I wanted to know more about it. She said, "I am here if you have any questions". I read a lot on accredited sites that the doctor recommended. I was troubled about one of the treatments and asked the doctor "What If I am exposed to serious bacteria and have an infection?
> *(Martin, male, 68)*

> My condition did not allow a second opinion. I had no time, I read about it all day.
> *(Moshe, 76)*

Patient's opportunities to lean about their disease and condition structured their time at the hospital and reduced their anxiety:

b. Carrying on a frank, respectful, eye-level talk – talking with participants about their diagnosis and their prognosis after they learned about their disease to provide them with additional explanations and reflect on room for improving their condition:

> It was late in the evening. The ward was quiet. We sat for a long time and talked about it. He (the doctor) looked at me and explained to me what is wrong with immense patience in simple words, I understood that the body creates new antibodies rapidly.
> *(Martin, 68)*

> The head of the Neurology Department wanted to know what was happening with me. He listened to me at length and then explained everything respectfully, at eye level. The relations I had with him were exceptional and greatly encouraged me. He and the nurse gave me a feeling that I would be OK. I felt in good hands.
> *(Koby, 74)*

c. Initiating updates for participants – providing them with information and creating a sense of control in the process. When participants knew what to expect next in the process and what is planned in the process, it made participants feel that they were safe. Sharing partial information and uncertainty with participants also enhanced the patients' sense of control, reducing anxiety:

> I kept falling, my legs would not hold me: the neurologist said, 'We read your CAT scan and there are definitely deficiencies, but we are not clear yet on the meaning.
> We'll hold a consultation and I'll let you know after the consultation if we recommend that you go into surgery today.' I felt in good hands. Despite my resistance to head surgery, I decided that if I needed surgery to come out of this, then surgery it is.
>
> *(Moshe, 76)*

Lack of communication for long periods created a sense of losing control and accelerated anxiety:

> I was taken to the Neurology Department in a wheel chair. I had never been this ill, it was very scary. I did not know what had gone wrong and what to expect. My worst fear was my next fall. What would I be doing when it happened again? I just sat there for ages. No one approached me, my head exploded with thoughts about what would happen ... I was hypoglycemic with heart fibrillation. Five physicians were around my bed. They did not talk with me. They didn't know what to treat first, my diabetes or my heart. Then one of them declared 'You are going into surgery'. No one answered my questions. At night I got another heart attack due to an infection. I had open heart surgery [long silence, sitting hunched over on the couch].
>
> *(Yoel, 81)*

Manageability

a. Instilling confidence – Participants attributed confidence to their interaction with the clinicians who treated them:

> One day the nurse announced: "Today we are standing". She sensed my fear and said, "Don't worry, I will hold you if you fall. I checked your leg strength – you should be able to stand up". She was a tiny 60-year-old woman. I was fearful of falling, but she held me. Eventually I succeeded. It felt amazing.
>
> *(Martin, 68)*

Clinicians' use of a professional jargon may have stimulated a sense of insecurity in elders, lack of self-efficacy in coping and a sense of objectification:

> The neurosurgeon came by to see me but didn't see me at all. He hardly spoke with me. When he turned to me he said: "You have excess fluid in your head that pressure your brain and explains your cognitive regression, loss of memory, and walking disorder. We will drill a hole in your head, insert a catheter, pull a tube from the brain

down through your stomach and regulate the fluids to decrease the pressure in your brain." [silence]. "I was scared to death. I felt intense cold throughout my body.

(Koby, 74)

Insecurity emerged from insensitivity of clinicians as well:

A resident invited me to the room, darkened it, and started talking to me about my farewell from life." [Silence]. "I understood that I would die soon, so I asked to sit on the bed and took out a cigarette. What did I care? I was dying anyway.

(Eli, 68)

The conduct of clinicians was unsettling and heightened anxiety.

b. Clinicians' reflection on perceived potential improvement – when clinicians reflected on their view of potential improvement, it positively affected participants:

I had no resources to deal with the news. I was on my way to surgery for the fourth time this year. I didn't want any hospital, any physician, nurse, or surgery.

When I shared my inability to accept my new medical reality the nurse had an interesting expression. She was quiet for a few minutes. Then she looked at me softly and said: "It is challenging, yes. There is nothing simple about this. But do you know how many people would change places with you? How many would want to detect their cancer early, remove it and move on with life?

(Michelle, 79)

"You are not dying on me", she said. "You will live". I told her that the previous doctor just clarified that I was dying… She said, "Oh, he knows nothing!" and yelled at him. At that moment, I had no doubt that I would stay alive [tears]. Participants whose physicians kept their spirits up persevered, patients who had a light condition but were depressed died because their disease spread. It is the biggest difference amongst physicians. I think 50% of the treatment is one's hope that they will live. It encouraged my determination to heal. [quiet]. I owe her my life.

(Eli, 68)

c. Allowing participants to reflect – time for reflection enhanced their perceived control enhancing a positive change in emotions and attitudes:

I was so sad. Then I felt fear. Friends and colleagues slowly drift away from you when you are that sick. The nurse would stay with me to talk about my fear of missing out on the weddings of our children and not knowing my grandkids. I was devastated. She would come with coffee and chocolate and I would share what I could not share with anyone in the world. It made a huge difference for me. I was lucky.

(Eli, 68)

Analysis of the experiences of participants stressed the existence of two groups with contrasting experiences. Koby, Eli, and Yoel experienced lack of emotional support. Martin, Moshe, and Michelle had, in their view, "exceptional" experiences. Eli distinguished between his experience with the resident physician versus his empowering experience with the nurse. Yoel elaborates on his experience, and how instead of feeling empowered, he felt diminutive:

> They did not fight for me. They were very technocratic. Basically, they did their job and that's it. They don't really care about me. If my fifth hospitalization this year taught me anything, it's that the hospital is a huge factory and I am just a kettle that needs fixing. No one talked to me. Not a surgeon, not a social worker, not a nurse or a psychologist [silent].
>
> *(Yoel, 81)*

Yoel interpreted the lack of communication as a lack of caring:

> When I was re-admitted again with excruciating pain, the staff recognized me but asked or said nothing. They didn't care about me and threw me away like a rag: "Go have a stomach, liver and kidney ultrasound in your local clinic and then come back".
>
> *(Yoel, 81)*

Interviews a month post-discharge - *psychological trauma versus resilience*
Meaningfulness

Two common subgroup themes emerged from the data (Spector-Mersel, 2010): "anxiety and helplessness" versus "determination to recover."

"Anxiety and helplessness": Staying in the psychological trauma zone (6)

Yoel, Moshe, and Koby felt anxious and helpless, and were traumatized by missing or partial communication and a lack of reflection from clinicians, which further stimulated their anxiety. Rather than gaining a sense of control, Yoel, Moshe, and Koby experienced further loss of control. Upon discharge, they felt victimized and degraded. They accepted their functional impairment, did not look forward to the future, and re-experienced traumatic degrading communication that added to their trauma of their progressive illness:

> It's not enough to know medicine if you don't understand the human soul.
> Clinicians have become technicians, they forgot to communicate and be healers. They don't know how to listen and they no longer hear anything. But, if they would at least communicate it could have been different. I am left with the sickness, and death is approaching me.
>
> *(Moshe, 68)*

> I was there so many times this year. They already know me by name. The experience was horrific. Hallelujah! I am home. I hope I stay home. I came out of there in a wheelchair, nothing will be the same. I just hope I am not readmitted again.
>
> *(Yoel, 81)*

[Yoel refused to be readmitted and died eight months after discharge].
Koby also felt helpless, but was determined to refuse future surgeries:

They were condescending and did not explain what I should expect. I decided that whatever happens to me, I would not go through any more surgeries. I expected the surgeon to come by after surgery and talk to me about how I was doing. Instead I was very anxious. I can hardly walk since the surgery. I am not active. People should stay away from hospitals.

(Koby, 74)

Common themes of "determination to recover"

Three participants (Michelle, Eli, and Martin) experienced inspiring communication that enhanced their perceived control, instilled confidence in them, and directed them to seek information, plan, reappraise their situation, and refocus on recovery. Clinicians encouraged them to learn about their disease and ask questions. Reflections of clinicians about their potential improvements lead them to re-assess their functional condition, plan, and take responsibility for their illness following the discharge. These participants were determined to bounce back to life despite the complexity of their illness.

Taking responsibility: meaningfulness and determination to recover following psychological trauma

Michelle, Eli, and Martin experienced communication that enables them to perceive that they are able to improve their health. They were determined to recover and get back to their routines. A month following her discharge, Michelle shared her view:

Now it's a long period of healing in order to renew my health. It's hard work. My body is under trauma, due to the surgery. Meeting my limitations is part of the healing process. I am less functioning, less able, have no strength or energy. I'm at the bottom of the climbing wall of my life. I need to climb up again and again. I need a lot of physical and mental strength to deal with such a transition. But who wants to stay down there? No one! I sure don't. I'm lucky that I can continue and play the "music" of rehabilitation.

(Michelle, 79)

Martin describes the hardship and his determination to walk again:

I told myself, "No matter how long it takes, you will walk again!" Every time some negative thought surfaces like – "you will never walk again" – I shove it away. It's tough but I am encouraged. Every day I force myself to take more steps than the day before, regardless of the pain or how long it takes.

(Martin, 68)

Meaningfulness and gratitude

Participants whose clinicians used communication to enhance elders' self-education, health-literacy, reflection, and perceived control, took responsibility for their recovery and bounced back to life:

I am slowly rehabilitating and getting back to a blessed routine. It's complex, but I have no complaints, I am lucky, I am so thankful. Every day I feel privileged to be alive.

(Eli, 68)

Martin shared his insights, while reflecting on his life before he was re-admitted and at present:

> You start off from the worst place, you don't know anything, you don't feel your legs, you cannot stand. All of a sudden, you wake up one morning with no motor senses. You just slowly assimilate that you have no control. We can only do the best we can.
>
> That's it. If anything happens, you cope with it. I understand that I have no choice but to manage myself.
>
> *(Martin, 68)*

Michelle shared her reflection as she was bouncing back to life after four readmissions in a year:

> On this whole journey we only have this moment, the here and now. When I reflect on the hospitalization periods, I remember the exceptional dedication of my clinicians during the four times I was hospitalized this year. All of them were so sensitive in their communication with me. I remember the entangled, intertwined roads of my journey. A ton of hours filled with my worry and their listening, encouragement, and support.
>
> Their beneficial presence undoubtedly encouraged me to return four times to the operating table for complex surgeries. Our presence is a gift. We really only have this moment.
>
> *(Michelle, 79)*

To sum, elder participants whose clinicians enhanced their health literacy, self-education, and held eye-level talks with them, felt valued. They had a higher comprehensibility of the complexity they faced and a higher sense of manageability. Participants who, a month following discharge were dedicated to their rehabilitation despite hardships, reported that their clinicians voluntarily updated them, instilled confidence in them and reflected on room for improvement. Discussion on room for improvement with elder participants enabled them to process their emotions and enhance meaningfulness.

Discussion

This study reveals that the conduct of clinicians in acute care with elder patients may impact their resilience by extending comprehensibility, manageability, and meaningfulness. Participants expected clinicians to address their distress throughout their hospitalization (Gabay, 2019; Tait & Hodges, 2013). The dimensions of SOC, if fulfilled, meet these expectations and promote resilience of elder patients following discharge (Antonovsky, 1991; Antonovsky, 1993; Mittelmark, Sagy, Eriksson, Bauer, Pelikan, Lindström, & Espnes, 2017).

By increasing the health literacy of participants, clinicians enhanced patients' sense of control. When participants felt respected and valued and when their clinicians were informative and honest with them, participants felt part of the process (Gaglio, Glasgow, & Bull, 2012; Kvåle & Bondevik, 2008). Feeling part of the process rather than simply sharing treatment decision made participants feel they were in control and enhanced both their comprehensibility and manageability (Antonovsky, 1991; Antonovsky, 1993; Mittelmark et al., 2017; Mittelmark & Bull, 2013; Trivedi et al., 2009; Vinje & Ausland, 2013). Participants whose clinicians enhanced their perceived control transitioned from psychological trauma in acute-care to resilience following discharge. This finding suggests that to promote resilience of elders, clinicians may enhance their sense of control in the process rather than in making decisions. In previous studies, communication that strengthened patients' perceived control lead to stress management, goal setting, gratitude, positive re-appraisal, and acceptance (Ezeamama, Elkins, Simpson, Smith, Allegra, & Miles, 2016). Communication that strengthened perceived control inspired participants, instilled confidence in them, and encouraged them to be determined to recover enhancing manage-ability (Loprinzi, Prasad, Schroeder, & Sood, 2011; Omeje & Nebo, 2011).

In severe illness, perceived control is modifiable through information and knowledge and is associated with overcoming health-damaging behaviors, preventing health problems, faster recovery, lower readmissions, and adherence to treatment plans (Berglund, Lytsy, & Westerling, 2014; Gabay, 2015). Participants who felt in control during the hospitalization expressed a stronger desire to live a month following discharge. This finding echoes a previous study in which communication of nurses with patients in acute-care influenced the self-management of illness by those patients six weeks following discharge (Vinje & Ausland, 2013). In contrast to previous findings, this study indicates that elders may be empowered through communi-cation with clinicians (Anderson & Funnell, 2010; Lubetkin, Lu, & Gold, 2010; Naaldenberg, Vaandrager, Koelen, & Leeuwis, 2012). By directing participants towards knowing more about their illness and towards information, clinicians built participants' ability to understand their treatment and to believe that they can improve their health.

This study supports previous findings that proposed that communication with patients might activate their engagement (Fridh et al., 2015). Findings stress that even the context of acute-care may provide clinicians with opportunities to activate and engage elder patients, leading them to trust their treatment following discharge resulting in: medication-adherence, satisfaction, and fewer re-admissions (Gabay, 2016; 2019).

Congruent to findings of previous studies, participants preferred face-to-face, clear, simple language conversations with clinicians, which reinforced the dimension of comprehensibility (Antonovsky, 1991, 1993; Mittelmark et al., 2017; Pearlin, Nguyen, Schieman, & Milkie, 2007; Slosser, McKibbin, Lee, Bourassa, & Carrico, 2015). Echoing previous studies, clinicians' who failed to avoid the use of professional jargon heightened the anxiety of participants who were already traumatized due to the re-admission (Lincoln, Arford, Prener, Garverich, & Koenen, 2013; Naaldenberg et al., 2012). Use of professional jargon in the acute-care lead to paralyzing anxiety, lower literacy, loneliness, sense of continued loss of control – all deepening trauma among participants. Similar to findings of prior work, impaired communication added stress that perhaps inhibited bouncing back to life (Maley et al., 2016).

Clinicians who encouraged participants to process their own feelings and their belief that they could improve their illness enhanced participants' self-esteem, well-being, and manage-ability (Antonovsky, 1991, 1993; Mears, 2009; Mittelmark et al., 2017; Mittelmark & Bull, 2013). Furthermore, clinicians who enabled participants to think about internal and external resources they can use in their recovery facilitated participants' self-efficacy regarding the management and coping with the complexity and the manageability of their illness. Participants whose clinicians provided them with information about their health status and supported them, reported that it helped them shape a positive outlook and to be hopeful and determined to bounce back to life (Antonovsky, 1991; 1993; Mittelmark et al., 2017).

Conclusion

Communication is essential to resilience of elder patients. Participants who believed that their efforts made a difference were more determined to achieve recovery goals despite hardships (Aloisio, Gifford, McGilton, Lalonde, Estabrooks, & Squires, 2018; Gabay, 2015). Clinicians often perceive elder patients as passive and frail, but in reality, many elders actively manage their life challenges. While clinicians frequently focus on negative repercussions of illness in elders (i.e., disability, loneliness, weight gain, falls), emphasizing limitations that the illness brings to older age (Jeste, Depp, & Vahia, 2010), elder patients focus on their supportive environments – their ability to use resources, manage their illness, and adapt to change (Huber et al., 2011). This focus of elders relates to the increasingly accepted definition of health as "the ability to adapt and self-management of illness reflecting resilience".

Clinicians may communicate with elder patients to enhance their comprehensibility of the complexity. Clinicians may also communicate with elder patients to provide them with a sense of coping with the complexity contributing to the meaningfulness that participants may attribute to the situation. Clinicians may motivate elder patients to take responsibility for their health, leading to resilience following discharge. Thus, clinicians may employ the dimensions of SOC with elder patients in hospitalizations, as illustrated in this chapter, to promote their resilience and well-being.

References

Aelbrecht, K., M. Rimondini, J. Bensing, F. Moretti, S. Willems, M. Mazzi, … & M. Deveugele. (2015). Quality of doctor–patient communication through the eyes of the patient: variation according to the patient's educational level. *Advances in Health Sciences Education, 20*(4), 873–884.

Aloisio, L.D., W.A. Gifford, K.S. McGilton, M. Lalonde, C.A. Estabrooks, & J.E. Squires. (2018). Individual and organizational predictors of allied healthcare providers' job satisfaction in residential long-term care. *BMC Health Services Research, 18*(1), 491.

Anderson, R.M. & M.M. Funnell. (2010). Patient empowerment: myths and misconceptions. *Patient Education and Counseling, 79*(3), 277–282.

Antonovsky, A. (1991). The structural sources of salutogenic strengths. In C. L. Cooper & R. Payne (Eds.), *Wiley series on studies in occupational stress. Personality and stress: Individual differences in the stress process.* John Wiley and Sons. 67–101.

Antonovsky, A. (1993). The structure and properties of the sense of coherence scale. *Social Science & Medicine, 36*(6), 725–733.

Aronson, E. (1992). The return of the repressed: Dissonance theory makes a comeback. *Psychological Inquiry, 3*(4), 303–311.

Atwal, A., K. Tattersall, S. Murphy, N. Davenport, C. Craik, K. Caldwell, & A. McIntyre. (2007). Older adults experiences of rehabilitation in acute health care. *Scandinavian Journal of Caring Sciences, 21*(3), 371–378.

Berglund, E., P. Lytsy, & R. Westerling. (2014). The influence of locus of control on self-rated health in context of chronic disease: a structural equation modeling approach in a cross-sectional study. *BMC Public Health, 14*(1), 492.

Browne, K., D. Roseman, D. Shaller, & S. Edgman-Levitan. (2010). Analysis & commentary measuring patient experience as a strategy for improving primary care. *Health Affairs, 29*(5), 921–925.

Eggly, S.S., T.L. Albrecht, K. Kelly, H.G. Prigerson, L.K. Sheldon, & J. Studts. (2009). The role of the clinician in cancer clinical communication. *Journal of Health Communication, 14*(S1), 66–75.

Ezeamama, A.E., J. Elkins, C. Simpson, S.L. Smith, J.C. Allegra, & T.P. Miles. (2016). Indicators of resilience and healthcare outcomes: findings from the 2010 health and retirement survey. *Quality of Life Research, 25*(4), 1007–1015.

Figueroa, J. F., K.E. Joynt, X. Zhou, E.J. Orav, & A.K. Jha. (2017). Safety-net hospitals face more barriers yet use fewer strategies to reduce admissions. *Medical Care, 55*(3), 229.

Fridh, I., E. Kenne Sarenmalm, K. Falk, I. Henoch, J. Öhlén, A. Ozanne, & E. Jakobsson Ung. (2015). Extensive human suffering: a point prevalence survey of patients' most distressing concerns during inpatient care. *Scandinavian Journal of Caring Sciences, 29*(3), 444–453.

Gabay, G. (2019). Patient self-worth and communication barriers to Trust of Israeli Patients in acute-care physicians at public general hospitals. *Qualitative Health Research, 29*(13), 1954–1966.

Gabay, G. (2016). Exploring perceived control and self-rated health in re-admissions among younger adults: A retrospective study. *Patient Education and Counseling, 99*(5), 800–806.

Gabay, G. (2015). Perceived control over health, communication and patient– physician trust. *Patient Education and Counseling, 98*(12), 1550–1557.

Gaglio, B., R.E. Glasgow, & S.S. Bull. (2012). Do patient preferences for health Information vary by health literacy or numeracy? A qualitative assessment. *Journal of Health Communication, 17*(suppl. 3), 109–121.

Hall, E. O. & B. Høy, B. (2012). Re-establishing dignity: Nurses' experiences of caring for older hospital patients. *Scandinavian Journal of Caring Sciences, 26*(2), 287–294.

Huber, M., J.A. Knottnerus, L. Green, H. van der Horst, A.R. Jadad, D. Kromhout, ... & P. Schnabel. (2011). How should we define health? *BMJ, 343*, d4163.

Jerofke, T., M. Weiss, & O. Yakusheva. (2014). Patient perceptions of patient- empowering nurse behaviors, patient activation and functional health status in postsurgical patients with life-threatening long-term illnesses. *Journal of Advanced Nursing, 70*(6), 1310–1322.

Jeste, D.V., C.A. Depp, & I.V. Vahia. (2010). Successful cognitive and emotional aging. *World Psychiatry, 9*(2), 78.

Josselson, R. (2013). *Interviewing for qualitative inquiry: a relational approach.* Guilford Press.

Karatsoreos, I.N. & B.S. McEwen. (2013). Annual research review: The neurobiology and physiology of resilience and adaptation across the life course. *Journal of Child Psychology and Psychiatry, 54*(4), 337–347.

Kvåle, K. & M. Bondevik. (2008). What is important for patient centred care? A qualitative study about the perceptions of patients with cancer. *Scandinavian Journal of Caring Sciences, 22*(4), 582–589.

Lincoln, A.K., T. Arford, C. Prener, S. Garverich, & K.C. Koenen. (2013). The need for trauma-sensitive language use in literacy and health literacy screening instruments. *Journal of Health Communication, 18*(sup1), 15–19.

Loprinzi, C.E., K. Prasad, D.R. Schroeder, & A. Sood. (2011). Stress Management and Resilience Training (SMART) program to decrease stress and enhance resilience among breast cancer survivors: a pilot randomized clinical trial. *Clinical Breast Cancer, 11*(6), 364–368.

Lubetkin, E.I., W.H. Lu, & M.R. Gold. (2010). Levels and correlates of patient activation in health center settings: building strategies for improving health outcomes. *Journal of Health Care for the Poor and Underserved, 21*(3), 796–808.

Luthar, S.S., D. Cicchetti, & B. Becker. (2000). The construct of resilience: A critical evaluation and guidelines for future work. *Child Development, 71*(3), 543–562.

Maley, J.H., I. Brewster, I. Mayoral, R. Siruckova, S. Adams, K.A. McGraw, ... & M.E. Mikkelsen. (2016). Resilience in survivors of critical illness in the context of the survivors' experience and recovery. *Annals of the American Thoracic Society, 13*(8), 1351–1360.

Manning, L.K., D.C. Carr, & B.L. Kail. (2016). Do higher levels of resilience buffer the deleterious impact of chronic illness on disability in later life? *The Gerontologist, 56*(3), 514–524.

Martin, L.G. & R.F. Schoeni. (2014). Trends in disability and related chronic Conditions among the forty-and-over population: 1997–2010. *Disability and Health Journal, 7*(1), S4–S14.

Malterud, K., V.D. Siersma, & A.D. Guassora. (2016). Sample size in qualitative interview studies: Guided by information power. *Qualitative Health Research, 26*(13), 1753–1760.

Mittelmark, M.B., S. Sagy, M. Eriksson, G.F. Bauer, J.M. Pelikan, B. Lindström, & G.A. Espnes. (2017). *The handbook of salutogenesis.* Springer.

Mittelmark, M.B. & T. Bull. (2013). The salutogenic model of health in health promotion research. *Global Health Promotion, 20*(2), 30–38.

Naaldenberg, J., L. Vaandrager, M. Koelen, & C. Leeuwis. (2012). Aging populations' everyday life perspectives on healthy aging: New insights for policy and strategies at the local level. *Journal of Applied Gerontology, 31*(6), 711–733.

Omeje, O. & C. Nebo. (2011). The influence of locus control on adherence to treatment regimen among hypertensive patients. *Patient Preference and Adherence, 5*, 141.

Pearlin, L.I., K.B. Nguyen, S. Schieman, & M.A. Milkie. (2007). The life-course origins of mastery among older people. *Journal of Health and Social Behavior, 48*(2), 164–179.

Pelikan, J.M. (2017). The application of salutogenesis in healthcare settings. In: Mittelmark M.B., Sagy S., Eriksson M., et al., (eds.) *The Handbook of Salutogenesis*, p. 261. Cham (CH): Springer.

Rosenberg, A.R., J.P. Yi-Frazier, L. Eaton, C. Wharton, K. Cochrane, C. Pihoker, ... & E. McCauley. (2015). Promoting resilience in stress management: A pilot study of a novel resilience-promoting intervention for adolescents and young adults with serious illness. *Journal of Pediatric Psychology, 40*(9), 992–999.

Sarmiento, T.P., H.K.S. Laschinger, & C. Iwasiw. (2004). Nurse educators' workplace empowerment, burnout, and job satisfaction: Testing Kanter's theory. *Journal of Advanced Nursing, 46*(2), 134–143.

Slosser, A., C. McKibbin, A. Lee, K. Bourassa, & C. Carrico. (2015). Perceived health status and social network as predictors of resilience in rural older adults. *Age, 1*(13), 806.

Spector-Mersel, G. (2010). Narrative research: Time for a paradigm. *Narrative Inquiry, 20*(1), 204–224.

Sürücü, H.A., D.B. Besen, M. Duman, & E.Y. Erbil. (2018). Coping with stress among pregnant women with gestational diabetes mellitus. *Journal of Caring Sciences,* 7(1), 9.

Tait, G.R. & B.D. Hodges. (2013). Residents learning from a narrative experience with dying patients: A qualitative study. *Advances in Health Sciences Education, 18*(4), 727–743.

Trivedi, R.B., J.A. Blumenthal, C. O'Connor, K. Adams, A. Hinderliter, C. Dupree, … & A. Sherwood. (2009). Coping styles in heart failure patients with depressive symptoms. *Journal of Psychosomatic Research, 67*(4), 339–346.

Trivedi, R.B., H.B. Bosworth, & G.L. Jackson. (2011). Resilience in chronic Illness. In *Resilience in Aging* (pp. 181–197). New York, NY: Springer.

Vinje, H.F. & L.H. Ausland. (2013). Salutogenic presence supports a health promoting work life. *Socialmedicinsk tidskrift, 90*(6), 890–901.

Uhrenfeldt, L., H. Aagaard, E.O. Hall, L. Fegran, M.S. Ludvigsen, & G. Meyer. (2013). A qualitative meta-synthesis of patients' experiences of intra-and inter- hospital transitions. *Journal of Advanced Nursing, 69*(8), 1678–1690.

25

AND THE ANTHROPOLOGIST MADE THE "EMOTIONAL NOTE"

Haris Agic

Introduction

The art of ethnography requires a certain degree of technical skill, most of which is usually associated with a variety of techniques for data-gathering and data-analysis. Success of any ethnographic enterprise is contingent to the ethnographer's ability to gather enough sufficiently thick ethnographic evidence and his/her dexterity of how to make sense of those data. To ensure a certain level of quality in ethnographic work, ethnographic tradition has forged a variety of rules and conventions, declaring what is to be regarded as "proper" techniques.

Consequently, research schools and scientific communities, as well as various literature on ethnographic research within or associated with the academic disciplines such as anthropology, sociology, ethnology, and social psychology, teach future ethnographers how to perform their fieldwork, how to fit in, how to notice and how to take notes, and how to follow up on informants' leads. Further, students are trained in how to capture their findings with the help of audio- and video recording technology, how to transform their field-notes and field-diaries into a particular format suitable for certain analytical techniques, how to transcribe the recorded material, how to feed these different forms of information into the computer programs specially designed for the storage, retrieval, and analysis of qualitative data, and so on and so forth…

And still, despite all the literature, classes and seminars about fieldwork methods and data analysis that I have read and attended, the particular nature of my fieldwork left me with a strong sense of working with a toolbox that, albeit extensive and intricate, still wouldn't suffice.

Each day as I left the site of my fieldwork I carried with me a big burden of painful emotional turbulence that would easily turn into a kind of numbness or vacuum. I do not write this to draw attention to myself or to angle for pity on my behalf. The people suffering from severe heart diseases, unbearable pain, uncertainty, and fear of dying are the ones worthy of compassion. My emotional burden was, perhaps, just the plain human response of caring. I got to leave the hospital and go home every day – most patients didn't. As this was having a heavy impact on me, I soon recognized that it would also affect my data gathering, interpretation, and analysis.

My field was a heart disease department at a large academic hospital in Sweden. This hospital is one of ten modern university hospitals in Sweden. It has several hundred beds and nearly five thousand employees. Besides being a place of advanced health care, it is also a place of research

313

and training. The part of the hospital dealing with cardiovascular diseases is composed of three large clinical departments: 1) the Department of Cardiology; 2) the Department of Radiology; and 3) the Department of Cardiothoracic and Vascular Surgery. Here, cardiology, diagnostic and interventional radiology, nuclear medicine, intensive care unit, thorax and vascular surgery, five wards of different specialties, and a reception area are all assembled into a highly modern part of the hospital. All this was a site of my fieldwork – a place I chose to call the Heartlands.

In my ethnographic exploration of cultural aspects of high-tech heart illness treatments (Agic, 2012), I found myself amidst a set of methodological challenges for which I, at the time a young, unexperienced, doctoral student, wasn't quite prepared. Perhaps the most important, albeit undoubtedly also the most wayward one, was the one about emotions.

The second I sat my foot onto the hard floor of the heart failure ward, it felt like entering the whirlwind of tense emotions such as fear, anxiety, loss, suffering, and uncertainty as well as their counterparts – hope, comfort, redemption, joy and confidence. The anthropologist in me realized that I won't be able to reach an adequate understanding of these people's reality – their practices and outlooks in the context of life-threatening chronic illness and promises of high-tech medical treatments – without getting involved with these emotions, my own included. I had a strong feeling that ignoring them would jeopardize my understanding of life in the Heartlands, leaving me with not only an incomplete but also a downright distorted picture. In other words, the comfort of protecting myself with professional emotional distancing from the emotions of my informants and also protection and regulation of my own emotions[1] wasn't mine to be enjoyed. So, I dropped all the shields and stepped right into the eye of the storm.

The aim of my study was to understand how the ways in which these practices are structured and performed tie into the shared understandings about life threatening chronic illness, the body, and medical technology. To do this, I have spent nine months of participant observation in the Heartlands, talking to people, attending their various meetings, following their daily routines such as ward rounds, conversations, examinations, and surgical treatments, and also corresponding with some of them by mail and telephone. This resulted in one thousand and eighty-five pages of typed fieldnotes, more than sixty-one hours of audio recordings of a variety of "episodes", and roughly two and a half hours of video-recorded open-heart surgery.

In this chapter I will start by explicating some of the "technical" keys I have used in analysis of ethnographic data. This will then be followed by critical discussion of "the technical" in anthropology with reference to the ethnographer's subjectivity and emotions as well as to the paradoxical character of field work itself. I will argue that the ethnographer's emotional experience of the field is a valuable, if not indispensable, tool in doing hospital fieldwork and, most importantly, understanding the field.[2]

I will argue for emotional notes as an ethnographic tool that, together with field- and mental notes, extends the anthropologists' reach where their diligence and curiosity alone cannot. I will also argue that, instead of jeopardizing the ethnographic endeavour, *feeling the field* adds to its validity. Amidst intense emotions, such as those dominating the world of hospitals, instead of rejecting our own emotional responses, we ought to embrace them as an often-neglected tool that can provide us with glimpses of things that are truly human.

I will also argue that emotional experience of the field and the people we study, especially the kind of emotional experience inherent in the fields of human misfortune and suffering, contains insights essential to our understanding of social, cultural, and emotional dimensions of human life. Above all, in situations where a researcher feels the *heartquake* being shared in those moments of "understanding and bonding in human suffering" (Van Dongen, 1998: 279), is when our understanding deepens beyond being merely intellectual.

Understanding the fieldnotes

Technically, then, in order to answer my research questions, I tried to look for the standardized daily routines in the field.[3] I also mapped people's action space.[4] Furthermore, I identified the ways in which people order and classify their worlds[5] and documented the metaphoric expressions that were in frequent use, in language as well as in practice.[6]

By paying close attention to the details of the ethnographic picture I have managed to gradually gather a large body of observational data containing detailed accounts of formalized practices and emic explanatory reflections which, when analyzed with the help of cultural analysis and ritual theory,[7] began to reveal certain repeating patterns from which I could draw certain blueprints – the analytical condensation. So, I continued looking for the standardized daily routines, only this time instead of looking in the field, I was looking in the fieldnotes.

The process of data analysis consists of systematic coding, auditing, interpreting, questioning, and intellectualizing of the content. For the first part of this process, organizing data, coding, and to a certain extent also analyzing, I used computer software specially designed for handling large amounts of qualitative data – Atlas.ti®. Hence, the total of one thousand and eighty-five pages of typed fieldnotes was fed into this software, the main purpose of which was to help with storage, retrieval, and the coding process. Coding means literally marking the text in order to label particular parts of that text and attaching code words to particular stretches of data, which allows the researcher to retrieve all instances in the data that share a code (Coffey, Holbrook, & Atkinson, 1996).[8]

By drawing on ritual theory[9] in my attempts to understand biomedical practices, I was inexorably also bound to use cultural analysis as a primary analytical key "… necessary to understand the symptomatic and explanatory idioms that actors put into practice" (Reynolds-Whyte, 1997: 4). As I take these medical practices to be primarily cultural processes, I turned to cultural analysis as a way of understanding them. By cultural analysis I mean a systematic probing of established views and "taken-for-granted's" among the people in question. The principle premise of this is that all social groups partake in the formation of their history, culture, and identity – the facets that are continuously being embodied through the routines and practices of everyday life (Ehn & Löfgren, 2001: 169).

First, with the help of a custom-designed search list I tried to map the social organization of the heart disease department.[10] Then I looked for phenomena or objects that are associated with strong sentimental values – symbols, myths, and legends. The main objective here was to capture cultural contexts and attitudes, emotional keynotes, and sentiments. The first (broad) search list consisted of general concepts such as chaos and order, individual and collective, nature and culture, human and machine, life and death, time and space, private and public, power, emotions, gender, moral, prestige, work, and cosmology. The second (narrow) search list aimed at discerning the particularities of how various cultural conceptions are organized in relation to technology, the heart, truth, knowledge/uncertainty, action-space, responsibility/obligations, hope/trust, borders/transgression of borders, spaces in-between, humor, routines, and regularities/exceptions. I have tagged several hundred codes according to these search lists, which were then organized into ten large code-families. In order to make further sense of the ethnographic data, I treated phenomena as cultural understandings and ideals. This way I could avoid the "taken-for-granted's" and understand what concepts of reality are brought about in practice.

Deployment of cultural analysis calls for the interpretative approach with an open character. In my case, this means that, while remaining primarily rooted in the anthropological tradition, I made use of fields of disciplines such as sociology, history, history of ideas, and philosophy.

I see the cultural perspective as a proper way of engaging in studies trying to understand human ventures. The challenge of contemporary scientific effort to bring together traditional academic disciplines was, in this study, I believe, acknowledged and approached with earnestness. My strategy was an answer to the Geertzian call for a particular kind of interdisciplinary approach – the one not proposing the total hybridization of (or total escape from) the separateness of traditional fields of study but rather demanding an openness where different disciplines embrace each other's findings and try to make use of them. Geertz told us that social sciences and humanities would benefit from establishing a common language where different types of theories and concepts can be integrated "… in such a way that one can formulate meaningful propositions embodying findings now sequestered in separate fields of study" (Geertz, 2000[1973]: 44). This way of looking at humanities and social science and its various fields resonates in more recent work of philosopher/ethnographer Annemarie Mol, who draws her inspiration not from "… a clear-cut discipline, but [from an] interdisciplinary, slightly undisciplined field" (Mol, 2007[2002]: 22). Mol describes this field as a flow of theory moving across the boundaries of disciplines. It is exactly the egalitarianism of this undisciplined discipline that I turn to when I think of inter- and/or transdisciplinarity. There is no hierarchy – no stratums among the different fields of study. There is no periphery and no core of human beings. Geertz has warned us of such a science by pointing out that culture, psyche, society, and organism must not be converted into divided scientific levels that are absolute and self-sufficient in themselves (Geertz, 2000 [1973]: 41).

And the anthropologist made the "emotional note"

Although necessary, this technical side of data analysis fell short of providing a more generic and comprehensive understanding of life in the Heartlands. Whatever I managed to squeeze out from the fieldnotes remained flat and square, forcing the colorful and vibrant life of the heart disease department into a far too narrow frame. There was something missing.

The missing element in my analysis was more systematically ignored on my part than it was ever simply undetected or overlooked. I felt as if I was playing a game of denial in order to fit into the rigorous frames of established conventions for scientific analysis. In the meantime, whenever I would let my emotional guard down while working with the fieldnotes, I was brought back, quite vividly, to the field itself. Just as I was swallowed by the avalanche of emotions – emotions of the people I studied but also my own emotions – during the field work, these emotions were easily evoked through the process of data analysis. Familiar bodily sensations – increased heart rate, a burning sensation on the surface of the skin, gasping for breath, anxiety often followed by fatigue – appeared as I went through certain episodes. I recalled – while analyzing, coding, questioning, and intellectualizing – the sentiment, the feeling… the frustration, anger, grief, indifference, happiness, joy. I felt it all once again… and again.

This made me wonder if this way of experiencing the field wasn't to some extent also what medical staff and patients felt in their dealing with vicious illnesses, uncertainty, and promising technologies? Isn't this the human way? Isn't there anything I can learn from my own emotional response to the things taking place in the field?

Soon enough I realized that my emotional response affected my research more than I was initially willing to admit. Should I be worried, I wondered, that my *feeling the field* will contaminate the purity of scientific objectivity? Is it a threat to reason? In the end, how am I to legitimize my own emotional relation to my field as valid ethnographic data? But then again, how can a quality that is so central to human ways of being in the world be ignored as a factor polluting our knowledge? In the following I will discuss this, suggesting that feeling the field opens up yet another dimension of understanding human ways. Instead of being dismissed, it can – and often should – be utilized as a tool in making sense of ever so intricate ethnographic data.

Emotional notes

Fieldnotes are the raw data in anthropological work – the ethnographic facts. Taken at face value, however, these facts might be deceiving. What they show is not equivalent with what they mean. Merely allowing the facts to speak for themselves would lead not to inference but to elusiveness. Hence, if any in-depth understanding of the cultural underpinnings particular to the field of study is desired, the meaning of the facts must be extracted through the process of interpretation. This means linking and bringing into balance the "… abstract concepts with the immediately perceived realities of everyday life" (Rabinow, 2007[1977]: 124).

Unsurprisingly, interpretation became the inevitable part of my attempts to understand life in the hospital. After all, the "facts of anthropology … cannot be collected as if they were rocks, picked up and put into cartons and shipped home to be analyzed in the laboratory" (Rabinow, 2007[1977]: 150). Each observable phenomenon is itself a product of culture. It is itself already an interpretation – it always has been – and is constantly in the process of becoming. What we encounter in the field as anthropologists is in the making.

The raw data, on the other hand, i.e. the fieldnotes, are but still shots of the observed flux of human life in a certain time and place. To make sense of the fieldnotes we need to bring them back to life. Nevertheless, to blow life back into this static picture is in no way an easy task – especially if we strive to retain our scientific stance. In what follows, I will try to get to the bottom of this problem and, based on my experience as an anthropologist in the Heartlands, also present some suggestions regarding how these problems could be circumvented.

We anthropologists take notes, i.e. we scribble them down in a notebook. Sometimes, however, some events, faces, places, and spoken words stick in our memory – so we make *mental notes* (Rabinow, 1977). Taking mental notes means that some things observed are, for various reasons, quite easy to remember, as if they were mental recordings of our observations. Mental notes form part of our overall field experience and are thus also influential on how we perceive, interpret, and analyze our transcripts and fieldnotes. Then again, some things are heartfelt. They move us and cut deep into our being. They leave their mark, adding to the sediment of our embodied cultural selves. Therefore, they have a particular way of influencing our perception of the people we study and how we go about gathering, interpreting, and analyzing our data. These are *emotional notes*. What sets emotional notes apart from the mental ones is that they are not only easy to remember – it turns out they might be rather hard to forget. Taking this into account, data gathered through the participant observation appears to be of three kinds:

1. Fieldnotes
2. Mental notes
3. Emotional notes

As one of them is a formal and acknowledged form of ethnographic data, while the other two are still very informal and generally mistrusted, the final ratio among all three types of notes that are used in each research situation is somewhat of a riddle. It depends, perhaps, on several factors, such as the deliberate individual preferences, tactics and choices of each ethnographer, his or her personality, background, and scientific environment.

In most conventional ethnographic accounts, however, the reader is not readily invited into this part of research. Perhaps engaging in such discussion is as exhaustive and demanding (both for the writer and for the reader) as it is generally dismissed and stigmatized amongst colleagues as irrelevant navel-gazing. Still, how can this part of our witnessing/understanding ever be open for critical scrutiny if we insist on systematically pushing it into the dark shadows of ethnographic research? Provided we really are able to detach ourselves from the objects of our studies and can limit ourselves to processing our data through the conventional filters, this should be no problem – although this situation would provide no room for the individual creativity of a researcher. But suppose we are not? Suppose we fail at being as "transcendent and clean" (Haraway, 1997: 36) as the ideal would want us to be? Even worse, is there a risk of damaging this particular kind of data when we perform as "detached" scientists – an ideal that belongs to the natural scientific paradigm? Or, in a word, is our ethnographic detachment creating the ethnographic blind spot?

In her analysis of Balinese construction of the self, Unni Wikan developed the concept of "double-anchoredness" (1990). In short, Balinese people view the self as anchored and continuously (re)created in two facets of a person – an inner self signified by the "heart" and an outer self-referred to as "face" (ibid.: 104–106). Drawing on Wikan's concept of double-anchoredness, anthropologist William Reddy emphasized the qualities of the situated cultural self, i.e. a part of our personality that most of the time stays hidden from our attention (Reddy, 1999: 266; 267). This kind of "heart", i.e. the situated cultural self, is made of a person's embodied social, cultural, political, class, and gender background giving us the kind of "thought material" that is not always directly accessible. Only a deliberate reflection, Reddy argues, enables us to pay attention and, ultimately, gain awareness of this level of our personality that is rather uncanny, unpredictable, and often escapes the firm grasp of reason (ibid.: 269).

In view of this argument, why we choose a certain subject to study, how we perceive it while observing it, and how we interpret and analyze the fruits of our observations depends to a large extent on this level of our personality. George Devereux argued that "The researcher's character structure ... radically affects both his data and his conclusions" (1967b: 197). Ruth Behar also concurred by stressing that "*What happens within the observer* must be made known ... if the nature of what has been observed is to be understood ... in anthropology everything depends on the emotional and intellectual baggage the anthropologist takes on the voyage" (1996: 6, 8; italics in original).

Clearly, these assertions are a call for a more reflexive approach in a more subjectivity-aware anthropology. In a word, as both our data and our way of analyzing it are filtered through our embodied "baggage", i.e. our cultural and idiosyncratic selves, we need to be open about our own influence.

An allegory might help here. Let's say we have a photo where everything appears bent or distorted in a circular motion. For those with a basic knowledge of the art of photography there is no doubt that this particular photography speaks more about the character of the fish eye lens that was used when it was taken than of the "truth" about the object or scene that is being portrayed. As long as this fact is taken into account, neither the photo nor the photographer can be accused of distorting the truth about the object/scene. The only thing distorted is the representation of the object/scene, with the aim of widening our experience of it by providing it with yet another dimension that is more stylistic and aesthetic. If, on the other hand, the photographer were to act as if no such lens was used, a photo might be regarded as a representation of truth about the object/scene and therefore also as a distortion of that truth. Similarly, anthropology does not claim to present the truth about people studied, simply because it is not a natural, positivist science searching for the ultimate objectivity through "exactness" by calculating and circumventing the "probable errors" (La Barre, 1967: vii). Provided that in anthropology there are as many lenses as there are anthropologists, in order to understand their ethnographic accounts, we also need to understand the authors. This is why Behar and Devereux suggest that subjectivity needs to be brought out of the dark and woven into the ethnography.

Why is this, then, so hard to implement in ethnographic work? Is it because we are concerned that any revelation of our subjectivity will distort our "scientific validity"? At the same time, how can we claim any scientific validity by simply avoiding and even discarding such an important aspect of our research? These questions obviously seem to lead back to the old dilemma of "value-free social science", i.e. the conflict between the ambition for scientific objectivity and the assumed impediment of scientist's subjectivity (Hollis, 1994). Behar asks this question: "How do you write subjectivity into ethnography in such a way that you can continue to call what you are doing ethnography?" (1996: 8, 9).

To what extent we refer to our field, mental or emotional notes while writing our ethnographies is perhaps not as much a matter of things actually taking place as it is of a tension between our personal inclinations and the conventions of our academic environments, which are still under the significant pressure of the natural science paradigm. In a word, some ethnographers will, unless they don't feel anything at all, ignore, repress, and/or deny whatever feelings they might experience in the field. Some others will be open about them and make themselves vulnerable to criticism by expanding them. Then again, some will sway somewhere between these polarities, tentative about what they should do with their emotional relations to their field. It appears that current conventions for doing ethnography fall short of providing the ethnographers with proper tools for dealing with their emotional notes. Instead, following the path of least resistance, it makes us shove our heads into the sand, pretending we either don't feel at all or, if we do, that we can easily put our emotions in brackets to ensure the sustained purity of our research. This needs to be changed.

It should perhaps be made clear that this call for emotional science is nothing of a novelty. Along with Devereux and Behar, mentioned above, philosopher James W. McAllister argued that emotions should no longer be considered to be antagonists of cognition and rationality and declares that "… reliance on emotional responses is a necessary condition for making sound inferences and decisions in many circumstances" (McAllister, 2007: 22). Sociologist Simon J. Williams found the historical – ever since the dawn of the enlightenment and onwards – view on emotions as "… the very antithesis of the detached, scientific mind and the quest for objectivity, truth and wisdom" to be erroneous and argues that it should no longer be regarded as the "embodied enemy of disembodied reason" (Williams, 1998: 748, 749). Williams also emphasized that emotions in fact are "… central to the 'effective deployment' of reason" (Williams, 1998: 749). Furthermore, with reference to his study of *Isoma* healing rituals among Ndembu in central Africa, Turner argued that "Man's 'imaginative' *and* 'emotional' life is always and everywhere rich and complex", (1997[1969]: 3, my emphasis) adding that it is "… the whole person, not just the Ndembu 'mind', [that] is existentially involved in the life or death issues with which *Isoma* is concerned" (ibid.: 42,43). Clifford Geertz also joined this emotion-praising quire with words of warning, saying that human sentiments should not be reduced "to a shadow of the intellect" (2000[1973]: 355). Perhaps some of the strongest and most recent voices propagating for the epistemological value of researcher's emotional experience in the field can be found in the edited volume *Emotions in the Field: Psychology and Anthropology of Fieldwork Experience* (Davies & Spencer, 2010). Here, a group of prominent anthropologists criticize, from various perspectives, the concepts of detached ethnographer and objective science while at the same time praising the subjectivity of researcher's emotional experience as indispensable for our understanding of human social, cultural and emotional life. However, the stigma of emotions in scientific work is deeply rooted and, as Behar expressed it, "… we still don't know whether we want to give it a seminar room, a lecture hall, or just a closet we can air now and then" (1996: 16).

The paradox of field work

The ethnographic field is by its very nature always rather weird and offbeat; it is almost real and far too real all at once. Or in other words, to an ethnographer a field is neither reality nor fantasy, but something in-between. It mocks the attempts at scientific objectivity and detachment, casts spells on our human selves, and seduces us into submission, while at the same time rejecting us as "strangers" (Agar, 1996) or as a temporary disturbance of the ordinary course of things (Devereux, 1967a), a violation of the daily lives of the people we study (Crapanzano, 2010), or as our own anthropological liminal phase (Jackson, 2010). Katz Rothman described this sense of being caught by the whirlwind of her field in the following words:

> Why was it so painful for me? For one thing, the women became so real to me; I came to know them, to care, to identify. Especially to identify. I had a baby at home. My second, born when I was 33 – too young in 1981, if not now, for amniocentesis. I was close, emotionally, and physically, to the pregnancy experience, to the terrible, urgent intimacy of that relationship.
>
> *(1986: 50)*

Behar highlights the contradictory nature of field work by listing some of the stopping points in each ethnographic voyage, asserting that for each ethnographer a field work will at some point evoke senses including being out of place, wishing to blend in, feeling clueless about how to do it, being scared of observing too coldly, being scared of observing too raggedly, feeling enraged because of this cowardice, not knowing what to do with the insight that is always arriving a second too late, and feeling unable of writing anything while at the same time feeling a burning desire to write something (1996: 3). In doing field work, we are expected to act as participants without forgetting to keep our eyes open. We should: "… get the 'native point of view', *pero por favor* without actually 'going native'" (ibid.: 5, italics in original). Ultimately, we should understand people's emotional lives, while at the same time renouncing our own emotions. This polarized symbiosis of incommensurabilities is the very paradox of ethnographic field work and especially of the method of participant observation.

In the meantime, blinded by our search for the ideal of scientific validity we seem to have forgotten that anthropological research can't be forced to fit the normative model of natural sciences. Anthropology, in words of Behar "is the most fascinating, bizarre, disturbing, and necessary form of witnessing left to us" (ibid.: 5). It is a kind of science which, besides being performed, also is lived and felt. It is, therefore, always more organic than it is ever synthetic; always more analog than it is ever digital. It deserves to be recognized and treated accordingly if we are to get the most out of it.

Deep encounters

During my fieldwork in the Heartlands I spent many hours talking to medical staff, patients, and sometimes also to their relatives. Somehow, despite the pretense of my white coat, I felt that I identified myself mostly with the patients. That depends, perhaps, on the fact that they were just as much outsiders in this context as I was. Compliant or not, they often didn't master the cultural codes of the hospital. The medical staff spent much time and effort in socializing them into the hospital culture and teaching them what is right and what is wrong and what the "ought tos", "dos" and "don'ts" are – until they reach the point of compliance and are ready to be integrated into Heartisan culture. Or perhaps I identified with the patients because of my background as a refugee. Specifically, the patients' crises brought by the disruption of their life narratives due to a life-threatening chronic illness rang a bell for me. I recalled my own fear of pain and death brought by the violence of war. I recalled shattered dreams. I recalled facing the end of life as I knew it. I once again saw myself enmeshed in an uninvited course of things, ending up in a new and unknown context full of uncertainties. I remembered new hopes and expectations. I remembered being different and misunderstood, being ignored and being taken care of, being worried and feeling comforted. To me, life with the chronic illness of end-stage heart failure looked a lot like a life disrupted by war. The rescue found in medical technology looked a lot like the rescue found in refuge. Should I have repressed this as an inappropriate and downright unscientific response? Is that what it really is?

As I became caught up in the intricate world of the power relationships, uncertainties, institutional frames, and a colorful diversity of vibrant human ways in the Heartlands, I also found myself deeply involved in understanding and bonding in human suffering. In the beginning, some of the patients turned out to be rather suspicious of me, not knowing quite where to place me. I wasn't a doctor, nor was I a nurse. Some of them stayed in the Heartlands for such a short period of time that I never got the chance to make real contact. Some, on the other hand, stayed longer and would still not talk to me in any other way than formally, briefly, and somehow as if they wanted me to leave them alone – which I of course also did. But most of them initiated contact with me, greeting me with big smile as I entered their room, and showed uninhibited signs of affection, warmth, friendliness, and appreciation. There were those who would confess to me, who would talk to me for hours and let me in, very close to the most private corners of their hearts, those who would hold my hand and let their tears pour out in cascades. This was the area of my strongest emotional involvement. This I could not ignore.

Before the field work, I was well aware of the dying and the human suffering that I was going to encounter. Was I really ready for this? Will I ever be? No, I wasn't! And no, I won't! I remember urging my supervisors to have a counselor on stand-by for me, in case I were to feel the need for debriefing while in the field. And I was right – my time in the Heartlands was one of the toughest things I've ever deliberately gotten absorbed into. The image of a man I shook hands with on my very first day in the Heartlands still haunts me – the next morning, when I came back to the ward, I was told that he had died during the night. This was my welcome to the field – and this wasn't the last time I encountered death while in the Heartlands.

Perhaps just as hard (if not harder) to handle as exposure to people dying was all the suffering I came to witness during my time in the Heartlands. These daily encounters with people in pain, people who seemed lost, became a constant reminder of how precious and how fragile life is. I can't say I felt their pain – no one really can! But I most certainly felt mine, raging through my whole body. I felt a huge lump of *nothing* growing inside me as if it threatened to burst my chest wide open. Often, while not in the field, I found myself unable to pay attention to whatever I was doing – talking to a friend or watching a movie, for example. I just drifted away as I pondered the hardships those I left behind at the hospital had to endure. While breaking a sweat on the treadmill running that extra mile, I would look at the little red lamp on the display showing my heart rate – and next thing you know I would find myself gasping for breath, haunted by uninvited images from the Heartlands. Prior to my field work experience, I was not bothered by these things. Of course, I knew that some people are less fortunate than others regarding their health and that there are a whole lot of heartbreaking stories taking place in the world. But I was never *this* aware of it. And, I admit, I wasn't so prone to intentionally engaging in any deeper thinking about these things. I was never exposed to this side of being human, not this close and vividly to those in despair. The images of these people became my shadow, following me everywhere even as I gathered with my friends over a cup of coffee, or attended family dinners.

Sometimes I would start talking about these people and the suffering they go through. Sometimes my friends and family would show interest and listen carefully. Yet, just as easily as the topics are avoided, so can also the people identified with certain topics be. I knew that these subject matters are heavy and could easily spoil the good atmosphere of any gathering. Therefore, I refrained from talking too much about this. I didn't want to burden the people around me. Nor did I want to commit social suicide. So, I wrote instead! And it also proved to be pretty good therapy. This was, among other things, the kind of thing that helped me make it through the whole nine months. I would put down almost anything on paper, never thinking of what specific significance this and that would have for the research – I just poured my guts out. Anger, frustration, anxiety, fear, melancholy, warmth, care, concern – I just put them down on paper or typed them onto the computer screen. And each time, it felt really good. I could feel a sense of relief grow with each word written, abating the *nothing*. However, I wasn't writing merely for therapeutic purposes. My feeling things, and my putting these feelings into words and phrases, was already having a huge impact on the way I perceived and interpreted fieldnotes. These two reasons were more than enough for me to recognize that these emotions ought to be embraced instead of ignored or repressed.

Seeing yourself in the "other"

> As I entered the room, I also felt that I was about to cry. This feeling, as I recall it, came over me as soon as I stepped into the dimly lit room, and is perhaps connected to the importance and awe ascribed to birthing and witnessing the seemingly consecrated practice of birthing.
>
> *(Jonvallen, 2010: 154)*

I have already mentioned the urge I felt to talk about these heavy subjects with my friends and family. Yet it was not always that easy. At the same time, many of the daily life situations would require that I explain myself to others – to explain why I might have been quiet at the dinner table, absent from a get-together, easily provoked, or touchier than usual. People around me would wonder what the matter was and I would feel that I must explain myself, to justify my behavior. However, once spelled out, these things would need to be negotiated. "It's getting to you", "It's all in your head", "Let's not go into that now", "You need to relax", or, worse, no response at all, were the most usual reactions to my whining. There was a paradox in this situation. Refraining from these negotiations left me short of desired recognition and empathy. Engaging in them made me unbearable to be around. This was one of those moments when I felt what I thus far had only read about in the scientific literature, describing how chronically ill people need to negotiate their experience of suffering on a daily basis – particularly the ones whose illness is not visible to others (Masana, 2010). My own experience, my emotional notes, have brought me closer to understanding the patients and the torment imposed on them by this situation.

The sensibilities I learned through my emotional experiences were, no doubt, strongest while still in the making, i.e. while I was still *in* the field – still among them. I remember one of the strongest examples of this emotional learning during an episode in which I *felt* the warmth of a man's hand as it stretched out to gently grab hold of mine only seconds before his chest was about to be split open – seconds during which the "see you later" and "good bye forever" sentiments are both paradoxically expressed in a squeak of cacophonic synchrony, a friction between forceful emotion and passionate reason caused by the "no warrant of success" character of any open-heart surgical procedure. I *felt* the gaze of his scared tear-filled eyes, and *felt* the sound of his voice saying, "Haris, I sincerely hope that you will get all that you need from all of this". It was a kind of inter-human emotional experience that provides the kind of understanding that intellect alone simply cannot. What's more, this emotional whirlwind was additionally boosted as it became clear that, to me, the hours to come meant staying focused, taking notes, and paying attention to details. But to this frail human being holding my hand, it meant a certain probability of finitude and uncertain probability of salvation.

And there we were, holding hands, looking at one another, sharing the moment – possibly his last – and yet belonging to two different worlds. In sharing this moment, the absolute difference between our destinies brought an acute and unmistakably emotional awareness of mortality to me. Desjarlais tells us: "One learns of another way of being and feeling through contrast, noting the differences that make a difference" (1992: 19). In similar fashion, this particular encounter with another human's finitude enhanced my sense of my own vitality in a rather absurd way. And that is when the absurdity of my vigor in the face of another human's misfortune rendered his destiny even more absurd and unjust to me. My body was positioned upright, his was lying down; I was looking down on him, he was looking up; I smelled of early morning shower, he smelled of hospital and alcohol-based hand cleaner; I had curiosity in my eyes, he had fear and doubt in his; I was frightened by his, was he encouraged by mine?

It was clear to me that the truth of any "fact" of life is always in the eye of the beholder. Therefore, I realized that people, in order to truly understand each other, need to learn to read the reflections of each other's "facts" of life, mirrored in each other's eyes, bodies and practices. In the eyes of this man I saw a bizarre image of myself – "a difference that makes a difference" *par excellence*. The ethnographer's emotional experience contains insights essential to our understanding of social, cultural, and emotional dimensions of human life. This power should not be neglected.

Fear, resistance, will, despair, hope – these sides of being human can never really be grasped solely through logical thinking and analysis, at least not in the same way as when a human is immersed in them. I didn't write this episode down. It is absent from my fieldnotes. And yet I can tell it by heart, in great detail, any time. I have seen it repeating in my head so many times now, both intentionally and unintentionally. There are plenty more of such heartfelt episodes that ended up as *emotional notes*. I know them all for a fact. And I don't think I can ever forget any of them. But even more importantly, I know these episodes *by heart*. The trick now is to pass on this sentiment to others, to evoke the readers' emotional responses by surrendering to a certain style of writing that allows them to "get it at the gut level" (Rothman, 1986). It seems as if "We lack the language to articulate what takes place when we are in fact at work. There seems to be a genre missing" (Geertz, 1995: 44). Doubting, nevertheless, that my writing skills could ever live up to these expectations I will make an honest attempt and still try not to turn this analysis into an instance of self-absorbed attempt at sensationalism. Be that as it may, I believe that it is unavoidable that the very fabric of this text is woven by the ways in which I have felt the field.

Similar to Rabinow's mental note, an emotional note is not easily forgotten. How could it be? My experience of the dark sides of the Heartlands proved to be rather painful, intense, and overpowering. There was no way of avoiding it. It lurked around each corner, in every room, in every encounter with anything and with anyone. At the same time, I believe that it is not possible, and neither would it be desirable, for an ethnographer to detach him- or herself from the field until he or she felt safe from feeling. At the risk of opening myself up to charges of engaging in sensationalism rather than serious scientific research, I argue that emotionally engaging in deep encounters provides insights into those areas of human life that cannot be grasped by reason alone. Unless we promote a complete expulsion of the "feeling" kind of ethnographers from the ethnographic community, we should at least consider giving them enough space so that they can make their unique contributions to the vast body of ethnographic knowledge about human life. Otherwise we might just end up with libraries of neatly made ethnographies behind which graveyards of disclaimed emotions lay hidden. Perhaps we can always try to hide our feelings, but we can never hide from them.

Still, an ethnographer is but a temporary visitor in his or her field, soon to be released from its burdening emotional grip. People spending their lives working in hospitals don't see their workplaces as "the field". Most of them are going to spend a significant part of their lives there. Perhaps it is a matter of time – medical staff, for instance, cannot afford to surrender to the emotional whirlwinds because sooner or later it would take its toll. Neither do the patients see the hospital as "the field", nor can they afford surrendering to their emotions – with the help of the medical staff they develop strategies to manage their emotions in order to cope with torment and uncertainty. Ethnographers are in no way an exception to this, although the extensive taking of emotional notes as suggested here might eventually leave us bloated and unprotected. And this is exactly what happened to me. During the last three months "in the field" my frequent nightmares about my field work became unbearable. I just felt that I had had about all I could take. It was time to leave the field. Nevertheless, in escaping the field I must not forget why I went there in the first place. Asking myself how I do anthropology, I often found myself answering another question of why I do anthropology, and vice versa. It didn't take long until I realized how intimately intertwined these two perspectives are for me – sentiment and reason, "heart" and "face", the emotional and technical hand in hand. The following assertion provides a rather precise answer to both questions, "The point is to make a difference in the world, to cast our lot for some ways of life and not others. To do that, one must be in the action, be finite and dirty, not transcendent and clean" (Haraway, 1997: 36).

Conclusion

My strong emotional response towards my field directed my attention closer to the emotional dimensions of high-tech medical treatments. By paying attention to my own emotional responses to the people, things, and/or events in the field I allowed my understanding of the ways in which they view human body, life, death, and medical technology to be less technical and more human. Drawing from this experience, I argue that the concept of "emotional notes" is a valuable asset for anthropological work, especially in trying to understand those sides of human life that border on issues of end-stage illness, death, and suffering. What's more, in the case of high-tech medical treatments of life-threatening chronic illness, the weight of the situation for each patient is, in its very core, emotional in that they are facing the probability of losing their lives and their loved ones, enduring physical and emotional pain by submitting to the extremely violent treatments, and coping with inescapable death-defying uncertainty. Paradoxically, one of the main properties of these treatments is that the emotions are bracketed in order for the treatment to be doable at all. To get to the bottom of such things, an anthropologist cannot afford to enter his/her field of study unemotionally.

Of course, a researcher's emotional response tells us something about the researcher him or herself – an observation often used as a critique of the role that emotions might have in science. Still, in each of researcher's emotional responses to his/her encounters with emotional dimensions of human life lies an important story about human ways that just can't wait to be told. In anthropology, emotional notes should be granted the status of a forest amidst the trees.

Notes

1 Common in professional training of physicians and nurses.
2 An in-depth account of other relevant topics – access to the field, dilemma of "closeness", the ethnographer's role and position, and keeping the fieldwork diary – won't fit into this chapter due to space limitations. For those topics I refer to my doctoral thesis (Agic, 2012).
3 What are the routinized practices? How are they done? When do they take place? How long do they last? In what context do they occur? What practices do they follow? What others do they precede? Which actors are involved in those practices? Which of them are central? What artifacts, texts, and technologies are used? What is their role? How do people relate to other people? To artifacts? Texts? Machines?
4 What do people say they can and cannot do and what do they in fact do? How do they do what they do? How do they talk about what they do?
5 Is there a repeated pattern of dualisms to be discerned in the discourses and the practices in the hospital – such as objective/subjective, mind/body, normal/pathological, health/illness, rational/irrational? What can we learn from those binaries?
6 Metaphors about the heart, the medicine, the body, the illness, and about the technology. The metaphorical expressions are treated here as a coded reflection of the encompassing cultural context and are indispensable in any serious attempt to unlock and understand the meaning of our actions.
7 Ritual theory was my main theoretical tool for this research. For more information on how I used ritual theory in my ethnographic work I refer to my dissertation (Agic, 2012).
8 The codes were grouped in code-families or code-groups. Analytic memoranda, or comments, were attached to some coded segments of the text. I have organized the process of coding according to a search list, i.e. a list of certain concepts and phenomena specially designed to help map the main themes in the data as well as the relation between different themes, and also to discern the emerging patterns.
9 Regarding the focus on rituals in particular, I tried to elicit from the data how the organization of ritual performance integrates people into the ritual action, what cultural ideas underlie ritual practice, and also what cultural ideas provide the interpretational logic for attribution of meaning to the misfortune of illness and to the technoscientific means of dealing with it.
10 The underlying structures, processes, the actors, their status positions, roles and relations, spatial organization/spaces, artifacts, and machines.

References

Agar, M. (1996) The professional stranger: an informal introduction to ethnography. San Diego: Academic Press.
Agic, H. (2012) Hope Rites: an ethnographic study of mechanical help-heart implantation treatment, Ph.D. Dissertation, Linkoping University Press
Behar, R. (1996) The vulnerable observer: anthropology that breaks your heart. Boston: Beacon Press.
Coffey, A., B. Holbrook, & P. Atkinson. (1996) Qualitative data Analysis: Technologies and Representations. Sociological Research Online 1(1).
Crapanzano, V. (2010) "At the Heart of the Discipline": Critical reflections on Fieldwork. In Emotions In the Field: The Psychology and Anthropology of Field Experience. J. Davies and D. Spencer, eds. Stanford, CA: Stanford University Press.
Davies, J., & D. Spencer. (2010) Emotions in the field: the psychology and anthropology of fieldwork experience, pp. xi, 276 p. Stanford, CA: Stanford University Press.
Desjarlais, R.R. (1992) Body and emotion: the aesthetics of illness and healing in the Nepal Himalayas. Philadelphia: University of Pennsylvania Press.
Devereux, G. (1967a) From anxiety to method in the behavioral sciences. New York: Humanities Press.
Devereaux, G. (1967b) From anxiety to method in the behavioral sciences. The Hague: Mouton & Co.
Ehn, B. & O. Löfgren. (2001) Kulturanalyser. Malmö: Gleerups Utbildning AB.
Geertz, C. (1995) After the fact: two countries, four decades, one anthropologist. Cambridge, MA: Harvard University Press.

Geertz, C. (2000[1973]) The interpretation of cultures. New York: Basic Books.

Haraway, D. (1997) Modest_Witness@Second_Millennium. FemaleMan©_Meets_OncoMouse™ : Feminism and Technoscience. New York: Routledge.

Hollis, M. (1994) The philosophy of social science: an introduction. Cambridge [England]; New York, NY, USA: Cambridge University Press.

Jackson, M. (2010) From anxiety to method in anthropological fieldwork: An appraisal of George Devereux's enduring ideas. *In* Emotions in the Field: The Psychology and Anthropology of Fieldwork Experience. J. Davies and D. Spencer, eds. Stanford, CA: Stanford University Press.

Jonvallen, P. (2010) Emotion work, abjection and electronic foetal monitoring. *In* Technology and Medical Practice: Blood, Guts and Machines. E. Johnson and B. Berner, eds. Farnham, Surrey: Ashgate Publishing Limited.

La Barre, W. (1967) Preface. In From Anxiety to method in the behavioral sciences, pp. vii–x. New York: Humanities Press.

Malinowski, B. (2002[1922]) Argonauts of Western Pacific: An account of native enterprise and adventure in the archipelagoes of Melanesian New Guinea. London: Routledge.

Masana, L. (2010) Invisible chronic illnesses inside apparently healthy bodies. *In* Of Bodies and Symptoms: Anthropological perspectives on their social and medical treatment. S. Fainzang and C. Haxaire, eds. Tarragona: Publications URV.

McAllister, J.W. (2007) Introduction: Dilemmas in science: what, why, and how. *In* Knowledge in Ferment: Dilemmas in Science, Scholarship and Society. A. in 't Groen, H.J. de Jonge, E. Klasen, H. Papma, and P. van Slooten, eds. pp. 13–24. Amsterdam: Leiden University Press.

Mol, A. (2007[2002]) The body multiple: ontology in medical practice. Durham: Duke University Press.

Rabinow, P. (2007) Midst anthropology's problems. Cultural Anthropology 17(2): 135–149.

Rabinow, P. (2007[1977]) Reflections on fieldwork in Morocco. Berkeley: University of California Press.

Reddy, W.M. (1999) *Emotional Liberty: Politics and History in the Anthropology of Emotions.* Cultural Anthropology 14(2): 256–288.

Reynolds-Whyte, S. (1997) Questioning misfortune: the pragmatics of uncertainty in eastern Uganda. Cambridge: Cambridge University Press.

Rothman, B.K. (1986) Reflections: On hard work. Qualitative Sociology 9(1): 48–53.

Turner, V. (1997[1969]) The ritual process - Structure and anti-structure. New York: Aldine De Gruyter.

Van Dongen, E. (1998) Strangers on terra cognita: authors of the Other in a mental hospital. Anthropology & Medicine 5(3): 279.

Wikan, U. (1990) Managing turbulent hearts: a Balinese formula for living. Chicago: University of Chicago Press.

Williams, S.J. (1998) Modernity and the emotions: Corporeal reflections on the (Ir)rational. Sociology 32(04): 747–769.

PART XI

Projective techniques

26

PROJECTIVE TECHNIQUES IN HEALTH RESEARCH

Taylor Malone and Paul M.W. Hackett

Introduction

Projective techniques are creatively-driven research techniques that work to engage participants, allowing them to share their natural and instinctive feelings about the research topic at hand. This form of research technique "seek(s) to uncover feelings, attitudes, beliefs, and motivations that may remain sub-conscious or difficult to express" (Donoghue, 2000).

Projective techniques in healthcare research are used to assist research participants in expressing their deeper emotions and motivations towards a wide variety of healthcare situations. By creating a situation where the participant is allowed to be open and innovative in their responses about healthcare experiences, responses may be shared about healthcare experiences that do not arise in direct questioning. While every projective technique is unique and will yield slightly different findings, at their core, each technique will provide insight into individual participant behaviors, and the subconscious, or unconscious, motives behind these.

Due to the flexible nature of these techniques, considerable planning of both the technique itself and the use of the technique by each research team is required. Without thorough planning, these creative techniques may not be effective. Projective techniques may be used in individual settings, or group settings, and are especially successful when used as part of a focus group. The participants selected for each study must possess a certain level of knowledge of the subject matter that will be discussed in your research; participants do not need to be considered "experts" in the field you are collecting data in, but they will need some kind of background or personal experience in order to be effective respondents.[1]

Projective techniques present stimuli that trigger emotions or thoughts in those taking part in their completion, which also opens up the participant to engage in deeper conversation. Projective techniques are generally and usefully divided into four non-exclusive categories. Thus, the individual techniques categorized based on the stimuli provided to the participants, are as follows: visual, verbal, imaginative, or text-based. However, some techniques may be a combination of two or more of these types of techniques. This chapter will outline examples in each category of projective techniques in their use in healthcare research; however, this is not an exhaustive list, and the parameters that each example provides are not the only mechanics that may be followed. Each technique can be adjusted or added to depending on the study and the intended outcomes of the research. In order to comprehensively disclose the participant's motivations and deeper feelings, more than the simple selection of a projective technique and planned execution is required. Due to the ambiguous nature of projective techniques, answers provided by participants are left to the researcher's interpretation. To fully discover what may lie behind a participant's censored thoughts and feelings, the expertise of a research professional is required to decode and delve deeper, providing the participant with a platform for expression. In the next part of this chapter we will briefly consider the use of some projective techniques in healthcare research.[2]

Text-based projective techniques

Text-based projective techniques are relatively easy and quick for participants to complete.[3] The five different, yet common, types of text-based projective techniques that will be discussed are *sentence completion, story completion, billboards, red pencil editing,* and *idea layering.*

Sentence completion

When using the sentence completion text-based projective, the participants are asked to, as the title would suggest, complete a sentence. The respondent is generally asked to complete the sentence with the first thought or word that comes to mind and isn't expected to respond with a perfectly crafted or grammatically correct answer. The expectation of a fast answer is in place so that the response provided isn't tainted by expectations from the group or researcher (if the technique is employed in a group setting), or any other influences (including wishing to maintain a positive status in reference to societal norms). This aids in eliciting subconscious feelings/responses. The sentence or sentences that the participant is asked to complete will differ between each study, as the information the researcher wishes to collect will vary between research topics and guiding questions.

Sentence completion is an easy technique to use as a minimal level of creativity is required by the respondent. This technique is also easily and appropriately used to initiate deeper responses from participants in an in-depth interview (IDI) or a focus group. The different questions or beginning phrases may be distributed on a paper worksheet or can be accepted verbally and noted by the facilitator. The questions are purposefully left very vague and ambiguous, in order to prompt the respondent "to 'project' their own feelings or reactions to a situation without any bias" (Kalter, 2016, p. 98). When crafting the sentence completion prompts, the researcher should consider using a combination of first-person and third-person sentence constructions, as by using the third-person approach this may allow for mental distance between the respondent, the situation proposed, and their answers. Conversely, the first-person construction will access more directly personal responses. Examples of sentence completion stimuli are as follows.

Sample sentence completion prompts

"When I suffer from a serious injury, I first _____ *"*
"Having a disability is _____ *"*
"People who use prescription antidepressants are _____ *"*

An example of the use of sentence completion in healthcare research is provided by Ødegård (2005) who investigated the perceptions of interprofessional collaboration in relation to children with mental health problems. Examples of the stimulus sentences Ødegård (2005) used are:

Children with mental health problems. . . . . .

When we are working with children with mental health problems, we have to…

Story completion techniques

Story completion is an extended version of sentence completion and is a strategy that may unearth previously unmentioned and unexamined beliefs, feelings, or thoughts about healthcare issues and practices. Instead of completing a sentence with one short word or phrase, the respondent completes several different-but-related sentence prompts to describe a situation or complete a story. These prompts may be very straightforward; however, they may involve deeper insights and more creativity on the part of the participant. This is generally an independent activity, done in an IDI or focus group setting. Once the stories are complete, the facilitator may ask a few of the respondents to share their completed stories. This strategy allows the facilitator to ask follow-up questions to the respondents, allowing for deeper development and expression of thoughts, feelings, and ideas about health-related issues. An example of such a use of story completion techniques in healthcare is provided below.

Sample story completion prompt

"When I was first diagnosed with breast cancer, my first choice when it came to my treatment options was_____. After being introduced to the option of [insert prescription treatment option here], I felt _____. This was/was not a good option for me because_____. When I am asked about my breast cancer diagnosis, I first feel_____. I feel that way because_____ _____ ".

An example of using story completion in healthcare research is provided by Tischner (2019), which explores constructions of weight-loss motivations and health using story completion. An example of this procedure is:

Version A (female stem):

    Catherine has decided that she needs to lose weight. Full of enthusiasm, and in order to prevent her from changing her mind, she is telling her friends in the pub about her plans and motivations.

    In as much detail as possible, please complete and expand on this story by describing Catherine to us, and telling us how the story unfolds…

(Tischner, 2019)

Billboards

Another text-based projective technique is that of billboards.[4] With the billboard projective technique, respondents are generally required to employ relatively little creativity. Just like a billboard that you would pass while driving along an American highway, the billboard pro-jective technique requires the conception of short, succinct phrases. This technique asks that the participants imagine that they are driving down the highway and see a billboard discussing or advertising the healthcare related product, issue, or topic at hand; what message would be written across it? They are then asked to explain why they have chosen the response they have. After they have created this image in their minds, respondents are asked to write their own three-word slogan or phrase. As with many other projective techniques, respondents are asked to begin this activity independently. After the activity is completed, they may be prompted to delve deeper through guided discussion with other respondents, or probing facilitated by the moderator.

Red pencil editing

In comparison to other projective techniques, red pencil editing requires almost no creativity. In this exercise, respondents are given a sheet with a prewritten explanation of a healthcare related issue, product, service, or concept. Their task, then, is to act as a stand-in editor of sorts and take a red pencil to the copy given to them. They are asked to cross out phrases or sentences that they find to be less crucial or desirable and circle the most important ones. Facilitators may even ask editors (respondents) to add commentary or other feedback in the margins of the sheet. After each respondent has completed the activity, the facilitator will open the group for further conversation. Generally, the conversation starts with respondents discussing the circled (positive) attributes of the healthcare related text they were given and then moving forward to discuss the negative (crossed-out) words and phrases. This conversation then is extended through further probing undertaken by the facilitator. Because of the minimal amount of materials required and the ease of material collection, the resulting responses are readily gathered and may be analyzed with little effort.

Idea layering

Idea layering is a group-based procedure and is the final text-based approach we will consider. Idea layering, whilst being a relatively straightforward procedure to use, does require a generous amount of respondent creativity. Each respondent is given a healthcare related prompt or topic, and they are asked to jot down a single idea that relates to said topic. From there they are asked to pass their single idea to their neighbor; when the idea is passed to the next person, they are then asked to add on to the previously supplied idea or suggestion. Each idea is then passed to all of the respondents in the study until it finally arrives back at the original participant who created the initial idea. Another variation of idea layering involves several respondents, each with their own whiteboard. Each respondent writes their idea or suggestion on their whiteboard, and each respondent following is asked to visit each and all of the other respondents' whiteboards. This variation allows respondents to have a more physical role in the process, as they are allowed to move out of a static seated position. This form of activity has been found to facilitate openness of expression. Once the rotation is complete, respondents may be asked to review the contributions that have been added by their fellow participants and select the contributions they believe to be most appealing or relevant to their original idea.

Verbal-based projective techniques

In verbal-based projective research techniques applied to healthcare, participants are asked to respond to various verbal prompts. In this technique, probing is essential to uncover deep insights and real meaning associated with healthcare issues, practices, etc. The three types of verbally based projective techniques that will be discussed in relation to healthcare research are *personification*, *word association*, and *word chain*.

Personification

Personification (see Belk, 2013), which is also referred to as anthropomorphism, is a technique that asks respondents to connect the healthcare concept that has been presented to a famous celebrity or well-known person. Because the individuals that each respondent may choose may be drastically different from one another in terms of background, preferences, celebrity, respondent knowledge, etc., the ways this technique can be used are large in number and extremely varied. Healthcare researchers should feel free to use personification-based approaches as they wish, tweaking and adapting its guidelines to fit their research study and goals.

Generally, when using personification approaches, when respondents are asked to select a current or historical celebrity, they are asked to do so quickly, as to collect honest and unfiltered responses. Once each respondent has answered, the moderator can begin a discussion that allows individuals to voice their reasoning behind their choice. Moderators may ask follow-up questions or for deeper insight from respondents. Using the approach in this way can reveal perceptions, understandings, feelings and emotions, and more details about the healthcare concepts, issues, practices, etc. There are many ways to alter, narrow, or modify this use of this method. For example, the researcher may decide to have a list of people that respondents are asked to choose from, or may provide parameters around the type of person the participant may select, such as choosing only celebrities, politicians, individuals related to healthcare, etc. The researcher may also even ask that participants choose animals to represent the issues or practices associated with the healthcare topic under investigation. Respondents could also be asked to relate the healthcare issue or concept to supplied or elicited human characteristics. The possibilities reach far and wide.

Word association

The word association task is a projective technique that asks respondents to respond with whatever first comes into their mind when a particular word or phrase is read aloud. The responses may be spoken aloud or written down. This depends on the design of a particular study, if the researcher wants public or private responses to be gathered, and the environmental factors associated with where the exercise is being completed. Word association is generally undertaken during an in-depth interview or in a focus group setting. This style of projective tries to avoid bias and the respondents fear of judgment by asking that they answer as quickly as possible. When a respondent hesitates or delays their response, it may be beneficial to note this, along with the reply itself, as this may provide additional insight. If word association tasks are given in a focus group setting, after the all respondents have completed the procedure and notes have been taken of their responses, the moderator can begin a discussion where respondents may reveal further answers, and provide insight into the thought process and biases that guided respondents' answers.

Word chain

A very simple description of a word chain procedure is as follows. Respondents are provided with a healthcare concept, issue, activity, etc., and are asked to write down several keywords and phrases that they associate with the idea provided. Once respondents have completed the initial keyword task, they are then asked to include their selected words in one or two sentences. From here, depending on the design of the procedure, respondents will share what they have provided as responses with one another, and the moderator will invite deeper discussion aimed at discovering additional insights.

Visual-based projective techniques

Using visually based projective techniques in healthcare studies may involve a significant time commitment for the researcher. This is because in order for the technique to provide useful information, and in order to successfully engage participants using a visually based projective technique, major and in-depth preparation is required. The four visually based projective techniques that will be discussed are *collaging, picture sort, talk balloon,* and *picture interpretation.*

Collaging

Collaging is an extremely successful technique in which respondents are asked to assemble collections of photos, illustrations, words, phrases, etc., on a board or paper. For each respondent, the collection has the specific aim of expressing their feelings and thoughts regarding the healthcare related subject being discussed. An example of the use of the collaging method in a healthcare research setting is provided in the writing of Cherrier (2012), who investigated health aspects of eating fast food. The images that are used by the respondent in their collage may be preselected by the respondent, or the moderators may provide computer-based images, pictures from magazines, or other image-based materials for the respondent to cut out and select for themselves. When selecting images, respondents are asked to avoid actual visual representations or images of the subject matter itself. For example, if a participant was assembling a collage on the subject of the transportation they received from an ambulance service, images that should be avoided are those of ambulances, drivers, cars, taxis, police cars, etc. Respondents are assisted in making the collage by the researcher asking them to think about making the collages based on their reactions, expectations, ideas, etc., as these relate to the subject of the research. Sometimes, respondents may be asked to create a story collage, and in this instance the collage would be narrative-based with a beginning, middle, and end.

The collaging technique may also be conducted electronically/virtually, on an "e-canvas". In this situation, a pool of images is also preselected by the researcher and then a selection of these are also chosen by respondents and submitted digitally. However, the digital version of the collaging procedure may be less engaging for respondents and less hands-on, resulting in less emotionally charged collages. Another type of collaging is the mood board. Here, respondents are provided access to a larger range of materials and can use fabrics, words, magazine images, and online photos. A similar procedure to the collaging technique is followed, as detailed above. Collages may be completed in a variety of ways including in-advance completion by the participants and completing collages in a focus group setting, or ahead of time in order to provide stimulus material for use in a future focus group, although this may have the perhaps undesired consequence of exposing respondents to the subject matter of a focus group prior to the focus groups itself. A collaging technique may be undertaken using any number of images, and the subject matter can be adjusted to fit most healthcare research topics. Moderators can also ask participants to explain their choices once the final collage has been produced, either verbally or through a written explanation, to analyze later for deeper understanding and meaning creation. A collage provides an excellent basis upon which to ask a respondent probing and often personal questions.

Picture sorts

When using the picture sort technique, respondents are asked to sort through a preselected assortment of photographs and images. Often the images are of people, but they may be of anything related to the topic being investigated. Respondents are then asked to group together the photographs or other images in terms of those appearing similar on some dimension or criteria, or because they fall into a particular category. An example of this form of sort procedure is to have an assortment of pictures or images that represent various health products or services available to the respondents. Then, ask respondents to group these photos together based on preselected categories. For example, items may be sorted into groupings that represent affordability, accessibility, etc. Once these sorting activities are completed, the moderator may ask respondents to start the procedure again and to provide different parameters for the sort (i.e., different categories).

The images-based sort technique can be significantly modified so that it fits the needs of researchers and research questions, and so that a sort is best able to unearth healthcare-related perceptions, emotional connections, perceptual differences, and much more. After the sort is completed, it is important that the moderator is able to probe the respondents by asking further questions in order to gain deeper insight and understanding. Uncovering these forms of underlying rationale is necessary for a more thorough analysis and to enable an interpretation of the data collected that is more accurate and meaningful to the person completing the sort.

Talk balloons

One of the more creativity-centred projective techniques is that of talk balloons. This technique requires respondents to complete a partially drawn cartoon. When using talk balloons, respondents are given one frame of a cartoon containing a scene and an empty dialogue balloon on a sheet of paper. Often, in the cartoon provided, more than one character is involved in the drawing and respondents are guided with a prompt or explanation of the storyline. For example, a moderator will give the respondent the pre-prepared sheet of paper with the cartoon on it and explain the context of the person or persons represented on the sheet. They may then ask respondents to complete the dialogue balloon and to state how they believe the character would respond in the specific situation with any other characters included in the cartoon. An example of this procedure would be to give a respondent a sheet with a stick-figure drawn upon it with three empty speech bubbles above the figure's head. The moderator would then assign the figure a specific function or role by saying something like, "The figure is you. You have just walked into your local doctor's surgery for your annual medical examination. What do you think and feel, and what will you do?" Alternately, two (or more) figures could be present in the stimulus material and the moderator would say "This figure is you, this is your partner. You have just walked into your local doctor's surgery to discuss your test results. What do you and your partner think and feel, and what will you do?"

It is important to note that the degree of artistry involved in the cartoon and the background of the cartoon is up to the research team. Sometimes, providing too much detail in the cartoon may be distracting or may influence the answers of the respondent, and the stick-figure, as in the above example, is sufficient to elicit meaningful responses. At other times, the lack of contextual or figure detail may confuse the respondent or leave them guessing. The characters in each cartoon may also vary in terms of the facial expression they display, or lack thereof. When no facial expression is provided, respondents may be asked to fill in the expression they believe to be appropriate. Talk balloon cartoons may be used to examine respondents' feelings towards a healthcare issue, possible treatments, or may allow researchers to evaluate how respondents feel in regard to recommending a treatment or approach to the care of a specific health issue. The talk balloon approach is an effective tool because it provides an avenue of expression without the respondents having to verbally communicate their thoughts and feelings.

Picture interpretation

The picture interpretation projective technique exposes respondents to multiple healthcare related photographs and images at once, and, in a way that is similar to the talk balloon procedure, these are left ambiguous and vague. This allows for the greatest amount of respondent interpretation. As little detail is provided, respondents are asked to imagine what the people in the images are saying or thinking and may even be asked to concoct a story about the events or conversations that took place before, during, and after the photograph(s) were taken. Respondents may also be asked to create a social story about one of the characters in the photos and images provided. They may be asked to discuss that individual's personal life, their beliefs and background, their job, etc., all based solely off of the character's image and the setting of the photo. Because respondents are creating their own stories, it is assumed that respondents will create these stories with their own biases and beliefs intertwined into them, and personal motivations or feelings will be exclaimed. This will provide researchers with deeper insight into the respondent's perceptions and assumptions about the focus of the research. In order to make sure each study will be as efficient as possible researchers may ask that these picture interpretations are undertaken by respondents in their own homes; this procedure is most commonly adopted when the respondents will be participating in a future in-depth interview or a focus group.

Imagination-based projective techniques

Another class of projective methods are those that are imagination-based. This form of projective techniques require the most creativity from respondents and can be challenging, for participants and researchers alike, when respondents lack that creativity. The five imagination-based projective techniques that will be discussed are *role-playing*, *guided fantasy*, *mock debate*, *the wish technique*, and *withdrawal*.

Role-playing

The role-playing projective technique involves a relatively simple procedure. However, role playing does require an immense amount of creativity on the respondent's part in order for the approach to be successful in terms of producing useful information in relation to healthcare research (e.g., Jacobsen, Baer, Lepp, & Schei, 2006). Creating a healthcare related role-playing exercise where all respondents will be able to create answers and meanings can be difficult and requires creativity on the researcher's end as well. In this technique, moderators present fictitious healthcare scenarios and ask the respondents to play specific roles in them. Because this can be awkward and difficult for respondents to complete, moderators are tasked with surveying the group to find the seemingly most expressive and creative person to begin the exercise. Generally, two respondents are asked to play two roles in a scenario (which could include roles such as: health provider; caregiver; patient; person inquiring about healthcare, and many other roles). After they have completed the task, another pair of respondents will be asked to complete the same role playing. This will continue until all of the members of the group have completed the exercise.

When using role playing to disclose respondents' understanding and personal meanings regarding healthcare the moderators also have the task of probing the respondents for further explanation and added meaning, either during the role-play scenario or immediately after the pair or group has completed the activity. It may also prove to be a useful addition if questions are asked of the respondents who are not actively involved in the role-playing scenario, and this may gather insights, opinions, and feelings regarding actions and responses to the actions provided by their group mates in the scenario. Deeper discussion amongst group members and the moderator may take place once the group has completed the role-playing scenario.

Guided fantasies

To use the guided fantasy technique in healthcare research, moderators ask respondents to use their imagination about a specific healthcare issue, event, etc., whilst they have their eyes closed. Respondents begin guided fantasy procedures by asking the respondent to imagine they are engaging in some form of imaginary task, activity, visiting an imaginary place, etc., that is in some way seen to be related to the healthcare topic of interest. The moderator then asks the respondent to state their feelings, visualizations, and reactions to the imaginary scenario. How the technique is taken further from this initial point is dependent on the healthcare research goals and questions at hand. Moderators may ask respondents to interact with different components of the fantasy scenario. For example, if the respondent is imagining being in a hospital, the moderator may ask the respondent to open doors into different parts of the building. Moderators may also ask respondents to interact with imaginary people in this location and describe them in detail along with their beliefs and their actions. Guided fantasies may be more abstract and may involve respondents being asked to enter an imaginary building and to open doors and to enter imaginary rooms that represent different healthcare related options, conditions, treatments, etc., and to report their feelings, etc., about their imagined experiences. Another avenue for completing this technique is to have the respondents imagine they are on a full voyage to different locations or planets where each location represents a different concept, activity, etc., related to the healthcare topic of research interest. In this situation, participants would be "guided" to each location and asked to explain the characteristics of the land, as well as the inhabitants. In whichever of the possible ways the moderator chooses to use the guided fantasy procedure they must take the time to probe the respondent at appropriate points during the exercise in order to draw out deeper understanding and meaning,

Mock debates

Mock debates are exactly as they sound—they are staged debates around the specific healthcare topic of research interest. In this procedure, groups of two or three respondents are first assembled, and each group is asked to represent one side of an issue or discussion topic; then, the groups come together to discuss the healthcare topic. When assembling a group, the researcher must consider the characteristics of each individual participant, and he or she must attempt to assemble some kind of balance between the groups assembled. Prior to the start of the debate, respondents are given a few minutes to meet and discuss how to best represent their side of the argument. The researcher may decide to assign respondents to the side of an argument that does not mirror their own personal beliefs or point of view, and whilst this may be a more difficult task for the respondents to perform, it may bring forth interesting and important data regarding their own interpretations or judgments of a healthcare, concept, issue, or idea.

Wish technique

The wish technique requires a very large amount of creativity on the participant's part. This technique asks that respondents imagine outside the realm of plausibility and possibility, in terms of the healthcare topic under investigation, and voice their deepest desires when it comes to the healthcare issue, event, etc., at hand. The moderator may begin by suggesting to the respondents that they open their eyes and their imaginations, to the possibilities beyond, and to their dreams, in relation to the healthcare topic. Having done this, the moderator may ask respondents to answer or respond to research-related prompts from this dream-like position. Respondents are asked to describe their most desired qualities, characteristics, and capabilities, while the moderator asks probing questions to further develop and explain these responses. The moderator continues to ask the respondent for more "wishes" regarding the healthcare topic, with the aims of gathering twelve different answers. Having achieved this number of answers, the moderator then asks respondents how they believe these more outrageous or dream-based thoughts and desires could be handled or achieved in a practical or realistic way. The answers that respondents provide can exemplify the unmet needs and desires of healthcare patients, professionals, relatives of patients, etc., and these may be adapted into practical solutions or an understanding of how a particular approach may help to meet healthcare needs.

Withdrawal/obit technique

Using the withdrawal technique can be very effective when looking for data relating to emotional connections to healthcare services, issues, etc. The withdrawal technique asks participants to imagine their lives without the healthcare topic that is the subject of the research: how would their lives and daily rituals change if it was suddenly non-existent? Another form of the withdrawal technique is writing an obituary for the healthcare issue at the heart of a piece of research. A very easily understood example would be to ask British participants in this exercise to write an obituary for the National Health Service! The obituary would describe various characteristics of the idea being discussed, what would be missed, and how this would impact upon their lives. This approach can again be useful in gathering data on the personal and emotional connections that respondents have with the healthcare concept, practice, etc., that is the subject of the research.

During this chapter, we have presented a wide and representative range of projective techniques that may be used in healthcare research. The examples are not exhaustive and, indeed, it is extremely common for a researcher to either adapt the above procedures or design completely novel projective techniques in order to answer the healthcare-related questions they have. The common characteristic of all projective techniques is that their main component is not a form of direct questioning of a participant, but rather, respondents engage in some other, perhaps neutral, activity. This activity will allow their more subconscious beliefs, values, etc., to be projected upon or displayed through their actions. Having gathered information using a projective procedure, the researcher is then faced with analyzing this in order to provide insight in terms of the research questions, and it is to data analysis that we now turn.

Results/analyses

Due to the creative, visual, and physical nature of projective techniques, the results collected by the researcher from a projective technique will often take the form of a sheet of paper or digital file that has been drawn or written on. Other common forms of data that are gathered are fieldnotes, video recordings, photographs, and recordings of the research setting that may be useful in the analysis of the data collected. Once data is collected, it must then be analyzed and reviewed several times in order to identify themes and key issues that were presented by the respondents. These themes and key issues can then be interpreted and presented to address the research question(s) proposed by the research team. We will not go into detail regarding the analysis of projective data, but rather we will refer the interested reader to the chapters regarding analysis (with emphasis on textual analysis) in this book.

Limitations

In this chapter we have advocated projective approaches for gathering unguarded information from participants in health research. However, as will all research techniques, the use of projective techniques has several limitations. For example, Pettigrew and Charters, (2008) criticized projectives for being ambiguous and vague, and the validity and reliability of the results arising from projective techniques may be questioned (e.g., Ramsey, Ibbotson, Bell, & Brendan, 2004). Another criticism is that these techniques uncover more about the psychological processes of the researcher interpreting the techniques rather than the participant (Boddy, 2005). As with qualitative techniques in general there is also the problem of attempting to generalize from results (Noble, Stead, Jones, McDermott, & McVie, 2007), however, the data from projective techniques does not lend itself to generalization but instead should be used to provide deep insight (Ramsey, et al., 2004). Projective techniques also take a long time to administer and analyze, and yield relatively little data (Langford & McDonagh, 2003).

Notes

1 This statement holds true for the vast majority of times a projective technique is employed. However, there are circumstances when a naïve sample of respondents is specifically selected in order to gain knowledge regarding the health care issue or practice from individuals with no existing knowledge of this.
2 For a more thorough coverage of this form of research in both health care and in a more general research setting, the interested reader is guided to: Belk, (2006); Bellack and Fleming, (1996); Cherrier, (2012); Mizuta, Inoue, Fukunaga, Ishi, Ogawa, and Takeda (2002); Tuber, (2018); Soley and Smith, (2008).
3 See Hackett, Schwarzenbach, and Jurgens (2016) for details regarding how to run some of these projective techniques.
4 It is worth noting that billboards are uncommon or non-existent in the UK, Europe, and many other countries.

References

Belk, R. (2006) Handbook of Qualitative Research Methods in Marketing. Cheltenham, UK: Edward Elgar.
Belk, R. (2013) Visual and projective methods in Asian research, Qualitative Market Research, 16(1): 94–107. DOI:10.1108/13522751311289721
Bellack, P. & J.W. Fleming. (1996) The use of projective techniques in pediatric nursing research from 1984 to 1993, Journal of Pediatric Nursing, 11(1): 10–28.
Boddy, C.R. (2005) Projective techniques in market research: valueless subjectivity or insightful reality? International Journal of Market Research, 47(3): 239–254.
Cherrier, H. (2012) Using projective techniques to consider the societal dimension of healthy practices: an exploratory study, Health Marketing Quarterly, 29(1): 82–95.
Donoghue, S. (2000) Projective techniques in consumer research, Journal of Family Ecology and Consumer Sciences, 28(1): 47–53.
Hackett, P.M.W., J.B. Schwarzenbach, & A.M. Jurgens. (2016) Consumer Psychology: A Study Guide to Qualitative Research Methods. Barbara Budrich Publishers.
Jacobsen, T., A. Baerheim, M.R. Lepp, & E. Schei. (2006) Analysis of role-play in medical communication training using a theatrical device the fourth wall, BMC Medical Education, 6: 51. doi-org.glos.idm.oclc.org/10.1186/1472-6920-6-51
Kalter, S. (2016) Using Projectives to Uncover "Aha Moments" in Qualitative Research, In Hackett, P.M.W. (ed.) Qualitative Research Methods in Consumer Psychology: Ethnography and Culture, pp. 98–108. New York and London: Routledge.

Langford, J. & D. McDonagh. (2003) Focus Groups: Supporting Effective Product Development. London: Taylor and Francis.

Mizuta, I., Y. Inoue, T. Fukunaga, R. Ishi, A. Ogawa, & M. Takeda. (2002). Psychological characteristics of eating disorders as evidenced by the combined administration of questionnaires and two projective methods: the Tree Drawing Test (Baum Test) and the Sentence Completion Test. Psychiatry & Clinical Neurosciences, 56(1): 41–53. doi-org.glos.idm.oclc.org/10.1046/j.1440-1819.2002.00928.x

Ødegård, A. (2005). Perceptions of interprofessional collaboration in relation to children with mental health problems. A pilot study. Journal of Interprofessional Care, 19(4), 347–357. doi:10.1080/13561820500148437

Noble, G., M. Stead, S. Jones, L. McDermott, & S. McVie. (2007) The paradoxical food buying behaviour of parents: Insights from the UK and Australia, British Food Journal, 109(5): 387–398.

Pettigrew, S. & S. Charters. (2008) Tasting as a projective techniques, Qualitative Market Research: An International Journal, 11(3): 331–343.

Ramsey, E., P. Ibbotson, J. Bell, & G. Brendan. (2004) A projective perspective of international 'e'-services, Qualitative Market Research: An International Journal, 7(1): 34–47.

Soley, L.C., & A.L. Smith. (2008) Projective Techniques for Social Science and Business Research. Soutshore Press.

Tischner, I. (2019) Tomorrow is the start of the rest of their life—so who cares about health? Exploring constructions of weight-loss motivations and health using story completion, Qualitative Research in Psychology, 16(1): 54–73. DOI: 10.1080/14780887.2018.1536385

Tuber, S. (2018) Using Projective Methods with Children: The Selected Works of Steve Tuber. New York and London: Routledge.

27

BEING CREATIVE USING PROJECTIVE TECHNIQUES

Paul M.W. Hackett

Researcher as detective

Sherlock glanced at the woman standing in front of him. However, to be glanced at by Sherlock Holmes was to be scrutinised in the most detailed manner possible. She was flustered and gently perspiring as if she had been walking briskly, a hypothesis supported by the slightly struggled way she was speaking, as if finding it a little hard to breathe. Noticing her slightly nibbled fingernails Holmes deduced she was of a slightly nervous disposition though the nails were not bitten to the skin, suggesting a mild level of anxiety rather than a severe psychopathology. He noticed the remnants of dandruff the one side of the collar of her jacket. Judging by the straight line the dandruff form it was apparent to Holmes that the woman had used an adhesive roller to remove the offending snow-like flakes. However, as she had not entirely completed the job, he deduced that whilst she was a person to whom her appearance was of importance, she had acted in haste and was not at the present time able to concentrate well on tasks at hand. This was confirmed by her shoes. She was well dressed in a coordinated shirt, jacket, and trousers, all of which were fairly new and expensive. However, the shoes she wore, whilst being new and of high quality, were practical rather than stylish, and most definitely did not fit with the rest of her attire. This mismatch suggest to the great detective that the shoes were chosen for the practical purpose of being able to run, or at least to walk briskly with ease, and for a woman who was otherwise so well dressed, Sherlock knew that this could mean only one of two things. Either she was suffering from paranoia and she fostered an unfounded belief that she was being stalked and she felt that she needed to be able to run from her pursuer. If this was true, Holmes knew that this was where his interest in the case would wane and he would be referring her to a psychiatrist. However, if it was indeed the case that she was being followed, then things were about to get a lot more interesting for the great man.

When employing projective techniques in research (see, Murstein, 1965), the person utilising such an approach may be forgiven for thinking of themselves as a psychoanalyst, a conjurer, or indeed as Sherlock Holmes. I believe that Holmes would have approved of the use of projective techniques in research and would perhaps even have thought of them as the only way to be able to enter into the deeper levels of the minds of research participants. I think he would also have enjoyed attempting to develop new techniques in order to penetrate the specific unconscious thoughts, feelings, and motives of those he was scrutinising. I fancy that Sherlock Holmes would also have been well aware of the limitations of projective techniques and the need for these approaches to be carefully and creatively thought through and well-designed. Holmes would similarly have been acutely aware that observations of a person's actual behaviour were the more reliable manner in which to ascertain if they actually committed the behaviour of interest. However, whilst observations may allow us to know if a person actually committed a given behaviour, observations alone tell us little about why they did what they did, and as all great detectives know, it is a person's motives that are central to understanding the criminal mind.

Background to projective techniques

Central to projective techniques is the idea developed by Sigmund Freud (1938) that a person may transfer feelings and thoughts about things to events and objects in the outer world and that they may do this without being consciously aware of the process. Freud thought of projection as a type of defense mechanism that was operated by a person ascribing to external events his or her own characteristics that were distressing or dangerous to him or herself. In this chapter I use the word projective (or projectives) to describe research techniques which are only tangentially related to the original use of the term by Freud (Francis-Williams, 2014). Projective techniques have very similar goals to many other techniques that may be used in health and well-being research. All of these methods attempt to identify the constructs that are being used by respondents when they relate to a specified area of interest. It is also the case that researchers are usually attempting to predict future behaviour from the information they have gathered. Furthermore, projectives try to bridge the gap between the behaviours we may observe a person commit and his or her mental processes (Rabin, 1968).[1]

In this chapter I will not be presenting a detailed account of projective techniques[2] but rather I will be taking a look at how if the health researcher adopts a curious and above all a creative perspective it may be possible for her or him to formulate a projective approach that is tailored to the needs of their specific health and well-being research study.[3] Projective research techniques are found in use in a wide variety of consumer and marketing research.[4] When projectives are designed into a study they have been incorporated with the explicit aim of attempting to reveal attitudes, motives, and such like that underpin a specific behaviour or belief that a person holds. The need for the penetrative use of the projective technique is rooted in the idea that we like to appear good or at least in a manner the researcher would approve of and that we thus may consciously or sub-consciously offer behaviours or statements that we think the researcher will approve of. Projective techniques are therefore designed to try to catch respondents to some extent unaware and to circumnavigate their psychological defenses.

In the next section I will start to describe the projective technique that I will be writing about in this chapter, namely, creative projective sessions.

Creative projective sessions

In the Boscombe Valley Mystery, whilst laughing, Sherlock Holmes said, "There is nothing more deceptive than an obvious fact" (Conan Doyle, 2011, p. 203). With these words Sherlock justified, unknowingly perhaps, the role of projective research techniques. These research techniques attempt to reveal that which is not obvious. One form of projective approach is the creative projective session, or just creativity session, which are intense activities most often conducted with groups of participants. These activities, with slight variations between each, are very similar to: working walls, research walls, design walls, research boards, ideation walls, and, slightly tangentially, inspiration boards, mood boards, pinboards, etc., and indeed, the names are somewhat interchangeable. In the creative projective (as in the other above-named techniques) these activities involve the act of physically drawing or writing on or pinning or sticking things to a large surface (see, Vyas & Nijholt, 2012). Moreover, creating and then having these displays in front of us is likely to allow us to reformulate ideas and concepts and to release new brainstorming and insights.

In this chapter, I will concentrate on creative projective sessions which usually take place over an hour or two but may take longer. These creativity sessions may be implemented to find answers specific health-related questions or objectives or for examining and revising practice. These are, in essence, sessions in which ideas are generated through creative interaction with materials which is focused or projected upon some neutral stimulus or activity and during which participants are encouraged to think out loud and to act openly (the Think-aloud approach can be found in Charters, 2003).

Creativity sessions can take many forms, and here we will concentrate upon sessions that rely on projection. As with other forms of projective techniques, creative projective sessions may employ verbal-, textual-, or image-based stimuli materials. Creativity walls are used in creative projective sessions and are related to the group-based technique of idea layering (see the chapter by Malone and Hackett (2020) in this volume) which in itself also requires participants to exhibit quite a lot of creativity. In idea layering, respondents are given some health-related concept or term and they are requested to write down a single idea based upon the stimulus. The paper, tablet, or whatever else the participant has written upon is then passed along to the next participant, who responds to the previous participant's offering. This procedure is repeated until all participants have made their offerings. Malone and Hackett (2020) note that a more physically involved variation on this approach employs the use of white boards, with one placed in front of each participant. Each participant writes down a word related to a stimulus term and then each participant moves around the room and writes a response to all other participants on each of the boards: being active has been found to help to facilitate response production.

In a creativity session, a creativity wall is employed as a supersized whiteboard. There are many ways that the moderator may start the session, and there are many variations in the activities that are performed. However, creativity is key to all of these variations, as is the notion that a group of individuals working together may produce ideas and responses that they would not have offered if they had been working alone or in an ordered manner. I will take one way a creativity session can be run as an example. Let us imagine that a group of participants are recruited on the basis of some experience of the health issue that is at the heart of the study. These people arrive at the research company's building, or at any other building that has been adapted to host the session. They will have the procedure in which they are about to engage described to them, and the broad aims of the research will also be specified. The description research aims should be carefully phrased in order to put respondent into a mindset that will help them produce results that will be useful to the researcher, but not too detailed as to guide what they will produce. The researcher using a creative projective technique will need to establish rapport with the participants completing the task. A non-prescriptive demonstration of what is required should be undertaken but it should be emphasised that what is being demonstrated is only one way in which the task may be completed. Furthermore, respondents should be encouraged to think outside of what was shown. The person administering the projective must also stress that there are several ways in which the creative projective task may be undertaken and that none of these are either inferior or superior to others.

When all of the participants are ready, the moderator may write on a wall a word, phrase, term, etc., or fix or create an image, that is indirectly related to the health topic under investigation. The wall they have created upon is white and provides a large area upon which participants may express their thoughts and feelings. If such a wall is not present, then the exercise may be undertaken on a large sheet of paper on the floor. The choice of stimulus is based upon the health concept under investigation and is planned in the research design. Having located the stimulus material centrally within the space available, the moderator asks participants to respond to this. How they respond is usually left open to the participants to decide. However, in all situations the moderator will choose the media that is available for participants to use; such as markers of a variety of colours, post it notes of various colours, images printed on paper, pens, pencils, etc. The list of possible materials is very long and again will be determined by the research question.

Participants are usually asked to write, make marks, fix images or interact with the stimulus on the wall at their own discretion. The moderator will typically act in a manner similar to a focus group moderator, that is they will encourage all participants to take part, probe, and question about responses and try to avoid some individuals "taking control" or dominating the procedure. They will also attempt to keep the process focused upon the health issue or question behind the session. Participants will not only react to the stimulus but also to other participants' offerings. They will also be encouraged to discuss their thoughts and feelings whilst they are participating and to produce, much like in focus groups, some joint and some individual offerings. This is similar to the idea layering technique, where participants are often asked to discuss all of the contributions made by the group and even to choose a favourite contribution and to explain their choice. However, in the creativity wall procedure, participants are asked to work together, if they choose and the whole of this procedure is video recorded. At the end of the session, the group is asked to describe what they have produced and the reasons for this. They will also be questioned about the extent to which the resulting wall images and textual offerings form a consensus of opinion or whether participants want to qualify this in some way.

During the creative projective session, asking participants to write words and phrases and to fix and create images on the wall produces a flow of associative activity. Starting from the central or key health-related concept that is written on the wall, participants are encouraged to radiate in all directions from this and to use lines to connect, in meaningful ways, the words and images that are offered. Participants produce a binge of ideas that are meaningfully arranged, though not necessarily sequentially ordered. By involving words and images, creative projective sessions engage all forms of thoughts and emotions and do not favour either between linguistically or artistically strong individuals. They may also help to provide a forum for those who do not feel they are strong communicators or who do not enjoy being asked to speak out in groups. The labelling of the links between images and words offered may also help individuals to notice other links that they were previously unaware of. Creativity sessions should, as much as is possible, be allowed to proceed in the way that participants wish. They should be allowed to notice and draw in their own connections, although it may help if the moderator asks a general question about the overall wall such as "are there any other relationships here?" It may also help to ask if there are any similarities or differences associated with any groupings of items or to ask for names or descriptions of linkages.

For creative projective sessions to be successful, they must be experienced as safe locations – settings in which participants are free to let loose their creativity and ideas, even absurd ideas, without fear of ridicule, intimidation or criticism. Creativity is at the heart of this approach and participants and moderators must develop a mutual trust in order to get the most out of the session. This is especially the case when the subject matter of the session is health, which is a personal topic and may be embarrassing. Creativity must be encouraged, which, dependent upon the participants, may require hard work by the moderator in order to achieve.

Above, I have presented the essence of a creative projective session and I have noted the importance of the moderator in making the session successful. Below I will note a few more characteristics of successful creativity sessions and suggest ways of achieving success. Returning to the idea of trust, one way to build trust within the group is for the moderator to discourage participants judging or being critical of each other and to encourage ideas being expressed that are even outlandish. During the session, participants should therefore be encouraged to accept each other's ideas and to discuss between themselves rather than criticising. However, critical debate may be engaged in at the end of the creativity session. The moderator may actively encourage openness amongst participants by commencing a creativity session with some activities that try to lessen barriers between participants. These may involve encouraging each participant to introduce themselves to the group and to share a funny anecdote about themselves. Another thing that can be done at the start of the session is for the participants to be given tea, coffee, cold drinks, and snacks, which should be available throughout the session and participants should be free to return to these as they wish.

The next practice that should be encouraged is for participants to produce as many creative ideas as possible rather than taking their time to edit their creative expressions to what they consider their best ideas. As well as encouraging participants to produce as many ideas as possible and to include these on the wall, those taking part should be encouraged to think outside of the normal and to offer what may be thought of as slightly mad or insane ideas. It should be remembered that what may initially appear a silly idea may be sensible when reflected upon, and even some of the most far-fetched ideas may later be adapted through group discussion. Indeed, encouraging the expression of somewhat wild ideas may facilitate the openness in others and increase their willingness to offer their ideas without embarrassment.

However, it will almost certainly be useful to place some bounds upon participants' activities, and it is the role of the moderator to make sure that the conversation and creative offerings are going in the desired direction. An important way of attempting to achieve this is by the moderator describing and elucidating exactly what the issue or question that is being addressed and for the aim or topic of the session to be written and placed in a position that is at all times visible. Rather than reprimanding or telling participants what to do, the moderator may keep participants on track by asking questions about what they create in order to get participants to nudge themselves back to the task at hand. Throughout the session the moderator should use the words we, us, etc., so as to not isolate any individuals. For example, if an idea is being discussed or proposed by one person that the moderator feels may be straying from the task at hand, they may ask the group, "How do we think this addresses the topic question?". Asking this question may get participants to reflect on their offering but it may also produce an answer as to why the person wrote something down that the moderator was unaware of.

Managing the session

Ultimately, it is the job of the moderator to create and manage the atmosphere of the creativity session so that it stimulates the unguarded expression of ideas. At the end of the session, participants and moderator engage in a discussion about what has been written, drawn, fixed to the wall, etc. This is the time for the moderator to be a little more direct in his or her questioning and even to be openly critical of the things that are on the wall in an attempt to draw out the reasons a participant had for offering what they did. The end of a session should also be used to get the group to ascribe assessments of usefulness and quality to the ideas that they came up with and the group should assess the quality to the ideas that have been produced in reference to the session's overall question or theme.

In health research, as in many other types of research, it may be the case that those involved in a new treatment, intervention, health message, etc. may concentrate upon achieving an end, for example, the acceptance of a new drug or treatment regimen. However, the stages that patients may have to go through in order to get to this point of acceptance may be neglected. Creativity sessions are excellent fora in which to address such processes. It may be helpful for the stimulus word or theme that is placed on the wall at the start of the session to include the phrase "and how to achieve this". Alternately, this may be written on the reminder board that is always present to attempt to keep participants on track.

If a moderator is looking for a way of encouraging the flow of ideas during a creativity session, they may suggest that the participants engage in reverse brainstorming. In this activity participants would be asked to think about what would make the health issue worse. For example, the group could be asked to think about how they could create a confusing or ineffective smoking cessation communication, or how they could design a treatment regimen that was difficult to comply with. Another tactic that may be used to encourage creative production in a creativity session is to take participants for a walk. Going for a walk often stimulates lateral thinking, allows participants to become clearer in their thoughts, and encourages participants to focus on the session's topic. Creative projective sessions may be used to solve health-related problems of a wide variety, and as such they operate at all stages of the problem-solving process. For example, they assist in: identifying problems, analysing the problem or issue, coming up with new ideas to solve the problem and evaluating the relative merits of these ideas, selecting a solution, determining the next thing to be done, and, finally, evaluating the success of the chosen procedure.

In marketing research SCAMPER (Serrat, 2017) is an acronym and a technique that is used to encourage novel thinking and the generation of new ideas. In the acronym, the S represents "substitute", and participants are encouraged to think about alternative solutions or aspects of the health-related issue that is the focus of the creativity session. C stands for "combine", and session members may be asked to think about how processes or other features that are suggested in the session can combine to answer the overall aim of the session. The letter A represents the word "adapt", and participants may be asked to think about how an existing health practice, etc., can be adapted to facilitate its improvement. M stands for the word "magnify" or "modify", and participants are asked to consider distorting the topic in an unusual manner of a process that will improve or help meet the health-related issue of the session. P stands for "put to other use", which is especially useful in a creativity session and asks participants to think of alternate uses for existing health-related treatments, etc. The letter E is used to signify "eliminate", and here participants are required to think of ways and things that may be removed in existing health practices in order to bring about improvements. Finally, R stands for "re-arrange" or "reverse", which asks participants to re-arrange existing health practices to achieve a new solution.

When using the SCAMPER approach as a stimulus within a creative projective session, the researcher may ask specific questions for each letter such as: Substitute: Who, what, which other things, people, places, etc., can be used to meet the health goal? Combine: Which treatments, approaches, messages, etc., can be combined to achieve the health-related goal? Adapt: Which of the practices, procedures, medicines, etc., that we have used in the past may be adapted, offer an equivalent, suggest an idea, may be copied, etc.? Magnify/Modify: What other health-related procedure, understanding, activity, product, etc., can I adopt or add? Put to Other Uses: What novel approaches may I make use of, what new ways may I adopt, in which new situations may I use, etc., in terms of the health-related procedure, concept, etc. Eliminate: What health-related procedure, product, etc., is it possible for me to get rid of, stop using, reduce, cut back on, etc. Rearrange/Reverse: What health-related service, procedure, product, etc., can I rearrange, change the layout, sequence, order, or pattern of, interchange the components of, or reverse the roles of the people, etc., involved.

I have thus far in this chapter described the creative project technique along with some ancillary tactics that may be adopted to get the most out of a session when used in health-related research. Before reviewing the approach and concluding, I will briefly mention what may be done with the procedure's results.

The data that is gathered in creative projective sessions is visual and therefore the output or results from such a session will usually take the form of a video, an audio recording, and still-frame photographs of the procedure. Recording the procedure will allow the moderator more time to manage the process, encouraging a free flow of ideas from or between participants. This information will come from the participants and also from the notes and observations that the moderator has made during the session. These datum will be transcribed and subjected to textual, narrative analysis to identify themes, commonalities, and unique aspects of the performances. I will not go into detail about these procedures but refer the interested reader to relevant chapters in this book.

Final thoughts

When using a creative projective technique, creativity on the part of the researchers designing the procedure is central to the development of a useful and productive creativity session.[5] The designing of a creative projective approach starts with ascertaining the issues or questions and the types of answers the researcher is attempting to gain from using the approach. For example, a health researcher may be interested in trying to understand the person's perception of a health-related concept, issue, practice, and so forth. Once the researcher has in this way clearly specified the aims of their projective procedure they must think of ways of getting the required information from participants. This is not as easy as it may at first sound and may involve a research team. The choice of stimulus materials that are not the actual concept, term, or thing that is of interest, but that is still related to these and will produce useful reactions is paramount to the success of a creativity session. Consequently, time should be taken to ensure that appropriate stimuli are used, and prior to running the session for real, at least one pilot run of the procedure should be undertaken with a group of participants who are similar to those who will be taking part.

Furthermore, a poorly designed creativity session may unintentionally prompt a participant to produce a certain answer, regardless of whether this is what they are actually thinking, feeling or whether their responses actually reflected their relationship with the issue at the heart of the research. A projective creativity session that has not been rigorously conceived and piloted may also run into the error of producing information that is only abstractly related to answering the research question and fulfilling a project's aims. However, projectives have been used in a wide range of research contexts and are particularly amenable to modification and to novel usage with the aim of revealing group insights. Projective creativity sessions also facilitate innovative brainstorming and may yield information that is deeper than a superficial, socially acceptable, and rationalized response.

Mr. Holmes is not the only detective who would have approved of the use of creative projective approaches, as there are many sleuths who have employed deduction and have attempted to go beyond overtly asking suspects about their behaviours and experiences. In health research, this approach may be used in an attempt to delve deeply into the subconscious mind of the participants. However, it should be noted that all forms of responses that a researcher gathers will be subject to bias either in terms of artificiality and/or inaccurate interpretation. The former of these error types refers to the behaviours (covert or overt) that are produced in a research setting not being the typical behaviours of respondents. The second of these error forms arises from the fact that the qualitative information that researchers gather will need to be interpreted in line with the research questions. Through attempting to subvert conscious alterations to participants' responses, projective techniques attempt to minimise the former of these error types.

Notes

1 Psychologists have used projective approaches in a wide variety of investigations, for example: as a general research technique in psychology (Hogan, 2018); with children (Gardner, 2004, Parente, 2019); for individual patient, groups, and family assessment and treatment in different health settings with different health-related issues (Jones, Magee, & Andrews, 2015, Ogden, 1992, Oster, 2004, 2016); and in personality assessment (Dana, 1982, Dritto, Tummineri, Moscuzza, Di Perri, Rizzo, Liotta, Merlo, & Cicciarelli, 2015, Tuber, 2014). Researchers have also applied projective techniques to investigate, for example: poverty (Mitchell, Loomis, Polillo, Fry & Mackeigan et al., 2018); criminality (Kroz & Ratinova, 2018), and political brand images (Pich & Dean, 2015) and it has even been used in teaching (Colakoglu & Littlefield, 2011).
2 Readers interested in a more comprehensive overview of projective techniques as they are actually employed to gain insights into respondents' motives, beliefs, attitudes, etc., are guided to Hackett (2016).
3 See Cherrier (2012) for an example of using projectives in health research.
4 See the following for illustrations of the approaches use in marketing and consumer research: Bradley, (2013), Buzan and Griffiths, (2014), Bystedt, Siri, and Potts, (2003) Ezan, Gollety, and Hémar-Nicolas (2015), Gámbaro, Parente, Roascio, and Boinbaser (2014), Iacobucci and Churchill (2015), Kujala, Walsh, Nurkka, and Crisan (2014), Leibowitz, (2014), Mason (1950), Morrison, Haley, Sheehan, and Taylor (2011), Soley and Smith (2008), Vidal, Ares, and Giménez (2013), Wassler and Hung (2014).
5 I have suggested how students may develop and use projective techniques in Hackett, et al., (2016).

References

Bradley, N. (2013) Marketing Research: Tools and Techniques, Oxford: Oxford University Press.
Buzan, T. & C. Griffiths. (2014) Mind Maps for Business: Using the Ultimate Thinking Tool to Revolutionise How You Work, Harlow: Pearson Educational Ltd.
Bystedt, J., L. Siri, & D. Potts. (2003) Moderating to the Max: A Full-Tilt Guide to Creative, Insightful Focus Groups and Depth Interviews, Ithaca, NY: Paramount Market Publishing, Inc.
Charters, E. (2003) The Use of Think-aloud Methods in Qualitative Research, An Introduction to Think-aloud Methods, Brock Education Journal, 12(2), 68–82.
Cherrier, H. (2012) Using Projective Techniques to Consider the Societal Dimension of Healthy Practices: An Exploratory Study, Health Marketing Quarterly, 29(1), 82–95.
Colakoglu, S. & J. Littlefield. (2011) Teaching Organizational Culture Using a Projective Technique: Collage Construction, Journal of Management Education 35(4), 564–85. Web.
Conan Doyle, A. (2011) The Boscombe Valley Mystery: Adventure IV, in The Adventures of Sherlock Holmes, pp. 200–216. San Diego, CA: Canterbury Classics.
Dana, R.H. (1982) Human Science Model for Personality Assessment with Projective Techniques, Springfield, IL: Charles C Thomas Pub Ltd.
Dritto, I.P., S. Tummineri, V. Moscuzza, M.C. Di Perri, A.S. Rizzo, M. Liotta, E.M. Merlo, & C. Cicciarelli. (2015) Type D Personality in Infarcted Patients a Study with the Rorschach Projective Technique. Mediterranean Journal of Clinical Psychology, 3(3).
Eberle, R.F. (1996), SCAMPER: Games for imagination development, Waco, TX: Prufrock Press.
Eberle, R.F. (2008), SCAMPER ON: More Creative Games and Activities for Imagination Development, Waco, TX: Prufrock Press.
Ezan, P., M. Gollety, & V. Hémar-Nicolas. (2015) Drawing as Children's Language: Contributions of Psychology to the Enrichment of Research Methodologies Applied to Child Consumers, Recherche et Applications en Marketing (English Edition), 30(2), 78–96.
Francis-Williams, J. (1968) Rorschach with Children: A Comparative Study of the Contribution Made by the Rorschach and Other Projective Techniques to Clinical Diagnosis in Work with Children, Oxford: Pergamon.

Freud, S. (1938) The Basic Writing of Sigmund Freud, (ed. By Brill, A.A.), New York: Modern Library Inc.

Gámbaro, A., E. Parente, A. Roascio, & L. Boinbaser. (2014) Word Association Technique Applied to Cosmetic Products – A Case Study, Journal Of Sensory Studies, 29(2), 103–109.

Gardner, R.A. (2004) The Psychotherapeutic Use of the Talking, Feeling, & Doing Game and Other Projective Techniques Book, Bohemia NY: Childswork/Childsplay.

Hackett, P.M.W. (ed.) (2016) Qualitative Research Methods in Consumer Psychology: Ethnography and Culture, New York: Routledge Publishers.

Hackett, P.M.W., J.B. Schwarzenbach, & A.M. Jurgens. (2016) Consumer Psychology: A Study Guide to Qualitative Research Methods, Barbara Budrich Publishers.

Hogan, T.P. (2018) Psychological Testing: A Practical Introduction (fourth edition), New York: Wiley.

Iacobucci, D. & G.A. Churchill. (2015) Marketing Research: Methodological Foundations, CreateSpace Independent Publishing Platform.

Jones, S.C., C. Magee, & K. Andrews. (2015) I Think Other Parents Might. …': Using a Projective Technique to Explore Parental Supply of Alcohol. Drug and Alcohol Review, 34(5), 531–39.

Kroz M.V. & N.A. Ratinova. (2018) Research of Psychological Features of Corruption Criminals with the Help of Projective Technique. Psychology and Law, 8(3), 135–49.

Kujala, S., T. Walsh, P. Nurkka, & M. Crisan. (2014) Sentence Completion for Understanding Users and Evaluating User Experience, Interacting with Computers, 26(3), 238–255.

Leibowitz, M. (2014) Interpreting Projective Drawings: A Self-Psychological Approach, London: Routledge.

Mason, H. (1950) Projective Techniques in Marketing Research, Journal of Marketing, 14(5), 649–656.

Mattimore, B. (2013) Imaginative Moderating: A Toolkit of Creative Techniques, QRCA Webinar, 12 August 2013.

Mitchell, T., C. Loomis, A. Polillo, B. Fry, & M. Mackeigan. (2018) Projective Technique Reveals Unconscious Attitudes about Poverty in Canada, Journal of Poverty, 22(6), 500–17.

Morrison, M.A., E.E. Haley, K. Sheehan, & R.E. Taylor. (2011) Using Qualitative Research in Advertising: Strategies, Techniques, and Applications, Thousand Oaks, CA: Sage Publications, Inc.

Murstein, B.I. (ed.) (1965) Handbook of Projective Techniques, Jackson, TN: Basic Books.

Ogden, T. (1992) Projective Identification and Psychotherapeutic Technique, London: Routledge.

Oster, G.D. (2004) Using Drawings in Assessment and Therapy, London: Routledge.

Oster, G.D. (2016) Using Drawings in Clinical Practice: Enhancing Intake Interviews and Psychological Testing, London: Routledge.

Parente, S.C. (2019) The Multiple Self-States Drawing Technique: Creative Assessment and Treatment with Children and Adolescents, London: Routledge.

Passuello, L. (2015), Creative Problem Solving with Scamper. litemind.com/scamper/

Pich, C. & D. Dean. (2015) Qualitative Projective Techniques in Political Brand Image Research from the Perspective of Young Adults, Qualitative Market Research: An International Journal, 18(1), 115–144.

Rabin, A.I. (1968) Projective Techniques in Personality Assessment: A Modern Introduction, New York: Springer.

Robertson, K. (2009) The ZMET Method: Using Projective Technique to Understand Consumer Home Choice, The Marketing Review, 9(2): 139–54.

Serrat, O. (2017) Knowledge Solutions: Tools, Methods and Approaches to Drive Organisational Performance, Cham, CH: Springer. pp. 311–314. DOI: doi.org/10.1007/978-981-10-0983-9_33

Soley, L.C. & A.L. Smith. (2008) Projective Techniques For Social Science And Business Research, Shirley, NY: The Southshore Press.

Tuber, S, (2014) Understanding Personality through Projective Testing, Lanham, MD: Rowman & Littlefield Publishers.

Vidal, L., G. Ares, & A. Giménez. (2013) Projective Techniques to Uncover Consumer Perception: Application of Three Methodologies to Ready-to Eat Salads, Food Quality and Preference, 28(1), 1–7.

Vyas, D. & Nijholt. (2012) Artful surfaces: an ethnographic study exploring the use of space in design studios, Digital Creativity, 23(3–4): 176–195. DOI: 10.1080/14626268.2012.658522

Wassler, P. & K. Hung. (2014). Brand-as-Person versus Brand-as-User: An Anthropomorphic Issue in Tourism-related Self-Congruity Studies, Asia Pacific Journal of Tourism Research, 20(8), 839–859.

PART XII

Focus groups

28

USING FOCUS GROUPS IN HEALTHCARE RESEARCH

Alicia Carlson and Paul M.W. Hackett

Introduction

The sun was pouring through the palm trees and into the beach-side bar under another cloudless San Marie sky. As the light breeze gently rippled the fronds of the palms, they cast shadows that animated an intoxicating dance. All four of the suspects had been gathered together and they were sitting drinking beers and cocktails and avoiding looking at the detective who had summoned them there. Richard was looking pleased with himself and he moved around the bar with the air of a man who was in control and was playing a game with those present, explaining how the murder happened and telling each of the suspects what they were doing at the time of the murder and how they could have committed the crime.

Richard had been talking for a few minutes when he said, "In front of you are a series of photographs of fingerprints we recovered from the scene of the murder of Daniel Evans", looking towards the fingerprints with an intensity of interest suggesting that he was seeing these for the first time. After a brief pause he continued, "I have conveniently arranged these into sets and labelled them 1 to 5. I am going to start with the final set, 5, as these are from Daniel Evans himself and we can ignore these for a moment. The prints in the other sets are from each of you and were taken from the baseball bat that was used to kill Mr. Evans". Checking to see that he had their attention he went on, "this shows that you all had held the bat, which we knew already from your statements, and from the testimony of witnesses". Richard paced around the room silently whilst the four suspects smiled and looked towards him with sincere faces. "I won't go into all of the sets of prints as they tell us very little, but the prints in set 3", he said, "are very interesting and you can see in the photographs that some of these prints are on top of other finger prints". Richard yet again paused for effect and then looked at the suspects, one by one. "And all of the finger prints they are on top are Daniel's. But you would know that, wouldn't you Sarah?" Richard said as he turned and stared at the woman who was sitting and smiling at Richard, apparently unmoved by the revelation. "I am assuming that you are saying that set 3 are my prints" said Sarah, "but that just means that Daniel touched the bat at some point before I did, not that I killed him". Richard had expected this retort and he now moved closer to Sarah and looked directly at her. His two officers, Dwayne and Camille moved to stand behind Sarah. "And that would be true if it were not for the brown smudge that you can see here, please come and have a look, Sarah" Richard directed Sarah to look more closely at one of the photographs.

"That smudge, you see there, is blood, it's Daniel's blood, and it is on top of your fingerprint, and as you only arrived on the island a couple of hours before Daniel was killed, I think we have you", Richard had a satisfied though resigned look as he walked behind Sarah and placed his hands firmly on the back of her chair. "I think we now know who killed Daniel Evans, don't we Sarah, arrest her please Dwayne".

Richard may well be an excellent detective, and one who always gets his man (or woman). However, it is quite likely that he would have been a terrible focus group moderator. It's perfectly fine for a TV detective to be the know-it-all quirky genius who knows the answer to who has committed the crime and has to guide one of the suspects to confess. But this is not the way a focus group interview should be conducted. In this situation, the set-up may appear somewhat similar to the one described above. A group of informed individuals are brought together along with stimulus materials, and maybe even drinks and snacks, and a conversation is facilitated by a knowledgeable moderator. However, the crucial difference between the crime scene collective and the focus group is that the person moderating the focus group should not be the one who does the most talking and it is not his or her opinions that are of importance.

When you think of healthcare research, you may think of scientists in labs working on discovering the next treatment for illnesses, or medical students at prestigious universities advancing research. However, there is a tremendous amount of value in gathering information directly from patients and their caregivers, and medical professionals who frequently interact with these populations as these individuals are in a position to provide peerless and unique insights. Focus groups can be a wonderful opportunity to learn about what health professionals, ancillary staff, those receiving care, and their families, friends and care-givers, etc., go through on a day-to-day basis. Furthermore, by gathering such information we are able to contribute the knowledge held by these people in order to advance the quality of patient care. Having made these bold statements we will start by considering exactly what a focus group is.

What are focus groups?

Focus groups, or focus group interviews, (see for example, Creswell & Poth, 2016; Hennink, 2007) are typically used in marketing and social sciences (Hackett, 2016; Hackett, Schwarzenbach & Jurgens, 2016; Potts, 2016). In these context they have been found to be a flexible way to easily gather quantitative information on a topic researchers are exploring. As well as being used in these areas, the focus group has also been used in many areas related to health and well-being. For example: sensitive health topics (Reisner et al, 2018); nursing (Cobb, Wolf, Shine, & Jadwin, 2018; Dunnachie & Story, 2019; Fung Yu, 2020; Kerr et al., 2020; Wong et al., 2018); sensory impairment (Anderson et al., 2018); cancer (Kim, Park, Kim, Hur, Lee, & Han, 2020; Lee & Lee, 2018; Shaw et al., 2018); health promotion and education (Egerod, Wulff, & Petersen , 2018); diabetes (Gardsten, Blomqvist, Rask, Larsson, Lindberg, & Olsson, 2018); mental health (Foley, Sheehan, & Jennings, 2018; Man & Kangas, 2020; Myklebust, Bjørkly, & Råheim, 2018); genomics (Viberg Johansson, Segerdahl, Ugander, Hansson, & Langenskiöld, 2018); public health (Robinson, Bottorff, Pesut, & Zerr, 2020; Royer et al., 2020); urinary tract disease (Kane Low et al., 2019); adolescents (Cotney & Banerjee, 2019); older adults (Bengtsson & Carlsson, 2006; Waterworth, Raphael, Gott, Arroll, Benipal, & Jarden, 2019); well-being (Hall, et al., 2018). Focus groups may also be conducted in a wide variety of settings. For example: in schools (Pawlowski, Tjarnhaj-Thomsen, Schipperijn, & Troelsen, 2014); nature reserve wildlife centres (Hackett, 2016); and online: (Ripat & Colatruglio, 2016; Jervaeus, Nilsson, Eriksson, Lampic, Widmark, & Wettergren, 2016).

Within any focus group, the diverse range of individuals recruited for a focus group have a common interest or a shared experience. They can also consist of people who fall into the same age range, live in the same geographical area, or have other shared characteristics. Focus groups are opportunities to produce and collect qualitative data and for researchers to explore what people think and why they have those opinions through collecting information and brainstorming on a topic. Focus groups are conversations between the focus group moderator and participants, within which all have the opportunity to make statements, ask questions, clarify questions, and explore the details around the participants' utterances. During these conversations, researchers can gain invaluable insights into the language used by patients, medical staff, or caregivers to describe the topic being researched. Researchers are able to gather a wide variety of insights during these sessions as focus groups are an excellent source of idea generation. When a discussion gains momentum within a focus group, new ideas can emerge, and in a well-run focus group, participants are made to feel comfortable sharing their opinions and experiences in more detail. These insights can lead to new or improved treatment plans, innovative support services, improved workflows for medical staff, and other things that could make the patient/caregiver or medical staff's experience a little easier.

However, there are some limitations to focus groups, especially in health care research. In a group setting, it is sometimes the case that conformity may dominate the session or participants may hold back their opinions. Facilitators may also encounter a dominant personality or two within the group, which may result in other participants withholding their own thoughts and ideas out of fear of being ridiculed or talked down. Focus group moderators need to take special care to control the flow of conversation, making sure everyone has equal opportunity to speak, that quiet participants are encouraged to participate through the use of positive reinforcement, and to encourage participants to speak their minds. If the moderator cannot properly control the conversation, data may skew in one direction that does not reflect the true opinion of the group. Healthcare is a highly personal topic for many people, and extra attention needs to be paid to creating a safe and comfortable space for everyone to participate equally.

If any participants in a focus group know each other, this may, to a large extent, defeat the purpose of a focus group as being a place where new ideas are generated and, in health research especially, anonymity may be required. While there is always a chance that someone may run into someone they used to work with, or grew up with, it is important for moderators to be aware of potential familiarity. If two people know each other and it is not possible to swap one of them out with another potential participant, moderators should ask the participants to sit separately and not directly across from each other. This will reduce the chance of side conversations occurring. A participant who is hesitant to share their own specific feelings may tend to agree more with what others are saying. In such situations moderators can navigate around conformity through managing conversations by asking good follow-up questions, such as: why do you feel that way; could you explain that further; earlier you mentioned _____; and it seems like you may be forming a different opinion, can you explain a bit about your thought process regarding this issue? Asking follow-up questions will reveal more information from the group, and may unveil a more truthful opinion. At all times, the moderator must avoid a focus group taking on the format in which he or she asks participants in turn to respond to a question, or respondents simply fall into answering in turn. If this happens, much of the spontaneity and novelty that could emerge from the group may be lost.

Confidentiality can be another influence on the success of the group, especially if the focus group consist of an assemblage of participants who fear what they will say will end up being reported back to their employer, their family, friends, or to other people in general. If the focus group participants are medical professionals, they may be fearful of other members discussing what they said to colleagues outside of the focus group, even to their superiors. These fears may result in employees not honestly and openly offering and explaining their thoughts and point of view, which damages the research. It is therefore very important to establish a confidentiality rule for the focus group at the very beginning of the session.

How to prepare for a focus group

Gathering information using a focus groups is not a quick process. A researcher must spend a considerable amount of time planning the focus group and preparing a focus group guide. The focus group guide is a structure that the moderator uses to run the group which consists of questions and probes along with a time schedule. After the session has finished, the recording of the focus group will need transcribing and the information analysed. The more prepared a moderator is, the easier it will be for the focus group to produce the innovative responses that were desired.

For focus groups in healthcare, a great amount of consideration needs to be given to making sure the location is comfortable for the participants. In any focus group situation, it is important to choose a location with a table and chairs where everyone can see each other as this will make it easier to facilitate a conversation and have participants interact with each other. A round or oval shaped table or chair setup may help bring about a conversation because everyone will be able to see and make eye contact with each other, encouraging participation and the sharing of ideas. A room with good lighting, moderate room temperature (or the ability to control the temperature), and close proximity to toilets is also important for general comfort. Good hospitality is also important to help participants feel comfortable and it is a good idea to provide water, tea, coffee, and a variety of snack options. It is also a good idea to ask about food allergies or diet restrictions when individuals agree to take part in the focus group so no one is excluded.

Beyond these details, it is really important to choose a location based on the group you are interviewing. Locations for patients and caregivers may need to be near their appointments, for instance, at a hospital or in a nearby building may be easier for them to get to. For example, if patients and caregivers are at a hospital multiple times a week for an appointment, the last thing they are going to feel up to is trekking across town to participate in a focus group. Empathy in designing a focus group for this population will result in a higher success rate. The same considerations regarding location are true for medical staff. However, they may not feel comfortable or relaxed participating in a focus group that is being held in their place of work and changing the setting to a neutral location that is near the hospital, surgery, etc., may encourage honesty and the expression of their private opinions.

Part of the setting of a focus group doesn't come in a physical form. The moderator is able to set a positive tone and atmosphere for the group, which creates a more positive experience for the participants. Happily greeting each person as they arrive, showing them where the refreshments and other facilities are, and thanking them for their time will show participants how their contribution is valued by the research team. A great sense of empathy for the participants should be developed by the moderator. The moderator viewing him or herself in the participants situation may help to avoid difficulties occurring in the procedure and will benefit the overall experience for the participants. Furthermore, this may also result in richer qualitative data because of the sense of trust between the moderator and participant.

Who to recruit for a focus group

In healthcare focus groups, there may be several layers of questions to ask to help narrow down the pool of potential participants for a focus group. These are:

- For whom is the focus of the research being conducted?
  - Patients?
  - Medical Staff (Doctors, Nurses, Medical Assistants, Administrators, Support Staff, etc.)?
  - Caregivers?
  - Medical authorities/companies?
- What is the reason for the research?
  - Improving systems for medical staff and/or patients?
  - Learning more about patient experience at a surgery or other medical facility?
  - Learning more about patient experience with an illness or condition?
  - Learning more about a caregiver's experience?
  - Learning more about what can improve a process for a member of a medical profession?
  - Gaining insights or feedback about a piece of medical technology in order to make improvements?
- Is there a specific condition, illness, etc., or level of professional experience needed for a participant to sign up for the focus group?
- Is there a specific age range or gender required for the research?

Note: Unless the research is targeting a specific age, gender, etc.,, it is always a good idea to build a focus group with a broad variety of demographics (age, ethnicity, gender, and geographic location, etc.). Diversity will allow for a variety of perspectives that will elevate the outcomes and increase the quality of data collected in a focus group.

Once the categories of people needed for the focus group have been determined, it is important to explore the possible power dynamics of people you will ask to participate. Patients may not provide honest opinions about their quality of care if they are participating in a focus group with any employee of a care facility, whether it is a doctor or member of the administrative staff. Patients and caregivers may not give honest opinions if they feel their opinions would be a burden to a loved one in the room and do not want to cause any more worry or distress to these individuals. Any medical professional may feel intimidated if their boss or another member of management is in the room. These are all important factors that need to be considered in order to ensure the success of the focus group and be able to gather the most authentic responses possible.

The ideal size of a focus group is not easily determined. As a rule of thumb, less than 6 participants may not provide a broad ranging discussion and more than 12 participants may be unwieldy and hard to keep on topic.[1] Once the researcher has selected 6–12 people for the focus group, the opportunity arises for the researcher to ask the participants to do a little homework to bring to the focus group. This homework may involve keeping a journal of specific experiences or symptoms over a period of time before the focus group. Preparation could also involve asking participants to take a few photos or short videos to share in the group. It could also involve bringing specific personal items to the group that are relevant to the topic.

Developing a focus group discussion guide and running the session

A moderator's role in a focus group is very much like a that of a reporter managing a debate, or a teacher facilitating a conversation amongst students about a piece of literature. In all of these settings, it's about staying neutral, setting a friendly tone for the group, and maintaining control of the conversation. Doing this will ensure that you can get through your discussion guide and get the information you need. It is important to have genuine curiosity and display kindness towards the participants because it will set the tone for the discussion and build trust.

Preparing a focus group discussion guide, as we briefly mentioned earlier, is essential to enable a moderator to remain organized, to make sure all questions are asked of the focus group participants, and to make sure that every participant has an equal opportunity to participate. It may sound strange but the discussion guide should attempt to create a framework for a conversation that will flow naturally in a structured group environment. The discussion guide should start with the beginning of the focus group and should include how you will welcome everyone, thank them for taking the time out of their busy day to participate, and although the participants know why they are there, it is good to explain again what the focus group is about. This is the best time to set the expectations and rules for confidentiality. By setting expectations and rules, trust is encouraged to form between focus group participants and the moderator, and begins to build amongst the participants themselves. It is important to remember that establishing trust will lead to more honest insights and richer information for the researchers. At this point, participants should introduce themselves to the group and say a few things that are relevant to the topic of the focus group. Some commonalities may arise, building trust among the participants. Each person should have about a minute of time for their introduction, so build this time into your discussion guide, whether you have 6 participants, or 12.

Questions can start off in a general, broad form to ease participants into a specific topic of conversation. It is important to keep the tone conversational because it will keep participants at ease. Approaching the focus group session from a point of authentic curiosity will put the participants at ease and encourage their participation, making them feel more positive about the whole group experience. Furthermore, this shows participants that their knowledge and experience with the topic is valuable, and their time is appreciated. Adopting a position of authority or as someone who needs to get a set of questions answered will tend to close down free and open conversations. If a participant provides an insight that could be valuable, but you need more information, the moderator should ask the individual open-ended follow up questions. Phrasing follow up questions in a positive way, such as "that is a really interesting point, could you tell me more about it" will yield information and insights that you may not expect, or prompt another participant to further explain their experience or point of view.

In any group situation, it is common for there to be people who dominate conversations as well as those who are quieter. It is the responsibility of the moderator to navigate these personalities and make sure everyone has equal time to participate in the conversation. This can be done by redirecting the conversation. If someone who is dominating the conversation pauses, it could be a good time to interject by thanking the individual for their opinion, and directly asking a quieter individual about their feelings or thoughts on the same topic. Kindly asking quieter individuals direct questions gives them the opportunity to contribute valuable insights.

With any discussion guide it is important to build in flexibility. The discussion guide is just that: a guide. If during the focus group you think of a question or want to ask a follow up question that is not in the guide, it is okay to ask those questions as long as you are able to get back on track and keep to time. Such managed tangential excursions are central to the success of a focus group and may be where much of the brainstorming and novel idea generation occurs.

Focus group materials

As well as the discussion guide, there are other materials that you will need to conduct a focus group. For example, you will need:

- Consent forms (*see Exhibit A at the end of this chapter for a sample consent form.*)
- Devices to record audio and/or video. It's a good idea to have a backup device in case the first one fails or malfunctions, and to have charging cables or extra batteries available.
- Pen, pencil
- Notebook
- Name tags / badges for the participants
- Clock
- Refreshments for the participants
- A drink for you

It is also recommended that you ask another researcher to sit in on the focus group and take notes on statements, reactions, and any non-verbal cues from participants. Having the support of a colleague allows moderators to stay focused on making sure each participant is able to contribute to the conversation equally and in meaningful ways. Having notes about how participants react to statements and ideas of others will support the conversation transcript and provide important insights that may make a significant difference in interpreting the transcript of the session and in forming research outcomes.

After a focus group concludes

At the end of a focus group session it is important to thank participants for their time, answer any questions they may have, and ask if it would be okay to follow up with them later, on an individual basis if it is needed.

It is important for researchers (the moderator and any other researchers present at the session) to debrief amongst themselves immediately following a focus group session whilst the experience is fresh in everyone's minds. Immediately following a focus group, researchers will have a lot of information to sort through and organize. The entire focus group conversation should be transcribed word for word, and notes on participant reactions and non-verbal cues need to be collated with each statement in the transcript. Themes will begin to emerge, and direct quotes from participants can be used as supporting evidence in a final recommendation report.

Conclusion

A focus group is a collection of individuals who have been selected and brought together to form a group because of their interest in or specialised knowledge about a health or well-being issue or problem. A focus group is an open discussion that seeks to explore alternative or completely new approaches or understandings about the topic. An example that would be extremely timely to my writing would be a focus group on possible ways to react to the coronavirus pandemic (COVID-19) that is at present hitting the world. It is likely that with such an important and deadly topic in which many different types of people are impacted in different ways, several focus groups may be convened. These focus groups could be comprised of: medical professionals' economists; local, national, and international law makers/politicians; drug manufacturers; families of people who have had the virus; individuals who have recovered from having the virus; and the list goes on. A moderator would need to be carefully selected, who would need to make her or himself thoroughly acquainted with the ideas. It would also be important, as with all focus groups, but especially with one into such an important though delicate health issue, that the moderator was comfortable working with a variety of different people and making them at their ease.

Focus groups are used in many settings in healthcare, public health, and other related areas to assist in elucidating suitable ways to tackle a problem. It can be seen from my description of the above focus group procedure that the approach is peerless in healthcare when it comes to generating novel and sensible ideas and solutions. Indeed, in this situation, and with a thoroughly divided and piloted discussion guide, it is possible that the focus group could develop a wide range of novel and innovative suggestions regarding the specific aspects of the disease that were the focus of the group, proposals and propositions that may not have been forthcoming through the use of any other research approach and which could be taken on for further scrutiny and investigation. However, the results of focus groups are always biased by the composition of the group and should not be thought of as definitive and should be viewed with some caution.

Note

1   6 to 12 people is only an approximate guide to the number of people in a focus group. Hennink, Kaiser, and Weber (2019) considered sample group size and response saturation in focus groups.

References

Anderson, M.L, T. Riker, K. Gagne, S. Hakulin, T. Higgins, J. Meehan, E. Stout, E. Pici-D'ottavio, K. Cappetta, & K.S. Wolf Craig. (2018) Deaf Qualitative Health Research: Leveraging Technology to Conduct Linguistically and Sociopolitically Appropriate Methods of Inquiry. Qualitative Health Research, 28(11). 1813–824.

Bengtsson, A. & G. Carlsson. (2006) Outdoor Environments at Three Nursing Homes: Focus Group Interviews with Staff. Journal of Housing for the Elderly, 19(3–4): 49–69.

Cobb, S., K. Wolf, C. Shine, & A, Jadwin. (2018) Involving Clinical Nurses in Evaluation of a Professional Practice Model: A Focus Group Research Study Approach. JONA: The Journal of Nursing Administration, 48(9): 466–68.

Cotney, J.L. & R. Banerjee. (2019) Adolescents' Conceptualizations of Kindness and Its Links with Well-being: A Focus Group Study. Journal of Social and Personal Relationships, 36(2): 599–617.

Creswell, J.W. & C.N. Poth. (2016) Qualitative Inquiry and Research Design: Choosing Among Five Approaches 4th Edition. Thousand Oaks, CA: Sage Publishers.

Dunnachie, G. & D. Story. (2019) Surgical Nurses' Perceptions and Experiences of a Medications and Oral Restrictions Policy Change: A Focus Group Study. Journal of Clinical Nursing, 28(17–18): 3242–251.

Egerod, I., K. Wulff, & M.C. Petersen. (2018) Experiences and Informational Needs on Sexual Health in People with Epilepsy or Multiple Sclerosis: A Focus Group Investigation. Journal of Clinical Nursing, 27(13–14): 2868–2876.

Foley, T., C. Sheehan, & A. Jennings. (2018) What Do Physiotherapists Need to Know about Dementia Care? A Focus Group Study. Age and Ageing, 47(5): V13–60.

Fung Yu, D. (2020) A Mixed Methods Study to Evaluate the Effects of a Teamwork Enhancement and Quality Improvement Initiative on Nurses' Work Environment. Journal of Advanced Nursing, 76(2): 664–75.

Gardsten, C., K. Blomqvist, M. Rask, A. Larsson, A. Lindberg, & G. Olsson. (2018) Challenges in Everyday Life among Recently Diagnosed and More Experienced Adults with Type 2 Diabetes: A Multistage Focus Group Study. Journal of Clinical Nursing, 27(19–20): 3666–3678.

Hackett, P.M.W. (ed.) (2016) Qualitative Research Methods in Consumer Psychology: Ethnography and Culture. New York: Routledge.

Hackett, P.M.W., J.B. Schwarzenbach, & U.M. Jurgens. (2016) Consumer Psychology: A Study Guide to Qualitative Research Methods. Opladen, Berlin, Toronto: Barbara Budrich Publishers.

Hall, L.H., J. Johnson, J. Heyhoe, I. Watt, K. Anderson, & D.B. O'Connor. (2018) Strategies to Improve General Practitioner Well-being: Findings from a Focus Group Study. Family Practice, 35(4): 511–516.

Hennink, M.M. (2007) International Focus Group Research: A Handbook for the Health and Social Sciences. Cambridge: Cambridge University Press.

Hennink, M.M., B.N. Kaiser, & M.B. Weber. (2019) What Influences Saturation? Estimating Sample Sizes in Focus Group Research. Qualitative Health Research, 29(10): 1483–496.

Jervaeus, A., J. Nilsson, L.E. Eriksson, C. Lampic, C. Widmark, & L. Wettergren. (2016) Exploring Childhood Cancer Survivors' Views about Sex and Sexual Experiences -findings from Online Focus Group Discussions. European Journal of Oncology Nursing, 20: 165–172.

Low, L.K., B.R. Williams, D.R. Camenga, J. Hebert-Beirne, S.S. Brady, D.K. Newman, A.S. James, C.T. Hardacker, J. Nodora, S.E. Linke, & K.L. Burgio, (2019) Prevention of Lower Urinary Tract Symptoms Research Consortium Focus Group Study of Habits, Attitudes, Realities, and Experiences of Bladder Health. Journal of Advanced Nursing, 75(11): 3111–125.

Kerr, D., S. Milnes, J. Ammentorp, C. McKie, T. Dunning, J. Ostaszkiewicz, M. Wolderslund, & P. Martin. (2020) Challenges for Nurses When Communicating with People Who Have Life-limiting Illness and Their Families: A Focus Group Study. Journal of Clinical Nursing, 29(3–4): 416–28.

Kim, S.H., S. Park, S.J. Kim, M.H. Hur, B.G. Lee, & M.S. Han. (2020) Self-management Needs of Breast Cancer Survivors After Treatment: Results From a Focus Group Interview. Cancer Nursing, 43(1): 78–85.

Lee, S.Y. & E.E. Lee. (2018) Cancer Screening in Koreans: A Focus Group Approach. BMC Public Health 18(1): 254.

Man, J. & M. Kangas. (2020) Best Practice Principles When Working With Individuals With Intellectual Disability and Comorbid Mental Health Concerns, Qualitative Health Research, 30(4): 560–571.

Myklebust, K.K., S. Bjørkly, & M. Råheim. (2018) Nursing Documentation in Inpatient Psychiatry: The Relevance of Nurse-patient Interactions in Progress Notes-A Focus Group Study with Mental Health Staff. Journal of Clinical Nursing, 27(3–4): E611–E622.

Potts, D. (2016) Focus Group Interviews, in Hackett, P.M.W. (ed.) (2016) Qualitative Research Methods in Consumer Psychology: Ethnography and Culture. New York: Routledge, pp. 118–130.

Pawlowski, C.S., T. Tjarnhaj-Thomsen, J. Schipperijn, & J. Troelsen. (2014) Barriers for Recess Physical Activity: A Gender Specific Qualitative Focus Group Exploration. BMC Public Health, 14(1): 639.

Reisner, S.L., R.K. Randazzo, J.M. White Hughto, S. Peitzmeier, L.Z. Dubois, D.J. Pardee, E. Marrow, S. Mclean, & J. Potter. (2018) Sensitive Health Topics With Underserved Patient Populations: Methodological Considerations for Online Focus Group Discussions. Qualitative Health Research, 10: 1658–673.

Ripat, J. & A. Colatruglio. (2016) Exploring Winter Community Participation Among Wheelchair Users: An Online Focus Group. Occupational Therapy in Health Care, 30(1): 95–106.

Robinson, C.A., J.L. Bottorff, B. Pesut, & J. Zerr. (2020) Development and Implementation of the Family Caregiver Decision Guide. Qualitative Health Research, 30(2): 303–13.

Royer, P.A., L.M. Olson, B. Jackson, L.S. Weber, L. Gawron, J.N. Sanders, & D.K. Turok. (2010) In Africa, There Was No Family Planning. Every Year You Just Give Birth": Family Planning Knowledge, Attitudes, and Practices Among Somali and Congolese Refugee Women After Resettlement to the United States, Qualitative Health Research, 30(3): 391–408.

Shaw, T., D. Ishak, D. Lie, S. Menon, E. Courtney, S.T. Li, & J. Ngeow. (2018) The Influence of Malay Cultural Beliefs on Breast Cancer Screening and Genetic Testing: A Focus Group Study. Psycho-Oncology, 27(12): 2855–2861.

Wong, R.K., J.Y. Lee, A.S. Surendran, K. Nair, N. Della Maestra, M. Migliarini, J.A. St Onge, & C. Patterson. (2018) Nursing Perspectives on the Confusion Assessment Method: A Qualitative Focus Group Study. Age and Ageing, 47(6): 880–86.

Viberg Johansson, J., P. Segerdahl, U.H. Ugander, M.G. Hansson, & S. Langenskiöld. (2018) Making Sense of Genetic Risk: A Qualitative Focus-group Study of Healthy Participants in Genomic Research. Patient Education and Counselling, 101(3): 422–27.

Waterworth, S., D. Raphael, M. Gott, B. Arroll, J. Benipal, & A. Jarden. (2019) An Exploration of How Community-dwelling Older Adults Enhance Their Well-being. International Journal of Older People Nursing, 14(4) e12267.

Exhibit A - sample consent form

(Disclaimer: All legal forms should be reviewed by your company's legal department before use.)

[NAME OF RESEARCH GROUP OR COMPANY]

CONSENT FORM FOR RESEARCH PARTICIPATION

Study Title: [INSERT TITLE OF THE FOCUS GROUP STUDY]

Principal Investigator(s): [ENTER NAMES AND CONTACT INFORMATION HERE]

We are planning to conduct a research study, which we invite you to take part in. This form has important information about the reason for doing this study, what we will ask you to do if you decide to be in this study, and the way we would like to use information about you if you choose to be in the study.

Why are you doing this study?

[ENTER A DESCRIPTION OF WHY THE STUDY IS BEING CONDUCTED.]

What will I do if I choose to be in this study?

You will be asked to:

- [ENTER EXACTLY WHAT ACTIVITIES WILL TAKE PLACE IN THE FOCUS GROUP. (e.g.; Participate in activities that will include completing sentences provided by the researchers, telling us what comes to mind when specific words are given to respondents, and a series of interviews.)]

Focus Group Duration: Study participation will take approximately [ENTER TIME HERE]

Focus Group Location: [ENTER LOCATION HERE]

Audio/Video recording: We would like to audio-record and/or video-record activities and interviews to make sure that we remember accurately all the information you provide. We will keep these recordings in [ENTER METHOD IN WHICH MEDIA WILL BE STORED] and they will only be used by members of the research team. We will destroy these materials [ENTER DATE].

We may quote your remarks in presentations or articles resulting from this work. A pseudonym will be used to protect your identity, unless you specifically request that you be identified by your true name.

What are the possible risks or discomforts?

To the best of our knowledge, the things you will be doing have no more risk of harm than you would experience in everyday life. Your participation in this study does not involve any physical or emotional risk to you beyond that of everyday life.

As with all research, there is a chance that confidentiality of the information we collect from you could be breached – we will take steps to minimize this risk, as discussed in more detail below in this form.

What are the possible benefits for me or others?

You are not likely to have any direct benefit from being in this research study. This study is designed to learn more about [ENTER RESEARCH GOAL HERE]. The study results may be used to help other people in the future.

How will you protect the information you collect about me, and how will that information be shared?

Results of this study may be used in [ENTER WHERE THE INFORMATION WILL BE USED HERE]. Your study data will be handled as confidentially as possible. If results of this study are published or presented, individual names and other personally identifiable information will not be used.

To minimize the risks to confidentiality, we will only share documents, photos, and videos with the research team. These materials will not be used in research presentations.

We may share the data we collect from you for use in future research studies or with other researchers – if we share the data that we collect about you, we will remove any information that could identify you before we share it.

If we think that you intend to harm yourself or others, we will notify the appropriate people with this information.

Financial Information

Participation in this study will involve no cost to you. [ENTER COMPENSATION INFORMATION HERE.]

What are my rights as a focus group research participant?

Participation in this study is voluntary. You do not have to answer any questions you do not want to answer. If at any time and for any reason, you would prefer not to participate in this study, please feel free not to. If at any time you would like to stop participating, please tell a member of the research team. We can take a break, stop and continue at a later date, or stop altogether. You may withdraw from this study at any time, and you will not be penalized in any way for deciding to stop participation.

If you decide to withdraw from this study, the researchers will ask you if the information already collected from you can be used.

Consent

I have read this form and the research study has been explained to me. I have been given the opportunity to ask questions and my questions have been answered. If I have additional questions, I have been told whom to contact. I agree to participate in the focus group research study described above and will receive a copy of this consent form.

_____

Participant's Name (printed)

_____

Participant's Signature   Date

29

FOCUS GROUP RESEARCH IN HEALTHCARE

Immy Holloway

Introduction: What is focus group research?

Focus group research is one of the ways to collect ethnographic, qualitative data. A focus group involves a number of people who participate in a discussion about a topic, generally in an informal setting. There is broad agreement among researchers about the characteristics of focus group research: Morgan (2019, p. 5), a prolific American writer in this area, describes focus groups as "a research method that collects qualitative data through group discussions", and he adds that focus groups rely on the interaction of its members. Barbour (2018, p. 171), a British academic, refers to a focus group discussion as "a group... convened for purposes that relies for data on the discussion generated between participants". This means that data will be collected from several people simultaneously. Although focus group research can stand alone, focus group discussions are sometimes just one source of data within ethnography and might complement individual interviews and observation. A study with homeless people and professionals about palliative care in the Netherlands (Klop, Francke, Van Dongen, & de Veer, 2018), for instance, demonstrates that focus group research can stand alone, while research by Arnold, van Teijlingen, Ryan, and Holloway (2014) in Afghanistan, with Afghan women, doctors, cleaners and midwives – is an example of complementary inquiry and includes both individual interviews and focus group discussions. The latter also entailed observations. (Focus group research can also be an adjunct to quantitative or multi-method research; for instance, researchers may generate findings which help in the construction of a questionnaire, or at the end of a survey to obtain more in-depth and open, candid data.)

Focus groups are set up to:

- elicit ideas, thoughts, and feelings about a particular topic
- find out about the shared experiences of group members
- explore a wide range of important issues
- generate a variety of rich and diverse data
- complement one-to-one interviews

The origin of focus groups

It is commonly believed that the sociologist Merton is the originator of focus group research in social science during the 1940s. Early focus groups were set up to show the social and mental influences of mass communication on the public – even in those days Merton considered health aspects (Merton & Kendall 1946) but also focused on army training and morale (Merton & Lazarsfeld 1950). At this time, they were called group studies. Initially, these groups were mainly used in market research to illuminate consumer attitudes, perspectives, and behaviour.

The term "focus group" has been attributed to Ernest Dichter, a Viennese Freudian psychologist. In the public health arena, focus group research was first used in family planning in the 1980s (Mitchell & Branigan, 2000), but other health researchers started to use it in the 1980s and it proliferated in the next decades.

The use of focus groups in health research

Focus groups as a research tool in the health arena have been used more frequently in recent years. Holloway and Galvin (2017) give some of the reasons for FGs in this field:

Researchers explore patients' experiences of their condition, treatment, and interaction with health professionals.

A group of Australian researchers, for instance, recruited focus group members from patients with chronic kidney disease in kidney dialysis and transplant centres of Australia (Tong et al., 2008). These patients were asked about their experiences and priorities. In Afghanistan, Arnold et al. (2014), for their critical ethnographic research, set up (among other interviews) two focus group discussions with women in a community, one with six members of a family, and another with women from a self-help group about care in Kabul maternity hospitals with interesting results (reported in Arnold et al., 2014).

Researchers wish to obtain the perspectives of health professionals about their roles and their patients' illnesses.

An example would be the research by Rasmussen and Ro (2018) who conducted focus group research with GPs (general practitioners) to understand medically unexplained symptoms that they encountered in their practice. Two focus groups were established whose members had varied clinical experience. There were a number of implications of this research which could help improve medical students' learning.

Focus group research has also been used in the evaluation of healthcare.

Mitchell and Branigan (2000), for instance, suggest that researchers, and in particular healthcare professionals, might use three types of focus group evaluation: formative, process, and outcome evaluation in different stages of a programme. They give some of examples for these, in formative research for instance to examine a draft of a programme or find out about the ideas of participants for a potential intervention; in process evaluation, to explore why patients might or might not want to participate; in outcome focus group research, to investigate perspectives of the effectiveness of the programme.

> Health professionals wish to obtain perspectives on public health issues through ethnographic
> focus group research.

A study by Thai, Taber, Oh, Segar, Blake, and Patrick (2019) showed how this might be done. They examined the perspectives of women from different ethnic backgrounds on health messages about physical activity and exercise and their responses to these messages.

Focus group discussions in health research are particularly useful because they often, though not always, deal with vulnerable people and focus on sensitive topics; research with homeless people, or those with HIV and AIDS, or even cancer patients undergoing therapy at the time of the research are examples of these groups. Occasionally, topics are inappropriate for focus groups, such as intimate personal experiences or life histories.

A critical appraisal checklist of focus group articles appeared in the European Journal of General Practice in 2002 (Vermeire, Van Roysen, Griffiths, Coenen, Peremans, & Hendricks, 2002). Although this article is not new, its contents is still valid.

Conducting focus group research

Recruiting a sample: Type of sample, sample size, and composition

Before forming focus groups, researchers need be clear about the topic or issue they wish to investigate and, of course, the context of the inquiry. They will have an overview of the broader questions for their study and consider the specific issues they wish to explore. Thus, the sampling is purposive as in all qualitative research; generalisability is not sought – though typicality might be found. The researcher will also be able to transfer emerging concepts to other settings and contexts (Morse, 2012).

One of the first steps in focus group research is the identification of potential participants. The research might be focused on a specific issue or on a variety of areas within the topic. Some people in the sample might have more information about this than others, some are more affected by it, others more indifferent to the topic. Therefore, researchers need clear criteria for the choice of group members. For instance, they might be small groups of older people with diabetes or groups of young people in physical work who have chronic back pain. There could also be groups of people who discuss the current state of particular health policies and strategies.

Recruitment of participants is often made through newspaper adverts, notice boards in hospitals or general practices – with permission of the institution of course – or through gaining access by having health professionals recruit the group members.

Choosing a sample is a complex task for the researchers, be they outsiders to the setting or insiders – an outsider could be a social science researcher, an insider a midwife who works in a particular hospital or in the community. The aim is of course, to gather a variety of rich and appropriate data for the study. Stewart and Shamdasani (2015) maintain that a sampling frame is useful. A sampling frame is the population of interest from which the sample is taken. In focus groups for health research, for instance, the population might be patients in a local general practice or consultants within a particular specialty. The authors above state, however, that in focus group research a sampling frame is less important than in survey research as researchers cannot generalise beyond the boundaries of the focus group(s). Group interaction generates not only discussion but also a variety and multitude of ideas, because of the varied experiences of participants. Occasionally, the sample is chosen because it includes individuals who are not typical for the group because the researchers need to have some "deviant cases" which enhance the dynamic of the interaction. Deviant cases are examples of comments that differ strongly from the general pattern that seems to emerge.

In general, focus groups are homogeneous, at least in their interests and experience. Morgan (2019) suggests the advantages of homogeneity are, indeed, a common interest and experience in the topic area. Thus, for instance, a researcher who is interested in the feelings about the birth of a first child of older mothers might form focus groups of older mothers who have had their first baby recently. The groups might include mothers who had a child in hospital and others who gave birth at home. It is obvious that a heterogeneous sample needs more recruits than homogenous groups. A project that, for instance, involves nurses, patients, and doctors should include more focus group members than a group of young people of a similar age who have diabetes.

Sometimes FG research in healthcare is used for convenience, where participants can be accessed with fewer resources where they occur naturally, for example, where the focus group takes place as part of, or after a meeting or assembly; it could be a team meeting of receptionists in a GP practice, or a meeting of nurse practitioners in a specific geographical area.

Group size and composition

Group size is quite important and challenging for the researcher. In market research in past focus groups, the groups tended to be quite large, but this would be difficult in healthcare research because large groups would be too complex and difficult. Hence the groups tend to be smaller. Participants in a small group with a sample size of four to six will find talking more comfortable and responding to each other easier. The researcher also finds the transcription and analysis much easier than that of larger groups. Goodman and Evans (2015) state that the sample is dependent on availability and the willingness to take part. The research usually will involve at least two to four groups, and sometimes more, depending on its topic and aim.

The groups might be pre-established or selected and constituted by researchers. Members, of course, need share common interests. *Pre-constituted groups* might consist of consultants in a particular specialty who meet regularly or nurses who get together often to discuss problems on a ward. The advantage is that the group members know each other, but that might also lead to preconceived assumptions. Where these participants are very familiar with each other, they might not disclose their deeper thoughts. Researcher-constituted groups allow researchers to search for specific participants and allow them to exert more control over the composition of the sample. The members are often strangers to each other, which has advantages and disadvantages – the advantage being that they are more open to disclosures, the disadvantage that they might be reserved with each other unless the facilitators have created a relaxed atmosphere.

Group members might be homogeneous or heterogeneous; the former have common interests and often share experiences; the latter could include individuals of different cultures and/or social or economic characteristics. They might also be of different ages, genders, or ethnicities. Of course, these groups overlap – the researcher might choose a homogenous group concerning conditions and treatment, but its membership might be heterogeneous in terms of age or gender. One might also have groups which are mostly homogeneous in terms of age or gender as well as experiences, such as for instance, a group of elderly women with breast cancer, or a group of newly trained oncology nurses.

Some practicalities of focus group research

In large focus groups which explore public health issues, members are sometimes rewarded or compensated for their time and effort, rarely with financial incentives as in market research but by a meal or tea and cake, for instance. In focus group research which is funded by research councils or large charities, members are sometimes paid for their time, as it often involves the public and working people.

Generally, however, researchers rely on good will in research with patients or health professionals. The researcher often finds difficulty in gaining access to the latter, particularly medical staff. In PhD and masters' projects there are few financial resources for participant payment.

The researchers also provide a pleasant environment, a room with the appropriate temperature and few distractions or interruptions, though the discussion can be stopped at an appropriate point, when group members wish to have a rest and refreshments or chat amongst each other.

The discussions

The concept of focus group interview does not reflect the reality of the situation. Discussions or conversations are not synonymous (although they are occasionally called group interviews) with interviews, because a discussion includes the interaction between participants, and the latter term is more often used (Barbour, has a detailed discussion in the introduction to her 2018 book). There may even be brainstorming rather than a completely structured discussion. The researcher, however, often uses some initial questions to relax the group members.

Damon and Holloway (2011), among others, suggest stages in focus group research:

- Introductory stage: warm-up and setting of ground rules
- The main discussion: aim and focus
- A more in-depth debate, instigated by the researcher
- The final stage: summary and thanks

The introductory stage consists of some small talk and perhaps a distribution of refreshments, especially when participants have come from further away. Researchers introduce themselves and the facilitator(s) explain their own task. They confirm the confidential nature of the discussions, which they promised in their recruiting letters. They also stress confidentiality which participants should keep about each other, and the reassure them that nothing will be repeated outside the group. This becomes particularly important when audio- or video-recorders are used. Researchers emphasise that the participants can withdraw at any time of their choosing and that the participation in the group is entirely voluntary. Then, the members of the group introduce themselves to each other. Participants give a short account of their background if they so wish, and this will put them at ease. Researchers will also assure the participants that they will not be judged and that there are no right or wrong comments, answers, or questions during the discussion. Finch, Lewis, & Turley (2014) suggest that researchers and facilitators make sure that everybody knows that they are free to express their ideas and whether they agree or disagree with what is said; indeed, conflicts and disagreements can deepen the research and enhance it, because topics might be investigated further. It is essential that participants have a time frame for the research.

In the main discussion, an opening topic covers the aim and purpose of the research, confirming the earlier letter to the participants. The initial question is of major importance and needs to be as open as possible. For instance: Today we might explore your experience of chronic illness. Can someone start off about their own feelings and thoughts on this? The outcome of one focus group might also provide an opening point for the next one.

The facilitators state that they welcome contributions from the participants and might sometimes produce some stimulus material such as photos, a vignette, a storyline or a video, but this is not always necessary because people are usually ready to discuss their experiences and expectations. Researchers and or facilitators listen carefully – probably one of their most important skills – to make sure that the discussion develops freely and to try to avoid the dominance of a few individuals (all writers on focus group research stress this).

A more *in-depth conversation* will probably follow. The researcher will ask for explanations if something is unclear or cannot be understood, or will prompt gently to develop more in-depth answers ("probing" is a word sometimes used, but one would advise against this, as it implies researcher control. It might also embarrass or hurt some group members). Researchers can also ask for more contributions when some members make relevant comments, and they are invited to ask questions or respond to others. If the participants repeat certain feelings and experiences often and emphatically, they become more important, and themes and patterns will emerge. When the conversation becomes irrelevant to the aim of the research, the facilitator tries to bring it back on focus and reminds the members of the purpose of its focus.

In *the final stage* the researcher or one of the group members - if they are confident enough to volunteer - summarises the discussion, in particular focusing on its purpose. Finally, the members are asked if they have any questions or further comments and thanked for their participation.

The tasks of researchers, moderators, or facilitators

The leader or guide to the focus group is the researcher, sometimes called moderator or facilitator. These terms are often used interchangeably (sometimes both a researcher and a moderator are present, but in qualitative health research this happens rarely because of lack of resources). Facilitator is probably the best label because it means that the discussion is less controlled and more open. It is important that the facilitators have people skills, can listen carefully, is non-judgmental and has the ability to manage the situation. Ground rules need be set at the beginning of the research which all members have to know. This helps prevent chaos and disorganisation. Establishing rapport and creating a relaxed atmosphere are important skills, especially if the group members are strangers to each other, in order to facilitate interaction. It is useful if facilitators develop a guide for the focus groups which they can use when the conversation flags, though the discussion should be as spontaneous and informal as possible.

They have the often difficult task of ensuring that dominant individuals do not take up too much of the discussion and that all individual group members have the opportunity to speak. They also need to ask stimulating questions when the conversation starts to flag or loses focus, diverting from the aim of the research. Indeed, facilitators promote the debate, steer the discussion so it keeps on course, and keeps it focused on the topic.

The timing of focus group discussions can vary depending on the topic, the participants' age, and other features. Older people or the very young might find concentration more difficult, and the duration is often shorter, for instance an hour, while some discussions take as long as three hours, although this is rare. Timing also depends on the importance, relevance or depth of the topic (Finch et al., 2014).

Online or virtual focus groups

Usually, FG research is conducted face-to-face in a room where the researcher, moderator, and group are located. In recent years, however, focus groups have often been conducted online. This means that group discussions take place online to debate a specific topic area for research purposes. This means, of course, that participants need to be computer literate. The research can occur through emails, on Facebook, through instant messaging, or in chatrooms, etc., or by audio-visual groups – through tablets, smart phones or Skype for instance. The advantage of online focus groups is that they allow researchers to gain access to hard-to-reach individuals, and that the group members can stay anonymous if they so wish. Online focus groups are often naturally occurring or pre-existing groups who share a common interest and experience that they discuss often, and researchers may attempt to gain access to these existing groups on the net, although they might also seek participants on Facebook or Twitter.

Online groups can be synchronous, occurring at the same time, or asynchronous, not occurring at the same, but at different times. In the European Journal of Oncology Nursing, Jervaeus, Nilsson, Eriksson, Lampic, Widmark, and Wettergren (2015) employed online focus group research with synchronous participation while investigating childhood cancer survivors' perspectives on sexual experiences and also on their potential needs for support from health professionals. The authors collected data on this as well as on fertility aspects through online focus group discussions in chat rooms. Ripat and Colatruglio (2016) on the other hand, reported from an asynchronous focus group about wheelchair use in winter. A website was left open for seven days and participants were able to communicate with each other as well as respond to ideas. The data were then transcribed verbatim by the researchers and analysed.

As in face to face groups, researchers and moderators help guide the groups by stating its topic and aim.

Recording, analysing and writing up focus group data

The main principles of focus group data analysis are similar to those of other types of qualitative research but they will be more challenging. In general, the researcher records the interviews, of course with the permission of the participants, and listens to them several times. The transcription follows. This is usually done by the researcher/facilitator but often the lack of time demands that another person is used who needs to know about the confidentiality of the discussion on the tape. It is better if researchers and/or facilitators do this themselves as they were present at the discussions and it is difficult to identify individuals' voices on a tape for someone who has not heard them. If the room contains four or more participants the tape recorder has to be in the right position. A poorly recorded discussion is hard to transcribe, and therefore extraneous noises should be cut out – even an open window can be a problem.

If the transcriber wishes to know the identities of the participants, video recording is sometimes used. Video recording also avoids the loss of nonverbal data such as gestures or facial expressions. Sometimes researchers take notes of the discussions without recording it verbatim. This is much more difficult and necessitates at least one other person to distinguish voices and comments. Some writers even recommend that in focus group discussions, a team of researchers should be involved (for instance, Rosenthal, 2016). This also helps the analysis, where team members can compare their own findings and interpretations.

As said before, it is easier to identify group members on video. Sim (1998) suggests that some group members might be reluctant to have the discussion recorded, particularly by video and especially when sensitive issues are involved; to give two examples: a group of vulnerable patients or hospital consultants who debate management issues.

Focus group research generates an even greater volume of data than individual interviews, hence a discussion of one to three hours might take a long time to transcribe, sometimes up to five or seven hours. The researchers label and date recorded files, fieldnotes, and memos. They leave a wide margin on the left on the transcript for comments and initial analysis which also includes observations made during the research, and unusual or contradictory occurrences which are noted. At the listening stage, relevant themes and patterns can be uncovered. The researchers follow through to saturation when no new ideas can be found in the data that are relevant to the aim of the research. Some writers call data saturation "the gold standard" for analysis in qualitative inquiry (Hancock, Amankwaa, Revell, & Mueller, 2016).

As in other types of qualitative research, the frequency of themes and patterns that are found is less important than relevance; some obviously have priority over others for the specific study. The analysts repeat the process with each focus group discussion and compare the findings. This means that they compare the participants' views both within and among groups. The main themes from each will overlap and the overlap might confirm or challenge the researchers' initial assumptions, or uncover new ideas. Once they have interpreted the meaning, they will initiate a debate with the relevant literature. This may corroborate or contest their own findings.

Articles on focus group discussions need a great deal of care. The methodology of these articles is of particular importance. Writers usually describe in detail how the participants were recruited, the number of focus groups, and their group members. Locations and dates might also be of importance as well as observations during the discussions. Typical comments can be quoted, especially if they are insightful and relevant to the aim of the research. Deviant cases and those that are atypical must also be discussed just as much as typical comments (see above and in chapter on QDA).

Ethical issues in FG research

Ethical issues in FG interviews are similar, though not the same, to those for other types of interview. (See chapter on ethical issues). They must be considered carefully before the research starts and negotiated with the group members.

Recruits take part voluntarily and informed consent is needed. This means that they cannot be compelled to take part and can leave at any stage or time in the research process. Participants are also able to refuse permission for their words being quoted, even for the final report.

Each individual agrees from the very beginning that words and interactions are kept confidential. This means that the researcher creates awareness of these issues particularly as confidential or sensitive areas might be uncovered. Group members are reminded of this before, during, and after the process of interviews. Although individual interviews might include more disclosures or discussion of sensitive issues, the interaction between group members means that disclosures are shared between more people and the danger of exposure is greater.

The safety of participants is paramount. The researchers might find this more difficult to achieve in focus group research than in other types of inquiry, especially that concerning emotional safety because more people are involved. Anonymity too can become a problem for this reason, especially when the group members know each other well.

Goodman and Evans (2015) also suggest that there may be unexpected consequences. People might become distressed when they disclose their own perspectives on an issue and researchers need give them time and space to recuperate. This, of course, is more likely in FG with patients.

Goodman and Evans add that the group members' opinions and feelings need be respected. A blog by the American author Kinsey Gimbel, who has been involved in qualitative focus group research in a variety of settings, adds advice for focus groups in health research. She makes a number of points, a few of which are given here:

- Researchers should speak respectfully about participants
- They should not point out mistakes to group members
- They avoid creating tensions
- They protect the privacy of participants

The advantages and problems of focus groups

The advantages of qualitative focus group research are similar to those for other types of inquiry, but differences also exist.

The main strength of this type of inquiry is, of course, the production of data through the dynamic of participant interaction. The participants listen to other group members and think about their own experiences, perceptions, and feelings in relation to those of others and respond to them. The answers might be broader and cover a wider variety of perceptions and feelings than those in individual interviews because of the input from a varied range of people. Some members are encouraged to talk because they feel that they are in a similar position as other group members and wish to contribute their own ideas. Focus group research does encourage spontaneity (Tausch & Menold, 2016).

Another advantage is that *new ideas will be generated in a shorter space of time* as the groups contain a variety of participants at one time. Researchers are able to clarify the ideas with additional questions.

Researchers have not as much control over the process as in in individual interviews, because they exert less influence on the participants. This gives more power to the participants which could be seen as an advantage. One might suggest, however, that weaker control might also be a problem as the discussion might become irrelevant for the purpose of the research and the members need some guidance for the conversation to achieve its aim.

Participants who feel shy might feel safer and more secure in a group of people with similar experience.

Some of the problems of focus group research start to become obvious. *The researcher has more difficulty managing and structuring the debate.* The organisation of focus groups takes time and space, and is often difficult to arrange. The time frame is difficult to judge as all members of the group should be involved. The researcher and/or facilitator must manage the setting and has to remember the original aim of the research, occasionally needing to remind the participants

If individuals of high status are involved, or even people who are very vocal, other, less confident members might be silenced. Those group members who have an alternative view also might be prevented from voicing their feelings, perceptions, and perspectives on the area of interest. Participants do not always wish to discuss controversial or sensitive topics within a group setting – although this could also be true for individual face-to-face interviews. Facilitators need give every individual an opportunity to verbalise their thoughts, and this is not easy, because some individuals tend to dominate the conversation; others may be too shy or introverted, or they could be in awe of the dominant individuals because they are members of an elite. A group of physiotherapists, for instance, might include some management staff members; a group of patients could consist of participants who seem to be well educated and others who feel disadvantaged as they are less articulate.

The researchers cannot investigate the topic in depth because individual ideas are not easy to follow up, and prompting might lead the group to follow their directions.

Final comments

Although focus group research in healthcare is a useful form of inquiry because ideas from a number of people can be gained at the same time, they are less personal than one-to-one interviews. Focus groups might be more superficial than in-depth, unstructured interviews.

Sometimes these interviews might be used because researchers feel this is an easy and popular way of gaining access to a larger sample, and funding agencies seem to welcome the convenience of focus groups. The complexities of setting up and facilitating focus groups are often forgotten. Although the article by Webb and Kevern (2001) was written almost two decades ago, they found rather unsophisticated and uncritical uses of focus group research in their early years and noted that their results were rather nonanalytical. Few articles contained empirical research, and furthermore, some of the discussions were superficial and nonanalytical. This research has improved very much: many more articles include empirical research and are analytical and not superficial. Holloway and Galvin wrote in 2017 that their search uncovered a large number of articles on focus group research in all areas of health research, and a number of books.

Summary of Key Points

- Focus group research is a form of inquiry where small numbers of people with similar experiences discuss a topic of common interest and share their thoughts about this.
- Several focus groups, each with a small number of individuals, are involved in a research project.
- Researchers/facilitators lead the group discussions in a relaxed atmosphere.
- Whilst the discussions are carefully planned, the facilitator needs the skills of flexibility, diplomacy, and tolerance.
- The dynamic and interaction of the group situation is intended to stimulate ideas.
- The data are recorded and analysed through qualitative analysis methods.

References

Arnold R., E. van Teijlingen, K. Ryan, & I. Holloway. (2014) Understanding Afghan healthcare providers: A qualitative study of the culture of care in a Kabul maternity hospital. *BJOG: An International Journal of Obstetrics and Gynaecology,* 22(2), 260–267.

Barbour, R. (2018) *Doing focus groups,* 2nd ed. London: Sage.

Daymon, C., & I. Holloway, (2011). *Qualitative research methods in public relations and marketing communications,* 2nd ed. London: Routledge.

Finch, H., J. Lewis, & C. Turley. (2014) Focus groups. In Richie, R., Lewis, J., Ormston, F., Nicholls, C. & Ormston R. (Eds) *Qualitative research practice: A guide for social science students and researchers,* 2nd ed. London: Sage.

Goodman, C. & E. Evans. (2015) Focus groups. In Gerrish K. & Lathleen J. *Nursing Research.* Chapter 29, pp. 401–412. Oxford: Wiley Blackwell.

Hancock, M.E., L. Amankwaa, M.A. Revell, & D. Mueller. (2016). Focus Group as saturation: A new approach to data analysis. *The Qualitative Report,* 21(11), 2124–2130. Retrieved from nsuworks.nova. edu/tqr/vol21/iss11/13

Holloway, I. & K. Galvin. (2017) *Qualitative research in nursing and healthcare.* Wiley.

Jervaeus, A., J. Nilsson, L. Eriksson, C. Lampic, C. Widmark, & L. Wettergren. (2016) Exploring childhood cancer survivors' views about sex and sexual experiences – findings from focus group discussions. *European Journal of Oncology Nursing, 20*, 165–172.

Klop, H., A.L. Francke, S. Van Dongen, & A.J.E. de Veer. (2018) The views of homeless people and health care professionals on palliative care and the desirability of setting up a consultation service: A focus group study. *Journal of Pain and Symptom Management, 6*(3), 325–336.

Merton, R.K. & P.I. Kendall. (1946) The focused interview. *American Journal of Sociology, 51*, 451–557.

Merton, R. and P. Lazarsfeld. (1950). *Studies in the scope and method of the American soldier.* Glencoe, IL: The Free Press.

Mitchell, K. & P. Branigan. (2000) Using focus groups to evaluate health promotion interventions. *Health Education, 100*(6), 261–268.

Morgan, D. (2019) *Basic and advanced focus groups.* Thousand Oaks: Sage.

Morse, J.M. (2012) *Qualitative health research.* Abingdon, Oxon: Routledge.

Rasmussen, R.B. & K.I. Ro. (2018) How general practitioners understand and handle medically unexplained symptoms: A focus group study. *BMC Family Practice, 19*: 50. doi.org/10.1186/s12875-018-0745-2

Ripat, J. & A. Colatruglio. (2016) Exploring winter community participation among wheelchair users: An online focus group. *Occupational Therapy in Health Care, 30*(1), 95–106.

Rosenthal, M. (2016) Qualitative research methods: Why, when and how to conduct interviews and focus groups. *Currents in Pharmacy Teaching and Learning, 8*(4), 509–516.

Sim, J. (1998) Collecting and analysing qualitative data: issues raised by focus groups. *Journal of Advanced Nursing, 28*(2), 345–352.

Stewart, D.W. & P.N. Shamdasani. (2015) *Focus groups: Theory and practice,* 3rd ed. Thousand Oaks: Sage.

Tausch, A.P. and N. Menold. (2016) Methodological aspects of focus groups in health research: Results of qualitative interviews with focus group moderators. *Global Qualitative Nursing Research, 3*, 1–12.

Thai, C.H., J.M. Taber, A. Oh, A., M. Segar, K. Blake & H. Patrick. (2019) "Keep it realistic": Reactions to and recommendations for physical activity promotion messages from focus groups of women. *American Journal of Health Promotion, 33*(6), 903–911.

Tong, A., P. Sainsbury, S.M. Carter, B. Hall, D. Harris, R. Walker, C. Hawley, S. Chadban, & J.C. Craig. (2008) Patients' priorities for health research: focus group study of those with chronic kidney disease. *Nephrology Dialysis Transplantation, 23*(10), 3206–3214.

Vermeire, E., P. Van Royen, F. Griffiths, S. Coenen, L. Peremans, & K. Hendricks. (2002) The critical appraisal of focus group research articles. *European Journal of General Practice, 8*(3), 104–108.

Webb, C. and Kevern, J. (2001) Focus groups as a research method: a critique of some aspects of their use in nursing research. *Journal of Advanced Nursing, 33* (6), pp.798–805.

Further reading

Barbour, R.S. & D. Morgan. (Eds) (2017) *A new era in focus group research: Challenges, innovations and practice.* London: Palgrave Macmillan.

Cyr, J. (2019) *Focus groups for the social science researcher.* Cambridge, UK: Cambridge University Press.

Flynn, R., L. Albrecht, & S.D. Scott. (2018) Two approaches to focus group data collection for qualitative health research: *International Journal of Qualitative Methods, 7*, 1–9.

Krueger, R.A. & M.A. Casey. (2015) *Focus groups: A practical guide for applied research.* Thousand Oaks, CA: Sage.

PART XIII

Multiple methods

30

BECOMING A PHYSICIAN OF THE PEOPLE IN A RURAL MOUNTAIN COMMUNITY IN MEXICO

Deirdre Guthrie

I didn't think twice when presented with the opportunity to do my social service year with (name of organization). I was part of the third generation of pasantes ... And I am now among the 90 percent of them who have decided to stay working with the team after the end of the social service year. That year exposed me to a transformative education: I learned to see disease as a social illness as well as a biological disturbance.[1]

~ *Excerpt from promotional article*

Introduction

An estimated 82 percent of rural primary care clinics in Mexico are under the purview of the Ministry of Health (MOH) and operated by "*pasantes*" who are often neglected by medical school and MOH officials because they are simply "passing by": post-internship, but not yet medical residents. They usually do not receive continuing education, training, or support. Meanwhile they face many challenges—medication stock-outs, black-outs, roads closed due to mudslides, or the expectation to provide care for complex illnesses without any functional team. As one supervisor explained, "to go to a marginalized community in the first place is a punishment. Those with the highest grades go to the larger, urban, better-equipped clinics. And those with the lowest grades are placed in the 'worst' clinics in the remote areas where people need medical care the most. And they don't want to be there. They see it as a punishment."

While Mexico has universal healthcare, resource-poor communities lack access to quality care. Hospitals and clinics, often located far away from rural mountain communities, are inadequately supplied and under-staffed. According to a supervisor, "The hospital here near base camp is always lacking medicines or they are expired. The personnel is often rude and dismissive with our community members. And the surgeon comes to work when he wants to, and often re-routes patients into his private practice [where he can charge them a higher fee]." CES seeks to reverse this national model, recruiting high-ranking students to work with clinical support and ongoing education in these high-need, remote, rural clinics, introducing them to the field of global health in the process. CES has expanded their primary care treatment for community residents to include patient referral and "right to health" programs, mental health services, along with a midwifery and maternal care center.

Healthcare practitioners readily admit to the challenges of living out their social justice values in daily practice during the *pasantia* but, for the majority who remain committed to the fraught process of social justice, their work remains a calling and source of inspiration. This chapter, drawn from practitioner field diaries and interviews across ten clinics in rural Mexico, analyzes how *pasantes*, with a newly politicized awareness from everyday experience with community members, begin to see themselves as not just physicians but global health providers.

From dehumanizing medical internship to humanizing accompaniment

When new *pasantes* arrive at the modest two-story building that serves as the organization's base of operations, with its cracked paint, iron bars to discourage thieves, and mosquito nets to lower the chances of getting chikungunya (a kind of "dengue-fever lite" most contract anyway), they have had little to no training on the political aspects of "global medicine," with its emphasis on structural violence and social determinants of health.[2] The majority have limited prior experience bringing medical resources or treatment to poor people in rural sites. And "some of them come with bad habits they've learned from the broader medical education system," admits one supervisor. While expressing an overall appreciation for medical internships' immersive learning, many were disturbed by the culture of privilege and entitlement that reproduced established hierarchies, which they later recognized in the clinics and hospitals that were supposed to serve community members.

"For me, the question as to what I really stood for began early on," said a supervisor, whose father had grown up poor and with a strong sense of justice and ethics. He described medical school as "traumatic" because cheating was rampant and instructors "did nothing." He took a semester off to backpack and read a lot of Carl Sagan and Mark Twain. A *pasante* who interned in the largest public hospital in Mexico was forthright. "I totally hated it. It was … huge …, pavilions with 100 meters of beds in rows … . Nobody cares about the patients. There is no place for imagination or critical thinking … like if you notice something that should be done in a different way you cannot say anything … . I really hated it."

Once they arrive, *pasantes* are assigned to a mountain community where they live and work out of one of the MOH clinics. They shadow former *pasantes* for two weeks and then work alongside *acompañantes* (trained community members) and a nurse. Clinical supervisors will visit at least twice a month to guide more complicated medical decisions. A U.S.-based supervisor explains, "I love my role … because … young physicians … are so open to learn … . We need to help them clinically but also socially and emotionally guide them to become better physicians."

But supervisors also know the support they are extending is limited, given the geographical and staff constraints. "In the U.S. system you're never turned alone on a patient. A supervisor is always 5–10 minutes away," continues the supervisor. "But … sometimes the best I can do is a WhatsApp or phone conversation during critical situations with patients. Just yesterday a clinician was texting me that a 2-month-old weighs only 6 pounds, is in real danger for malnutrition and needs surgery. The parents have given up on the public system … and the *pasante* was frustrated and faulting them. And this happens. The young physician doesn't know how to deal with parents who don't understand the implications of not following through with a procedure. Navigating them through all of this via text isn't sufficient."

Another recalls what it was like before supervisors or a referral system existed. "There were times when I was completely alone and the only option was to call [a founding member of the organization] and he would call somebody else or search on the Internet for answers. We didn't have connections within the hospital. And so mostly people didn't get what they needed. And well, I think a lot of *pasantes* still sometimes feel abandoned and complain that we didn't help them solve this problem. For me, I realized that I was [the organization's representative] within my community, and that problem had to be solved within the community, with my help. And gradually you start to feel more confident about your qualifications. So it just gets better with time."

Ultimately, the *pasantes* who "make it" exhibit a few consistent qualities: adaptability, flexibility, an ability to deal with uncertainty, and an openness to integration with their communities. It also helps to have had some previous experience living in a rural setting, including lights out by 9 p.m. and a deafening nocturnal silence amidst the dizzying panorama of mountains and stars, an atmosphere many twenty-something urbanites on their first extended journey away from home find initially unnerving.

Others thrive in the isolation. "I have never devoted this much to a community or to myself," said another *pasante* who described the experience like a kind of retreat. "I've never been able to read this much or play my cello. I have had time to think, to live in a peaceful environment, to fight my own demons [smiles]." This *pasante* recalled "highlights" as more quotidian moments. "Like one day we brought a brigade of medicine to a community of ranch workers during our free days. It was very rewarding to be with these people. They didn't need any critical treatment but they were so grateful. On the drive back I remember feeling *lleno* [full]. My heart was warm, the night was falling. It was a little thing we did but I felt satisfied. I still remember that feeling, *lleno*." For many *pasantes* the prospect of accompanying community members through disease and healing re-instills a sense of purpose; they become not merely physicians but global health activists.

Catalyzing meaning

Humanitarian work is often described as a vocation, where, in the abstract, meaning is bound up with human-rights values that affirm a belief in the dignity of the whole person, and practiced, in the case of *pasantes*, in daily life to guide the medical encounter. Historically the term "vocation" includes an ethic of public service and renunciation which morally fuses service work with one's life. It may be distinguished from a "career," which is often motivated more by gaining compensation in various ways: power, title, authority, and salary.[3] "Vocation" and "career" may overlap or supersede one another at different life stages. But humanitarian workers who seek to redress global health disparities must align work and their core values, affirming moral motives in addition to craft and compensation motives, to sustain their commitment. In other words, these young professionals are motivated by actualizing deep levels of meaning in their work, in addition to refining their technical skills as clinicians or acquiring the social status that coincides with being a physician or specialist.

A key feature that catalyzes this meaning-making process for *pasantes* is "transformative education," a humanistic curriculum facilitated at the end of each month by organizational leaders, which contextualizes both the broader sociopolitics and their own positions. *Pasantes* return from their communities to bunk at headquarters and reunite with their colleagues for an intensive weekend before enjoying a few days off. In addition to processing case studies and gaining clinical education, they explore the psychosocial aspects of medical care and begin to make sense of what they are experiencing with patients. Documentary films prompt discussions about becoming change agents in a society marked by structural violence and suffering.

According to one supervisor, "We have a term for what we know is coming, when they will have to face their limitations in terms of what they can do in service, and they face the enormity of need from those they serve. It often happens early, around the third month of the internship. We call it … facing *la enormidad,* the enormity." Another supervisor explained, "… when you begin to understand the complexity of the system, and all the people and institutions involved in its failures and those gaps … from the colonies to the World Bank and structural adjustments to the impact of global warming and the coffee markets on local coffee producers to the current health system and bureaucracies and all the power structures, you realize, you just have to concentrate on what you *can* do."

Despite the challenges of confronting *la enormidad,* a founder says, "We see our transformative education program as a way to re-humanize what is often experienced as a dehumanizing internship. We hope it will help *pasantes* regain their faith in humanity by introducing them to this exciting new field of global health." Global health, as defined by *pasantes* and leaders, means:

> **Health as a human right:** "It is absolutely unacceptable and unethical to have different qualities of healthcare, especially if these different qualities are offered according to the purchase power of the individual or patient … ."
>
> **Quality of care:** "Providing patients with the best evidence-based medical option without regard to cost, and delivering that care with empathy. Seeing the person as a whole. What I'd want for myself or my family."
>
> **Humane treatment with respect and dignity**: "This means these souls are human beings and deserve a lot. Respect means 'a little bit of empathy' to try to understand them but to also know we are not the same and to recognize the differences too, that we won't always be able to understand or stand with them … ."
>
> **Preferential option for the poor through accompaniment:** "Solidarity, a focus away from 'compliance' with our treatment prescriptions and, instead, using medical intervention as a statement of solidarity for those who are entitled to healthcare but disenfranchised by the broader social political system."

If the transformative education is a key formative space, a second feature that catalyzes meaning-making and fulfillment during the *pasantia* is *the container of the field.* For *pasantes,* this consists of mostly rural coffee-plantation communities, resource-poor, geographically isolated, and often lacking infrastructure like paved roads or reliable electricity. But as professionals are promoted they find themselves distanced from the field. As one founder put it wryly, recalling the days when he used to deliver medicine up in the Sierras by caravan, sleeping under the stars on the bed of his pickup truck, "I used to find meaning every day in my work. And now I spend all my time assuring that others have meaning." Clinical supervisors worry they will "forget" the truths they assimilated as they advance their medical careers.

Accompaniment in theory

For *pasantes,* "accompaniment" translates into living for one year in highland communities, sleeping in clinics or a neighbor's home. This "container of the field" in which they work and practice accompaniment, combined with the transformational education weekends that create a discursive space to reflect upon and analyze their own positions in the medical encounter, creates a dynamically unstable and productive *pasantia* experience.

In many ways "accompaniment," derived from a theological vocabulary, combines all the values of the humanistic work *pasantes* are engaged in and may be seen as the latest relational model of care that aspires to incorporate iterative dialogical processes and community voices in medical practice. An indispensable feature of the *pasantia* is the involvement of *acompañantes*, respected women from the community who have the social skills and authority to broker and translate medical knowledge to community people. "More than this, they are 'knowledge with legs' or 'walking knowledge,'" says their coordinator, "visiting families daily at their homes to discuss their health." *Acompañantes* fill a critical gap in a model "designed around patients and communities rather than disease and medical systems."[4]

During diagnosis, as part of the doctor-patient interaction, accompaniment calls upon relational capacities such as empathy and what Humanistic Nursing refers to as enacting "presence," a mode of being available or open in a situation with the wholeness of one's being. In this way accompaniment represents a move toward a more empowered doctor-patient interaction and away from paternalism. As an ideal, it may set up the conditions, a discursive space, in which a patient might construct her identity and represent herself.[5] Accompaniment may include active listening, the laying on of hands, emotional support, moral solidarity and responsibility, and affirming the patient's humanity, and is inherent in those who are "called" into their work from a private to public space of caretaking. According to Arthur Kleinman (in a 2015 lecture to my students at Western Michigan University), those who enact "presence" in accompaniment feel alive and are energized: "It's what makes care non-mechanical, gives care a vividness, a fullness."

According to Paul Farmer (2006), accompaniment involves "an element of mystery, of openness … . I'll go with you and support you on your journey wherever it leads." In its enactment of liberation theological principles, which ask that practitioners "opt for the poor" and thereby "place ourselves *there,* to accompany the poor person in his or her life, death, and struggle for survival," it breaks from colonial-era development and aid models that reified the power of the medical establishment, intellectual community, or organized religion as rescuer-benefactors.[6] But this type of interaction also requires a physical proximity in which to actualize accompaniment.

Farmer quotes theologian Roberto Goizueta (2009) to illustrate this critical point of proximity: "As a society, we are happy to help and serve the poor, as long as we don't have to walk *with* them where they walk, that is, as long as we can minister to them from our safe enclosures. The poor can then remain passive objects of our actions, rather than friends, *compañeros* and *compañeras* with whom we interact. As long as we can be sure that we will not have to live with them, and thus have interpersonal relationships with them … we will try to help 'the poor'— but, again, only from a controllable, geographical distance" (192).

Physical proximity to those *pasantes* serve in the field catalyzes a kind of "truth process."[7] It allows for certain encounters between doctor and patient that would be impossible in a traditional clinic setting where one retreats each evening into one's (upper-middle class) home and community. The field, to paraphrase Jacques Lacan, punches a "'hole' [trouée] in one's [institutional truth] knowledges" (Legrand, 2018, 43) and may even threaten to unmoor one's previously coherent identity. The truth process can be uncomfortable, painful, or even intolerable. When faced with social injustice or the arbitrariness of one's own social position, there is no retreat, so one is forced to reconcile with the revelation of complicity in an exploitative system.

After two years in global health a clinical supervisor observed, "it is hard because … you realize that you're part of this oppression and unequal mechanism. And I was really trying to not harm in any way … And then I go back and I see how my family is in a whole different reality within that privileged society, and that mechanism. At first it was hard for me to connect with them and even to love them. Not that I didn't love them, but it was a conflict that—how can I love these people so much if they are harming these other people that I love so much too? And I mean, not that I am the good one, but it's just like, how can these two realities coexist?

And being in the middle of both realities also. It was hard." However, those who can hold this space of discomfort and contradiction and not retreat into apathy or cynicism may enter a new field of possible lived-relationships.

Accompaniment in practice: the art of medicine

Accompaniment in practice in resource-poor contexts is hard. As any humanitarian or social justice community organizer knows, simply informing people of their human rights doesn't result in automatic empowerment. In fact, patients may actually insist upon traditional hier-archies. Female *pasantes*, for example, were often frustrated when their female patients ignored family planning advice and deferred to the decision-making leadership of their husbands. Another *pasante* felt "between deflated and angry" when his patients "begged" for care. "I try to tell them respectfully, 'You don't have to beg me because your health is your right and you deserve it. So I'm going to stand with you'... . And well, it shows me how much they've been mistreated."[8]

"Breaking bread and walking with" community members is further challenged when they refuse or disregard a prescribed course of treatment. When asked for an estimate of how many patients are medication-compliant, a clinical supervisor said, "I think it's less than half. Even less than a third. But they're compliant with treatment in that they receive visits from *acompañantes* and they go to their appointment at the clinic, even if they don't take the medicine all the time. So when that happens I'm okay as long as the patient is progressing."[9] It makes sense that *pasantes* struggle when community members disregard their medical advice or seek outside opinions from shamans or healers who promise cheap, instant cures or symptom-alleviation. It undermines *pasantes'* fledgling confidence as authoritative practitioners and exposes the contradictions between a biomedical system and the humanist model of care espoused by global health ideology. Ideally, a *pasante* has the time and sensitivity to guide each patient to an informed treatment decision. But accompaniment in practice may involve a softening of the sometimes heroic expectations surrounding the "change agent," while not necessarily relinquishing the agent's intention to change systems. A "good enough" accompaniment approach allows *pasantes* to negotiate a treatment plan with patients while accepting limitations as they try to bridge the gulf between lay and biomedical knowledge systems and administer treatment with whatever resources are on hand.

A commonly used modern version of the Hippocratic oath states: "I will remember that there is art to medicine as well as science, and that warmth, sympathy, and understanding may outweigh the surgeon's knife or the chemist's drug." In this vein, *pasantes* learn creativity. For example, a supervisor writes prescriptions for pharmaceuticals along with traditional remedies prescribed by folk healers (herbal teas or compresses, etc.) as long as they are not contraindicated. And a *pasante* describes in his field diary how he prescribed that an ill and isolated older man should "eat with his daughter daily and receive a hug," then demonstrated by taking the man in his arms (much to his surprise). His daughter later thanked the *pasante* for brokering this oppor-tunity for her to embrace her father before he died.

Community members have their own ways of describing physical and emotional pain. People spoke in terms of "hot" and "cold" illness, or symptoms ranging from fever, insomnia, to diarrhea caused by "susto," a kind of spirit attack which may lead to "chronic somatic suffering stemming from emotional trauma or from witnessing traumatic experiences lived by others" (Razzouk, Nogueira, & de Jesus Mari, 2011). A *pasante* recalls how a woman who complained of lethargy placed her hands on her heart and explained, "I have too small of a heart. It does not have enough strength." He realized she had depression. Other illnesses were believed to originate inside the navel. "Inside the umbilical cord there's a tendon which goes from the belly button to the liver" explained one supervisor with Maya relatives. The Maya see this inner opening as a portal connecting a person with the universe and one's mother.

In order to bridge these gaps in knowledge systems, the *acompañantes'* coordinator taught basic medical components of chronic disease in a way that community members would understand and be able to translate to patients. And he had to instruct *pasantes* to let go of many of the models they memorized in school: "For example, with…diabetes it is not important for the patient to know about interceptors. We don't talk much about insulin and the pancreas because you don't see the pancreas so how are you going to understand? So when we explain diabetes, we use the metaphor of a house. The house is your body and the sugar is the rain, and the ceiling is your pancreas. So after a lot of rain, water begins to fall into your house…so how you can restore the ceiling? Well you need a new one but there is no new pancreas so how do you make patches to the ceiling? Well, with medication, and trying to not eat too much sugar and tortillas which is the rain… ."

But he admitted that convincing patients of this diagnosis, when symptoms may subside for a time and then re-occur, is difficult. "With patients, sometimes talking to them about disease is a slow process, and it takes time for a patient to be ready to hear you. Also there are respected people in the community, midwives, shamans, who say chronic disease such as diabetes and hypertension are curable with a certain kind of vitamin … . People tend to believe what they experience, which is pretty understandable, and who wants to give up their tortillas and coffee with sugar?"

Another clinical supervisor, who self-identified as "mestiza," offered some unique insight into this area of compliance and the doctor-patient interaction. Her indigenous aunt and uncle had told her, "'Half that you do with the medicine will heal them, but the other half will be the faith that they put in you.' And actually, at the end of the year working there, I used to go and drink coffee with Don Andres, the shaman, and after a while he would refer patients to me. He would write simple notes which said, 'Doctor, I already did this and that and I think he has this and this syndrome … .'"

I asked her how *pasantes* she mentored struggled with accepting a lay view of the body and health. One of her mentees had earlier expressed strong frustration with his patients' noncompliance. He was now six months into his service year. She grinned and said, "A few weeks ago he texted me and said, 'You are not going to believe this, but I have started to write on my prescriptions your psycho-magical stuff [the vitamin and herb drinks] along with the medicines and it works! They are taking it.'" She grabbed her iPhone. "And look at this!"

She showed me a photo of an older woman sitting like a guardian on the edge of the *pasante's* bed, pressing a hot compress to his forehead. "He had a terrible migraine that day and none of our injections gave him relief. This woman, she waited quietly in the back of the clinic waiting room until we were done and then asked, very humbly, if she could apply these hot compresses, bathed in herbs, to his forehead. I looked at him and he shrugged weakly and agreed. Within 20 minutes he was feeling better. I took this photo of her watching over him. He told me later, 'Maybe it helped because it reminded me of my mom taking care of me.'"

Stories like this remind us of the kind of *intercambio* or reciprocal exchange that can take place in the context of community when both parties are open to benefitting from the exchange. The *acompañante* coordinator, who hosts a local radio/TV show and volunteers at a rehab clinic in his off hours, often tells *pasantes* that "If you create a safe space for community people, play with their kids, make tortillas in their kitchens, spend time with their families, you will see they are full of ideas for how to improve their health and lives." He goes on, "And we see clearly that the better connection a *pasante* has with his/her community, the higher the level of community member investment, *confianza* (social trust), mutual respect, *acompañante* participation, and the better the community health outcome."

La enormidad: hitting the wall and confronting limitations

Treating the "whole person" and "meeting a patient where they are at," when opportunities for patients to escape extreme poverty are severely limited and forces of structural violence are institutionalized and hegemonic, is also very difficult. Sometimes *pasantes* "hit the wall" from sheer exhaustion after months of fifteen-hour days. But often the break comes from emotional stress and ethical worries over diagnosing a patient, particularly when there is no clear referral option or treatment means/resources.

The physical geography of the mountains and remote locations of these communities are a constant limitation that *pasantes* and supervisors must reconcile as they attempt to refer patients with serious conditions. Even when *pasantes* and supervisors are able to manage [through the "right to health" system] a referral, the patient may say "enough." A *pasante* described how difficult it was for him to accept when a patient, a man in his 30s, finally refused treatment for colon cancer. The *pasante* learned secondhand that the young man had decided after four years of fighting the cancer and making eight-hour drives to dialysis that he was tired. The specialist believed he would die within a few months without surgery. "I was angry at first that we had put so much effort and resources on him, that he didn't want to fight for his life … it's difficult, you really want to see the outcome, to see that they want to fight for their lives and overcome this disease … but with every patient you have, you treat, they are the final decision-maker, you have to respect that … all you can do is give them choices so they can make an informed decision and that's it … .We did everything at our disposal. We searched for the doctor, we searched for the labs, for the appointments, for everything. We told him about all the options but at the end he decided not to go through with any of these."

From rupture to calling

Accompaniment can seem like a futile or weak gesture some days. And recognizing one's limits when faced with the enormity of need in a seemingly unfair and arbitrary system may lead to a kind of apathy or cynicism which *pasantes* (and leaders) must struggle through. One of the most moving stories I heard was about a supervisor and *pasante* who spent a night driving an HIV-positive patient through the mountains, taking turns with a hand ventilator to keep him breathing ("when my hands cramped up, I'd hand the ventilator to her and get back on the phone trying to find a place that would admit him") to various clinics where he was denied because they were either closed or didn't have functioning equipment, until finally the patient died. "She [the *pasante*] was crying and I told her, listen, the system here in Mexico is closed to poor people, there is no social justice for them. You have an opportunity to interrupt this. And now she's an amazing right-to-health coordinator. And that's what still inspires me, that I feel I'm part of a world global movement where we have the opportunity to change the lives of people, and we must take it."

According to one of the organization's founders, most medical staff eventually re-gain faith, either motivated by spiritual beliefs or the global health justice movement (or both). "I think there are two ways in which you can live," he says. "One is guided by your belief the universe has an order and the other is that it's based on chance. They provide very different life experiences. The problem when you think things happen by chance is you can never eliminate fear." He felt that most of us believe somewhere in between order and chance, but that those who believed that life was random were more fearful, and therefore more apt to try to control the uncontrollable, a sure exercise in frustration.

He continued: "The social global health movement itself is founded on liberation theology. Personally I believe people who do not have a spiritual background have a much harder time doing this kind of work. From the materialistic point of view there is no point in trying to realize this work, to get a return on your investment. It's a waste of time when you could be gathering other experiences." But those who did not describe themselves as believers still found inspiration in the work, in remarkable mundane moments that were life-affirming and led to feeling *lleno*. One clinical supervisor recalled, "There was a day when I had a patient that had a tumor in his hand, an enormous bone tumor … . He hadn't been able to get it treated … because, even though the doctors were willing to do it, there weren't beds available inside the hospital. So for two days we, the patient, the driver, and I, were there at the hospital, waiting and asking for help … . We were running all over the hospital talking to people from social work and the director … . Finally we spoke to the doctor who said, 'Bring him in.'

"Meanwhile," she went on, teary-eyed at the memory, in their absence "the patient was sitting on the floor of the waiting room until something shook him and he stood up, alone, and said, 'I'm not going to move from here until somebody gives me a bed.' He crossed his arms and said that he wouldn't move … . So, when I got back to tell him that I had … found a doctor who would treat him, I saw him already wearing a blue robe because he had defended his rights … . That's one of the most important achievements of the Right to Health program. Sometimes we can be very paternal with patients, and there are patients that literally ask you to hold their hands or get in line for them, or demand things for them, be like their mother. So, when a patient acknowledges … that their health is their right and they have to defend it, for me it's one of the biggest achievements … ." This patient recovered.

Conclusion

One *pasante* wrote in his field diary that the service year created "a space to both lose and find yourself." There are few festivities or distractions and *pasantes* are privy to so much suffering and aspiration that sometimes *la enormidad* comes rushing in. At times the needs seem Herculean in their scope. *Pasantes* know that much is beyond their control, due to the effects of structural violence, structures that implicate them, structures, that, previous to their education in global health, may have seemed so ordinary they often appeared invisible. And one must reckon with the meaning of it all.

But *pasantes* are deeply humanized through their unique and imperfect yet remarkable caring work. The life-affirming way they learn to identify with their work in the space of community and transformative education elicits a kind of hope much needed in the world that resonates with the aspirational concept articulated by Rebecca Solnit (2016): "It's important to say what hope is not: it is not the belief that everything was, is, or will be fine. The evidence is all around us of tremendous suffering and tremendous destruction. The hope I'm interested in is about broad perspectives with specific possibilities, ones that invite or demand that we act. It's also not a sunny everything-is-getting-better narrative, though it may be a counter to the everything-is-getting-worse narrative. You could call it an account of complexities and uncertainties, with openings" (xiii).

In the bardo of the existential unknown there is faith that what *pasantes* are doing matters even when medical outcomes are inconsistent or unclear. After that HIV-positive patient died in the truck, despite all the nocturnal efforts of the supervisor and his *pasante*, the family of the young man embraced them. "They were moved by how much effort had been made to try to save their son," said another supervisor. The way practitioners buoy one other as comrades in the struggle cannot be underestimated. Seeing the tireless commitment of each other's efforts was cited often as a source of inspiration among *pasantes* and leaders alike. One *pasante*, after a difficult day, received a surprise visit from a fellow volunteer which warmed her spirit:

> And even though I look outside my window and sometimes I'm scared of the enormity in which I'm in, I see mountains and mountains, and I feel like I'm lost in the middle of nowhere, suddenly these things happen and make you see that, after all, you are not alone and that far away. And … well, it makes you feel like you're part of something bigger than you think, and you're part of a team that is really a team. Many times at school you work in teams or doing surgery at a hospital, but it's only for a short time. Here it's all the time, it's constant, like knowing and being convinced that if something happens, your team is going to be there to support you. Because the number one thing, the most basic thing is that we share the vision and the ideals that we are here for, fighting for equality, for social justice, to bring high quality health services that gives preference for the poor. I think that's something that unites us all; all of us here share those ideals and vision.

Transcendence, a connecting with something greater that allows us to rest in the knowledge that we are all in this together, that the seeds we are planting will indeed grow and bear fruit, even if we may not see it within our lifetimes, can be a powerful social glue and anchor. Solnit (2016) uses the metaphor of the mushroom to describe how this incubating evolution towards a higher purpose can spread from the shadows: "After a rain mushrooms appear on the surface of the earth as if from nowhere. Many do so from a sometimes vast underground fungus that remains invisible and largely unknown. What we call mushrooms mycologists call the fruiting body of the larger, less visible fungus … . Uprisings and revolutions are often considered to be spontaneous, but less visible long-term organizing and groundwork—or underground work— often laid the foundation" (xv).

Perhaps the best definition of accompaniment I have heard to date, which might inform not just the doctor-patient interaction but all ways of affirming human connection, came from the "mestiza-doctor" I interviewed, who was describing Mayan notions of personhood: "The Mayan greeting 'In Lak'ech Ala K'in' means 'I am you, and you are me' or 'You are another Me'. Both are ways of honoring the other." There is a cultural underpinning of personhood that agrees we are all one, connected, though we've cut the cord and forgotten. In this way, the service year of the *pasantia* is a gift of remembering.

Acknowledgments

Special thanks to the Director, Supervisors and Pasantes from Companeros en Salud for sharing their struggles, aspirations and experiences with me with such thoughtfulness and candor. There is no need to mention Spore Studios as I was still working at the University at this time..

Notes

1 The Lancet Commission for Health Professions Education called for efforts at medical education reform to be guided by two main principles: transformative (rather than only informative or formative) learning, and interdependent and interdisciplinary education.
2 Structural violence is a term coined in the 1960s to describe social structures that result in disparate access to resources, political power, education, healthcare, and legal standing. These structures seem so ordinary they are often invisible (Farmer 2006).

3 A third motive is "craft," which centers around honing one's skills and experiencing the pleasure of work for its own sake. This motive is increasingly threatened by market and bureaucratic forces (see Overell 2018).

4 *Acompañantes* have been written about extensively elsewhere. They have carved out respected roles within the communities, wearing their official shirts and carrying medical bags, and do most of the critical follow-up with patients to encourage their participation in improving their health. In October 2015 there were fifty *acompañantes* across six communities, focusing on education about chronic disease, nutrition, and mental health. In January 2016 they were learning psychosocial models and cognitive therapy strategies to support mental health, including their own. According to the mental health coordinator, a large percentage of *acompañantes* were diagnosed with depression themselves when they first joined the program.

5 A dialogic encounter between doctor and patient is understood as a conversational transaction or negotiation that has taken place between the doctor's initial hypothesis and the patient's opportunity to unfold the narrative according to her own explanatory system. The result of this dialogic process is discursive space for the patient to construct her identity and to represent herself (Delbene, 2015, 5).

6 This is captured in Rosario Castellanos's 1950–60s writings about the doctor and his assistant at the Indian Aid Commission, the anthropologist at the Mission of Charity, and the linguistic expert brought in to translate the Bible into Tzeltal for the "organization" in the Sierra highlands.

7 For Badiou "a truth-process" is heterogenous to the instituted knowledges of the situation. So the revelation of a truth is a kind of break or rupture—one is jolted out of what one knew or lived, into a new place, a new series of possible lived-relationships. Hence, how one responds to this opening is what counts, because often (if not even "normally") these openings are foreclosed upon.

8 Culturally, *pasantes* were uncomfortable with behavior they viewed as sexist, homophobic, and cruel to animals (many were vegetarians). Still, many were able to carve out a professional niche from which to work and negotiate friendships with individuals who, in some cases, even became close enough to be considered family.

9 This estimate of non-compliance raises questions around how effective these medicines will be for the chronic conditions like diabetes, hypertension, and depression for which they are prescribed.

References

Delbene, R. 2015. "Listening to 'How the Patient Presents Herself': A Case Study of a Doctor–Patient Interaction in an Emergency Room." *Journal of Education and Training Studies* 3(10), 5–6.

Farmer, P. 2011. "Accompaniment as Policy." Kennedy School of Government, Harvard University, May 25, 2011, www.lessonsfromhaiti.org/press-and-media/transcripts/accompaniment-as-policy.

Farmer, P. 2011, October 24. Re-imagining accompaniment: Global health and liberation theology – Conversation between Paul Farmer and Father Gustavo Gutiérrez. Ford Family Series, Notre Dame University, South Bend, IN, USA.

Goizueta, R. 2009. *Christ our Companion: Toward a Theological Aesthetics of Liberation.* Maryknoll, NY: Orbis Books.

Legrand, D. 2018. "The Violence of the Ethical Encounter: Listening to the Suffering Subject as a Speaking Body." *Continental Philosophy Review* 51(1), 43–64.

Overell, S. 2018. "Inwardness: The Rise of Meaningful Work." *Provocation Series* 4 (2), nanopdf.com/download/inwardness-the-rise-of-meaningful-work_pdf.

Razzouk, D., B. Nogueira, & J. de Jesus Mari. 2011. "The Contribution of Latin American and Caribbean Countries on Culture Bound Syndromes Studies for the ICD-10 Revision: Key Findings from a Work in Progress." *Revista Brasileira de Psiquiatria* 33(Suppl 1), S5–20, doi:10.1590/S1516-44462011000500003.

Solnit, R. 2016. *Hope in the Dark: Untold Histories, Wild Possibilities.* Expanded edition. New York: Nation Books.

31

BREAKING DOWN SILOS

The value of interdisciplinary production of knowledge for (health) innovation

Tamira Snell

To study a culture,… means not to analyse the habits, customs, beliefs, ideas and arts in an enclosed and isolated place, but to investigate the connections and disconnections, the circulations and movements, the ups and downs that make a culture a living culture above and beyond its singular location

(Oswell, Culture and Society, p. 9)

The struggle over meaning and the power of language

The first time I started working with social science methods in a corporate setting was in a management consultancy specialised in growth strategy. I had been hired to integrate qualitative methods, primarily ethnography, as well as to develop a framework for applying mega trends into the strategic advisory processes of the company, and I remember spending the first months participating in meetings where unknown words and concepts seemed like they were flying through the air. I was constantly trying to grasp them and make meaning of them.

From the beginning I had turned to the husband of a close friend of mine who was partner in a competing consultancy firm, asking him for books that could guide me in this new field, clearly sensing I had entered a culture where I did not yet know the cultural codes, nor the language. Different fields of work are often rooted in different theoretical and academic disciplines, whereby different cultures accompany them, and require different forms of capital.

In order to fit in I was trying hard to learn the new language, but at the same time I knew that I would always have an accent that would tell my corporate colleagues that I was not one of "them". Language, as we know from Foucault (1972), is closely linked to knowledge and discourse and the construction of power, and I quickly understood that most work cultures rest on the need of an *imagined community* (Anderson, 1991), where other ways of sense and meaning-making can be experienced as destabilising discourse. I was the minority trying to implement change, and in that process, I learned that it was crucial to know and communicate clearly the specific value of the qualitative and explorative methods (and ways of thinking) I was bringing to the table in order to be accepted by corporate culture. Just as important, I myself had to open up to other ways of seeing the world. I had to apply my own methods-toolbox on myself and explore and question my own perceptions, construction of knowledge, and prejudices to allow other views in. In the words of Clifford Geertz, it became an (self)interpretive analysis in search of meaning:

> ... man [sic] is an animal suspended in webs of significance he himself has spun and I take culture to be those webs, and the analysis to be therefore not an experimental science in search of law but an interpretive one in search of meaning.
>
> *(Geertz, 1973: 5; cited in Walsh, 2004: 227)*

As such, my entry into corporate life became an ethnography in itself. An ongoing process of understanding its culture, its people, and how different cultures of knowledge and meaning-making can manage to co-exist and allow space for one another.

However, the most important lesson is by far the experience that the potential of working interdisciplinary with various methods can succeed in translating the manifold of knowledges into more valuable in-depth deliverables. Especially working with innovation and strategy within a health context where the understanding of people, their behaviour, values and beliefs, patterns of consumption, and lifestyles is moving more and more into the centre of attention.

In recent decades there has been an increasing focus for businesses in general on the user of their products, services, or offerings, which has been just as present working in the field of health and healthcare. It might have helped to create a pull and demand from corporate organizations to acquire more knowledge from various perspectives and disciplines. As such, the shift that has occurred is a movement towards an interdisciplinary orientation within different spheres of applied academic research practice in both public and private arenas with a shared approach to driving insight, problem solving, and creating solutions that increasingly seeks mixed research methods and analytic processes.

It is this journey I am a part of, where my own ethnography on the triangulation of methods unfolds and the source of my experiences into the struggles over meaning-making takes its beginning.

In this field, methods play a vital role, because it is exactly through the use of methods that we can create insights and knowledge about a specific field. But it is also exactly in these methodological decisions and processes that the meaning made can be challenged, especially when the cultures of knowledge, that have to work together and have to move from theory into practice, are different. However, when meaning is challenged, a space also opens up for deeper insights that can provide us with the ability to actually move forward and change something.

In the context of this chapter, I wish to reflect on the application of ethnography and other exploratory methods within corporate settings, and how this has created an interdisciplinary platform to engage in new forms of knowledge and meaning-making that have proved to be extremely valuable to the user-centric and interdisciplinary turn, even in the digital big data era.

A turn to interdisciplinary approaches and integrated methods

As part of this user-centric and interdisciplinary turn within the fields of innovation, design and business strategy is an increasing focus on the value of social situatedness in everyday life. Moreover, the development seems closely linked to the rise of consumer culture and popular culture, both within academic disciplines as well as within corporate contexts where the power of the consumer has become ever more present. To understand society, we must understand the consumer. As Mike Featherstone points out in Consumer Culture and Postmodernism:

> To use the term 'consumer culture' is to emphasize that the world of goods and their principles of structuration are central to the understanding of contemporary society. This involves a dual focus: first, on the cultural dimensions of the economy, the symbolization and use of material goods as 'communicators' not just utilities; and second, on the economy of cultural goods, the market, principles of supply, demand, capital accumulation, competition and monopolization which operate within the sphere of lifestyles, cultural goods, and commodities [... .] The concern with lifestyle, with the stylization of life, suggests that the practices of consumption, the planning, purchase, and display of consumer goods and experiences in everyday life cannot be understood merely via conceptions of exchange value and instrumental calculation.
>
> *(1991: 82–84)*

Along with the rise of consumer culture, another interesting thing has occurred: the blurring of the perception of "the patient", where patients are moving into the arena of health consumption and becoming consumers of health. This does not entail that the healthcare system has developed into a complete consumer market economy. However, it encapsulates that "the patient" is behaving increasingly with a consumer logic or mindset, and that the healthcare system, along with "the patient", are slowly moving away from a siloed position and into the flow of everyday life, integrated with other institutions and identities of self.

Consumer expectations and decisions related to the healthcare system as well as its products and services have become more parallel to those applied to consuming other products and experiences than previously observed. "Patient-centric" and "consumer-centric healthcare" are other terms that point towards the same development, where patient and consumer are being applied interchangeably. This is an interesting discussion in itself and embodies many challenges which have been discussed by several scholars and academics (i.e. Goldstein & Bowers, 2015, Gusmano, Maschke, & Solomon, 2019). What I would like to establish here is the link between the pull for qualitative, explorative, ethnographic methods I have experienced from the business side and the development of consumer culture and patient-as-consumer perspectives. In some ways, that combination has been my *raison d'être* as corporate ethnographer and cultural analyst. My fundamental methodological model or base was therefore right from the beginning formed from cross-disciplinary fields that could help me address a topic from both a theoretical and a practical point of view.

To be able to move continuingly between theory and practice has been a process of accepting movement, uncertainty, and the paranoia of letting go of some of the control. It has been a basic requirement when working with innovation, futures thinking, and strategic decision-making. It has also been a question of being able to question my own knowledge discourse, and to be curious and reflective about my own reactions in the research field.

In order to navigate this uncertainty and the premise of being constantly challenged by other knowledge discourses, I found stability in both theoretical and methodological perspectives, especially within applied ethnography (Cefkin, 2009; Kusenbach, 2003; Pink, 2007, 2008), design-research (primarily design-anthropology (Halse, Brandt, Clark, & Binder, 2010; Sanders, 2002, 2006)), and then of course my own theoretical backpack from my Sociology and Cultural Studies degree. Very early on, this was accompanied with other exploratory methods from within trend research, future studies, and scenario planning, which I will address further on in this chapter in relation to the potential and value of triangulation of methods.

All these theoretical and methodological perspectives together form my interdisciplinary frame-work to develop from and enter the practical field of exploration and the unknown. What I wish to unfold here, is that an essential part of these perspectives is the integration of a practical element into research and development contexts, manifested in an interest in "the social", "everyday life", and an engaged and situated involvement in order to create meaning and knowledge about the world.

Ethnography becoming a part of the corporate zeitgeist

To my luck, applied ethnography has become a popular field and a tool used in various forms of research practice (Malefyt, 2009: 201). It has evolved in new directions, from virtual, mobile, and visual ethnographies, to corporate, industrial and business ethnographies (Cefkin, 2009; Hine, 2000; Jordan & Lambert, 2009; Malefyt, 2009; Pink, 2007). According to the corporate ethnog-rapher Melissa Cefkin (2009), it is socio-economic currents that have been leading the way in this development as they have led to the emergence of a growing cultural perspective. Here, consumption, as already mentioned, is one example of a driving need, where the importance of understanding the consumer and the social relationships and interactions that affect them have been increasingly acknowledged by businesses, and therefore the demand for competencies that can open up this field of insight has increased.

Many academic disciplines and professions have been and are still a part of this ethnographic development/evolution – from anthropology, sociology, and cultural studies, to computer-human interaction, psychology, and business, among many others. I will propose that it is within this multidisciplinary framework that the field both provides a common basis to work and research from, and at the same time establishes an opportunity to renew itself through collaborations between the academic world and private and public institutions (Jordan & Lambert, 2009; Cefkin, 2009: 6–8). In other words, it is through its practical application that the field has also developed and evolved, as well as the ways in which it dynamically relates to culture and theory. Cefkin points out that it is precisely the theoretical, conceptual and methodological dimensions of ethnography that can contribute as a positive framework in various research contexts:

> In many ways, the notion of 'practice' forms the third leg of a stool, together with 'ethnography' and 'culture', upon which much of this work sits. Informed through trajectories ranging from attention to performance and self-presentation found in the symbolic interactionism of Erving Goffman (1956, 1961, 1967, 1974), to both Michel de Certeau's (1984) and Pierre Bourdieu's (1984, 1990) notions of everyday practice and habits, theories of practice have provided ethnographers in the industry a theor-etically nuanced yet empirically resonant object of analysis by which to frame and ground their work.
>
> *(Cefkin, 2009: 12)*

In my experience, this became evident through almost every phase of the research processes I have been part of. These theories of practice became a grounding element to develop the research design – from the initial scoping of a project, to the theoretical perspectives that would ground the field books I had to create in order to approach and explore the research fields and the respondents, to the internal pattern recognition discussions and insight analysis within my corporate team. The foundation for each project was a field book with the entire research design that discussed the the-ories that could help frame and analyse the topic along with the chosen methods and structure. It became an essential part for myself as a researcher, but just as much for my colleagues and my clients, who would sometimes join me in the field to grasp some of these approaches to knowledge and insight-creation that were new to them. In these situations, it sometimes became evident how distant and detached a traditional development or innovation process can be.

Just recently, I had the opportunity to assist a start-up that had developed a cutting-edge DNA technology. In order to develop their product further they had approached it from a market logic point of view and researched for the largest patient group that could quickly scale their market. However, through meeting with a healthcare professional, not even a patient, who introduced and shared a very different kind of insight – the professional experience of being situated within the field – it quickly became evident that they possibly had to approach their innovation differently and look towards a completely different patient group.

The field books have in many ways been my kind of theories of practice and as I was situated in a corporate context it provided me with a feeling of freedom to experiment and combine theories and methods in new ways that might not have been so easy elsewhere.

Adding design research to the formula

Design research covers a broad variety of perspectives and traditions (Sanders, 2002; 2006; Sanders & Chan, 2007), and the field has been shaped by psychologists, anthropologists, sociologists, and engineers, among others over the years. One direction has been formed by a participant-oriented approach that highlights the situatedness within research and design processes and the need to be present together with the users in their everyday lives in order to better understand their needs and design better solutions (together). In this way, designing becomes a joint action where people engage themselves in the everyday to create solutions to smaller or bigger challenges (Jönsson, Svensk, Malmborg, & Anderberg, 2005: 1).

The link between design and applied social sciences has, since the 1980s, become more and more integrated and has moved towards more active involvement from users (Halse, 2010a: 13; Sanders, 2002: 1). Another established field within design research is user-centred design, where practitioners gather, analyse, and interpret data in order to develop products, services, concepts, and prototypes that are focused on the users' needs (Sanders, 2006).

The field of design anthropology has emerged out of participant-oriented design but integrated elements from user-centred design as well (Cefkin, 2009: 6). Design anthropology is defined in *Rehearsing the Future* (Halse et al., 2010) as a design-anthropologic innovation model where openness and inter-discipline lays at the heart in relation to designing new solutions and new ways to approach a field. As such, it provides a way to theorise and experiment with theory (and methods) through practice and activity, where dialogue and interaction is at the centre of developing and practicing new knowledge:

> Theorizing is itself a particular practice. The kind of research practice that we are advocating here, as a form of learning, is fundamentally a social activity, not purely an intellectual one. There are two important consequences to this. First, the process of researching is dialogical. Second, the knowledge emerging from interactions in the field is to be evaluated less in terms of epistemological criteria (is this a true representation?) than in terms of practical, ethical, social, and aesthetic demands of the world that our research subjects and we both share (how will this affect our lives?).
>
> *(Halse, 2010c: 148)*

Design anthropology was a natural evolution and next step for my applied ethnographic work. Being a part of a corporate agenda, the implications of an innovation on the lives of the users was evidently at the forefront.

I was first introduced to the field of design research through a large research project that was a joint collaboration between smaller companies and the municipality of Copenhagen, along with a couple universities.

During a period of four months we spent a great amount of time in a senior residential complex in order to focus on the everyday lives of senior citizens. For the research we designed different methodological tools to help us structure our insights and map the needs of the seniors. We wanted to develop specific propositions through an in-depth understanding of the seniors in order to better enable them to build relations, use technology, and establish new opportunities for social interaction.

One primary insight that emerged from our study was that the seniors' activities were strongly driven by the state of their individual health. It was almost as if their health was the underlying and tacit game board upon which they made their choices as to how they would play and move their pieces in the game that was their everyday life.

Through our field work, we could see that health was a clear identity marker that we had to understand and incorporate in every insight in order to design for the lives of the seniors. The seniors' health condition played not merely a physical role but posed a great influence on their image and perception of selves. It influenced the way in which they related to their surroundings and at the same time how their surroundings related to and understood them.

It was the seniors' health, felt and embodied, that situated them in life and decided how they could or would engage themselves in different parts of their everyday lives. Influenced by the term "situated elderliness" (Brandt, Binder, Malmborg & Sokoler, 2010) we came to frame this identity marker as *situated health* (Boysen & Snell, 2012). A situational and embodied knowledge that affects the seniors and their everyday choices. We could see that, within this field, there existed an opportunity for innovation and for developing new products and services successfully. By understanding the seniors' situated health in the process of designing new technological and practical aid, there existed a real possibility of helping them in maintaining the everyday and continuing their practices, physically as well as emotionally.

Through this research project, we theorised through practice, learning, and experiencing knowledge emerge through social activity and in finding different, novel ways to talk about their everyday lives.

Tools, tools, tools

In order to create this dialogical and interactive sphere of meaning-making there is a need to open up a space where we feel safe and can talk about our lives, needs, feelings, thoughts, worries, hopes, and dreams in new ways. One of the ways to do this is through the use of "thinking tools" (Sanders, 2002: 4; 2006) that are designed to make people express themselves through emotional or cognitive toolkits:

> With "emotional toolkits," people make artefacts such as collages or diaries that show or tell stories and dreams. We have found that these tools are extremely effective in accessing people's unspoken feelings and emotional states. With "cognitive toolkits"; people make artefacts such as maps, mappings, 3-D models of functionality, diagrams of relationships, flowcharts of processes, and cognitive models.
>
> *(Sanders, 2002: 5)*

According to Sanders, the emotional toolkits facilitate a way to tell stories about feelings, dreams, worries, and hope, whereas cognitive toolkits can help understand how people perceive and understand things, events, and places (Sanders, 2002: 5). As such, these toolkits create a new language because they add to the interaction and communication between the various parties involved (ibid).

These toolkits and research tools are closely linked to the concept of *cultural probes*. Coined by Gaver, Dunne, and Pacenti (1999), its focal point is about being able to engage the users in a design research context. Cultural probes act as a collection of thinking tools typically provided to users or respondents in a research situation to help generate reflections or depictions that can provide insight into everyday practices (Gaver, Boucher, Pennington, & Walker, 2004: 53). Another way of generating knowledge in design research, especially participant-oriented design, has been in the form of design games (Brandt, Messeter, & Binder, 2008: 51). Since the 1990s, there has been a rising interest in games and dramaturgy as an explorative platform in the interaction and collaboration between designers and users and sometimes other stakeholders. The tools within this development range from theatre and performance, to games and scenario development as future-oriented, narrative-creating research methods to investigate problems and opportunities and to map potential solutions (ibid).

Before I move into the future-oriented methods, I wish to stress how this way of talking about things though games or performances can make certain topics less intimidating and easier to approach. Especially when it comes to exploring emotional and difficult topics like disease, death, and sex, the true value of these thinking tools has become ever so clear to me. Once, working on a project that dealt with young people's perception of sexually transmitted diseases, their relation to their own health, and their future outlook, I designed a game to make some of these themes more approachable. The respondents had to imagine a scenario of being someone else in a specific situation and then describe what they would do themselves if they were put in the same situation. Through the game, the respondents would feel more and more comfortable talking about personal and intimate parts of their lives. It became a way of opening up and establishing trust about a theme that would have been challenging otherwise for a stranger to ask questions about. The outcome was a much more in-depth understanding of the problem that needed to be addressed.

From proof of concept to proof of problem, and the value of trend research

Popular approaches to innovation where applied ethnography has been a part have a tendency only to focus on solving a single problem as quickly and as efficiently as possible. This creates at least two challenges in relation to meaning-making and knowledge creation: Firstly, there is a risk that the problem is not explored exhaustively. If we are too solution-focused, the research phase will quickly become a matter of execution instead of exploration. We need to understand the problem, unfold it, and explore its dynamics, before we can solve it. This means everything from understanding the client's need and investing time in creating the research design, taking into account theoretical and methodological perspectives, to fieldwork with the users. However, it also means mapping the underlying structures and the web of culture surrounding the problem. Secondly, if we do not invest time to understanding the problem but simply hunt for the first solution we discover, we risk creating a vicious cycle of innovation, where the solution to one problem merely leads to the creation of several others.

I have witnessed this corporate mindset and behaviour towards applied ethnography and qualitative design research methods many times. When it comes to innovation and business (strategy) development, there is a focus on *proof of concept*. I will suggest that a focus should be dedicated to *proof of problem* too. We need to know the problem in order to develop the right solution. In my opinion, innovation in a business context, and health innovation belongs here as well, these need to be re-invented to cope with the increasing complexity of our world today. To *proof* a problem, in my view, means exactly opening up to its connections and disconnections, its movements and the living culture it is a part of, and thereby exploring its innovation potential. We need to engage ourselves with people, patients, or consumers, as well as the larger systems that surround them. We need to think about innovation in a more systemic way too.

Trend research – bridging the gap

I started working with trend research while I was still studying, so one could say that this approach to innovation has been ingrained in me right from the beginning. I fell instantly in love with qualitative methods, especially ethnography, and I was mesmerised by all the cultural theories and ideas on structure and agency that I was introduced to. At the same time, I experienced first-hand how I could apply much of what I learned to the various projects I was working on at the trend companies where I freelanced.

I was studying changes and behaviour in modern society and how this was happening in order to advise the different clients on how to navigate, how to develop their products and services, how to renew and innovate their offerings, and how to change our ways of working. I did not have a theoretical or methodological framework for trend research at the time as it was quite a new field, both academically and professionally, but I learned everything from being a part of the field of work and applied my own academic discipline of sociology and cultural studies, the theories and methods I was studying. Some years later I discovered the term *trend sociology*,[1] and I remember that I felt a slight relief to have something to cling to that was not completely "unacademic" when it came to my profession as a trend researcher. This feeling was a part of a struggle going on inside me, which continued as I progressed in my career and moved in the direction of working with strategy development and management consulting. A struggle of fitting in. The power battle over knowledge and meaning. In the beginning this struggle concerned the pragmatic way of working with academic methods within a corporate setting. Being extremely devoted to validity and representativeness, I had to open up to combining ways of knowledge creation and, as an example, allow different fields of thought to mingle and blend. As I moved on and up the corporate ladder, I remember feeling a sorrow to leave academia, because I feared that I would probably not fit back in again. Later on, this struggle continued as a feeling of not fitting in with all the management consultants, economists and statisticians as they had been formed by a different positivistic discourse and informed by linear analysis and fast problem solving. I called it the paradigm of the economic man. In some way, trend research became a bridge to solve this battle within and also a way to communicate together with "the other", in order for my prejudice to finally be put to shame.

The field of trend research is large and complex and spreads over more creative trend forecasting, to futures studies and foresight. It stretches over possible futures (what might happen), which are move explorative, over the probable future (what will likely happen) which is more predictive and linear, to the preferable future (what we want to happen), a normative approach of thinking and analysing the future ahead.[2] I have worked in the intersection of these branches, however most of my experience lays within the explorative approach, accompanied by the framework of mega trends[3] where some are more measurable than others, their expressions and implications, and the method of scenario planning which is a structured way of working collaboratively and interdisciplinarily with possible futures in order to map opportunities and risks and to be able to make strategic decisions about the road ahead. As I mentioned, my work has been largely defined by working in interdisciplinary teams, where each individual with their discipline has added value to create a fuller picture, however my own contribution is founded in trend sociology and my constant insistent demand to invest in the in-depth understanding of people's behaviour in the context of accelerated complex change rather than just technological progress (as one example). It is change in people's behaviour, values and needs, not so much technology in itself that is hard to predict.

Martin Raymond, one of the most acknowledged trend researchers and co-founder of the Future Laboratory has defined a trend as,

> the direction in which something […] tends to move and which has consequential impact on the culture, society, or business sector through which it moves […] A trend is about difference and the direction along which that difference travels […] A trend can also be described as an anomaly – an oddity, inconsistency, or deviation from the norm, which becomes increasingly prominent over a period of time as more people, products, and ideas become part of that change […] Trends are […] a fundamental part of our emotional, physical, and psychological landscape, and by detecting, mapping, and using them to anticipate what is new and next in the world we live in we [trend researchers] are contributing in no small way to better understanding the underlying ideas and principles that drive and motivate us as people.
>
> *(2010: 14–15)*

A trend can therefore be both part of a greater picture, so called macro trends (where mega trends belong) which refer to longer time horizons and global scale, and a trend can also be part of a smaller picture, so called micro trends, that have a shorter life span. Whereas mega trends are very visible, i.e. ageing population, urbanization, etc., micro trends are often detected through *horizon scanning* which refers to a method for spotting early signs of a potential important development by scanning and observing curious novel events in the present. Horizon scans help us ask questions about curiosities that we observe: What does it tell us about changing attitudes and values towards health and wellbeing when the New Zealand government introduces the world's first national wellbeing budget to measure the population's quality of life? Or when we start collecting incidents of senior citizens committing petty crimes in South Korea and Japan, what can this be a sign of? And can it, for instance, be connected to a global implication of demographic changes and the rise of loneliness amongst seniors that we can expect to see in various other forms around the world?

Connecting the dots is what comes next. It is this cross-cultural analysis across cultures and different industry sectors that can help determine if an observation could become a long-term trend and how influential it might become (Raymond, 2010: 35). But the cross-cultural analysis of trends can also help create a better understanding of an implication of a trend, identify a shift in zeitgeist or unfold a problem that then opens up an opportunity space for innovation.

The American forecaster Faith Popcorn coined the term *cultural brailing* to explain how doing trend research is about feeling the bumps in culture, across cultures, sectors, industries, geographies etc. (ibid.: 37).

However, these cultural bumps or cross-cultural insights can also prove imperative when it comes to engaging various stakeholders. My work with the future health agenda has put me in contexts of multi-client scenario planning projects, where stakeholders from public and private arenas, representatives from patient organizations, multinational medico companies, and NGOs jointly had to explore future health challenges, opportunities, and risks in order to find a common ground and explore possible common recommendations. Here, the incentives present were manifold, each participant was firmly placed within different cultures, discourses, and understandings of the truth regarding the health system. The collaborative process of developing a common meaning also became an exercise in understanding the multifaceted layers of our health culture from an intimate, personal, individual, local, and global point of view, and in creating a space for difference in order to be able to see some of the possible similarities for interaction and engagement.

What has become evident to me over the years in relation to the value and power of combining applied ethnographic and design research methods with trend sociology and futures studies perspectives, is the ability to understand the nuances and differences that happen between systems and people, structures and agency, across different locations, cultures, and points in time. I have experienced the strength of triangulation,[4] where more methods are used in a research process in order to arrive at a more precise and valid conclusion. Especially when working with the unknown future and new innovations within health, it has been a prerequisite to be open to the exploration and sometimes experimentation of methods and the combination of methods, moving from inductive to deductive frameworks and meaning-making in order to establish, de-establish, and create a fuller picture.

Enter big data

Over the years, I have often had to argue for the value of qualitative and explorative insights as I was situated within a quantitative discourse. It has made me sharp to the edges in my argumentative logic about *why*, but I have also been blessed with curious colleagues close to me, and I have been carried on a corporate wave of consumer culture that made this corporate meeting more welcoming. Happening alongside this development has been the rise of digitization of consumer culture, and with it the ascent of big data. As marketing professor Craig J. Thompson argues:

> Big data is a direct consequence of the digitization of consumer culture. Consumers' social media posts, web browsing and on-line shopping histories, smart phone apps, fit bit self-monitoring, GPS tracking, video and music streaming services and 'smart home' devices, such as Alexa, all create a dispersed digital record that can be aggregated, searched, and cross-referenced.
>
> *(2019: 3, referring to Deighton 2018)*

This has been reinforced even further in health consumption. Now patients can self-monitor their own big data, and thereby in some cases self-manage their health. Big data has become a myth within quantitative discourse with its ability to collect data sets at a scale and pace that has not been available or possible before, and thereby "[conveying] an aura of truth, objectivity, and accuracy" (ibid.: 4, referring to Boyd and Crawford 2012, 663). With action comes reaction, and with *big* data came *thick* data, inspired by Geertz's *thick description* 1973),[5] as the qualitative response or defence (Thompson, 2019; 15). It seems like the ever present struggle over meaning and knowledge-making between quantitative and qualitative fields of research, also in the realms of corporate ethnographies, continues. And in this struggle over who provides the truth, little dialogue between big data and thick data is actually taking place, mostly because they often exist in different work cultures or industries.

Lately, this is starting to shift. Big data has started working with ethnographic approaches. With the acknowledgement of how an in-depth understanding of people is evermore essential for successful strategies and product/service innovation, there has been a rising interest in combining the *what* with the *why*, and thus integrating several research methods, including ethnography, into various processes.

This became clear to me recently while running a prototype app test on young students to explore how physical and mental wellbeing, along with social community building can be facilitated through a digital solution. The app could collect vast amounts of data from the students interacting with it, however it could not explain why some of the patterns occurred, like why one entire class all of a sudden did not interact with the app activities anymore. An anthropologist and I ran several visits to the schools, engaged with the students, talked with the teachers, and discovered a lack of trust between the classes had occurred by using the app. The ethnographic findings became an equally important insight for the further development of the innovation.

Ethnography lies in the heart of everything – working within the health agenda with a network of important stakeholders, an ethnographic approach is not merely crucial when exploring users, citizens, and patients, but just as much when navigating stake holding health professionals, health innovators, boards, funding partners, etc. Even when working with big data. It becomes valuable in every aspect of a successful outcome.

Concluding

Having by now navigated quite a few different knowledge arenas, different discourses of meaning, and fields of power it has become quite clear to me, as a cultural analyst in a corporate and commercial setting, that there is a struggle going on. A struggle over knowledge and a struggle of the construction of meaning and sensemaking. A struggle which often resides between the quantitative and qualitative epistemologies, and ways of working. It is experienced as a continuing paradox of being situated in a context driven by hypotheses and at the same time attempting to open up for the value of working inductively. A context that is dominated by deadlines and fast paced decision making. Put simply, it can be a challenge for an ethnographic researcher to have to maintain the importance of dedicating time and attention to establishing the component of the problem in a culture that is solution-driven and, per definition, will invest more time in executing problem solving, not problem investigating.

Knowledge is a complex entity, and it is a true art to grasp a concept that can feel as slippery as sand flowing through your fingers. Being curious and open as to how knowledge is being created and how meaning is continuingly formed and shaped in new ways and in new contexts through various methods is an imperative requirement for working with explorative and qualitative research methods in a corporate setting. Because it is exactly through the use of methods that we can create insights and knowledge about a specific field. There exists an inherent potential in interdisciplinary approaches when working with research in a corporate context. So instead of closing around a simple discipline's approaches to creating knowledge, we should be interested and motivated in combining and experimenting, in letting ourselves become challenged and conflicted, and in enjoying the ongoing construction of knowledge from a lived and situated perspective.

Notes

1 Trend sociology is the discipline of doing trend research and trend analysis and the knowledge of seeing contexts and currents in a constantly changing world. It is a generalist discipline involving politics, economics, marketing, psychology, history, ethnology, anthropology, cultural studies, and sociology.
2 Copenhagen Institute for Futures Studies
3 The Copenhagen Institute for Futures Studies' Mega Trend Perspective:

> Mega trends are long term complex aggregation of trends that form societies globally today and in the future. Mega trends have a lifetime of at least 10–15 years. They are interconnected, which

means there are synergetic opportunities where they intersect. While mega trends are expected trajectories, do not expect the development to occur linearly.

4 By triangulation I wish to refer to both data triangulation in terms of different data sources where the same phenomenon is examined at different places and through different persons (Denzin, 1989 in Mason, 1996: 148–149), as well as theory and method triangulation found in the different theoretical perspectives and the combination of methods (Flick, 1998: 68, 229–230).

5 The anthropologist Clifford Geertz has played a significant role in relation to the reflexive approach and analysis of data. Through the concept of thick description, ethnographic analysis for Geertz becomes a matter of the many layers of meaning that can describe the complex relationship between cultural structures, knowledge and meaning. Thick description is a way of approaching the process of analysis in which in-depth descriptions of an event or observation can contribute to broader interpretations of cultural contexts (Walsh, 2004: 227).

References

Anderson, B. (1991), *Imagined Communities*, London: Verso.

Boysen, L. & T. Snell, (2012), 'Med helbredet som spilleplade' in Brandt, E., Mortensen, P.F., Malmborg, L., Binder, T., Sokoler, T. (eds.), *SeniorInteraktion, Innovation gennem Dialog*, Det Kongelige Danske Kunstakademis Skoler, pp. 90–93.

Brandt, E., J. Messeter, & T. Binder. (2008), 'Formatting Design Dialogues – Games and Participation' in Binder, T., Brandt, E., Gregory, J. (guest editors), *Codesign – International Journal of CoCreation in Design and the Arts*, 4(1), 51–64.

Brandt, E., T. Binder, L. Malmborg, & T. Sokoler. (2010), 'Communities of everyday practice and situated elderliness as an approach to co-design for senior interaction', OZCHI '10: Proceedings of the 22nd Conference of the Computer-Human Interaction Special Interest Group of Australia on Computer-Human Interaction, available at *portal.acm.org/ft_gateway.cfm?id=1952314&type=pdf*, downloaded d.16.04.11.

Cefkin, M. (2009), 'Introduction: Business, Anthropology, and the Growth of Corporate Ethnography', in M. Cefkin (ed), *Ethnography and the Corporate Encounter, Reflections on Research in and of Corporations*, Berghahn Books, pp. 1–40.

Featherstone, M. (1991), *Consumer Culture and Postmodernism*, London: Sage.

Flick, U. (1998), *An Introduction to Qualitative Research*. London: Sage.

Foucault, M. (1972), *The Archaeology of Knowledge, And the Discourse on Language*, New York: Pantheon Books.

Gaver, W., A. Dunne, & E. Pacenti. (1999), 'Design: Cultural Probes', *Interactions*, 6(1), 21–29. Available online: doi.acm.org/10.1145/291224.291235

Gaver, W., A. Boucher, S. Pennington, & B. Walker. (2004), 'Cultural Probes and the value of uncertainty', *Interactions*, XI (5), 53–56.

Geertz, C. (1973), *The Interpretation of Cultures*, London: Fontana.

Goldstein, M.M. & D.G. Bowers, (2015), 'The patient as consumer: empowerment or commodification? Currents in contemporary bioethics', *Journal of Law Medicine & Ethics*, 43(1), 162–5, available at: www.ncbi.nlm.nih.gov/pubmed/25846046, assessed: 31 October 2019.

Gusmano, M.K., K.J. Maschke, M.Z. Solomon, (2019), 'Patient-Centered Care, Yes; Patients As Consumers, No', *Health Affairs*, 38(3), available at : www.healthaffairs.org/doi/abs/10.1377/hlthaff.2018.05019?journalCode=hlthaff, assessed: 31 October 2019.

Halse, J., E. Brandt, B. Clark, & T. Binder. (Eds), (2010), *Rehearsing the Future*, Copenhagen: The Danish Design School Press.

Halse, J. (2010a), 'Manifesto / Introduction' in J. Halse, E. Brandt, B. Clark, T. Binder (Eds), *Rehearsing the Future*, Copenhagen: The Danish Design School Press, pp. 12–17.

Hine, C. (2000), *Virtual Ethnography*, London: Sage.

Jordan, B. & M. Lambert. (2009), 'Working in Corporate Jungles: Reflections on Ethnographic Praxis in Industry', in M. Cefkin (ed), *Ethnography and the Corporate Encounter, Reflections on Research in and of Corporations*, Berghahn Books, pp. 95–136.

Jönsson, B., A. Svensk, L. Malmborg, & P. Anderberg. (2005), 'Situated Research and Design for Everyday Life', in T. Binder and R. Maze (eds.) Proceedings of the NORDES Conference 2005, pp. 1–11, available at: www.tii.se/reform/inthemaking/files/p1.pdf.

Kusenbach, M. (2003), 'Street Phenomenology, The go-along as ethnographic research tool', *Ethnography*, 4(3), 455–485.

Malefyt,T.D.W. (2009),'Understanding the Rise of Consumer Ethnography: Branding Technomethodologies in the New Economy', *American Anthropologist*, 111(2), 201–210.

Mason, J. (1996), *Qualitative Researching*. Sage Publications cited Denzin NK (1989) *Qualitative research methods*. Vol 17. Interpretive biography. Sage.

Oswell, D. (2006), *Culture and Society*, London: Sage.

Pink, S. (2001), *Visual Ethnography*, London: Sage.

Pink, S. (2007), *Doing Visual Ethnography*, London: Sage.

Pink, S. (2008), 'An urban tour – The sensory sociality of ethnographic place-making', *Ethnography*, 9(2), 175–196.

Raymond, M. (2010), *The Trend Forecaster's Handbook*, London: Laurence King Publishing Ltd.

Sanders, E.B.N. (2002), 'From User-Centered to Participatory Design Approaches', in J. Frascara (Ed.), *Design and the Social Sciences*, New York: Taylor & Francis Books Limited, pp. 1–8.

Sanders, E.B.N. (2006),'Design Research in 2006', *Design Research Quarterly*, 1(1), Design Research Society.

Sanders, E.B.N. & P.K. Chan. (2007), 'Emerging Trends in Design Research - changes over time in the landscape of design research', available at www.maketools.com/articles.../EmergingTrends1_Sanders_Chan_07.pdf, downloaded 17.05.2011.

Thompson, C.J. (2019), The "Big Data" Myth and the Pitfalls of "Thick Data" Opportunism: On the Need for a Different Ontology of Markets and Consumption, *Journal of Marketing Management*, 35(3–4): 207–230.

Walsh, D. (2004), 'Doing Ethnography', in C. Seale (ed), *Researching Society and Culture*, London: Sage, pp. 225–238.

PART XIV

Analyzing data

32

ANALYZING THE DATA

Conditions, meanings, and reasonings analysis

Tine Aagaard

Introduction

The method of analysis in a research project is not chosen according to random preferences. The method of analysis relates to the research problematic, the character of the empirical material, and the theoretic concepts. Still, the choice of method sometimes seems to be more or less unreflected, simply chosen because the methods are widespread within the research tradition in question. For example, the epistemological foundation of choice of method is seldom thematized in research publications (Carter & Little, 2007).

Humanistic health research is engaged in understanding people's experiences and actions through qualitative research. The methods of gathering empirical material are, among other things, qualitative interviews and participant observations. This approach prompts the informants' own perspectives on problems and opportunities as they appear from *their* location. This kind of research seeks knowledge about patients' subjective perspectives on health practice. The interview questions influence what kind of knowledge is produced this way. It is questionable whether qualitative interviews always produce knowledge that enables the researcher to gain insight in subjective perspectives. For example, the concept of "context" in studies of patients' perspectives is often limited to the institutional context (see e. g. Launsø, Olsen, & Rieper, 2011). Focusing only on the institutional context, the researcher risks to exclude knowledge about the patients' more comprehensive conduct of everyday life, including their resources to overcome health problems in everyday life and their own views on relevant professional support. I have discussed these problems concerning the production of knowledge about patient perspectives elsewhere (Aagaard, 2015 and 2017). The reason I mention it here is that the character and the quality of the empirical material also influences the analysis because the empirical material is produced on the same epistemological grounds as the analysis.

In the presentation of the conditions-, meanings-, and reasonings analysis I use my research project "Everyday life with illness – patients' cultural perspectives on health practice in Greenland" (Aagaard, 2015) to give concrete examples of the method. In the project, the researcher perspective is moved from professional practice to the patients' everyday lives, e.g. work, family and friends, place of home and local community, leisure interests, and institutional contexts when they are hospitalized. The empirical material was produced through ethnographic fieldwork in the patients' home and local community and during hospitalization over a period of three years. The methods used were single interviews with patients, interviews with patients and their spouses, focus group interviews, participant observations, and document analysis. Also, care professionals in the health system were interviewed about their professional practice. The study showed how patients' values and resources are anchored in their conduct of everyday life and how institutional health practice is connected with patients' conditions and opportunities for handling the everyday life with illness.

Background
Critical psychology

The analysis of the project builds on a critical psychological approach to research in social practice. Critical psychology is a theoretically argued conceptual frame of analysis. The ontological approach is that human beings have the potential to change and develop social practice for the common good (Holzkamp, 1998 and 2005; Dreier, 1996 and 2008).

A fundamental category in critical psychology is the concept of *Conduct of Everyday Life* (CEL). In the 1980s, the German psychologist Klaus Holzkamp and his colleagues developed the concept CEL out of a fundamental critique of the experimental psychology for studying psychological phenomena isolated from the contexts in which they arise in everyday life. Psychological experiments cannot catch how people handle their life situation outside the experiment and this creates problems with the use of experimental findings. In order to overcome these problems, Holzkamp developed the concept of CEL as a way to conceptualize the subject's endeavors to make the everyday life hang together concerning time, practical organization, and personal relations. Because of the shortage of time the demands of the various life areas (work, family, leisure activities, etc.) must be integrated by the subject through prioritizing, compromising, and conflict resolution. The demands are interpreted by the subject in terms of their relevance for maintaining the everyday life (Holzkamp, 1998). In this way, the concept of CEL mediates between subjective conduct of everyday life and social structures. Through our conduct of everyday life, we handle our social conditions on the basis of their meaning for us, and thus we give reasons for our conduct in the problems and opportunities we see.

The idea of subjectivity presented by the concept CEL points out that people are participants in social practice. Participation emphasizes that we are connected with each other in social practice. We participate from different locations and positions, with different knowledge and interests and different opportunities to influence the common practice (Dreier, 2008). In research analyses, when we presuppose that people act situated in connected practices, then the concrete personal thoughts, feelings, and actions can teach us about institutional structures. When personal perspectives are related to the more comprehensive structures of practice that the person participates in, then the understanding of problems and opportunities are moved from personal characteristics to ways structures are arranged. This understanding is not only obtained through what we call "analysis" in a thesis; understanding is a dynamic process throughout the whole research project, that is, production of empirical material, description, gathering results, and publication (Højholt & Kousholt, 2011). But in order to be able to handle the composition of a thesis it can be appropriate to write a separate chapter of analysis.

Method of analysis

In critical psychology, the analysis of social practice is called a "conditions-, meanings-, and reasonings analysis". It suggests how an understanding of people's situations can be obtained by analyzing the connections between life conditions, their meaning for the individual, and the individual's reasons for action grounded hereon. Thus, the purpose of the analysis is to gain insight in connections, not in detached "factors" or "variables".

Life conditions are both the conditions of everyday life and the conditions made by the health system. As participants in social practice we also form conditions for each other. In the contexts we participate in, we each handle our conditions from our experience of them and our actions are influenced by and have consequences for other participants in the same context. Conditions are historically and culturally developed and can be influenced and changed by the participants.

"Everyday life with illness" – scientific problematic and analysis

The overriding problematic of the project is about opportunities and dilemmas in the relationship between, on the one hand, patients' conditions and prerequisites for handling the everyday life with illness and, on the other hand, structural and institutional conditions for providing professional support for this. The problem was illuminated through the following research questions:

1. Contexts of personal participation in everyday life.
2. How the disease has changed the conduct of everyday life.
3. How people handle life with illness.
4. How people experience and use professional interventions.

Therefore, the first step in the analysis was to structure the empirical material in each case according to the research questions.

Five patients were followed over a period of one to three years. Among these, I chose three courses for deeper analysis. As a basis for the analysis, these courses were reconstructed according to the research questions. The purpose was to show the patients as subjects of their own lives and as embedded in historical, cultural contexts. This illustrates the theoretical approach to the concept "perspective": We participated in social practice from different locations and positions; location and position is something entirely concrete, the place we live, the activities we are engaged in, the people we are related to etc. (also during hospitalization). To elaborate these concrete contexts as seen from the perspectives of the patients facilitates the understanding of her or his ways of acting. At the same time, it facilitates the discovery of other possible ways of acting because, as a researcher, one has other and different, more overriding perspectives (Thorgaard, 2013). In this project, these overriding perspectives included insight in other forms of knowledge and practice like professional, administrative, and political practice. The point here is not that patients should be educated about their opportunities. The point is that patients' handlings of their lives with illness can inform the researcher about opportunities and problems in the conditions. These opportunities and problems can be challenged and discussed by the researcher (possibly in dialogue with the participants in the research) in order to expand the ideas of how to act – still with point of departure in the perspectives of the patients.

The course of analysis in a research project can be constructed in many ways and must be determined in each case according to the scientific problematic, etc. The purpose of this chapter is not to present a prescription for that. Instead, I will give some examples of conditions-, meanings-, and reasonings analyses from the project "Everyday Life with Illness". But first a short description of Greenland as context of the research.

Greenland as context of the research

Greenland is the world's biggest island, more than one-fourth the area of the United States. Most of the land is covered by ice. The population of 56,000 is spread along the ice-free coastline in 17 towns and about 60 settlements. The capital Nuuk holds 18,000 inhabitants. There are no roads between towns and settlements, most transportation is done by boat, flight, or helicopter which are sensitive to the weather. Economic production comes from fishing, hunting, herding, tourism, and service. Greenland was a Danish colony from 1721–1953 and a county in Denmark from 1953–1979. In 1979, home rule was established and since 2009 Greenland has had self-rule in commonwealth with Denmark. Especially in the time as a county in Denmark, a welfare system was built based on a model of Danish institutions. This means that Greenland is a welfare society, with free access for all to education, social welfare, and treatment of disease. Greenlandic institutions still look to Denmark for inspiration, and a constant flow of Danish administrators, working for a period in Greenland, bring Danish systems to Greenland and maintain them.

The course of John – a reconstruction[1]

Contexts in the conduct of everyday life

John is in his mid-fifties and lives with his wife Alice in a town. John is an educated blacksmith and works as a manager in the municipal's technical service department. He is fond of his job which he finds meaningful because it is useful for the community and gives him professional satisfaction and many social contacts. Alice is also working fulltime. Besides this, she takes care of the housework. They spend their spare time with family and friends.

How the disease has changed the conduct of everyday life

John has gone through a course of several years in the health system where he has been treated for a heart disease. During the course he has been fired from his job because of too many days off and therefore he has taken early retirement. After the treatment he is back in good shape and he actually could have continued his work for a couple of years. Besides the heart disease, John has diabetes. In the outpatient ward of the local hospital, John has been instructed to change his lifestyle. He and Alice have stopped smoking, changed their dietary habits, and started exercising. This causes sacrifice, but is effective concerning physical condition, weight loss, and normal blood sugar values.

How life with illness is handled

When John loses his job, he loses his motivation to execute a healthy lifestyle. He becomes increasingly passive and depressed. He won't hear about exercise or the municipal's offer of occupational therapy in the local day center for the unemployed (he calls it "useless pastime"). He seldom leaves home and has started smoking again. He is looking for a new job, but in vain. Alice, who has supported him throughout the course of his illness and treatment, tries to motivate him to take up the healthy lifestyle again, but without success. She is now worn out and has symptoms of stress. The situation affects their relationship negatively.

The experience of professional intervention

During hospitalization, John expresses satisfaction with treatment and care. He keeps his problems to himself and has no expectations that the professionals are interested in them. Alice, on the contrary, spending many hours at his bedside, frequently tries to engage in a dialogue with the staff about the difficult situation at home, but without success. The staff is busy and she is reluctant to take up their time. When John visits the outpatient ward for check-ups, the professionals there only ask about his smoking and dietary habits. He feels that they moralize over his life style and he is bitter because they do not follow up on his condition as chronically ill – yet he is not able to express his needs apart from the need for physical exercise by a physiotherapist.

Conditions-, meanings-, and reasonings analysis

The purpose of the analysis is to go behind immediately visible phenomena in the meeting between patients and professionals in order to find opportunities for professional actions that can support patients in expanding their opportunities for handling their everyday life with illness in a way that is meaningful in their own perspective. A prominent dilemma in John's case is that he damages his health by dropping the healthy lifestyle, but his reasons for this are not spotted by the professionals and therefore they cannot support him by for instance talking with him about his occupational situation. The professionals only reprimand his lifestyle, hoping that he will "pull himself together" and change it. According to the problematic of the project one could ask: What are John's conditions and prerequisites in everyday life for handling life with chronic heart disease and diabetes, and what do the conditions mean for his way of handling his situation? What are the professionals' structural and institutional conditions for providing support for John and what do the conditions mean for the way the professionals make decisions?

Table 32.1 Overview of conditions-, meanings-, and reasonings analysis

Conditions	Overriding societal conditions:
	– Societal and institutional perceptions of knowledge and health
	– Political strategies
	– Administrative structures
	– Perceptions of health among the population
	Individual conditions in everyday life:
	– Influential social relations, work, and other activities
	– Changes as consequences of the disease
	– Institutional health- and treatment interventions.
Meanings	The meaning of the conditions for the individual person:
(with a focus on that	– Action possibilities and -limitations provided by the conditions
conditions can have	– How does the person her-/himself perceive the conditions – what
different meanings for	possibilities and limitations does the person see her-/himself
different persons)	
Reasonings	What forms of conduct of everyday life come out as a consequence of
	the conditions and their personal meanings for the individual person
Action possibilities	Change in conditions and personal ways of handling them

Conditions

In the analysis, the conditions must be embedded in their historical, cultural contexts. Besides, preunderstandings of disease and health must be questioned. For example, how come the professionals focus on lifestyle as the only way to health and wellbeing? What does it tell us about prevailing perceptions of health in the health system? How are the perceptions expressed in political strategies and in health practice? And how are these health perceptions related to perceptions among patients? These fundamental questions concerning the conditions arose in all the patient courses in different ways. The questions caused closer studies of the development of the Greenlandic health system and of various historic and contemporary health perceptions in the Greenlandic community and how they are embodied in practice. As a consequence, the chapters in the thesis about the structural framework for the project's problematic were a starting analysis of the conditions, because already here the conditions were assessed in relation to opportunities and limitations for including patients' perspectives in practice.

The studies of the development of the health system showed, among other things, that the Greenlandic system is built on a model of the Danish system and builds on the same concepts of health as absence of disease in the individual. Looking to the development of the disease pattern in Greenland, which resembles the one in the Western world, according to this perception of health there is focus on disease prevention through strengthening the body, that is, a focus on diet, exercise, no smoking, and minimizing alcohol consumption. As a prerequisite for this kind of health, professional knowledge must be transferred to the patients. In line with this, the research shows that during hospitalization, nearly all institutional procedures aim to exercise diagnostics and treatment of physical disease and to give patients information about it.

The studies of health perceptions showed that widespread notions among the Greenlandic population about a healthy life are related to the opportunities for maintaining a good life in local communities. For example, people do not talk about "exercise" and "diet", but about enjoying nature, breathing fresh air, gathering supplies by hunting, fishing, picking berries etc. and having good relations with family and friends. These kinds of health perceptions are not expressed in the structures of the health system.

The studies of political strategies showed that social problems, not surprisingly, are relegated to the social sector. Consequently, there are few procedures in health practice for including knowledge about patients' social problems in connection with illness or for the handling of such problems.

The overriding structural conditions for the meeting between John and the professionals in the outpatient ward can be outlined like this:

- The prevailing perceptions of knowledge and health in the health system.
- In line with these, the political strategies and institutional procedures for professional contributions.
- Health perceptions among the population.

John's conditions in the everyday life include family and other participants in his life contexts, first of all his wife who is his most important support, but who is now having trouble with solving the problems related to John's illness. Also, work and leisure activities are important conditions for John's opportunities for living a meaningful everyday life. In the present situation, he has to deal with having lost his job and finding new forms of meaningful occupation – and maybe new ways of contributing to the family's economy. The disease and its consequences, such as reduced level of function and the actions he must take to maintain his current level of function, are also conditions. Moreover, the health system and the opportunities it provides in cases with chronic illness are important conditions for his conduct of everyday life.

John's conditions for the conduct of everyday life can be outlined like this:

- Important social relations, work and other activities.
- The changes that the disease has caused.
- Institutional health- and treatment interventions.

It should be pointed out that the overriding structural conditions and John's conditions in everyday life are separated here for analytical reasons. In social practice, the conditions are connected with each other; for example, the health contributions for individuals are influenced by prevailing perceptions of health.

Conditions, meanings, and reasonings

The conditions, the meaning of the conditions for the individual, and the individuals' reasons for action grounded in the meaning of the conditions are closely woven together in practice. Therefore, conditions, meanings, and reasonings all appear in the following example. They are marked with italics.

For the health professionals in the outpatient ward, the task is to support John's endeavors to maintain a healthy lifestyle. The doctors have informed him about the consequences of an unhealthy lifestyle, the dietitian about dietary changes, the physiotherapist about exercising, and he has been referred to a municipal social worker in order to find occupation. According to the health system's procedures, the professionals have done what is possible for them within the institutional framework. When John attends the outpatient ward for check-up and smells of cigarette smoke and admits that he does not follow the professionals' counseling and the professionals see no more opportunities for support, then they understand the situation as a consequence of John's lack of will or ability to follow their advice. The limited *conditions* that are available for John within the health system *mean* for the professionals that their interventions are not successful. Based on their subjective experience of not being able to help John, they explain John's misconduct as a question of his personality. They *reason* that their powerlessness is grounded in John's lack of will to cooperate.

For John, *conditions* such as illness and unemployment have a negative *meaning* for his opportunities for maintaining a meaningful life, and this causes depression and passivity. This situation affects his companionship with Alice. Alice has stood by John's side throughout the course of his illness, but as he loses his motivation for a healthy lifestyle she stands alone with trying to motivate him. This is a threat against their relationship and thereby a threat against John's opportunities to handle his situation. Alice and John each try to handle the problems in their own way. John tries to find a new occupation. Alice tries to contact the health personnel in order to gain their support for the problems at home. Their different attempts to solve the problems are grounded in their different *reasonings* about a good solution: John wants an occupation that corresponds with his own perspectives on a meaningful occupation. Alice wants John to follow the professional counseling because she is mostly concerned about his health.

Thus, behind the immediate picture the professionals get of John in the outpatient ward there are several activities going on between John and Alice in order to handle the health problems. The professionals know about the health problems, but they don't know John's *conditions* for handling them and what the conditions *mean* for his conduct of everyday life. Therefore, they see John's resignation as a consequence of his personality (he is "irresponsible", "non-cooperative"), not as *reasoned* by the opportunities and limitations the *conditions* provide and what they *mean* to him.

A focus on differences

The overriding societal and institutional conditions are more or less the same for all patients. But the conditions can have different meanings for different patients.

An example is another patient I followed through some years, Julie. Like John, she suffered from a chronic disease causing a loss of physical functions and the loss of her job. But besides having a wage-earning job, Julie was also a housewife. She was still able to do some work at home in spite of her illness, so she had no problem with lack of occupation. This differs from John's situation. John's professional work was of vital meaning for him, and when he lost it, it left an empty space in his life. Besides, his work experiences were limited to wage-earning work, so his abilities to imagine other kinds of occupation (like e.g. domestic work) were also limited.

These examples show that the same conditions, chronic disease and loss of work, can have different meanings for different patients, because they have different prerequisites and different conditions for handling their situations. This kind of analysis does not explain patients' different handlings as mainly related to their personality, but as related to societal structures like cultural life modes, such as employee or housewife. For Julie it was a life mode to sustain the home through picking berries and herbs, taking care of the children, cooking, producing clothes etc. Therefore, it was meaningful for her to continue this occupation after the loss of job. In contrast to this, for John, the wage-earning job gave content to life, it was in the job he realized his abilities and skills and established meaningful relationships. When he could not maintain this life form, he lost meaning in everyday life.

The insight in patients' different ways of handling their situations emphasizes the importance of embedding patients' personal situations in more comprehensive societal structures such as cultural life forms with different ethos, should the professionals be able to understand individual patients' situation with illness (see also Højrup, 2013).

Action possibilities

Elaborating conditions, meanings, and reasonings for patients' conduct of everyday life and professional practice is a method of analyzing health practice as an intersubjective concern. Finding action possibilities to realize the aim of health practice, namely to support the patients in handling their life with illness, demands an understanding of both the patients' life conditions and the professionals' working conditions. Action will often include changes both in the individual patient's everyday life and its conditions and in institutional procedures for professional practice and the professionals' handling of them.

The conditions-, meanings-, and reasonings analysis of patients' situations will often point to new and unseen action possibilities, like, for example, involvement of relatives' knowledge and experiences in professional support or meaningful occupation for chronically ill patients. The results of the analysis clarify that development of professional practice not only is a question about what is going on between the individual patient and professional. Professional interventions are embedded in and spring from established forms of practice building on specific perceptions of health, economic and administrative rationales, theoretic traditions, work cultures, etc. Therefore, the development of interventions is a common concern in the professional community of practice and involves the perspectives of patients and relatives.

The description and elaboration of health practice by means of the conditions-, meanings-, and reasonings analysis can be the first step to identifying problems and opportunities for action and change. The description itself can be transformed in practice on various levels. First, the description can be integrated in the way the patient's situation is understood in a dialogue between patient and professional (the individual level). Second, the description can be a common task in the professional community of practice by being a method of deciding on principles for a good quality of practice (the institutional level). Third, an institutional gathering of analyses of patient courses can facilitate political initiatives, such as those concerning occupation that include the perspectives of chronically ill patients (the societal level).

Distribution of knowledge in practice, insight in coherency, and the researcher's self-reflection

As mentioned in the introduction to this chapter, conditions-, meanings-, and reasonings analyses demand that the empirical material of the research project is gathered with this method of analysis in mind. Moreover, it demands of the researcher a high level of self-reflection about her own conditions and their meaning for her decisions and actions. Just like the informants in the research, the researcher herself is influenced by conditions such as prevailing perceptions of health and wellbeing and institutional epistemology. A conditions-, meanings-, and reasonings analysis is critical of practice simply as a precondition for finding opportunities for a constructive development.

When we as researchers or students initiate an empirical study we are "naïve" – our preunderstandings are limited. A way to overcome this is to question our own preunderstandings and prevailing understandings in practice. This critical and self-critical approach to examining practice can easily lead to a point of disconcertment – how to pose questions, what to observe, in which direction to move on with the project, etc. The methodological approach presented in this chapter points to a way out of the problems: The solution lies in a thorough and respectful exploration and description of the research participants' concrete practice coupled with an ongoing questioning and challenging of one's own and common assumptions.

As shown earlier in this chapter a conditions-, meanings-, and reasonings analysis will often reveal problems that are not immediately solvable. But as researchers or students we do not have to cave in under the pressure for proposals for action. The description of problems and opportunities as seen from the participants' different perspectives will often in itself be an encouragement for the professionals in practice to intervene for the sake of improvement (Dreier, 1996). An important aspect of the description is to follow what the participants in practice point out as important *for them*.

Everyday life and institutional practice is complex and conflictual. Conditions-, meanings-, and reasonings analyses are designed to catch the complexity and conflictuality and connect individual conduct of everyday life with contextual conditions. The method of analysis demands a clear stand of the researcher to what kind of knowledge she is after, that is, the epistemological basis. The method of analysis builds on an explicit perception of knowledge: All knowledge springs from practice, but has different forms in scientific practice, in professional practice, and in the everyday life of the citizens, respectively. But all forms of knowledge influence common practice (like welfare-institutional practice) and therefore have relevance for researching practice. It demands an involvement of all forms of knowledge in the studied practice – societal, institutional and individual, citizens' and professionals'. The researcher who wants to use a conditions-, meanings-, and reasonings analysis must reflect on this epistemology.

Conditions-, meanings-, and reasonings analyses break with traditional ideas about research as either inductive or deductive (Jartoft, 1996). This method of analysis creates a dialogue between theory and practice through the critical reflection about practice and about personal preunderstandings. We do not go out and explore the human world cleansed of theory and other prerequisites, so what is our implicit theory and preunderstanding? It is crucial for the researcher to reflect on that. Likewise, theories are not plucked out of the air, nor are they expressions of universal truths, so the researcher must reflect on where theories come from, for what purpose they have been developed, what interests they are created to serve, and what they can be used for and not be used for in practice.

Thus, conditions-, meanings-, and reasonings analyses present various challenges. First of all, it takes a reflected stand to knowledge as distributed among different participants in practice. Second, it takes thoroughness. For instance, it is not enough to pluck out quotations from empirical material and analyze them isolated from the context in which they were put forward, or from the context in which the content of the quotations took place. People's conduct of everyday life must be analyzed in their complex connections to other people and to overriding societal conditions. This method of analysis provides the researcher with knowledge about *coherency,* that is, coherency in individuals' conduct of everyday life and how it is connected to overriding societal contexts such as welfare institutions and discourses of health and wellbeing.

Conflict of interest

The author has no conflict of interest. This chapter is based on my chapter in a Danish anthology about qualitative methods of analysis in health research (Gildberg & Hounsgaard, 2018). The publishing of this English version has been agreed with the Danish publisher Klim.

Funding and grant-awarding bodies

The author thanks the following for providing support for the research: The Government of Greenland, Greenland's Nursing Organization and the Danish State.

Note

1 All details concerning name, education, occupation etc. are anonymized.

References

Aagaard, T. (2015). Hverdagsliv med sygdom: Patienters kulturelle perspektiver på sundhedspraksis i Grønland [Everyday life with illness: Patients' cultural perspectives on health practice in Greenland]. *Inussuk – Arktisk forskningsjournal, 1,* 1–221. Nuuk: Naalakkersuisut/ Grønlands Selvstyre.

Aagaard, T. (2017). Patient involvement in healthcare professional practice in hospital – A question about knowledge. *International Journal of Circumpolar Health,* 76: 1, 1403258, www.tandfonline.com/doi/full/10.1080/22423982.2017.1403258

Carter, S.M. & M. Little. (2007). Justifying Knowledge, Justifying Method, Taking Action: Epistemologies, Methodologies, and Methods in Qualitative Research. *Qualitative Health Research,* 17(10), 1316–1328.

Dreier, O. (1996). Ændring af professionel praksis på sundhedsområdet gennem praksisforskning [Changing professional health practice through practice research]. I: Jensen, U. J., Qvesel, J. & Andresen, P. F. (red.): *Forskelle og Forandring – bidrag til humanistisk sundhedsforskning.* Aarhus: Philosophia.

Dreier, O. (2008). *Psychotherapy in Everyday Life.* New York: Cambridge University Press.

Gildberg, F.A. & L. Hounsgaard. (2018). *Kvalitative analysemetoder i sundhedsforskning [Qualitative Methods of Analysis in Health Research].* Aarhus: Klim.

Holzkamp, K. (1998). Daglig livsførelse som subjektvidenskabeligt grundkoncept [Conduct of everyday life as basic concept of a science of the subject]. *Nordiske Udkast 26*(2), 3–31.

Holzkamp, K. (2005). Mennesket som subjekt for videnskabelig metodik [The human being as subject for scientific method]. *Nordiske udkast 33*(2), 5–33.

Højholt, C. & D. Kousholt. (2011). Forskningssamarbejde og gensidige læreprocesser: Om at udvikle viden gennem samarbejde og deltagelse [Research cooperation and reciprocal learning processes: Developing knowledge through cooperation and participation]. I: Højholt, C. (red.): *Børn i vanskeligheder – Samarbejde på tværs.* København: Dansk Psykologisk Forlag.

Højrup T. (2013). Kulturelle livsformer og helbred [Cultural life modes and health]. I: Niklasson, G. (red.): *Sundhed, menneske og samfund.* Odense: Samfundslitteratur.

Jartoft, V. (1996): Kritisk psykologi: en psykologi med fokus på subjektivitet og handling [Critical Psychology: a psychology with focus on subjectivity and action]. I: Højholt, C. & Witt, G. (red.): *Skolelivets socialpsykologi: Nyere socialpsykologiske teorier og perspektiver.* København: Unge Pædagoger.

Launsø, L., L. Olsen, & O. Rieper. (2011). *Forskning om og med mennesker: Forskningstyper og forskningsmetoder i samfundsforskning [Research about and with human beings: Research types and research methods in social research].* København: Nyt Nordisk Forlag Arnold Busck.

Thorgaard, K. (2013). Critique of influential epistemological presuppositions in clinical reasoning. *European Journal for Person Centered Health Care 1*(1), 124–28.

33

COMPUTER-ASSISTED QUALITATIVE DATA ANALYSIS SOFTWARE (CAQDAS) AND ETHNOGRAPHIC HEALTH RESEARCH

Áine M. Humble

Introduction

Qualitative research methods are effective for answering health-related questions such as "How do people think about their own health and that of their communities? What do they do to maintain health, or deal with illness? How do health practitioners relate to their patients, and to other professionals?" (Green & Thorogood, 2018, p. 4). As a form of qualitative research, ethnographic health research focuses on data that occurs in natural settings, such as a palliative care unit, and involvement (i.e., observation) in the everyday lives of participants is a key feature (Prentice, 2010).

To understand what is occurring in a field of interest, ethnographers often collect large amounts of data, and this data may be collected in various ways and exist in varying formats (see Table 33.1 for examples). Observational methods are key, in the form of videotaped recordings or recorded notes in various formats such as jotted notes in a notebook, a digital audio file generated from a mobile phone's voice memo function, or typed notes in a Microsoft Word document. However, some ethnographers might not actually use observation (Pool, 2017). The following are examples of additional forms of ethnographic data, many of which could be in the same study:

- Interviews
- Focus groups
- Visual techniques such as photovoice
- Documents such as "reports, case-notes, death certificates, etc." (Prior, 2010, p. 425), and policy documents, which may be of particular importance in institutional ethnographies (Kearney, Corman, Hart, Johnston, & Gormley, 2019)
- "Naturally-occurring data, such as [previously existing] video-recordings of consultations" (Green & Thorogood, 2018, p. 176)
- A researcher's personal reflections (Pool, 2017)

- Social media data (Coffey, 2018)
- Questionnaires (quantitative data)

The sheer amount of data that can be generated in ethnographic research raises questions of how best to organize and analyze it. Moreover, additional factors can affect the complexity of a qualitative study in terms of how it needs to be managed and how it can be analyzed, such as how structured or unstructured the data are and whether data are collected at one point in time or over time, by one person or multiple people, or at one site versus multiple sites (Gilbert, Jackson, & di Gregorio, 2014).

It is clear that effective management of data in ethnographic studies is key (Angrosino, 2007), and toward that end, various authors have suggested that computer-assisted qualitative data analysis software (CAQDAS) can greatly facilitate the management of such large amounts of data (e.g., Angrosino, 2007; Coffey, 2018; Fetterman, 2020). CAQDAS also, of course, assists with data analysis, and it can speed up very time consuming tasks (Fetterman, 2020). This chapter, thus, explores the role that CAQDAS can play in ethnographic research, using health research as examples.

I first define CAQDAS and briefly describe its history. How CAQDAS can be used to manage and analyze ethnographic data is then discussed. Three examples of health ethnographies that have used CAQDAS programs are presented. The chapter concludes with identifying—and challenging—some fears around CAQDAS use and reiterating the importance of reflexivity.

Definition and history of CAQDAS

A simple definition of CAQDAS is that it is a program meant to support the work of qualitative researchers (Gilbert et al., 2014). Lewins and Silver (2009) emphasize that the main purpose of such a program must be to *qualitatively* analyze *qualitative* data, which means interpreting data "through the identification and linking or coding of themes, concepts, processes, contexts, etc., in order to build explanations or theories or to test or enlarge on a theory" (p. 3). Some programs may have quantitative functions that assist with mixed methods research, but the main purpose should be qualitative analysis.

CAQDAS can assist with both management of a project and analysis of the data. For management, researchers can store their data in one project file and organize it in ways that fit their needs. Some programs may allow researchers from different geographical areas to easily assess the data and/or access it simultaneously. To assist with analysis, CAQDAS has functions for tasks such as coding, writing memos, linking data together, data retrieval, diagramming relationships, querying the data, and generating various reports and other outputs (Silver & Lewins, 2014). Retrieval of data is fast and easy. Many other features have developed over the years, such as the ability to import social media data, transcribe, and connect transcripts directly with audio or video files.

Davidson and di Gregorio (2011) describe the history of CAQDAS. For example, they note how these programs first emerged in the 1980s as independent researchers—unaware of similar efforts being carried out in different parts of the world—sought to find better ways to manage their data. The 1980s and early 1990s saw researchers critically examining the software programs as well as the methodological backgrounds on which they were developed. The "Era of Competition" in the early 1990s to 2000 saw three programs emerge as leaders in the field: (a) ATLAS.ti, (b) MAXQDA, and (c) NVivo. Researchers became more critical in their evaluations of the programs, and the first textbooks about CAQDAS were published. A key resource developed during this time was the CAQDAS Networking Project, which was created in 1994. It is based in the UK and provides non-partisan, unbiased reviews of software programs as well as training. New opportunities and issues have emerged from 2009 onward as a result of Internet and digital advances (Davidson & di Gregorio, 2011; Silver, 2018).

Although the CAQDAS Networking Project currently reviews 12 programs, the estimated number ranges from 20 (Fielding, Fielding, & Hughes, 2013) to 40 (Frietas et al., 2018). Free programs and cloud-based programs have emerged. Some cloud-based programs are standalone ones, such as Dedoose, whereas other developers have added cloud-based versions to their already existing desktop versions (e.g., ATLAS.ti). Additional versions of the same software exist. In recent years, for example, Mac-based program versions have emerged, but they are not always fully compatible with PC versions of the same software, which may create issues for those wanting or needing to move from one platform to another. Additionally, some programs also offer multiple versions with different capabilities. MAXQDA (version 2020), for example, has three different versions: Standard, Plus, and Analytics Pro. All three versions support qualitative and mixed methods data analysis, but Plus and Analytics Pro add quantitative and statistical analysis capability.

Data management with CAQDAS

Researchers typically use CAQDAS for data management, and a program's underlying architecture is important to understand before setting up a project file. As the software programs have advanced over the years, they have become more similar to each other in many ways, which Evers (2018) refers to as *creeping featurism*. A common situation is one in which a software developer creates a new function and then other software developers quickly develop a similar function. Yet, each program still has its unique underlying structure and subtle differences, which can influence its perceived functionality (Evers). A software program's underlying structure influences aspects such as (a) what kind of ethnographic data can be imported; (b) the various ways in which the data can be stored, which influences a project's portability; (c) how many people can access a project file at the same time; (d) how analyses are carried out; and (e) what kind of output can be generated. In this section, I briefly describe some issues related to the importing of data into CAQDAS, portability of project files, and the impact of data organization on analysis.

Knowing what kind of data formats can be imported into a program for analysis is important, but the initial format of such data should not necessarily limit a researcher from importing it into a CAQDAS project file. Handwritten field notes, for example, can be scanned and imported as PDF documents. Digital audio or video recordings from the field can be directly imported in, and can be linked to their transcripts, which supports closeness to one's raw data. Some CAQDAS programs also directly support field work. MAXQDA, for example, has a mobile app that allows a researcher to take notes, record audio, code, and write memos on their mobile phone, all of which can be easily transferred later into the project file.

Portability is an issue if researchers need to share a project file with others, and the concepts of internal and external databases are important to understand for desktop programs in which only one person can work on a project file at a time. Some desktop programs use an internal database in which data imported into a "project file" are located within that file. This means that the file can be easily moved from one location to another (not just between two computers but also from one folder to another on the same computer) without losing any data. In contrast, programs with external databases create *links* to the data. The data appear to be in the project file, but they are actually retained in their original location (e.g., a different folder on the computer). The project file can still be moved from one location to another, but additional steps must be taken to ensure the linked data moves with it. Some software programs also use a combination of internal and external databases, depending on the data being analyzed. An internal database might be used for text documents and images and an external database used for larger audio and video files.

Cloud-based programs in which the data are located in the Internet rather than on a desktop computer approach data storage differently. The data do not need to be moved for different researchers; researchers can easily access the one project file from different geographical locations, and may be even be able to access it simultaneously. This may appeal to ethnographers working in large teams across geographical regions. Salmona, Lieber, and Kaczynski (2019), who provide instruction on the cloud-based program Dedoose, note that "the challenges faced with file sharing, platform compatibility, and version control cannot be understated" (Chapter 1). However, ethnographers should be familiar with both their institution's policies regarding data storage and with where cloud data are stored for particular CAQDAS programs before they decide to use a cloud-based program. All "clouds" are located somewhere, and a cloud could be located in a country different from the researcher's location and possibly not allowed by their institution.

One of the main functions of a CAQDAS program is to organize the data (Gilbert et al., 2014), which is key when working with the large amounts of data that can be generated in ethnographic studies. Data organization can occur in many ways, such as by type of data (e.g., separating interviews, observations, and healthcare documents into separate folders), date, or data collection site. Data can also be categorized within itself: field notes, for example, can be separated according to their format (e.g., observation, speculative, personal reflections), and links created between related field notes. The effective organization of field notes helps inform analysis (Fetterman, 2020), and clear—but flexible—data organization in CAQDAS "enables the researcher 'to see' the data more clearly" (Gilbert et al., 2014, p. 225).

The way in which the data are stored can also affect what kind of analyses are possible. In my role as a CAQDAS consultant, I have occasionally been asked questions about how to carry out particular analyses, and in doing so, I have helped researchers understand that the initial set up of their project files is critical. Two examples are provided here.

In the first situation, a researcher who was collecting longitudinal qualitative research was planning on having each year's data in a separate project file. However, she planned to compare the data across the different times, and I pointed out that this would be difficult to do if the yearly data were stored in different project files. I recommended she use one project file with different "folders" for each year's data. Luckily, this question was asked before the study commenced.

In a different situation, however, a researcher had copied all of his interviews into one Word file, imported that Word file into his CAQDAS program, and two people had completed an initial round of coding on the data (over 5000 codes—a very large amount of coding). He now wanted to compare the analyses of the interviews with each other as well as carry out intercoder agreement analysis, but realized he could not do these because all the data were in one file. The correct set up of the project file would have been to import each interview in a separate Word file rather than all of the interviews in one Word file. Thus, if there were 20 interviews carried out, then 20 different Word documents—each consisting of one interview—would be imported in rather than one Word file containing 20 interviews. Unfortunately, there was no easy fix to this problem, and the researcher was now spending a great deal of time recoding the data in order to continue with his analysis.

Data analysis with CAQDAS

In addition to organizing data, Gilbert and colleagues (2014) describe how CAQDAS assists with three general data analysis activities: (a) exploring the data (e.g., becoming familiar with the content, searching for content, and retrieving it); (b) interpreting and reflecting on the data (e.g., writing memos, creating diagrams); and (c) integrating the data (e.g., linking the data to other pieces of information). These activities help support the development of *thick description*, the cornerstone of powerful ethnographic research, as well as the identification of verbatim quotes, which are important features of ethnographic research (Fetterman, 2020). In this section, I focus mainly on coding, but also provide examples of other features helpful to ethnographic data analysis, and end with a commonly reiterated caveat about the capabilities of CAQDAS.

Coding is commonly used in ethnographic research (Willis & Anderson, 2017), and it is the central feature of CAQDAS programs, which typically provide multiple ways to code textual, visual, and audio data, and various ways to easily and quickly retrieve the coding. A code is "most often a word or short phrase that symbolically assigns a summative, salient, essence-capturing, and/or evocative attribute" (Saldaña, 2013, p. 3, cited in Miles, Huberman, & Saldaña, 2014, p. 72) to a piece of data. For example, in their ethnographic study of surgical teams in operating rooms, Tørring, Gittell, Laursen, Rasmussen, and Sørensen (2019) created a code for "relationship dynamics", with three subcodes underneath it: shared goals, shared knowledge, and mutual respect.

However, this kind of *topic coding* (Richards & Morse, 2013) or *first cycle coding* (Miles et al., 2014), which stays close to the raw data, is not analysis, per say. Rather, it is the *first step* of an analysis (Serry & Liamputtong, 2017) that leads to the identification of broader themes in the data. Researchers look for similar codes across the data points, and cluster certain codes together to create broader analytical themes (Miles et al., 2014). Such identification of categories and themes is an acknowledged manner of analyzing ethnographic data, which can either be conducted on its own or combined with a narrative format (see Willis & Anderson, 2017).

CAQDAS has other features that assist researchers in moving away from the originally collected data toward higher levels of analysis or abstraction, such as MAXQDA's "Summary Grid" and "Summary Table" functions. *Descriptive coding* (Richards & Morse, 2013), in which pieces of pertinent information are attached to data items, can also be carried out in CAQDAS. No interpretation occurs with this type of coding, but it allows the researcher to ask questions about the data (Richards & Morse, 2013). For example, in a multi-site ethnography, transcripts could be classified by their healthcare site to see if there are any different topic coding patterns based on where patients or health practitioners are located.

Many other CAQDAS features support interpretation and reflection on one's ethnographic data, and familiarity with a program's features is required for the researcher to understand how these tools can be harnessed. Memos are another key component. They assist researchers in recording key insights about the data (Roper & Shapira, 1999) and can be assigned to different parts of the data (e.g., codes, documents, document groups, segments of data, and "free standing" memos). Diagrams, matrices, and other visual tools can be created to show the relationships between codes, and facilitate new insight into "lengthy, unreduced text" (Miles et al., 2014, p. 108), but these kind of functions are typically underused (Woods, Paulus, Atkins, & Macklin, 2016). Some ethnographers may collect quantitative data (Fetterman, 2020), and CAQDAS programs support mixed methods research. Data from online questionnaires, for example, can be saved in Excel format, imported in and linked to the qualitative data. This integration can be more helpful than using separate software for the quantitative analysis (Annechino, Antin, & Lee, 2010).

It is very important for researchers to know that although software programs assist with data analysis, the programs do not "do" the analysis for the researcher (Coffey, 2018; Roper & Shapira, 1999; Serry & Liamputtong, 2017). Rather, it is always the researcher who is in control of the analysis and who decides how the software is used (Coffey, 2018; Gibbs, 2013; Humble, 2012). For example, the researcher—not the program—chooses what to code, what to name a code, whether to merge codes together, what to select for a coded segment, how much detail to enter into a memo, what code occurrences to search for, what content to insert into a diagram and how relationships are identified, and what kind of content is exported. Shortcuts such as autocoding content from searches should be used carefully, and it is the researcher who ultimately decides whether the output generated by such automated functions is helpful. The ideal user is a *critical appropriator* (Mangabeira, Lee, & Fielding, 2004) who uses a CAQDAS program but is reflexive about how it is used.

So what does it look like when CAQDAS is actually used in ethnographic health research? The next section highlights three examples.

Examples of health ethnographies using CAQDAS

I searched for recently published journal articles of health-focused ethnographies that used CAQDAS to see how such use was described (many ethnographies are published in monograph format; however, it was not possible to carry out this kind of search in books). Few examples were found, which may mean that the majority of health ethnographers are not using CAQDAS. However, it is also possible that some researchers are using CAQDAS but not mentioning that they do so. Very little detail is typically provided in journal articles about how CAQDAS is used (Humble, 2012; Paulus, Woods, Atkins, & Macklin, 2017; Woods et al., 2016), and, indeed, this was the case with what I found.

I therefore invited first authors of some of these articles to provide me with additional detail about how they used their programs. I deliberately sought out health ethnographies that used different types of CAQDAS, and three researchers (Jo Turnbull, Martin Charette, and Birgitte Tørring) kindly agreed to participate. The following programs were used: (a) ATLAS.ti (Turnbull, Prichard, Pope, Brook, & Roswell, 2017); (b) QDA Miner (Charette, Goudreau, & Bourbonnais, 2018); and (c) NVivo (Tørring et al., 2019). Table 33.1 lists each article's title, data sources used for the health ethnography, and direct quotes from the article about CAQDAS use.

As seen in Table 33.1, the original quotes briefly refer to using CAQDAS for data management and/or data analysis. However, the additional detail provided to me showed that each researcher used a number of functions in ways similar to other research (see Silver & Rivers, 2014) and also reflected on how they used their software. Below, I summarize their comments into three categories: (a) data management, (b) data analysis, and (c) critical reflections regarding CAQDAS use.

In terms of data management, all three researchers noted that they used different folders for each of their data sources. Turnbull also created a folder for the digital audio files of her interviews and focus groups, which were imported into her project file in addition to the transcripts. She noted that having such easy access to the audio files "sharpened [her] memories of the interview situations" (J. Turnbull, personal communication, October 13, 2019). Both Tørring and Turnbull also noted how they backed up copies of their files: Tørring, for

Table 33.1 Examples of CAQDAS use in health-focused ethnographies

Ethnography	Data Sources	Software mention in article (direct quote)
Factors influencing the practice of new graduate nurses: A focused ethnography of acute care settings (Charette, Goudreau, & Borbonnaise, 2018)	• Field notes from 40 hours of observations in three acute care units • 11 semi-structured interviews (transcripts) • Two focus groups (transcripts) • Clinical documentation (35 pages from nine documents)	"The analysis was done using QDA miner[a] (version 4.1.16)." (p. 3623)
Communication and relationship dynamics in the operating room: An ethnographic study (Tørring, Gittell, Laursen, Rasmussen, & Sørensen, 2019)	• Field notes from 240 hours of observations of surgical teams in orthopedic operation rooms (based on *grand tour* and *mini tour observations*) • 15 semi-structured interviews (transcripts and audiofiles) • Two focus groups (transcripts and audiofiles)	"Fieldnotes and transcriptions from the interviews were organized as verbatim text in the qualitative data analysis software program NVIVO[a]." (p. 3)
Risk work in NHS 111: The everyday work on managing risk in telephone assessment using a computer decision support system (Turnbull, Prichard, Pope, Brook, & Roswell, 2017)	• Field notes from 356 hours of observations of call-handling staff in an urgent care service and observation of other staff/activities (e.g., clinical nurse/paramedic advisors, training) • Six focus groups (transcripts)	"We imported the field notes into Atlas.Ti software 6.2 (Scientific Software Development GmbH, Berlin) to facilitate data archiving and retrieval and facilitate analysis." (p. 195) "Each researcher read a sample of transcripts independently identifying topics and issues. We then compared and discussed the different ways in which each researcher had coded their transcripts and sought to create an agreed set of codes which were then applied to the rest of the data using Atlas.Ti [a]." (p. 196)

a Spelling of software's name in the quote differs slightly from the software developer's spelling.

example, used NVivo's "Copy Project" function to store different copies of her project file when experimenting with different ways of coding.

All three researchers used their program's basic functions, and noted that other advanced features such as visual functions and intercoder agreement, as well as transcription, were not used. All of them used their program's coding functions and mentioned carrying out more than one stage of coding, such as Charette, who followed a 5-stage analysis framework suggested by Roper and Shapira (1999). His analysis began with topic coding, which was later regrouped into code categories. Specific CAQDAS functions can be used to create code groups: Turnbull used ATLAS.ti's "Code Group Manager" function to do this. Functions that supported malleability in coding were utilized, such as the "merge" function in QDA Miner and the "Code Manager" function in ATLAS.ti. All three described the importance of using their program's memo functions to keep track of the analysis. In Turnbull's project, the memos were particularly important for two researchers to communicate with each other about their interpretations and decisions. Query functions to search for specific words and sentences and code segment retrieval functions were also used.

The importance of flexibility in using CAQDAS was apparent in Turnbull, Charette, and Tørring's comments. As noted, not all of each program's functions were used, and they also described how they sometimes used functions that did not make it into their final analyses. For example, Tørring used NVivo's "case classification" function for descriptive coding, where she assigned pieces of information such as unit and gender to her participants, with the intent to use these to examine the topic coding patterns. However, she did not use this coding in her analysis ultimately. Similarly, Turnbull used an autocoding function, but the results did not inform her final analysis.

Second, not all of the data analysis took place within the CAQDAS programs. Export functions were used to relocate content out of the CAQDAS programs and save in other formats for further examination. This was done for two reasons. The first reason was that it allowed the researchers to share their data with others who were not familiar with the software program or did not have access to it. Charette, for example, exported codes and coded segments to share with his PhD supervisor, whereas Tørring shared her coding in a Word file with other team members. An additional reason was that the carrying out of some analyses, such as the development of matrices, was seen as easier to complete in other programs such as Excel (although one person noted that it could also have been related to simply not knowing how to use the matrix function in their CAQDAS program). Again, these non-CAQDAS files were easier to share with team members. Turnbull summarized how "much of the 'thinking'/analytical work took place outside ATLAS.ti—we held team data clinics to discuss emerging codes and then translated these discussions back to ATLAS.ti" (J. Turnbull, personal communication, November 5, 2019), a point that I return to in the next section.

Fears about using CAQDAS

Some ethnographers may resist using CAQDAS because they fear it will negatively affect their analysis or that it does not suit ethnographic research. Yet such resistance may be based on misconceptions that have persisted over the years (Jackson, Paulus, & Woolf, 2018). Constructive debates about CAQDAS are ongoing (Davidson & di Gregorio, 2011; Gibbs, 2013) and good for the field, as they signal that researchers are thinking critically about the interface between technology and data analysis. Ethnographers should be cognizant of the issues raised in these conversations (Coffey, 2018), and this final section summarizes some of these issues, with an emphasis on the concern about CAQDAS promoting distance from one's data.

Jackson et al. (2018) categorize criticisms of CAQDAS into four main areas: "Separation/Distancing, Homogenization/Standardizing, Mechanization/Dehumanizing, [and] Quantification/Decontextualizing" (p. 74). These criticisms may have had relevance early on in the history of CAQDAS, but CAQDAS advocates argue that these limitations have been addressed with later versions of programs (Silver, 2018). Research shows that these concerns can be managed when researchers become more experienced and critical users of CAQDAS, and experienced users report many benefits of using the programs, particularly for complicated projects (Gilbert et al., 2014). Moreover, alarmist concerns fail to acknowledge the researcher's agency and that poor qualitative research can occur in both "manual" and CAQDAS-assisted analysis (Gilbert et al., 2014).

Take, for example, the issue of separation/distance. This concern emerged with early programs, where researchers felt that CAQDAS created a barrier between themselves and their raw data. Programs have changed significantly from the 1980s, yet 20-year old concerns that were relevant at the time continue to be cited in recent research (Jackson et al., 2018). Current CAQDAS programs offer many ways of being close to the data and of linking analysis with the raw data. Coded segments, for example, can be easily viewed within the broader context (e.g., transcript) from which they were drawn, and time stamps applied to transcription can take the researcher immediately to a specific section of audio or video to listen to it.

Moreover, coding is so easily carried in CAQDAS that it can result in *too* much coding, which Gilbert et al. (2014) refer to as a *coding trap*, in which "users engage in nonproductive coding because they do not know when enough is enough" (p. 18). The nonproductive coding may also, however, represent a lack of training in qualitative research that results in researchers not knowing how to advance their analysis beyond their initial round of topic coding. Regardless of the reason, unproductive coding suggests too much closeness to data, and the example provided earlier of a researcher creating more than 5000 codes likely represents this level of coding. A balance between closeness and distance can be achieved, and it takes time to develop strategies to manage this (Gilbert et al., 2014). Moreover, there may be times when it is helpful to temporarily step away from the computer to gain a different perspective on the data (Silver, 2018), which was demonstrated in Turnbull's comment in the previous section.

As noted earlier, the researcher is always in control of the analysis, and reflexivity occurs in many ways. A critical appropriator (Mangabeira et al., 2004) will think carefully and realistically about how and when their program is used. CAQDAS programs have become more complex over the years, and not all of their functions need to be used (Allen, 2010; Humble, 2012). Moreover, analysis can and should be moved away from the software when relevant, and this does not mean that the CAQDAS has become irrelevant or has been discarded.

Conclusion

The CAQDAS field has changed greatly from its inception in the 1980s in response to user feedback and technological advances, and current programs can help with managing and analyzing ethnographic research data, as demonstrated by the three examples of health ethnographies provided in this chapter. A number of factors will assist health ethnographers in using CAQDAS effectively. First, it is helpful to know about the types of software available (Coffey, 2018), and the CAQDAS Networking Project can help in this regard. Second, if CAQDAS is used, scholars should mention it in their publications and provide detail about its use (Humble, 2012). Third, they can benefit from understanding the debates about CAQDAS, and about how early concerns about CAQDAS are no longer present in current software versions. Finally, health ethnographers can engage in reflexivity, which involves elements such as critically reflecting on what features to use and when to use a program—or when to temporarily step away from it, and remember that they are always in control of the analysis. CAQDAS offers many benefits, but it does not supply researchers with the "creativity, imagination, intuition, curiosity and evidence" (Trigueros-Cervantes, Rivera-García, & Rivera-Trigueros, 2018, p. 390) that is required when carrying out qualitative data analysis.

References

Allen, D. (2010). Fieldwork and participant observation. In I. Bourgeault, R. Dingwall, & R. de Vries (Eds.), *The SAGE handbook of qualitative methods in health research* (pp. 353–372). Thousand Oaks, CA: Sage.

Angrosino, M. (2007). *Doing ethnographic and observational research.* London, England: Sage.

Annechino, R., T.M.J. Antin, & J.P. Lee. (2010). Bridging the qualitative-quantitative software divide. *Field Methods, 22,* 115–124. doi:10.1177/1525822X09360760

Charette, M., J. Goudreau, & A. Bourbonnais. (2018). Factors influencing the practice of new graduate nurses: A focused ethnography of acute care settings. *Journal of Clinical Nursing, 28,* 3618–3631. doi:10.1111/jocn.14959

Coffey, A. (2018). *Doing ethnography.* London, England: Sage.

Davidson, J. & S. di Gregorio. (2011). Qualitative research and technology: In the midst of a revolution. In N. K. Denzin & Y. S. Lincoln (Eds.), *The SAGE handbook of qualitative research* (4th ed., pp. 627–643). Thousand Oaks, CA: Sage.

Evers, J.C. (2018). Current issues in qualitative data analysis software (QDAS): A user and developer perspective. *The Qualitative Report, 23*(13), Art. 5, 61–73. Retrieved from nsuworks.nova.edu/tqr/vol23/iss13/5

Fetterman, D.M. (2020). *Ethnography: Step-by-step* (4th ed.). Thousand Oaks, CA: Sage.

Fielding, J., N. Fielding, & G. Hughes. (2013). Opening up open-ended survey data using qualitative software. *Quality & Quantity, 47,* 3261–3276. doi:10.1007/s11135-012-9716-1

Freitas, F., J. Ribeiro, C. Brandão, F.N. de Souza, A.P. Costa, & L.P. Reis. (2018). In case of doubt see the manual: A comparative analysis of (self)learning packages qualitative research software. In A. P. Costa, L. P. Reis, F. N. de Souza, & A. Moreira (Eds.), *Computer supported qualitative research: Second international symposium on qualitative research (ISQR 2017)* (pp. 176–192). Cham, Switzerland: Springer. doi:10.1007/978-3-319-61121-1_16

Gibbs, G.R. (2013). Using software in qualitative analysis. In U. Flick (Ed.), *The SAGE handbook of qualitative data analysis* (pp. 277–294). Thousand Oaks, CA: Sage.

Gilbert, L.S., K. Jackson, & S. di Gregorio. (2014). Tools for analyzing qualitative data: The history and relevance of qualitative data analysis software. In J. M. Spector, M. D. Merrill, J. Elen, & M. J. Bishop (Eds.), *Handbook of research on educational communications and technology* (pp. 221–236). New York, NY: Springer. doi:10.1007/978-1-4614-3185-5_18

Green, J. & N. Thorogood. (2018). *Qualitative methods for health research* (4th ed.). Thousand Oaks, CA: Sage.

Humble, A.M. (2012). Qualitative data analysis software: A call for understanding, detail, intentionality, and thoughtfulness. *Journal of Family Theory & Review, 4,* 122–137. doi:10.1111/j.1756-2589.2012.00125.x

Jackson, K., T. Paulus, & N.H. Woolf. (2018). The walking dead genealogy: Unsubstantiated criticisms of qualitative data analysis software (QDAS) and the failure to put them to rest. *The Qualitative Report, 23*(13), Art. 6, 74–91. Retrieved from nsuworks.nova.edu/tqr/vol23/iss13/6

Kearney, G. P., M.K. Corman, N.D. Hart, J.L. Johnston, & G.J. Gormley. (2019). Institutional ethnography? Why now? Institutional ethnography in health professions education. *Perspectives on Medical Education, 8,* 17–24. doi:10.1007/s40037-019-0499-0

Lewins, A. & C. Silver. (2009, April). *Choosing a CAQDAS package.* Retrieved from www.surrey.ac.uk/sites/default/files/2009ChoosingaCAQDASPackage.pdf

Mangabeira, W.C, R.M. Lee, & N.G. Fielding. (2004). Computers and qualitative research: Adoption, use, and representation. *Social Science Computer Review, 22,* 167–178. doi:10.1177/0894439303262622

Miles, M. B., A.M. Huberman, & J. Saldaña. (2013). *Qualitative data analysis: A methods sourcebook* (3rd ed.). Thousand Oaks, CA: Sage.

Paulus, T., M. Woods, D.P. Atkins, & R. Macklin. (2017). The discourse of QDAS: Reporting practices of ATLAS.ti and NVivo users with implications for best practices. *International Journal of Social Research Methodology, 20,* 35–47. doi:10.1080/13645579.2015.1102454

Pool, R. (2017). The verification of ethnographic data. *Ethnography, 18,* 281–286. doi:10.1177/1466138117723936

Prentice, R. (2010). Ethnographic approaches to health and development research: The contributions of anthropology. In I. Bourgeault, R. Dingwall, & R. de Vries (Eds.), *The SAGE handbook of qualitative methods in health research* (pp. 157–173). Thousand Oaks, CA: Sage. doi:10.4135/9781446268247.n9

Prior, L. (2010). Documents in health research. In I. Bourgeault, R. Dingwall, & R. de Vries (Eds.), *The SAGE handbook of qualitative methods in health research* (pp. 417–432). Thousand Oaks, CA: Sage. doi:10.4135/9781446268247.n22

Richards, L. & J.M. Morse. (2013). *ReadMe First for a user's guide to qualitative methods* (3rd ed.). Thousand Oaks, CA: Sage.

Roper, J. M. & J. Shapira. (1999). *Ethnography in nursing research.* Thousand Oaks, CA: Sage.

Salmona, M., E. Lieber, & D. Kaczynski. (2019). *Qualitative and mixed methods data analysis using Dedoose.* Thousand Oaks, CA: Sage.

Serry, T. & P. Liamputtong. (2017). Computer-assisted qualitative data analysis (CAQDAS). In P. Liamputtong (Ed.), *Research methods in health: Foundations for evidence-based practice* (3rd ed., pp. 437–450). Sydney, Australia: Oxford.

Silver, C. (2018). CAQDAS at a crossroads: Choices, controversies and challenges. In A. P. Costa, L. P. Reis, F. N. de Souza, & A. Moreira (Eds.), *Computer supported qualitative research: Second international symposium on qualitative research (ISQR 2017)* (pp. 1–13). Cham, Switzerland: Springer.

Silver, C. & A. Lewins. (2014). *Using software in qualitative research: A step-by-step guide* (2nd ed.). London, England: Sage.

Silver, C. & C. Rivers. (2014). *Learning from the learners: The role of technology acceptance and adoption theories in understanding researchers' early experiences with CAQDAS packages.* 2013 ATLAS.ti User Conference. Retrieved from depositonce.tu-berlin.de/handle/11303/5139

Tørring, B., J.H. Gittell, M. Laursen, B.S. Rasmussen, & E.E. Sørensen. (2019). Communication and relationship dynamics in the operating room: An ethnographic study. *BCM Health Services Research, 19.* Advance online publication. doi:10.1186/s12913-019-4362-0

Trigueros-Cervantes, C., E. Rivera-García, & I. Rivera-Trigueros. (2018). The use of NVivo in the different stages of qualitative research. In A. P. Costa, L. P. Reis, F. N. de Souza, & A. Moreira (Eds.), *Computer supported qualitative research: Second international symposium on qualitative research (ISQR 2017)* (pp. 381–392). Cham, Switzerland: Springer. doi:10.1007/978-3-319-61121-1_32

Turnbull, J., J. Prichard, C. Pope, S. Brook, & A. Roswell. (2017). Risk work in NHS 111: The everyday work on managing risk in telephone assessment using a computer decision support system. *Health, Risk & Society, 19,* 189–208. doi:10.1080/13698575.2017.1324946

Willis, J. & K. Anderson. (2017). Ethnography as health research. In P. Liamputtong (Ed.), *Research methods in health: Foundations for evidence-based practice* (3rd ed., pp. 121–137). Sydney, Australia: Oxford.

Woods, M., T. Paulus, D.P. Atkins, & R. Macklin. (2016). Advancing qualitative research using qualitative data analysis software (QDAS)? Reviewing potential versus practice in published studies using ATLAS.ti and NVivo, 1994–2013. *Social Science Computer Review, 34,* 597–617. doi:10.1177/0894439315596311

34

ETHNOGRAPHIC AND QUALITATIVE DATA ANALYSIS

Immy Holloway

The nature of qualitative data analysis

To interpret and make sense of the data, the researcher has to analyse them. Data analysis is an important part of ethnographic health research; it is the process of examining the raw data in detail in order to transform them into meaningful information and give insight into the perspectives and understandings of the participants in the research. In this book, ethnography is used as an "umbrella term" for a number of qualitative approaches, some of which have different ways of analysing data. There is no rigid single type of analysis, but it needs to have its roots in the data generated by the participants and coherence with the specific method used (for instance grounded theory, narrative inquiry, and other methods). In some methods, data collection and analysis interact (GT for instance). In others, such as narrative research or phenomenology, data are collected first and consequently analysed. For beginners, a clear text such as Harding (2019) will be useful, as are relevant chapters in introductory texts such as that of Green and Thorogood (2018) or Ritchie, Lewis, Nicholls, and Ormston, (2014). At a later stage there might be a progression to more complex books like that of Miles, Huberman, and Saldaña, (2020). Most approaches to analysis are not linked to a particular discipline. Many of these overlap and are not unambiguous; they also have their own variations – examples are Straussian, Glaserian or Constructivist grounded theory and hermeneutic, descriptive, or interpretative phenomenology. Depending on which textbook researchers read, they might find a different version of the specific approach; no approach is strictly prescriptive, and many are not as "pure" as some of their originators would wish, although novice researchers are advised to follow a clear, specific approach.

In this chapter, we shall attempt an overview of data analysis in ethnographic health research and discuss the most frequent types: constant comparison (including coding and categorising), analysis of phenomenological and other narrative data, and thematic analysis. Initially however, it will be shown how researchers can prepare, transcribe, and organise their data.

Silverman (2017) discusses the status of interview data in particular, which must be taken into account before the process of data analysis can start. These data are rarely raw, he states, but have already been processed through the mind of the researcher. In observations too, fieldnotes sometimes show how environments shape interaction, and highlight other features such as the setting and context.

Preparing the data for analysis

The data need protection and storing. All tapes, notes, and transcripts are locked in a safe place and anonymised. It is advisable to keep several copies. The pseudonyms and real names of the participants are held in separate places.

Listening

The first step in analysis involves playing and listening to audio or video-tapes of interviews or observations. Parallel to this, researchers need to read their notes for each recorded item. At this stage, they also comment not only on the ideas that emerge but also on any queries, problems, or potential misunderstandings. It seems useful to summarise individual interviews and observations for potential future comparison. Gibbs (2018) claims that researchers often use textual data as a basis of analysis; therefore, they need transcripts of interviews and other data.

Transcribing tapes

Researchers prepare the data for analysis by transcribing them, if audio- or video-tapes exist. The transcripts should be *verbatim* (word for word) but gestures, facial expressions or laughs and coughs are taken into account as well as setting and context.

If researchers transcribe their own tapes, they become familiar with the data. Transcription takes time: One hour of tape could take four to six hours of transcription or longer for novice researchers. Sometimes researchers engage a typist to do this, because it saves time, and researchers use the time instead for listening and analysing. Anybody who transcribes must be advised on the confidentiality of the data.

Early audio or video-taped interviews should be fully transcribed so that the researcher has a basis for further analysis. Novice researchers should transcribe all tapes, while more experienced people can be more selective in their transcriptions and transcribe that which is linked to their developing ideas. (In certain language-based approaches such as discourse analysis or conversation analysis it is necessary to transcribe all the tapes.) There is a danger that researchers who fail to record the interviews will overlook significant issues, which they might meet on reflection when listening to the tape or considering the transcript. The front sheet of each transcription should contain name (pseudonym), date, location and time of interview as well as the code number for the informant and important biographical data (but no identifier). Convention dictates that researchers number each line of the transcript so that they can retrieve the data quickly when needed. Space is left for analysis and comments.

Although researchers number their transcripts line by line, they do not always use symbols in transcribing the data; however, well-known transcription systems do exist and are used mainly in discourse and conversation analysis, that is, language-based research, "naturally occurring data". The best known of these is by Gail Jefferson who uses symbols for non-verbal actions such as coughing, pausing, emphasising. Braun and Clarke (2013: 165) adapted Jefferson's system. Silverman (2017: 539) too gives a list of simplified transcription symbols which could be helpful in conversation analysis or discourse analysis. For many approaches, however, these systems would be inappropriate, for instance for phenomenology or other types of narrative research.

Of course, researchers transcribe in detail, and as accurately as possible as they choose sections from the data which answer their research questions. The focus needs be on the perceptions and words of the participants, not on the assumptions of the researcher.

Observations can be video-taped but only with the permission from those involved (unless they are done in a public space where everybody sees what is happening). Fieldnotes and diaries are as important in observation as in interviews. The mere act of transcribing means also a transformation of the data

Note taking and memoing

Researchers take notes all through the work. (Participants' facial expression, gestures and interviewers' reactions and comments during interviews can be recorded or noted, if they do not disturb. This can be done when interviewees do not wish to be tape-recorded, for instance in research with sensitive topics. Notes can also be taken immediately after the interview. This should be done as soon as possible after the interview without the presence of the participant to capture the flavour, behaviour and words of the informants and the ideas of the researcher. During interviews without recording on tape, the researcher can only write down a fraction of the sentences, and they only note down important sentences. It is always better to record the interview. When reading transcripts and writing memos, researchers also collect a series of significant quotes, which have relevance for use in the study to show the ideas and perceptions of the participants)

Notes do become an important part of the analysis. Listening to the tapes and making notes will sensitise researchers to the data and uncover not only ideas but also ambiguities within them. Indeed, the process of writing fieldnotes and memos is in itself an analytic process and not just data recording. It helps the researcher to interact with the data.

Ordering and organising the data

Qualitative researchers generate large amounts of data consisting of narratives from interviews, fieldnotes, and documents, as well as a variety of memos about the phenomenon under study (Bryman, 2016). Many use the relevant literature as data. Through organisation and management, the researcher brings structure and order to the unwieldy mass of data. This will help eventual retrieval and final analysis. All transcripts, fieldnotes, and other data should have details of time, location, and specific comments attached. The use of pseudonyms or numbers for participants prevents identification during the long process of analysis when the data might fall into the hands of individuals other than the researcher. Everything has to be recorded, cross-checked, and labelled. Then the material has to be stored in the appropriate files for later retrieval.

From the very beginning of the study, health researchers recognise significant ideas and themes. On listening to tapes, reading transcriptions and other documents, or looking at visual data, common themes and patterns will begin to emerge and become crystallised.

Different types of qualitative research have different approaches to data analysis. Even within one approach, researchers sometimes adopt a variety of analytic strategies. There are, however, some steps which most approaches have in common. They all start with listening, examining the data in detail, and eventually gaining a holistic view and extracting meaning.

These are some of the common features in QDA:

1. *Data analysis starts from the beginning of data collection*
   From the very first interview, observation, or document, the researchers have thoughts and gather ideas which they note down in their fieldnotes or memos.

2. *Data analysis is an iterative process*
   This involves "tacking", moving back and forth from collection to analysis several times, ensuring accuracy and being able to refine the questions and answers gained from the data.
3. *Fieldnotes, researcher diaries, and memos form not only part of data collection but also of analysis.*
   We have heard before, that researchers need to make notes and comments while gathering the data. This in itself is the start of analysis. While doing analysis, the researcher has to take the notes into account as they often help to focus.

At all times the researcher is aware of ethical issues, not merely during data collection. In health research, analysis too has ethical elements, not least the accuracy of the data as obtained from the participants.

The constant comparative method

Although difficult and sometimes confusing, the constant comparative method is one of the oldest and most often used. It has its origin in Grounded Theory, particularly in the book by Glaser and Strauss (1967), although other types of analysis also use codes and categories (see for instance, thematic analysis or IPA, and occasionally Narrative Analysis). The book by these authors has influenced generations of qualitative researchers, although not always in its original form.

The three main strands of GT analysis are the so-called Straussian, Glaserian – or Classic, as Glaser named it – and Constructivist. Examples for these can be found in the articles by Miller, Waring, Bolton, & Sloane, (2019) for Straussian; Roddis, Holloway, Galvin, and Bond (2019) for Constructivist GT. The preceding authors provide instances of coding and categorising and contain an emerging theory. The three approaches differ in various ways, but they also share a number of tenets. They rely on constant comparison; they use coding and categorising, and they have a core category (or core variable as Glaser and Strauss call it in their original book). As well as theoretical sampling, they all demand theoretical sensitivity and generate theory which is grounded in the data. Gibbs (2018) also suggests that GT needs a focus which becomes clearer as the research progresses. The emerging theory is explanatory. This means that it establishes causal relationships. To give an example: "When patients with a chronic illness have detailed knowledge of their condition, they are better at coping with it".

Most other types of qualitative analysis do not include explanation. *Memoing* – writing memos – is an important process in most constant comparative analysis, although other qualitative approaches do this too. (For specifics of these approaches, Glaser's numerous books and articles written in the last two decades, or Charmaz' more easily accessible texts should be read). Dunne (2011) suggests that GT constantly develops, it is "evolving".

Constant comparison is the result of the interaction between data collection and analysis. It is generated by *coding and categorising* and cannot be separated from these procedures. In their original book, Glaser and Strauss required comparisons between codes and categories, hence the name "constant comparative method". A very simple example of coding and categorising might be the following:

Codes

I felt seriously ill and didn't know what to do
The nurse came and helped me into bed
The doctor then examined me and prescribed medication
My family members visited, and I felt better with them around me

Pulling these codes together, getting them to a higher level might turn into the following:

Categories

Searching for answers
Help from professionals
Social support

A code is a label given to sections or segments of data. This might be a word or a phrase which represents the essence of the data (Saldaña, 2016). These – often numerous – codes, are compared with each other and reduced to main concepts and ideas, indeed they are examined for similarities and differences. Relationships between these are found, and they are grouped into categories and patterns, from which eventually the theory emerges. At every stage of the data collection and analysis process, codes and categories are compared with each other. *Theoretical sampling* occurs when researchers develop and improve the ideas in the tentative categories by searching for further instances of codes or categories. From the start of the data collection and analysis, researchers decide what and where to collect the next set of data. This is an ongoing process. Charmaz (2015) insists that this type of sampling makes the categories more accurate and specific. This might mean looking for more sites or ideas which lead in the direction of the developing theory. Theoretical sampling goes on until saturation, that is, when nothing new – of importance for the emerging theory (!) – can be found. A *core category* helps to establish a theory of a model. This category is a concept or a phenomenon at the centre of the categories and that integrates them.

Memoing, another common trend in constant comparative approaches, starts at the very beginning of data collection, indeed it is one of the early steps of analysis, when the researchers interact with the data and write notes on their observations and thoughts.

Much grounded theory research starts with *in vivo* coding which uses the actual words or phrases of participants showing the meanings which they give to their experiences; for instance, a new nurse might disclose that on her first day on the ward she was thrown in at the deep end. This comment then becomes a search for further instances of this code, which are then examined and summarised. This will help in the search for more data. The category at another level might then become "sink or swim", which demands explanation.

A Straussian grounded theory is described in a paper by Johnsson and Nordgren (2019) who investigated Swedish GPs' different responses to the pressure of divergent norms and built a model of responses towards a theory. An example for so-called classic grounded theory is that by Flenedy et al. (2017) which aimed to develop an explanatory theory of Emergency Department nurses' reasoning when reporting respiratory rate observations, while Andrews, Tierney, and Sears (2020) employed a constructivist approach to their research into self-care and self-compassion in nursing.

Thematic research and interpretative phenomenology also include coding and categorising, as does some narrative analysis.

Thematic analysis (TA)

Thematic analysis is a popular and straightforward, generic way of analyzing qualitative data, a method without a deep philosophy base. Novice researchers will find it useful. Braun and Clarke (2006, 2013) helped to make this type of approach popular and developed it. As they suggest, it is a research tool and need not be located within a specific theoretical or philosophical approach. It is often applied to psychology, sociology, healthcare, and also in education because of its flexibility and ease of use. According to Braun and Clarke (2006:79) TA is "a method for identifying, analyzing, and reporting patterns (themes) within the data". Most researchers use the approach developed by Braun and Clarke; however, other versions do exist. One of the earliest books for this is that by Boyatzis (1998), and many others, including Guest, MacQueen, and Namey (2012). Saldaña (2016) in text books, and Vaismoradi et al. in a nursing article write about it. TA is not a "pure" or sophisticated type of analysis, and it has some critics (see later); certain features can be found in other approaches – such as coding and categorising GT and also in IPA – but it is relatively easy to use, and if applied appropriately, can lead to a good research study.

Braun and Clark constructed a guide to TA which includes the following: After becoming familiar with the data and transcribing interviews or other material, researchers have already generated thoughts and major ideas. They then suggest the main phase, namely coding the data. A code, which is a label which summarises an element in the data of significance to the researcher, represents a small section of some of the material which the researcher collected. The coding system they use is similar to that in Grounded Theory (see the above).

An example of thematic analysis is given by Grogan, Turley, and Cole (2018) in research with women who have endometriosis. This study adopted open-ended questioning, during which women disclosed their thoughts about their condition. The data were coded and several themes emerged. An instance of one of these is "a constant struggle with pain and fatigue". Grogan et al summarised and discussed these themes and linked them to previous studies which they found in the literature.

Template analysis

Thematic analysis (TA) is not a single rigid approach to the data, and several versions exist. Template analysis for instance, is a type of TA which imposes a degree of structure on the data (Brooks, McCluskey, Turley, & King, 2015).

As with all analyses, this strategy demands familiarisation with and in-depth knowledge of the data. The initial steps include preliminary coding, and Brooks et al. (2015) suggest that the researcher is allowed to start with "a priori" themes that can later be changed when new ideas arise. Unlike other types of analysis which are inductive – deriving directly from the data – this contains an element of deduction in which the researcher sometimes imposes the themes after an overview of the data. As usual, of course, researchers search for links and relationships between the themes and organise them into clusters. An initial coding template is created which derives from early and varied interview or diary data. This template is applied to the rest of the data and redefined if necessary, adding new themes or discarding others. In the latter stages of template analysis, researchers use the final template for all the data and do not discard any which are important for the answers to the research question (Brooks et al. 2015). The template analysis by Brooks et al. (2015) was connected to "the integrative model of uncertainty" which included "uncertainty", "cognitive, emotional, and behavioural domains", and their influencing factors. This was the template for the research interviews of the authors. They also developed a hierarchical list of themes, categories, and codes.

Some researchers do not code or categorise because they wish to perceive the essence of the phenomenon as a whole, a *Gestalt*. Breaking the data into codes may lose this holistic view of the phenomenon and fragment the ideas contained in the data. Examples of this type of analysis can be found in phenomenology in all its forms as well as in other types of narrative research (more often called 'narrative analysis').

Analysis in phenomenology and other narrative research

As in grounded theory, there are a number of approaches in phenomenology, the main types being descriptive, hermeneutic, and interpretative phenomenology (IPA). The latter is considered easier, and many data have been analysed through IPA. However, in its purest form, descriptive phenomenology is one of the earliest. The best-known authors in this field are Giorgi and Colaizzi who wrote in the 1970s. Although much of their work has been authored decades ago, Giorgi is still writing at this time.

Descriptive phenomenology explores the "lived experience" of human beings, hermeneutic (or interpretive) phenomenological analysis focuses on the interpretation of texts – oral or written stories. Both have their foundation in philosophy. It is unfortunate that often researchers who claim to use this method of analysis (with which this chapter is concerned) do not base their work in philosophy. The terminology in phenomenological methods is different from that of other qualitative research.

Giorgi's approach has its origin in the philosophy of Husserl and Merleau-Ponty. When exploring his method of analysis, researchers realise that his main concern is the 'Gestalt', the whole. Broadly, descriptive phenomenologists take the following steps to analyse the data:

- "Bracketing" one's own assumptions about the phenomenon.
- Getting a sense of the whole, the "Gestalt".
- Describing "meaning units", that is, "intuition" is used to get the sense of each description.
- Translating the meaning units into insights and highlighting common themes.
- Going from concrete examples to consistent statements and to the essence of the experience.

The steps thus include "description, reduction, and construction" of essential structures. They become much clearer when looking at examples of descriptive phenomenology such as that of Fry (2016) or Broomé (2011). Broomé discusses the methodology of his thesis, and Fry gives examples of meaning units and their transformation in one of her appendices. Colaizzi's approach is similar though he breaks it down into seven steps. Sugden and King (2019) used this in their work about the experience of blood donation and described Colaizzi's steps in detail.

Van Manen in his *hermeneutic or interpretive phenomenology* takes the following steps according to Rodriguez and Smith (2018: 91 – directly quoted from their book)

- Turning to a phenomenon, a commitment by the researcher to understanding that world.
- Investigating experience as we live it rather than as we conceptualise it.
- Reflecting on the essential themes, which characterise the phenomenon.
- Describing the phenomenon through the art of writing and rewriting.
- Maintaining a strong and oriented relation to the phenomenon.
- Balancing the research context by considering the parts and the whole.

Sommer (2019) wrote a thesis, using van Manen's hermeneutic phenomenology, on support from the social and welfare services for young persons with mental health issues in a small Norwegian community. Her findings were uncovered by this method and helped understand these problems.

Interpretative phenomenological analysis (IPA) is one of the most popular ways of collecting and analysing data, particularly in qualitative health research. It was developed by Jonathan Smith from 1996, with Flowers and Larkin in 2009, later with his colleague Virginia Eatough (2019) and others. An article by Aldridge, Fisher, and Laidlaw (2019) explores the experience of shame in people with dementia. This shows some of the processes of analysis that are often used in IPA which uses both coding and searching for themes. IPA has an underlying philosophy, but it resembles GT and TA in its coding and thematising.

Narrative research or narrative analysis has a number of ways in which data are analysed. In this chapter, we are not so much concerned with the early classic texts by authors such as Clandinin and Connelly (2004), Lieblich, Tuval-Mashiach, and Zilber (1998) or Andrews, Squire, and Tamboukou (2013) but more with those focusing on analysis in social or health care specific-ally. One of the latest books in the latter field is that by Lucius-Hoene, Holmberg, and Meyer, (2018). Although all of these texts mention analysis, none of them discusses it in detail, hence here the focus is specifically on the well-known writings of Kohler Riessman (1993 and 2008) and the text by Bold (2012, Chapter 7) which describe types of analysis. Riessman, in particular, describes three types of analysis: thematic, structural, and dialogic/performance. Thematic or holistic analysis focuses on content (story and plot). Structural analysis – initially discussed by Labov and Waletzky in 1967 – considers the form and structure of the narrative, while dialogic/performance analysis takes into account all of these and includes the interaction of people in the tale and its context. In her M.A. dissertation, Stanley (2019) used a narrative thematic ana-lysis about communicating health among methadone patients in an area of the US during their recovery from opioid addiction. Wong and Breheny (2018) give an example of structural ana-lysis in narrative research in psychology. They researched stories of older people in residential care concerning their involvement in animal therapy and other aspects of health. Their article shows how structural analysis can be used with personal stories of individuals. Research on dia-logic/performance analysis is more difficult to find. Thakrar (2018) however, managed to use this as well as the other ways of analysing in a thesis on men's narratives of planning to go back to work after a burn injury.

The process of analysis and interpretation

In his book, Silverman (2014) discusses the interpretation of data. In all types of QDA it is important that researchers stay as close to the data as possible and look at everything connected with the phenomenon under study. Their data have primacy. A completed study is never a "mere" description of the participants' experience, and even "pure" description involves inter-pretation because researchers have choices. It is important to remember that the final product of research depends on the collaborative effort of participants and researcher. While those observed and interviewed are active agents in their world rather than passive participants and construct their social reality, researcher and participant also construct meaning together. The reader of the study too, will eventually be involved in construction of meaning.

Problems of QDA

Because of the complexities of QDA, a number of problems might arise. Li and Seale (2007) list several, and one of these relates to not knowing where to start the process. This might be solved by asking novice researchers to analyse short sections of data. Many find the resulting themes or codes ambiguous, and of course, there is sometimes overlap of meaning. Reporting or recording problems can be overcome more easily. These issues are often connected with forgetting to note down the identifier of the participant or not being able to retrieve ideas that had previously been discovered. Some new researchers over-interpret – everything has meaning for them – or they report inaccurately and give no evidence where ideas have their roots.

Computer-Assisted (or Aided) Qualitative Data Analysis (CAQDAS)

In ethnographic research, computers are seen as a useful tool. Most researchers use them for entering, storing, and retrieving data, as well as for various other tasks, such as making notes, keeping diaries, etc. In this chapter, there is a short discussion of computer analysis of qualitative data.

Computers are particularly popular for analysing large amounts of data more quickly. Funding agencies, which are used to computers in quantitative inquiry, seemed to be more impressed when qualitative researchers suggested a computer package for analysis. Computers have been used in the analysis of qualitative data mainly since the 1980s. The University of Surrey is well-known for its courses and textbooks in this field, and members of the CAQDAS team (Computer-assisted or aided Analysis Qualitative Data Software) also advise on the appropriate computer package. Computers can and do make the process of qualitative research easier, as they can order, organise, and manage the data, particularly in complex studies where different research teams work together.

It must be said, however, that the computer is merely a tool, if a useful one, especially for a lengthy study with a large number of participants and/or several researchers. The computer shortens routine and mechanical tasks and can be a device make the task less time-consuming (a warning however: a novice researcher might spend a long time learning to use a computer package, and it is essential to become familiar with it). Holloway and Galvin (2017) warn, however, that while computers can be useful, the use of technology does not replace the "intellectual reflective process" of the researcher which is so important in qualitative analysis.

Several types of computer-aided QDA software exist, of which the best known are NVivo, NUDIST (Non-numerical Unstructured Data Indexing, Searching and Theorising), ATLAS. ti and HyperResearch (for a list and advice for best uses of the various programs, see Silver and Lewins, 2014). The packages have slightly different functions (for advice see the relevant texts).

For further information and details on particular programs, we advise researchers to refer to up-to-date text books such as Silver and Lewins (2014) Jackson and Bazeley (2019), and the various writings of Lyn Richards and Janice Morse (2013, 2015). Lewins and Silver (2007) have written a step-by-step guide updated to Silver and Lewins in 2014 (Silver & Lewins, 2014). In some of these books, programs and addresses can also be found.

The reasons for computer use (taken from Holloway and Galvin, 2017)

Tesch (1993) listed tasks which can be performed by computers but can also be carried out manually, and his is still the clearest advice for these tasks.

- Storing, annotating, and retrieving texts
- Locating words, phrases, and segments of data
- Naming or labelling
- Sorting and organising
- Identifying data units
- Preparing diagrams

- Extracting quotes

Tesch (1991) describes three main approaches to QDA (described below) but acknowledges that these groupings and their subgroups are not neat and discrete; they overlap and do not reflect reality. Both the content of the text and the process of communication are seen as important.

Language-oriented

These types of analysis are used by researchers who are primarily interested in language and its meaning – examples are conversation and discourse analysis. These approaches focus mainly on words and verbal interaction.

Descriptive/interpretive approaches

These deal with narratives and give descriptions of feelings and actions. Examples are life histories and certain types of ethnography as descriptions and interpretations of a culture. There are also approaches to narrative inquiry and to various forms of phenomenological research.

Advantages of computer use

Harding (2019) claims that the use of computers is more efficient than manual analysis, (one must note that computers also allow cutting and pasting).

Data are more accessible and computer analysis is less time consuming for an experienced computer user – (as stated before, it takes time to learn to use computer analysis programmes and packages). More time can be given to thinking about the data. The process of qualitative analysis becomes more manageable with large amounts of data.

The disadvantages of computer analysis

Certain problems emerge, however, when using computers. Apart from national studies and social policy issues, qualitative research projects are generally not large, but computer use might tempt researchers to collect more data than necessary and analyse them too quickly, and deeper meanings could be missed.

Some researchers believe that computer analysis is not necessary, and it might change qualitative research's intimate nature. Computers might distance researchers from the data, and while this might be appropriate in business research, in health research it could be detrimental. Researchers need keep close to the data and actively interact with them.

Developing a dialogue with the literature

Literature related to the topic is part of all stages of ethnographic research. At its start, it shows the gaps in knowledge that the researcher aims to fill. It can also become part of the theoretical perspective of the research, and plays an important role to explain the specific methods used. The place of the literature in a qualitative research study is ambiguous, nevertheless, and qualitative experts have a variety of perspectives. Relevant articles and books can be found, such as, for instance, Dunne (2011), Holloway and Galvin (2017) or Harding (2019). Here we do not focus on the problematic issues but on the important place of the literature in the analysis of data. In the analysis, researchers have developed major themes (categories, etc., depending on the research approach). These findings form the basis for a dialogue with the relevant literature. In some approaches, such as some forms of GT and thematic analysis, the link to the literature starts at the very beginning, in others such as in narrative research, the connection to the literature begins after the data have been collected. Each main idea is linked to findings of others in a similar area and discussed in relation to it. This action might confirm, validate or challenge the researcher's own findings. It also assists in gaining a deeper understanding of the research problem. Concepts emerging from the study can be compared with those generated by the literature. Strauss and Corbin (1998) also state that the literature can be used as an added source of data (but is questioned by some). Nevertheless, the literature linked directly to the main findings might produce new ideas which could be followed. The researcher's own data, however, always have primacy in a qualitative research study.

Summary

Data are analysed in various ways which depend on the approach, the type of data and the philosophical stance researchers adopt.

- QDA is complex, and takes time and care.
- It often interacts with data collection.
- Many approaches use thematic analysis, coding, and categorising, from a basic to a more abstract level, while others apply a holistic approach and are more descriptive.
- Data analysis is flexible but needs to be rigorous.
- Computers can be a tool in the analysis of data, especially in data retrieval and management, but they are not absolutely necessary for qualitative research unless there is a huge amount of data.

References

Aldridge, H., P. Fisher, & K. Laidlaw. (2017) Experiences of shame for people with dementia. *Dementia,* 18(5): 1896–1911.

Andrews, H., S. Tierney. & K. Seers. (2020) Needing permission: The experience of self-care and self-compassion in nursing. *International Journal of Nursing Studies,* January 2020, article103436.

Andrews, M., C. Squire. & M. Tamboukou. (2013) *Doing narrative research.* 2nd ed. London: Sage.

Bold, C. (2012) *Using narrative in research.* London: Sage.

Boyatzis, R.E. (1998) *Transforming qualitative data: Thematic analysis and code development.* Thousand Oaks, CA: Sage.

Braun, V. & V. Clarke. (2006) Using thematic analysis in psychology. *Qualitative Research in Psychology,* 3(2): 77–101

Braun, V. & V. Clarke. (2019) Reflecting on reflexive thematic analysis. *Qualitative Research in Sport, Exercise and Health,* 11(4): 589–597

Braun, V. and V. Clarke. (2006) Using thematic analysis in psychology. *Qualitative Research in Psychology,* 3(2): 77–101.

Braun, V. and V. Clarke. (2013) *Successful Qualitative Research: A Practical Guide for Beginners.* London: Sage.

Broomé, R (2011) Descriptive phenomenological psychological method: An example of a methodological section from a doctoral dissertation. Saybrook University. works.bepress.com/rodger_broome/9/

Brooks, J., S. McKluskey, E. Turley, & N. King. (2015) The utility of template analysis in qualitative psychological research. *Qualitative Research in Psychology,* 12(2): 202–222.

Bryman, A. (2016) *Social Research Methods,* 5th ed. Oxford: Oxford University Press.

CAQDAS Networking Project, University of Surrey. Available at caqdas.soc.surrey.ac.uk/index.htm

Charmaz (2015), Charmaz, K. (2015). Teaching theory construction with initial grounded theory tools: A reflection on lessons and learning. Qualitative Health Research, 25, 1610–1622.

Clandinin, D.J. & F.M. Connelly. (2004) *Narrative inquiry: Experience and story in qualitative research*. San Francisco: Jossey-Bass.

Colaizzi, P. (1978). Psychological research as a phenomenologist views it. In: Valle, R. S. & King, M. *Existential Phenomenological Alternatives for Psychology*. New York: Open University Press.

Dunne, C. (2011) The place of the literature review in qualitative research. *International Journal of Research Methodology* 14(2): 111–124.

Fielding, N. and R. Lee. (1998) *Computer analysis and qualitative research*. London: Sage.

Fielding, N., Lee, R. & Blank, G. eds. (2017) Online research methods. 2nd ed. London: Sage.

Flenady T, Dwyer T, Applegarth J. Accurate respiratory rates count: So should you! Australas Emerg Nurs J. 2017 Feb; 20(1): 45–47. doi: 10.1016/j.aenj.2016.12.003. Epub 2017 Jan 7. PMID: 28073649.

Fry, J. (2016) A descriptive phenomenological study of independent midwives' utilisation of intuition as an authoritative form of knowledge in practice. PhD thesis, Bournemouth University.

Gibbs, G. (2018) *Analyzing qualitative data*. 2nd ed. (from the Sage Qualitative Research Kit). London: Sage.

Giorgi, A. (1970) *Psychology as a human science: A phenomenologically based approach*. New York: Harper & Row.

Glaser, B.G. (1978) *Theoretical sensitivity*. Mill Valley, CA: Sociology Press..

Glaser, B.G. & A.L. Strauss. (1967) *The discovery of grounded theory*. Chicago, Ill: Aldine.

Green, J. & N. Thorogood. (2018) *Qualitative methods for health research*. 4th ed. London: Sage.

Grogan, S., E. Turley, & J. Cole. (2018) So many women suffer in silence: A thematic analysis of women's written accounts of coping with endometriosis. *Psychology and Health*, 33(11) 1364–1378.

Guest G.S., K.M. MacQueen, & E.E. Namey. (2012) *Applied thematic analysis*. Thousand Oaks, CA: Sage.

Harding, J. (2019) *Qualitative data analysis: From start to finish*. 2nd ed. London: Sage

Heinonen, K (2015) van Manen's method and reduction in a phenomenological hermeneutic study. *Nurse Researcher*, 22(4): 35–41.

Holloway I and Galvin K *Qualitative Research in Nursing and Healthcare,* 4th Edn. 2016. Wiley-Blackwell.

Jackson, K & P. Bazeley. (2019) *Qualitative data analysis with NVivo*. London: Sage.

Johnsson, L. & L. Nordgren. (2019) How general practitioners decide on maxims of action in response to demands from conflicting sets of norms: A grounded theory study. *BMC Medical Ethics*, doi.org/10.1186/s12910-019-0360-3

Kelle, U. (ed.), (1995) *Computer-Aided Qualitative Data Analysis: Theory, Methods and Practice*. London: Sage.

Labov, W. & J. Waletzky. (1967) Narrative analysis: Oral versions of experience. In Helm, J. (Ed) *Essays on the verbal and visual arts,* pp. 12–44. Seattle: University of Washington Press.

Lewins, A. & C. Silver. (2007) *Using Software in Qualitative Research: A Step-by-Step Guide*. London: Sage.

Li, S. & C. Seale. (2007) Learning to do qualitative data analysis: an observational study of doctoral work. *Qualitative Health Research*, 17(10): 1442–1452.

Lieblich, A., R. Tuval-Mashiach, & T. Zilber. (1998) *Narrative research: Reading, analysis and interpretation*. Thousand Oaks, CA: Sage.

Lucius-Hoene, G., C. Holmberg, & T. Meyer. (2018) *Illness narratives in practice: Potentials and challenges in health-related contexts*. Oxford: Oxford University Press.

Miles, M.B., A.M. Huberman, & J. Saldaña. (2020) *Qualitative data analysis: A method sourcebook*, 4th ed. Thousand Oaks, CA: Sage.

Miller, P.K., L. Waring, G.C. Bolton, & C. Sloane. (2019) Personnel flux and workplace anxiety: Personal and interpersonal consequences of understaffing in UK ultrasound departments. *Radiography*, 25(1): 46–50.

Richards, L. (2015) *Handling Qualitative Data: A Practical Guide*, 3rd ed. London: Sage.

Richards, M.G. & J.M. Morse. (2013) *Readme First: A User's Guide to Qualitative Methods*, 3rd ed. Thousand Oaks, CA: Sage.

Riessman, C.K. (1993) *Narrative analysis*. Newbury Park, CA: Sage.

Riessman, C.K. (2008) *Narrative methods for the Human Sciences*. Thousand Oaks, CA: Sage.

Ritchie, L., J. Lewis, C.M. Nicholls, & R. Ormston. (2014) *Qualitative Research Practice: A Guide for Social Science Students and Researchers*. London: Sage.

Roddis, J., I. Holloway, K. Galvin, & C. Bond. (2019) Acquiring knowledge prior to diagnosis: A grounded theory of patient experiences. *Patient Experience Journal*, 6(1): 10–18.

Rodriguez, A. & D. Smith. (2018) Phenomenology as a healthcare method. *Evidence-Based Nursing*, 21(4): 96–98 (from the series *Research made simple*).

Saldaña, J. (2016) *The coding manual for qualitative researchers*, 3rd ed. Thousand Oaks, CA: Sage.

Silver, C. & A. Lewins. (2014) *Using Software in Qualitative Research: A Step by Step Guide*, 2nd ed. London: Sage.

Silverman, D. (2017) *Doing Qualitative Research: A Practical Handbook*, 4th ed. London: Sage.

Silverman, D. (2014) *Interpreting Qualitative Data*, 5th ed. London: Sage.

Smith, J.A. (1996) Beyond the divide between cognition and discourse: Using interpretative phenomenological analysis in health psychology. *Psychology and Health,* 11(2): 261–271.

Smith, J.A., P. Flowers, & M. Larkin. (2009) *Interpretative phenomenological analysis.* London: Sage.

Smith, J.A. & V. Eatough. (2019) Introduction. Looking forward: conceptual and methodological developments in interpretative phenomenological analysis. *Qualitative Research in Psychology,* 16: 163–165. *doi.org/10.1080/14780887.2018.1540620*

Sommer, M. (2019) Support as possibility Lived experiences of support of young persons with mental health problems: A hermeneutic phenomenological study. PhD thesis. University of South-Eastern Norway

Stanley, B.L. Communicating health: A thematic narrative analysis among Methadone patients. Graduate Theses and Dissertations. scholarcommons.usf.edu/etd/7953

Strauss, A.L. and Corbin, J. (1998) Basics of Qualitative Research: Grounded Theory Procedures and Techniques, 2nd edn. London: Sage.

Sugden, N. & N. King. (2019) A descriptive phenomenological analysis of the experience of blood donation as a regular donor. *Journal of Health Psychology.* Nov 29 doi.org/10.1177/1359105319890014

Thakrar, S. (2018) Challenges in the present, storied for the future: Men's narratives of planning to return to work after a burn injury. PhD thesis. The University of Manitoba, Canada.

Tesch, R. (1991) Software for qualitative researchers. In N.G. Fielding and R.M. Lee (Eds) *Using Computers in Qualitative Research*, pp. 16–37. London: Sage.

Tesch, R. (1993) Personal computers in qualitative research. In M.D. LeCompte, J. Preissle and R. Tesch (Eds) *Ethnography and Qualitative Design in Educational Research*, 2nd ed., pp. 279–314. Chicago, IL: Academic Press.

Wong, G. & M. Breheny. (2018) Narrative analysis in health psychology: A guide for analysis. *Health Psychology and Behavioral Medicine*, 6(1): 245–261.

Further Reading

Creswell, J.W. & C.N. Poth. (2018) *Qualitative inquiry and research design.* Thousand Oaks, CA: Sage.

Gibson, B. & J. Hartman. (2014) Rediscovering grounded theory. London: Sage.

Kenny, M., & R. Fourie. (2015). Contrasting Classic, Straussian, and Constructivist Grounded Theory: Methodological and philosophical conflicts. *The Qualitative Report,* 20(8): 1270–1289. Retrieved from nsuworks.nova.edu/tqr/vol20/iss8/9

Flick, U. ed. (2014) *The Sage handbook of qualitative data analysis.* London: Sage.

Langridge, D. (2007) *Phenomenological psychology.* Harlow, UK: Pearson/Prentice Hall.

Salmons, J. (2016) *Doing qualitative research online.* London: Sage.

Zahavi, D. (2019) *Phenomenology: The basics.* Abingdon, Oxon: Routledge.

35

ETHNOGRAPHIC CREATIVE NON-FICTION

The creation and evolution of *Lily's Lymphedema*

Elise Radina

Lily's Lymphedema is a work of ethnographic, creative non-fiction in the form of a short story for children. In this chapter, I begin by explaining the origins and utility of creative nonfiction as a method of communicating ethnographic research findings. I explain the basic elements of lymphedema, a chronic condition that is the focus of *Lily's Lymphedema*, in order to provide the reader with context for the story. In so doing, I also provide an overview of the methods my research team used to collect qualitative interview data from parents of children with lymphedema. I conclude by detailing data analysis processes and how those processes, as well as my 20 years of knowledge accumulation about lymphedema (LE), informed the creation of *Lily's Lymphedema* (Appendix A) as a work of ethnographic, creative nonfiction.

Ethnographic creative non-fiction

Creative nonfiction, as a literary genre, has its beginnings in journalism (Gutkind & Fletcher, 2008) in that it is grounded in fact (i.e., research data), while also employing "literary conventions" (Smith, McGannon, & Williams, 2015; p. 59). Leavy (2013) connects ethnography and creative nonfiction by stating, "ethnographic writing, at its best, involves storytelling" (p. 31). The result of combining these two storytelling techniques is ethnographic, creative nonfiction – a "novel way for representing work done in this qualitative tradition [ethnography]" (Smith et al., 2015). Works of ethnographic, creative nonfiction are fictionalized renditions of empirical data collected from or about real people and their unique lived experiences (Clayton, 2010). By employing the technique of creative nonfiction, ethnographers and other qualitative researchers are able to succinctly show a number of research findings as well as represent the experiences of multiple participants in one cohesive story (Smith et al., 2015; Gutkind & Fletcher, 2008). At the same time, the presentation of ethnographic or qualitative research findings in the form of a story allows the researcher to share research findings beyond a purely academic audience (Smith, Papathomas, Martin Ginis, & Latimer-Cheung, 2013).

In considering the use of ethnographic, creative nonfiction, the terms *creative* and *fiction* may understandably give those pause who are familiar with more positivist perspectives on research criteria. These terms can evoke assumptions about fabrication and lack of authenticity as well as concerns that the work does not conform to strict notions of positivist, scientific rigor (e.g., objectivity, validity, and reliability). Gutkind (2012) argues that the term *creative* as it is used in creative nonfiction, "doesn't mean inventing what didn't happen [or] reporting or describing what wasn't there" (p. 7). Indeed, the facts of the story, or in the case described here, data from qualitative interviews, serve as the backbone of the work of creative nonfiction. These facts "constitute the important teaching element, the informational content introduced throughout the story that leads to the reader's sense of discovery" (Gutkind & Fletcher, 2008; p. 53). Echoing this perspective, Leavy (2013) notes that verisimilitude, or truthfulness or likeness to "real life" (Smith et al., 2015), is an essential element of both nonfiction and fiction writing. The same is true for ethnography (Humphreys & Watson, 2009). Both ethnographic writers and writers of creative nonfiction share the same goal of recreating the *real*-life experiences of *real* people in a form that is both informative and engaging (Gutkind, 2012; Leavy, 2013).

Smith and colleagues (2015) offer several reasons that qualitative researchers may choose to employ the technique of creative nonfiction. Beyond those discussed above, they also note that by reading the story, readers are called on to "become a witness of others" or to see others' perspectives in new ways (p. 63). The creative nonfiction writer's use of everyday language, descriptive technique, representation of emotions, and the humanization of research participants allows the reader to not only be engaged but also to "inhabit the lifeworld of participants and/ or researchers" (p. 63).

Basic elements of lymphedema

Lymphedema (LE) is a condition involving an accumulation of interstitial fluid. LE results from the malformation or malfunction of the lymphatic system and has been estimated to occur in 140–250 million individuals worldwide (Mendoza, Li, Gill, & Tyring, 2009). LE is chronic, progressive swelling of the affected body parts, which can have an impact on quality of life (e.g., physical disability, psychological distress; Smeltzer, Stickler, & Schirger, 1985). LE that develops at birth or before three months is referred to as congenital or primary lymphedema. Primary LE tends to occur in the legs, feet, genitals, and trunk. When lymphedema develops between four months and adulthood it is referred to as lymphedema praecox (Smeltzer et al., 1985).

The use of specially fitted compression garments is the preferred method of treatment to manage lymphatic swelling in children. This includes the use of compression stockings and a specialized wrapping that use Ace-type elastic bandages (Maclellan & Greene, 2014; Smeltzer et al., 1985). This use of compression may follow or be used in conjunction with a specific type of massage called manual lymph drainage, which is designed to move fluid out of the affected area to elsewhere in the body (Maclellan & Greene, 2014).

In order to avoid the very real risk of cellulitis, a serious skin infection, which can make lymphedema symptoms worse, parents are advised to ensure that their children avoid disruptions to the skin including the use of sunblock to avoid sunburn, bug spray to avoid bites, and wearing clothing to keep the skin covered when compression is not being used (Maclellan & Greene, 2014).

Ethnographic work behind *Lily's Lymphedema*

The creation of *Lily's Lymphedema* (Appendix A) involved many years of qualitative data and information collection about the chronic condition of lymphedema. My research regarding lymphedema initially began in 1999 with the study of lymphedema in breast cancer patients. I have continued to pursue this line of research and as a result, I have attended many national and international conferences where I presented this work, attended instructional sessions and presentations about lymphedema diagnosis and treatment and how to prevent the exacerbation of symptoms. I spoke with seemingly countless patients and medical professionals about their experiences with lymphedema. I attended community-based support groups and had the privilege of observing a patient as her specially trained massage therapist conducted manual lymph drainage. I informally interviewed an adult who developed lymphedema as a child and engaged in informal conversations with parents of children who had been diagnosed with lymphedema. In 2016, my team of undergraduate research assistants and I conducted a study of parents of children with lymphedema, which I describe in more detail later in this chapter. It is the culmination of my experiences in learning about lymphedema as well as the stories from the parents in this study that informed the creation of *Lily's Lymphedema*.

Data collection methods

Participants (n=27) were biological parents of children with LE who were diagnosed between the ages birth to 18 years. The decision to limit participation to biological parents was based on the genetic connection that can sometimes explain the occurrence of lymphedema (Schlögel, Brouillard, Boon, & Vikkula, 2015). Participants were recruited from The National Lymphedema Network and The Lymphedema Treatment Act Advocacy Group through newsletters, listservs, and web-based interfaces. We also created a Facebook page for the study. Potential participants were encouraged to contact me as the principal investigator so that I could screen them for eligibility.

Participants were between 25 to 64 years of age, primarily white (92.3%), and female (96.3%). Participants were from Canada, US, UK, New Zealand, Australia, South Africa, and Ireland. Approximately 67% of the participants' children were diagnosed with LE before age two. Two-thirds of the children displayed LE in their legs while the remaining were affected in their genitals, their feet and hands, their face, chest, or their full body.

Semi-structured interviews were conducted via video or audio call and transcribed by undergraduate research assistants. Interview questions were open-ended and focused on the experiences and diagnoses of participants (e.g., "How has your child been treated for lymphedema?"), parenting challenges (e.g., "What unique challenges have you experienced as a parent of a child with lymphedema?"), participants' advocacy on behalf of their children (e.g., "What unique challenges have you experienced as a parent of a child with lymphedema?"), how they explain LE to their children and to others (e.g., "How have you explained what lymphedema is to your other children, if any, who do not have lymphedema?"), how they cope with the stress of parenting a child with LE (e.g., "Who has provided you personally with support as a parent of a child with lymphedema?") and family dynamics (e.g., "How does your family feel about taking on the challenges of lymphedema?").

Data analyses

We began by summarizing each interview and basic demographic data (e.g., age and gender of child and parent, age of onset of lymphedema, country of residence) in the form of an excel spreadsheet that we referred to as case summaries. We created a codebook that included codes we identified as being of interest to our overall aim of exploring the lived experiences of parenting children with LE. The codebook included such codes as the care of compression garments, children's engagement in leisure activities (including outdoor activities), child's socialization, challenges in finding clothing, child/peer interactions related to LE, and parents' thoughts on depriving their children of a sense of normalcy. We coded each interview using

NVivo. After coding each interview, we deliberated on the coding and made adjustments using a process of creating consensus. It was the voices of these parents among these codes that provided inspiration and were then woven into the story that Lily tells in *Lily's Lymphedema*; a work of ethnographic creative non-fiction as a method of depicting the lives of these parents' children.

Creating *Lily's Lymphedema*

The motivation to represent these data as a work of creative nonfiction grew out of informal conversations that my research team and I had with study participants as well as medical professionals who attended conference presentations of our initial findings. During those conversations, we learned that there was only one book aimed at children that explained lymphedema in a developmentally appropriate way. That book, *The Big Book of Lymphedema* by Jacqueline Todd, was published by Drewton Publishing in 2009. Because the book is no longer in print, I relied on the kindness of a participant who owns a copy, to take digital photographs of the book and email them to me. *The Big Book of Lymphedema* is a non-fiction interactive work-book. In comparison, *Lily's Lymphedema* provides readers with a fictional story about a child living with lymphedema. Thus, *Lily's Lymphedema* fills a gap in children's literature in that there are no other books or stories in print about lymphedema that are written for young readers and their families. Given the number of children impacted by lymphedema, the need is great for these children to see themselves in a children's book. Seeing their life experiences represented in literary form aimed at people their age may help children to cope with the stigma and lone-liness that they may experience in living with a chronic condition such as lymphedema (Egert, Egert, Vitman, & Costello, 2017).

While reviewing our initial coding of the interview data with my research team, we noticed specific passages and stories that stood out to us as particularly powerful. I made notes of these during our discussions with the intention of ensuring that, if appropriate, these passages appear in our presentations of findings (e.g., the nicknaming of compression garments, parents' quoting their children). At the same time, I noted recurring themes that seemed to flow across the codes (e.g., concerns about their child feeling normal, coping with questions and stares from children and adults, the particular challenges of going swimming). All of these notations along with the coded data and my accumulated knowledge about lymphedema served as the "facts" that made up the backbone of *Lily's Lymphedema*.

I set out to craft a story, told by a child to other children, that incorporated as much of this information as possible. This allowed me to create composite characters (e.g., Lily; her little brother Liam; her mom, dad, and nana; her teacher Mr. Garcia, and her physical therapist Paige). This technique is particularly useful in creative nonfiction when the researcher wishes to ensure the anonymity of participants and protect participant confidentiality (Gutkind & Fletcher, 2008; Smith et al., 2015).

In order to develop Lily's voice in the story, I drew on my own knowledge of young chil-dren that I acquired from my role as the mother of a daughter who was around Lily's age as well as five years of part-time work in early childhood education during my undergraduate and graduate studies. In drawing on these personal experiences, as well as what I have learned while researching lymphedema, I am incorporating my positionality and defining my role within the telling of Lily's story. That is, "truth is personal – it is what we see, assume, and believe, filtered through our own lens and orientation…there are many truths to a story and many versions of the same story" (Gutkind, 2012; p. 19).

Table 35.1 show the relationship between elements of the story, qualitative interview data, ethnographic data, and research-based information sources upon which they are based.

Table 35.1 Comparison of coded quotations to passages in lily's lymphedema

Element	Passage from/Elements in Lily's Lymphedema	Representative quotes from Qualitative Interview Data	Ethnographic Data Source	Research-based information source
Bandages	I need those bandages sometimes. When my leg and my foot get really big, I need them to help my body calm down. Those bandages that my brother likes to play mummy with are important too. After the massage she wraps my leg and foot up in the bandages. I have to wear those for a while before I can put My Precious back on.	"When the garment's not quite doing it, we'll wrap at night." (23LEP) "For about two months we did wrapping up to his calves and feet. Right now we are not doing wrapping except for as needed when it gets really tight. Like yesterday his legs were really bad so we wrapped yesterday." (34LEP)	Notes from an observation of manual lymph drainage and subsequent wrapping treatment.	"Bandaging at night was a key priority for many. Children were often frustrated at this and parents sought to normalize this with routines and fun activities." (Moffatt et al., 2019a, p. 249) Maclellan & Greene (2014)
Challenges with (Mis)diagnosis	I had to wear a big cast for a bit. I have pictures of me in a cast... I guess the doctors thought I broke my leg. But they were wrong!	"We first noticed a problem at seven months old. She wasn't diagnosed ... for 11 months. She had a lot of diagnoses that we knew were not correct ... obviously it's really nerve wracking." (23LEP) "He was hospitalized and we didn't know what was wrong with him ... We thought he might have allergies ... he went through a week's worth of tests in the hospital. [The] doctors had no idea. He was having blood drawn just about every day." (22LEP) "She was given an orthopedic boot to wear." (33LEP)	Observation of breast-cancer related lymphedema patient support groups.	Radina & Fu (2011)

Basic Elements of Lymphedema	What makes my leg and my foot big is called swelling. It's not like the swelling you get with a fat lip… It doesn't just go away on its own. Usually it doesn't really hurt. It is pretty much there all the time. Lymphedema happens because the parts of my body didn't develop in the same way as it does in other kids. Lymphedema isn't just something that can happen to kids. Grown-ups can have it too. It's not contagious — you can't get it by touching me. It also doesn't ever go away.		Maclellan & Greene (2014)
Use of Compression Garments	One thing that I have to do all the time is wear this long sock that covers my whole leg and foot. It sort of keeps everything in. They try and make it look like my skin but it really doesn't. I can tell.	"[The] majority of lymphedema is in his foot and then from the ankle to the knee. He wears a compression garment up to his knee during the day and in the evening he wears a different garment that goes to his thigh." (22 LEP)	Maclellan & Greene (2014), Deng et al. (2015)
Care of Compression Garments	We have to be really careful with it. Dad says that it is so expensive so I have to take good care of it – keep it clean, don't scrape it up. Dad calls it "My Precious" because we have to take such good care of it.	"…you're wearing a 500, 700 dollar piece of medical equipment. Try not to, you know, jump off your bike and scrape your knee and tear up your garment." (25LEP)	Maclellan & Greene (2014)

Observations of/interactions with compression garment vendors at LE conferences

(continued)

Table 35.1 Cont.

Element	Passage from/Elements in Lily's Lymphedema	Representative quotes from Qualitative Interview Data	Ethnographic Data Source	Research-based information source
Treatment Using Manual Lymph Drainage	Every day I have to have Mom or Dad (or sometimes Nana does it) give me a massage. I have to sit on the couch and let Mom rub my leg and foot.	"It is a sequence, a systematic sequence of massage starting from his neck all the way down his body and then back up front and back. A light, gentle massage to increase lymphatic flow." (06LEP) "We watch TV for about 45 minutes while I wrap [him] because that's what keeps him entertained while he's laying on my lap while I'm doing massages and wrapping him." (07LEP)	Notes from an observation of manual lymph drainage and subsequent wrapping treatment.	Maclellan & Greene (2014)
Treatment Using Night Garments	Before bed I have to put on a long sock-like thing that looks like an oven mitt for your leg. Sometimes it gets hot. I don't like it so I take it off.	"… and they have nighttime compressions, but they aren't fun either… they're like wearing oven mitts." (33LEP)		Radina, Watson, & Faubert, (2008)
Treatment Administered by Physical Therapist	Sometimes when my lymphedema gets out of control, I have to go see Paige. She is my physical therapist and she gives me an extra, super, special massage.	"I think having a supportive therapist has really been life-changing for us." (07LEP) "… whenever her legs started to swell we went to the physical therapy [who] helped with everything." (25LEP)	Notes from an observation of lymphatic massage conducted by a certified lymphedema therapist.	Radina & Fu (2011)

Challenges with Footwear	*Sometimes my foot can get so big that I have to wear two different size shoes. Sometimes my shoe hurts.*	"… but some department stores will actually sell you shoes in two different sizes for medical reasons …" (02LEP) "… with shoes they'll only fund their shoemaker and I've had two pairs of shoes from the shoe guy before and he likes to make them in leather and leather doesn't work for her … it doesn't sort of mold to her foot and it doesn't stretch with her because she does go up but she does go down as well as it needs to be something stretchy and they don't do that." (03LEP) "…just shoe shopping…you almost need a different size for one foot or the other…" (10LEP) "And then I anticipate within the next year we'll probably start having to buy two pairs of shoes …" (30LEP)	
Bullying Interactions With Other Children	*Other kids point and giggle and hold their noses like my foot stinks or something.* *Sometimes at swim meets other kids will say something about my lymphedema or My Precious.*	"… there will always be kids teasing her somewhere …" (03LEP) "… they just stare and then you get kids that say 'Oh, look at her ugly legs' and stuff like that." (03LEP) "People have been kind of insensitive towards us though. People have comments like, 'Oh, he has such fat feet'…" (07LEP)	"Parents expressed a deep concern for their child to experience friendships and normal adult relationships. A number of children shared their experience of addressing bullying at school and the way they addressed this." (Moffatt et al., 2019a, p. 250)

(continued)

Table 35.1 Cont.

Element	Passage from/Elements in Lily's Lymphedema	Representative quotes from Qualitative Interview Data	Ethnographic Data Source	Research-based information source
Knowledgeable Teacher as Advocate	Mr. Garcia, my teacher, knows all about lymphedema. At the start of the school year, my mom had her usual talk with Mr. Garcia about it.	"We have a 504 ... one of the reasons why we have all those in place ... I just want to make sure that everybody that's in her life understands her situation ... from her teachers, to her coaches, and to her friends." (18LEP)		
Challenges with Clothing	No long pants that are too tight on my one leg and make me hot and uncomfortable. Shorts rock! Except when people notice My Precious and ask silly questions.	"... he rarely wears pants because the leg doesn't fit." (19LEP) "The frustration and trouble that we have with clothing with her is now it's summer and my son didn't care, he would wear shorts with [his compression stocking]." (37LEP) "Even no in the summer she wants to wear shorts and doesn't want to wear her compressions." (37LEP)	Observation of breast–cancer-related lymphedema patient support groups.	Deng et al. (2015)
Precautions to Avoid Cellulitis	Things like bug bites, bee stings, sunburns, or scraping my knee can all mean a stay at the hospital. I've gone twice and it is no fun! If the skin on that leg or foot gets hurt, it could mean that I get a bad infection. Because of my lymphedema I can't just put a Band-Aid on it. I have to be extra careful to clean it and not get hurt in the first place. Sometimes the infection makes the swelling worse and we have to start all over.	"... we use bug spray more often and the Neosporin and we worry about the sun more." (17LEP) "... [if] he hurt the leg or cut or bruised the leg we can treat it immediately." (22LEP) "... we are extra careful. She just seems so prone to infection compared to other kids." (23IEP) "... you know, wear your sunscreen and put your pants on ... wear long pants and ... where's the Off!?" (30LEP)		

| Child as Self-Advocate | *What helps the most is telling people like you about my lymphedema. Sometimes when people stare, I get so mad that I walk right up to them and say, "Excuse me. I wear this because I have lymphedema, and lymphedema is a build-up of fluid in my leg, but it doesn't make me different!"* | "… he's so proud that he knows how to explain it because he will … jump in first …" (02LEP)

"… he goes around and he explains … he will go right up to them and say, 'Excuse me, I wear this because I have lymphedema, and lymphedema is a build-up of fluid in my leg, but it doesn't make me any different." (06LEP)

"… she basically just says 'Oh, my leg doesn't work right and so it swells' and … most of the time that's a perfectly good answer for people." (18LEP)

"… he'll just say sometimes if he's in really polite mood, 'I have lymphedema and that is all I care to share.'" (19 LEP) | "[Adolescents with lymphedema] also showed they viewed themselves as being useful advocates and mentors for younger children." (Moffatt et al., 2019b, p. 243) |
| Child-like Response to Questions | *If I am not feeling as polite or kind of silly, I might say something silly like, "Oh what? I battled a dragon and won! He got me though."* | "Trying to find simple explanations for them, you know, so they're not scared of him or scared of the gloves or anything like that … So, we try to explain it pretty simple." (07LEP) | Suggestion from parent of two children with LE (not a study participant) |

After drafting *Lily's Lymphedema*, I began the process of seeking feedback from beta readers. I began by identifying those participants who have children of the approximate age-level of my anticipated audience for *Lily's Lymphedema*. That is, I reviewed the case summary notes for each participant and selected those who had children between the ages of 5 and 10 years old. I then contacted those participants and asked them if they would be interested in receiving a copy of *Lily's Lymphedema* and then be willing to provide me with their thoughts and feedback. I also posted a call for beta readers in a closed Facebook group for writers and other creative people. Lastly, I shared *Lily's Lymphedema* with a writing group for nonacademic writers (e.g., novelists, poets, essayist) and received their feedback. I utilized this feedback, which took place over a period of nine months, to gradually revise and refine the story toward what appears in Appendix A.

Conclusion

The outcome of this processes described above is a work of creative non-fiction inspired by both qualitative data and the collection of information and experiences related to lymphedema over almost 20 years of studying LE. By writing up findings from qualitative interview data, ethnographic data, and research in the form of a children's book, I was able to see the combined stories of these families in new ways. Specifically, I was able to visualize their lived experiences as parents coping with the fears, precautionary behaviors, and realities of parenting a child with a chronic illness. As a parent, I was also able to reflect on my own perspectives on the general parenting challenges of protecting children (e.g., telling Lily to be careful), encouraging compliance (e.g., using silly voices to introduce that it is time for massage), advocating for child's needs (e.g., meeting with Mr. Garcia), and worry about their social development (e.g., references to bullying and child self-advocacy).

Lily's Lymphedema is intended for young children but may be of interest to early middle-school readers as well. LE may appear at any time but is most likely to appear before the age of 2 or around the onset of puberty (Levinson, Feingold, Ferrell, Glover, Traboulsi, & Finegold, 2003), both elementary and middle school readers may find such a story informative and helpful. Such a text would be useful in school-based contexts in order to explain lymphedema to a child's peers. While *Lily's Lymphedema* has not, at the time of this writing, been published as a standalone children's book, I anticipate continuing to pursue appropriate outlets that will facilitate getting Lily's story in the hands of children, teachers, social workers, child life specialists, and others who may benefit from Lily's message. Future work in this area includes exploring the creation of another work of creative non-fiction about primary LE for middle-grade readers. The need for such a book is high given that female children are more likely than male children to experience the onset of LE during puberty (Levinson, et al., 2003).

Appendix A: *Lily's Lymphedema*

Hi! I'm Lily and I am 9 and a half. Pretty soon I will be 10!

We are already planning my birthday party. My Nana is going to make my cake to look like a swimming pool! Complete with a diving board and a slide. I drew a picture for her so she knows just how I want it.

I have a brother, Liam. He's 5 and VERY annoying. He's always taking my bandages so that he can pretend to be a mummy. I don't think it is very funny.

You see … I need those bandages sometimes. When my leg and my foot get really big, I need them to help my body calm down.

You see, I have what is called lymphedema. It's a big word and it took me a long while to say it right. I thought it was limp-a-dema for the longest time. Maybe because when my leg and foot get too big I limp when I walk.

I've had lymphedema for as long as I can remember. My mom says that she noticed almost right away that something seemed different with me. It took almost two years for the doctors to figure out what it was. I had to wear a big cast for a bit. I have pictures of me in a cast – my Grandpa drew all kinds of funny cartoons on it to make me laugh. I guess the doctors thought I broke my leg. But they were wrong!

Now I am an "expert" about lymphedema. At least that is what Mom says. So, I want to tell you all about it.

Lymphedema means that parts of my body – mostly my leg and my foot – are bigger than they should be. Sometimes I look a bit lopsided. What makes my leg and my foot big is called swelling. It's not like the swelling you get with a fat lip (from little brothers throwing their trucks at you. So annoying!!). It doesn't just go away on its own. Usually it doesn't really hurt. It is pretty much there all the time. Lymphedema happens because the parts of my body didn't develop in the same way as it does in other kids.

Lymphedema isn't just something that can happen to kids. Grown-ups can have it too. It's not contagious – you can't get it by touching me. It also doesn't ever go away. Someday I will be a grown-up with lymphedema.

One thing that I have to do all the time is wear this long sock that covers my whole leg and foot. It sort of keeps everything in. They try and make it look like my skin but it really doesn't. I can tell. We have to be really careful with it. Dad says that it is so expensive so I have to take good care of it – keep it clean, don't scrape it up. Dad calls it "My Precious" because we have to take such good care of it. The way he says it always make me giggle.

Every day I have to have Mom or Dad (or sometimes Nana does it) give me a massage. I have to sit on the couch and let Mom rub my leg and foot. I try not so squirm but sometimes it tickles!

When Mom does my massage she always starts by talking in a funny accent and asking me, "M'lady, are you ready for your very fancy massage?" That used to make me laugh but not any-more. I hate the massage. It's so boring and I would rather be doing something else. Anything else! I still laugh sometimes because Mom's trying to make it fun. I still think it's funny when she calls me "ma-lady." Before bed I have to put on a long sock-like thing that looks like an oven mitt for your leg. Sometimes it gets hot. I don't like it so I take it off. Mom doesn't like it when I do that.

Those bandages that my brother likes to play mummy with are important too. Sometimes when my lymphedema gets out of control, I have to go see Paige. She is my physical therapist and she gives me an extra, super, special massage. (She's SOOO much better at it than Mom). After the massage she wraps my leg and foot up in the bandages. I have to wear those for a while before I can put My Precious back on.

Sometimes my foot can get so big that I have to wear two different size shoes. Sometimes my shoe hurts. When it feels like that at school, I kick my shoe off under my desk.

Mr. Garcia, my teacher, knows all about lymphedema. At the start of the school year, my mom had her usual talk with Mr. Garcia about it.

Mr. Garcia doesn't mind if I take my shoe off. Sometimes the other kids see me do it. Most of them don't care either – we have been going to school together forever so they get it. Other kids point and giggle and hold their noses like my foot stinks or something. (It doesn't, by the way). I get really embarrassed. And sometimes I get mad. Usually Mr. Garcia notices and tells them to "Knock it off!" I like knowing that Mr. Garcia gets it.

It's summer now. Summer is complicated. What should be a super awesome time of year can be a total pain for me.

There are three things that make summer great.

1. No long pants that are too tight on my one leg and make me hot and uncomfortable. Shorts rock! Except when people notice My Precious and ask silly questions like "Did you burn yourself?" or "Wow, what did you do to your leg."
2. Swim team!!!!! Coach Miranda is so cool! I love my swim friends!!
3. No school – lots of time to play with friends and read and nap and play video games and annoy my brother …

But … summer is terrible for me for one HUGE reason … everyone is telling me to BE CAREFUL. Mom, Dad, Nana, Grandpa, my swim coach, other parents, the lifeguards. Things like bug bites, bee stings, sunburns, or scraping my knee can all mean a stay at the hospital. I've gone twice and it is no fun! If the skin on that leg or foot gets hurt, it could mean that I get a bad infection. Because of my lymphedema I can't just put a band-aid on it. I have to be extra careful to clean it and not get hurt in the first place. Sometimes the infection makes the swelling worse and we have to start all over.

So, summer for me has lots of rules.

1. No bare feet!
2. Sunscreen. Always. No excuses.
3. Bug spray. Always. No excuses.

Mom tried the "no running" rule but I just couldn't help it. Now that rule is "run smart." So, I can run in places that are safe where I am less likely to fall down. I still do sometimes …

The best part of summer is swim team! My swim friends are the best. We have been friends forever and they don't care about my stupid big leg. They even say that my big foot gives me an advantage.

Sometimes at swim meets other kids will say something about my lymphedema or my Precious. My swim friends always stand up for me. I love them.

I love to swim because my WHOLE body feels lighter and stronger in the pool. And, I don't have to where the Precious. I feel like a super hero. Or maybe I just feel like what normal kids without lymphedema feel like.

Sometimes I wish I didn't have lymphedema. I can get pretty mad about it. All the being careful and the precious and the fancy massage. Usually Mom or Dad will hug me and just say "I know." It helps, sometimes.

What helps the most is telling people like you about my lymphedema. Sometimes when people stare, I get so mad that I walk right up to them and say, "Excuse me. I wear this because I have lymphedema, and lymphedema is a buildup of fluid in my leg, but it doesn't make me different!" If I am not feeling as polite or kind of silly, I might say something silly like, "Oh that? I battled a dragon and won! He got me though."

If I tell you what it's like to be me, maybe you will be nicer to me, and people like me, now that you know what it's all about? You get it now!

Maybe one day someone will figure out how to make lymphedema go away. Until then though I plan to work hard on being me, Lily. I'll still chase my brother around when he plays mummy with my bandages. I'll still complain about being careful (and I will probably try and be careful). I'll still be a kid who loves to swim and hang out with good friends who don't care about my big leg and foot and the precious and all of that. I'll keep working hard on being a Lymphedema Expert. But most of all, I will work hard on being me.

References

Clayton, B. (2010). Ten minutes with the boys, the thoroughly academic task and the semi-naked celebrity: Football masculinities in the classroom or pursuing security in a 'liquid' world. *Qualitative Research in Sport and Exercise, 2*, 371–384.

Deng, J., E. Radina, M.R. Fu, J.M. Armer, J.N. Cormier, S.R. Thiadens, … & S.H. Ridner. (2015). Self-care status, symptom burden, and reported infections in individuals with lower-extremity primary lymphedema. *Journal of Nursing Scholarship*, 47(2), 126–134.

Egert, T., Y. Egert, R. Vitman, & W. Castello. (2017). Educating young children, parents and doctors through the medium of an illustrated children's book. *Annals of the Rheumatic Diseases*, 76, 1556.

Gutkind, L. (2012). You can't make this stuff up: The complete guide to writing creative nonfiction – from memoir to literary journalism and everything in between. Philadelphia, PA: Da Campo Press.

Gutkind, L. & H. Fletcher. (Eds.). (2008). Keep it real: Everything you need to know about researching and writing creative nonfiction. London, England: W.W. Norton & Company.

Humphreys, M. & T.J. Watson. (2009). Ethnographic practices: from 'writing-up ethnographic research' to 'writing ethnography'. *Organizational Ethnography: studying the complexities of everyday life*, pp. 40–55.

Leavy, P. (2013). Fiction as research practice: Short stories, novellas, and novels. Walnut Creek, CA. Left Coast Press.

Levinson, K.L., E. Feingold, R.E. Ferrell, T.W. Glover, E.I. Traboulsi, & D.N. Finegold. (2003). Age of onset in hereditary lymphedema. *The Journal of Pediatrics*, 142(6), 704–708.

Maclellan, R.A. & A.K. Greene. (2014, August). Lymphedema. *Seminars in Pediatric Surgery*, 23(4), 191–197.

Mendoza, N., A. Li, A. Gill, & S. Tyring. (2009). Filariasis: diagnosis and treatment. *Dermatologic Therapy*, 22(6), 475–490.

Moffatt, C., A. Aubeeluck, E. Stasi, R. Bartoletti, C. Aussenac, D. Roccatello, & I. Quere. (2019a). A Study to Explore the Parental Impact and Challenges of Self-Management in Children and Adolescents Suffering with Lymphedema. *Lymphatic Research and Biology*, 17(2), 245–252.

Moffatt, C., A. Aubeeluck, E. Stasi, S. Mestre, S. Rowan, S. Murray, & I. Quere. (2019b). A Study Using Visual Art Methods to Explore the Perceptions and Barriers of Self-Management in Children and Adolescents with Lymphedema. *Lymphatic Research and Biology*, 17(2), 231–244.

Radina, M.E. & M.R. Fu. (2011). Preparing for and coping with breast cancer-related lymphedema. *Novel Strategies in Lymphedema*, 53–88.

Radina, E., W. Watson, & K. Faubert. (2008). Lymphoedema and sexual relationships in mid/later life. *Journal of Lymphoedema*, 3(2), 21–30.

Schlögel, M.J., P. Brouillard, L.M. Boon, & M. Vikkula. (2015). Genetic causes of lymphedema. In A. Greene, S. Slavin, & H. Brorson, (Eds.) *Lymphedema*. Champaign, IL: Springer. https://doi.org/10.1007/978-3-319-14493-1_3

Smeltzer, D.M., G.B. Stickler, & A. Schirger. (1985). Primary lymphedema in children and adolescents: A follow-up study and review. *Pediatrics*, 76(2), 206–218.

Smith, B., K.R. McGannon, & T.L. Williams. (2015). Ethnographic creative nonfiction: Exploring the whats, whys and hows. In G. Molnar & L. Purdy (Eds), *Ethnographies in sport and exercise research* (pp. 73–88). New York, NY. Routledge.

Smith, B., A. Papathomas, K.A. Martin Ginis, & A.E. Latimer-Cheung. (2013). Understanding physical activity in spinal cord injury rehabilitation: Translating and communicating research through stories. *Disability & Rehabilitation*, 35, 2044–2055.

PART XV

Novel approaches

36

MAPPING NETWORK DISTURBANCES

Case studies that demonstrate the use of an ethnographic approach to health and well-being research

Maria Louise Bønnelykke

The Anthropocene – disturbed human-environment relationships

The Great Barrier Reef along the north-eastern coast of Australia in the Coral Sea is the largest and most complex coral reef system in the world. It stretches for more than 2300 kilometres and includes some 3000 coral reefs, 600 continental islands, 300 coral cays and approximately150 inshore mangrove islands. Here, 1500 species of fish, 411 types of hard coral, one-third of the world's soft coral, 134 species of sharks and rays, six species of marine turtles, and over 30 species of marine mammals live.[1] However, the Great Barrier Reef has lost half of its coral since 1985 because of coral bleaching, cyclones, and an endemic star-fish, the crown of thorns, that feeds on coral tissue (Miller et al., 2015). During 2016–2017, the Great Barrier Reef suffered two consecutive coral bleaching events for the first time in recorded history.[2] Marine biologists studying the impact concluded that the number of new corals had decreased by 89% after the back-to-back bleaching events and that the intervals between bleaching events have declined from 25 years in the 1980s to 5.9 years since 2010 (Hughes et al., 2019).

This was the context against which I carried out one year of ethnographic fieldwork in Far Northern Queensland, in the towns of Cairns, Townsville, and the Whitsundays during 2016–2017 among scientists, activists, and political actors. The predicament on the reef sparked discussions about whether the Great Barrier Reef was dying and placed it among the landscapes that are now known to be Anthropocene.

The Anthropocene is labelled as the era when humans became a global geophysical force (Steffen, Crutzen, & McNeil, 2007; Monastersky, 2015; Clark 2014), and this concept frames this ethnographic study, in which I examine how ideas and practices of wild and Anthropocene landscapes are shaped by and shape science, civil participation, and politics. The Anthropocene describes the time we live in as a period in which humans are capable of destroying the earth. By causing climate change, pollution, and mass extinction, human disturbance to the earth even exceeds the role that glaciers have historically played (Tsing, 2014). The human impact at multiple planetary levels is now so significant that humans have ushered in this new geological epoch. The Anthropocene is a young and disputed concept with roots in geology, philosophy, theology, and social science (Latour, 2015). Going beyond such concepts as environmental degradation, the Anthropocene warns us that the responsibility lies with human actions and processes (Crutzen, 2002). Ecologies that are self-correcting, self-balancing, and self-healing are replaced by "a new phase in the history of the Earth, when natural forces and human forces [are] intertwined, so that the fate of one determines the fate of the other" (Zalasiewicz, Williams, Steffen, & Crutzen, 2010).

The Anthropocene deals with environmental injustice, the gravity of the human dominance of ecosystems, and how humans can take responsibility for our current predicament (Seary, 2015; Ogden, Heynen, Oslender, West, Kassam, & Robbins, 2013; Latour, 2017). However, critics point out that the risk of the concept is that anthropos, mankind itself, becomes everyone and no one, fostering an external view of the earth's changing chemical cycles (Haraway, Ishikawa, Gilbert, Olwig, Tsing, & Bubandt, 2016; Malm & Hornborg, 2014). Donna Haraway points out that the Anthropocene discourse places Anthropos in the center, which distracts from the view that we ought to care for and pay attention to the ways we are connected to other forms of life (Haraway, 2016). While the Anthropocene announces the human destruction of the planet, Haraway reminds us that the sky has not fallen yet and proposes that we tell multispecies stories of tentacular modes of living and making with (Haraway, 2016).

For the purpose of this research, the Anthropocene is not only a task of naming a new geological epoch, it is a task of making new kinds of labour for new kinds of nature as the Anthropocene comes into being through knowledge practices, truth claims, and heterogenous landscapes of disrupted human-environment relations. This chapter addresses some of the urgent questions of our time: How can ethnographic fieldwork be retooled to study human-environment relationships when the world we inhabit is changing in dramatic ways? And how do we capture the particular experience of each landscape as well as a global system in crisis?

Coral-like ethnography

Worldwide, coral reefs occupy only 284,300 km², yet they are home to one fourth of all marine species (Spalding in Bruckner, Alnazry, & Failsal, 2011). In anthropology, coral is theorised as a figure used to "think with" (Haraway, 1995; Roosht, 2010) and a boundary organism of flesh and stone generating "speculation about the living and non-living" capable of challenging notions of subjectivity, agency (Helmreich, 2010), and heterosexuality (Hayward, 2010). Helmreich proposes that corals attune humans to epistemological questions. He reveals ambiguous versions of the reef through three concepts: emergency, emergence, and immersion. Coral conjures up images of *emergency*. The suffering reefs make them a warning sign of poor planetary health. Corals' growth and decay reflects larger social and environmental conditions across scales. *Emergence* describes corals' generative capacities; corals' stony structures can be likened to the social work that makes social constructions durable. *Immersion* shifts the focus to the soft coral bodies to reveal that corals are not only stony sculptures, but alive in assemblages of polyps and tentacles. Immersion in coral life offers new perspectives and potential for cultural critique (Helmreich, 2010). In this chapter, coral plays a role, both as a figure "to think with", but also as a figure to "conduct fieldwork with". Coral not only makes the Anthropocene visible and tangible it can also ground and connect ethnographic work. By exploring aspects of coral life, I propose three ways in which coral-like ethnography can inform the study of disturbed human-environment relationships.

Transcending scale

To study the impact of the Anthropocene, ethnography needs to capture both the situated experiences of human environment relations as well as environmental systems in crisis. Coral-like ethnography permits the ethnographer's attention to be stretched and bent so that seemingly diverse scales (from situated experiences to global systems in crisis) become part of the same story.

The coral reef stretches for thousands of kilometres. It is the largest single thing made by one living organism. However, each coral animal is almost too small for the eye to see. My fieldwork began in late 2016, and, in a way, so did coral life. In mid-November, the Great Barrier Reef spawned, a mass event cued by environmental factors where eggs and sperm are released from the coral. Even with the reef located some 40 km off the coast, the beaches turned milky from spawn. This is how corals begin their life, as miniscule larva swimming in large numbers among the microscopic world of plankton. If the ocean current moves the larva to a suitable environment, they attach themselves to the ocean floor. Each larva develops into a polyp – a tiny sea anemone, one to two centimetres in size, with a cylindrical body crowned by a ring of tentacles and a central mouth. The polyp secretes calcium carbonate to form its stony white skeleton, and the exposed tissue of the polyps gives the coral its bright colours (Sapp, 1999, p. 3). The stony skeleton forms the coral reef, which protects the coral animal from predators and offers a substrate on which new coral polyps can grow. The Great Barrier Reef is not only massive in space but also in time, as coral reefs are the most spectacular, exotic, and crowded ecological communities that have "slowly evolved over a period of almost fifty million years" (Sapp, 1999, p. 4). It is easy to assume that because of the size of the Great Barrier Reef, as well as its depth in time, we are dealing with an endpoint on a scale of complex natural phenomena. However, Hastrup clarifies this notion when writing about climate change in Northwest Greenland:

> It does not hold that the more you zoom out, and the more the ground you cover, the more you know. It is not a matter of more or less, but of different points of perception. This implies that the local and the global are not endpoints on any absolute scale; empirically, they are enfolded in each other.
>
> *(Hastrup, 2012, p. 148)*

The Great Barrier Reef is a complex phenomenon, not because of its size or age, but because it is richly entangled. The complexity is similar at any point on a scale from small to large. The endless stretches of reefs cannot be separated in any meaningful scalar fashion from the tiny faceless coral animals – empirically they are enfolded in each other (see Hastrup, 2012, p. 148). Hastrup describes the ethnographer's access to a world that is at once local yet not circumscribed by local boundaries: "There is a constant moving about and bending and stretching particular perspectives, which it is for the anthropologist to write forth from immersement in conversations, connections and concerns in the field" (Hastrup, 2012, p. 161). The near and the far intermingle and contribute to a particular figuring of the world (Hastrup, 2012, p. 149; Tsing, 2010, p. 48). Coral reflects social and environmental conditions across scale, and the practitioners of coral-like ethnography can study the impact of the Anthropocene by immersing themselves in richly entangled conversations and connections.

In March 2017, a category 4 cyclone, Debbie, formed in the Coral Sea. It made landfall in Airlie Beach, a small tourist town of about 1200 inhabitants where I was conducting fieldwork. From inside my apartment, I observed the cyclone rage. As the eye of the cyclone came through Airlie Beach, it brought strangely calm weather. I could even make out a group of cockatoos in the rainforest and heard other birds chirping. Yet the winds from the tail gained terrifying strength – this weather system was intense and slow moving. Trees in the rainforest snapped like match sticks, and heavy debris flew through the air as if almost weightless. I saw trees in the rainforest snap like match sticks, and heavy debris flew through the air as if almost weightless. Debbie's fury left the area transformed. The following day, it seemed as if wildlife had been driven out of the rainforest. Pythons were crossing the streets, and I almost stepped on a huntsman spider in my kitchen. I saw pythons crossing the streets, and I almost stepped on a huntsman spider in my kitchen. A praying mantis had taken residence in my hallway, and a golden silk orb-weaver spider spun an impressive web in my garage – unusual even for the tropics. We were told that it could be weeks before running water and electricity would be reinstalled, the once lush rainforest quickly turned brown, and we began to hear news that coral colonies had been knocked over by the wind. One victim, Debbie the Cockatoo, gained surprising attention. While the eye of the cyclone made landfall, bringing a moment of clarity from the strong winds, a local photographer found a group of cockatoos clinging to a tree after battling the cyclonic winds. On the ground, he found Debbie. The cockatoo was naked because the winds had stripped her from her feathers, leaving her unable to fly. Bringing the cockatoo home, the photographer could only offer her cyclone emergency food, dry crackers and sun-flower seeds. For a while, she seemed to be on the mend and was given the name Debbie. But after a few days, she was found lifeless in her box, probably losing her battle to survive to internal injuries. Pictures of the wet naked bird went viral, and local and international media told the story of the rescue and death of Debbie. The life and death of the featherless, wet, and battered cockatoo transcended scale. The near and the far intermingled to consolidate the cockatoo's fate. It was a situated account of a bird fighting for its life but entangled in forces and events that resisted being localised – the warming of oceans and the forming of cyclones. Debbie became a figure of and a way to think about the non-human victims of the cyclone, which would have included Debbie the coral polyp and Debbie the bull shark,[3] among other Debbies. Telling the story about Debbie was telling a story about liveability on a damaged planet.

Tracing patchy stories

Coral life, emerging in a state between tissue and stone, animal and plant, singular and plural, destabilises the divisions between nature and culture, human and non-human. In the same vein, coral-like ethnography encourages a critical engagement with concepts such as the Anthropocene, raising questions about how it is defined, made visible and knowable and to what effect.

A coral organism contains anything from a single coral polyp to thousands of polyps, all genetically identical and embedded in one common body (Chen, Stiefel, Sejnowski, & Bullock, 2008). Once the larva has settled and developed into a polyp, coral grows by reproducing itself. While it divides, each new coral polyp remains attached to the originator by a thin membrane. This is known as *budding* (Szmant,1986). Thus, colonies of coral typically consist of numerous animals all linked by a common body and gastrovascular system so that food consumed by one is circulated to neighboring polyps (Muller-Parker, D'Elia, & Cook, 2015, p. 100). Corals' growth and their asexual reproduction remind us to be critical of standard categories of being. Coral challenges ideas about subjectivity, holism, and boundedness and encourages us to explore and understand how biological and social life come to be, function, and matter.

Doing coral-like ethnography includes transcending scale by immersing in conversations and connections as described above. However, the conversations and the connections are equally constituted through bifurcation and emergence, and this ethnographical approach deals with how to trace them. The coral is at the same time complete, intact, and operating while it is also emerging, partial and unfinished. At first glance, the coral appears solid, such as the concept of the Anthropocene, but by tracing its growth and examining how the parts and the wholes are constituted, we recognize how it is in fact dynamic and partial. When it comes to truth claims about phenomena such as the Anthropocene, we must pay attention to the way they are constituted and how they achieve their integrity. This can be done by examining how they are constructed and circulated and how they bring new realities and relations into being. Swanson et al. describe this as *noticing*: "Living in a time of planetary catastrophe thus begins with a practice at once humble and difficult: noticing the world around us" (2017, p. 7). They argue that noticing draws inspiration from scientific observation alongside ethnography and critical theory (2017).

During my own fieldwork, the act of noticing could be asking the deceptively simple question: How is the reef? Usually located more than 40 km off the coast, most of the reef rarely, if ever, gets human visitors, while other reefs are visited daily by tourism operators. Then where is it appropriate to look for answers to this question? During fieldwork, two seemingly contradictory truth claims circulated about the state of the reef: the reef is dying, and the reef is *not* dying. In the same way that we notice how polyps reproduce and grow and how the reef reveals itself to be simultaneously part and whole, we can notice how these truth claims are constituted, fractional, and circulated.

Obituary: Great Barrier Reef (25 million bc-…). This is the name of an article that went viral in late 2016, bringing news of the Great Barrier Reef's recent death and details about its life and achievements:

> To say the reef was an extremely active member of its community is an understatement. The surrounding ecological community would not have existed without it. (…) No one knows if a serious effort could have saved the reef, but it is clear that no such effort was made.
>
> *(Jacobsen, 2016)*

The article, authored by Rowan Jacobsen, otherwise known for contributions on food and the environment in magazines such as *Harper's* and *Outside*, had journalists across the globe and the most renowned marine biologists commenting on it. It was criticized for being flawed and no more than a joke (see D'Angelo, 14 October 2016). Whether the article was sincere or a joke remains unknown, but it was one attempt at answering the question: How is the reef? Shortly after the article was published, Pauline Hanson, the leader of the nationalist right-wing party One Nation, donned a wetsuit, a mask and a snorkel to visit a reef off the coast of Rockhampton. She wanted to disprove claims that the reef was dying. Inquisitively studying pieces of coral at the ocean's surface, she announced that the reefs were in pristine conditions and that "they are growing all the time" (*ABC News*, 25 November 2016). The trip was widely criticized as Hanson took her senators and the media to a healthy section of the reef some 1000 km from where the severe bleaching took place (*Sydney Morning Herald*, 27 November 2016). Hanson's announcement of the pristine reef demonstrated that statements about whether the reef is dying or not, were less a matter of fact and more a matter of opinion, where stories and sections of the reefs were drawn together to justify a particular position.

Science, of course, was also expected to answer this question. At the Australian Institute of Marine Science (AIMS), the Long-Term Monitoring Program has run for three decades.

This program has the only long-term, comprehensive data set covering the health of the Great Barrier Reef. Asked about the history of the program, a scientist from the community explained:

> The director of AIMS waking up in the middle of the night thinking: if the Minister of Environment asks me "What's the state of the reef?" Then what will I tell him? That is supposedly one of the ways it came about. We have 47 reefs that we have been studying since the 1990s. On each reef, there are three sites; they are marked with iron bars. Each site has five transects, they are about 300 meters long. We also photographed the coral, and then we did a manta tow survey around the entire reef.

A manta tow involves towing a snorkel diver at a constant speed behind a boat. The observer holds on to a manta board attached to the boat by a 17-metre long rope. The diver makes a visual assessment of specific variables during a two-minute manta tow and records these on the manta board when the boat stops. I wanted to know more about how these 47 reefs were selected, and the head of the program explained the following:

> They were selected because they were in bands of latitude around centres of population, so in high-use areas. They also have this cross shelf transect. That's the big gradient from the ocean to the coast. Beyond that, AIMS had a history of studying things there, so they were selected for the practical reason that they had good anchorage.

What answer can three decades of data from 47 reefs provide? The 2017/18 Long-Term Monitoring Report concludes that coral cover has declined across the entire Great Barrier Reef. The north showed the biggest decline in coral cover because of severe bleaching, ongoing crown of thorns outbreaks, and two severe cyclones. The central region showed lower coral cover for the longest time, compared to the other regions. As the coral began to show signs of recovery after cyclone Yasi in 2011, the reefs were severely impacted by bleaching in 2016 and 2017. The southern region experienced no severe cyclones or crown of thorn outbreak from 2009 to 2016, giving the coral a window to recover from cyclone Hamish in 2009. However, it was severely impacted by cyclone Debbie and the crown of thorn outbreaks in 2017, causing dramatic coral cover declines in some areas (Sweatman, 2018). This regionalization of the reef shows that the reef is not a homogenous organism; it is uneven, and our understanding of the reef is partial. A scientist on the program explained the condition of the reef in his own words:

> The barrier reef is a big place. Some bits are good; some bits are not so good. Right now, after the bleaching, in the far north, there's less than 5% coral cover. It's awful. The reefs off Townsville haven't looked better since the program started. What do you say? People want you to *tweet* the state of the reef. What do you say?

We *notice* how the reef appears uneven through these contradictory and inconclusive answers to the question: "How is the reef?" The notion of the patchy Anthropocene has been developed by Anna Tsing and her colleagues to imagine the Anthropocene as broken into uneven and unequal patches (Tsing, Mathews, & Bubandt, 2019, p. 186). The Anthropocene is patchy because it is composed of varied assemblages of livability, and it exists only in and through these patches. Patches are formed in vernacular histories "which tie them to the contingencies of encounters and the peculiarities of place" (Tsing 2016, p. 5). Landscape patches are socio-ecological constellations with unique histories and forms of interaction between humans, plants, and other species. Every patch is unique but simultaneously connected to other patches;

they mutually transform and create one another (Tsing et al., 2019). Tsing uses the plantation to exemplify patchiness. She refers to the plantation as a machine manufacturing proliferation (Tsing, 2016). The plantation aims to reduce the number of living things to just one kind, and such ecological simplifications nurture and spread disease (Tsing et al., 2019). Bubandt demonstrates a patchy landscape where people create lawns and lawns create people through the lawns' constant need for attention through nurturing, fertilizing, and weeding (2019). Even if the Great Barrier Reef is rich in biodiversity and not "boxed off" like a plantation or lawn, the patchy Anthropocene might prove helpful for examining truth claims about the Anthropocene. AIMS scientists are uneasy answering questions about how the reef is, and the reef is at once declared dead and thriving. Such truth claims can coexist because the reef consists of varied assemblages of livability. The reef could be considered a patchwork where every patch is historically unique and has a unique constellation of species inhabiting and influencing it. A patch might be in proximity of a catchment area where nutrients from agriculture are washed into the sea. A patch might be in a high use area, receiving hundreds of tourist visitors each day. A patch may survive high ocean temperatures from being in a cool current or a shady spot. A patch may be exposed to bleaching, cyclones, and crown of thorns starfish. Every patch is unique yet woven into other patches, and all patches respond to and modify each other. Tsing and her colleagues use the concept of the patchy Anthropocene to examine how environmental degradation is linked to social inequality (Tsing et al., 2019). I elucidate how the stories of the Anthropocene are patchy in themselves. Claims that the reef is both dying or not dying demonstrate that the Anthropocene is not unified or homogenous. Rather, patches are woven into stories about our environment. Each patch can become the object of ethnographic studies that reveal how it is constituted and how the Anthropocene is uneven and unequally distributed.

Studying the ethics of earthly survival

The interspecies relationship between the coral animal and zooxanthellae is a reminder to anthropology of finding ways to overcome anthropology's conventional focus on humans to show the multiple ways that earthly survival is already attempted.

At night, corals extend their stinging tentacles to catch small floating animals called zooplankton, and the prey is pulled into the corals' mouths and digested. However, the waters surrounding coral reef ecosystems are known to be nutrient poor, so corals need other ways to supplement their diet. They have entered into a unique relationship with single-celled plant-like organisms called dinoflagellates. Also known as zooxanthellae, the algae live inside coral cells, and here they get energy from photosynthesis. Instead of preserving the organic carbon the algae make, they release up to 95% to their host. The coral animals use this energy to grow, reproduce and build their skeletons. In return, the zooxanthellae receive inorganic nutrients from the waste metabolism of the coral. The coral relies on photosynthesis by zooxanthellae and are thus limited to inhabiting the shallow photic zone where sufficient light is available. This relationship between plant and animal is referred to as mutualistic endosymbiosis because the algae live inside the coral body and both plant and animal benefit from their mutual exchange. It is the microscopic zooxanthellae that live in the translucent tissue of the coral that give the reef skeletons their characteristic brown, green, and purple colors. (Hoegh-Guldberg & Dove, 2019, p. 97; Hopley & Smithers, 2019, p. 10).

However, this interspecies relationship breaks down in some circumstances. Stressors, such as reduced salinity or high temperatures, cause the coral animals to respond by ending their partnership with the algae and their mutual sharing of energy and nutrients. When water temperatures reach 30°C, the algae develop heat stress and produce toxic waste which poisons the coral (Fujise Yamashita, Suzuki, Sasaki, Liao, & Koike, 2014). The coral has no choice. To survive, the coral has to expel the zooxanthellae from its tissue. As a result, the coral changes rapidly from a colored pigmented appearance to pale or white. This is known as coral bleaching (Hoegh-Guldberg, 2019, p. 150). Bleached coral is not, per definition, dead, but it is starving. If the stress is mild, coral can recover its zooxanthellae populations in the months following an event; otherwise, the coral will die (p. 151).

For more than 70 years, small patches of coral reef bleaching have been observed, but it was not until the 1980s that it was understood that it was zooxanthellae being expelled from the animal which caused bleaching (p. 146). More recently, *mass* bleaching refers to events that affect reefs over hundreds or thousands of square kilometers. Mass bleaching has affected almost every reef worldwide since the 1980s (pp. 150–151).

To envisage the relationship between coral and zooxanthellae, it is not sufficient to imagine nodes and edges of discrete individuals engaging. Rather, the species are mixed up with each other – their biologies interwoven. Meanwhile, the bleached corals make visible that transforming conditions, in this case increasing temperatures, make repercussions ripple. When conditions shift, once life-sustaining relations turn deadly (Swanson et al., 2017, p. 5).

In "Staying with the Trouble – Making Kin in the Chthulucene", Donna Haraway raises questions about what it takes to live well together in the Anthropocene, or the Chthulucene (Haraway's term). Haraway's project involves learning to be in multispecies entanglements and thoughtfully responding to them in these current times of devastating events and extinction (2016, p. 1). This is achieved by "a making together", in a similar way to the zooxanthella and the coral, but also between the artists and scientists who are inventing new ways of working together and with other species (Haraway, 2016, p. 25). While Haraway advocates methods for earthly survival, I propose that we simultaneously study the attempts of ensuring earthly survival that are already taking place and that we critically question what earthly survival is. The coral polyp attempts to ensure survival by expelling the zooxanthella, a risky but necessary action, which suggests that survival is a complex relational event that, in this case, includes starvation, poisoning, and maybe death.

Here, I return to the crown of thorns starfish by introducing a version of the starfish that emerged during my fieldwork – *the salt and vinegar crown of thorns*. Marine biologists still have an incomplete understanding of how human disturbances drive the outbreaks of crown of thorns. However, nutrient runoff from agricultural practices is in particular singled out as a driving factor (Pratchett, Caballes, Rivera-Posada, & Sweatman, 2014, p. 159, 168). If such a causal relationship exists between human disturbances and outbreaks, the most effective way of preventing them would be to change land use practices. However, the existing management strategy is systematic culling of the starfish once outbreaks occur. The Association of Marine Park Tourism Operators manages a control program where disadvantaged youths are trained as crown of thorns divers. The program is currently equipped with two vessels, so reef-wide protection is not feasible, but outbreaks can be controlled at significant tourism sites (see ampto.org). James Cook University developed the killing method used on the Great Barrier Reef – a single-shot lethal injection with bile salt (see Rivera-Posada, Pratchett, Aguilar, Grand, & Caballes, 2014), but other scientists are developing less expensive methods that can be implemented across the Pacific region. In these studies, vinegar, a common household item, is used to kill the starfish. I interviewed a scientist working in this field. Before inviting me into the office, they offered me a tour of the lab where they had prepared a tank with a crown of thorns starfish. I was excited; this was my first encounter with a crown of thorns. The animal was crawling across the wall of the tank from where I could clearly see it from below through the glass. For the first time,

I could see its mouth, feet and small tentacles. Seeing it there before me, slowly moving around the tank, I felt compassion for what it was about to endure in the lab. While I studied the starfish, the scientist explained the following:

> Here you see the poisonous spines. On the bottom, you see the little tube feet, and the hole you see at the centre is the mouth. It pushes its stomach out when it eats. Along the edges you see the little eyes, or that might be a bit much, but these little tentacles are light sensitive, so it can navigate. You know, it has no brain.

I asked them to tell me about her vinegar project, and the scientist explained to me:

> Vinegar has been tried before; I didn't invent the wheel. They tried it in Japan in the 1960s with limited success, but I tweaked the method a bit. They used big needles and different concentrations. They only had a 70% success rate, and you need a 100% success rate for it to be worthwhile.

"What did you do differently?" I asked. "Thinner needles", they answered, showing me the needle. "The needles used in Japan were thick agricultural tools used to inject banana plants with pesticides. That created a big hole, and my theory was that the solution ran back out. I did experiments with dye, and it did run straight back out. I then used smaller needles". I examined the needle and noticed it was short, probably 2 cm. The scientist explained,

> This is another advantage because when you inject this (pointing at the big needle) it goes straight through the animal. With a shorter needle, that doesn't happen. The Japanese used high concentrations. If you inject something strong, they just drop that arm and heal or one starfish splits into two. I used lower concentration, but higher volumes so that it fills the whole thing. Then – I'm just speculating – if you sneak it in, they don't notice before it's inside their entire system, and then it dies.

Curious about how the vinegar kills the starfish, I asked: "And what's the process of actually dying?" Pointing at a science poster on the wall with pictures of a dying starfish: The headline is "Salt and Vinegar Crown of Thorns" on a bag of chips. "They go through multiple stages. They are hyperactive for about 45 minutes – basically, they're stressed out. Within an hour they stop moving and flip upside down. They are functionally dead; they don't eat anymore, and the spines start drooping."

The interspecies relationship between the coral animal and the zooxanthella demonstrates that survival is a complex relational event; it involves risk, it demands sacrifices, and it does not benefit all. To ensure survival, the coral animal attracts the zooxanthella, and the two organisms both benefit from their relationship, but given certain circumstances, the coral animal expels the zooxanthella from its tissue, risking starvation and death. It was not until the 1980s that coral bleaching was understood, and it was the tangled interdependence between species that delayed the understanding of this survival strategy. To ensure survival of selected reefs, scientists, environmental managers, divers, and boat crews collaborate to inject starfish with bile salt and vinegar. The age of the Anthropocene requires us not only to learn to be in and respond thoughtfully to multispecies entanglements as Haraway suggests but also to continue to scrutinize what survival is and how it takes place. This requires paying careful attention to how all living relationships are valued, which includes the relationships that are protected and nurtured and the ones that are ignored or poorly understood.

Concluding remarks – ethnographic approaches to studying disturbed human-environment relationships

The management strategies on the Great Barrier Reef aim to protect coral from humans and to strictly regulate interaction between humans and the reef.[4] The underlying reasoning suggests that coral animals are beings outside of human history. Yet, with the onset of the Anthropocene, the fate of the reef seems to be ever-more closely tied to human actions that concern both the degradation of the reef and its restoration. This chapter offers ethnographic approaches in the light of this change, and it attempts to experiment with different ways of carefully exploring human-disturbed landscapes without causing more damage. The ethnographic approaches that I write forth are inspired by Haraway's project on how to live together well in the Anthropocene, which involves learning to be in and thoughtfully responding to the multispecies entanglements of which we are part (2016, p. 1). I have attempted this by carefully considering what our other animal earth companions can teach us about conducting ethnographic fieldwork in disturbed environments. Coral makes the Anthropocene visible and tangible, but in this chapter coral also grounds and connects ethnographic work. I have proposed three different ethnographic approaches by focusing on different aspects of coral's life worlds: an approach of *transcending scale* where I argue that we have to capture both situated experiences and a global system in crisis to study the impact of the Anthropocene, and we can achieve that by immersing ourselves in richly entangled conversations and connections. However, the Anthropocene and the stories we tell about are often uneven, contradictory and inconclusive, because the Anthropocene is not unified or homogenous. By *tracing these patchy stories,* we can make each truth claim about the Anthropocene an object of ethnographic inquiry to show how the Anthropocene is constituted and how it achieves its integrity. Finally, we need to learn to live together well, but I suggest that we also need to *study earthly survival* by questioning what survival is and examine how scientific and political work ensures particular kinds of survival by creating and protecting certain relationships and ignoring others.

I feel compelled to mention the unprecedented bush fires that, at the time of writing this, are destroying bush land, farming land, and residential areas, in particular in New South Wales, Victoria, and South Australia. Without mentioning the catastrophic losses experienced by humans and other animals, ethnographic approaches similar to the ones proposed in this chapter may shed light on how these socio-natural landscapes are transformed and negotiated. For this – and to understand the impact of such an event – we need approaches that can transcend scale to uncover how social and environmental conditions are connected across scale. Secondly, in the wake of the fires, patchy stories about causality, climate change, and responsibility are flourishing, and we have the opportunity to study how these stories are constituted, and how they achieve their integrity. And as the bush fires die out, we should critically question what survival is, how it takes place and who it benefits.

Notes

1 www.wwf.org.au/our_work/saving_the_natural_world/oceans_and_marine/priority_ocean_places/ great_barrier_reef/
2 See information from GBRMPA: www.gbrmpa.gov.au/about-the-reef/reef-health.
3 In the town Ayr, north of Airlie Beach, a bull shark had washed up on land during the cyclone and was found dead in a floodwater puddle on a road.
4 See Reef 2050 Long-Term Sustainability Plan (2018).

References

ABC News. (2016) Pauline Hanson visits healthy reef to dispute effects of climate change. Retrieved from www.abc.net.au/news/2016-11-25/pauline-hanson-visits-the-great-barrier-reef-climate-change/8059142

Bruckner, A.W., H.H. Alnazry, & M. Failsal. (2011) A Paradigm Shift for Fisheries Management to Enhance Recovery, Resilience and Sustainability of Coral Reef Ecosystems in the Red Sea. *Sustainable Fisheries: Multi-Level Approaches to a Global Problem*, pp. 85–111.

Chen, E., K.M. Stiefel, T.J. Sejnowski, & T.H. Bullock. (2008) Model of Traveling Waves in a Coral Nerve Network. *Journal of Comparative Physiology A* 194(2), pp. 195–200.

Clark, N. (2014) Geo-politcs and the Disaster of the Anthropocene. *The Sociological Review,* 62(1), pp. 19–37.

Crutzen, P.J. (2002) Geology of Mankind. *Nature – The Weekly Journal of Science*, 415(23), pp. 23.

D'Angelo, C. (2016) *Great Barrier Reef Obituary Goes Viral, to the Horror of Scientists*. Retrieved from www.huffpost.com/entry/scientists-take-on-great-barrier-reef-obituary_n_57fff8f1e4b0162c043b068f?guccounter=1&guce_referrer=aHR0cHM6Ly93d3cuZ29vZ2xlLmNvbS88&guce_referrer_sig=AQAAABWhDB8PR9duwWIFksy5kHzGdpoIkLPo2nd8nfrEWPkhlLjaJUATGmEc3VUddBYggcCzeSlDGZqMS5Tim8-9ztnGi13xztXm55rwdRkhuiADc1LS-ieNb66SHkC0a-BZUdW3RPsrRR3KIFSt3N2o4-lr0nQ94lOr0T18nirTioc

Fujise, L., H. Yamashita, G. Suzuki, K. Sasaki, L.M. Liao, & K. Koike. (2014) Moderate Thermal Stress Causes Active and Immediate Expulsion of Photosynthetically Damaged Zooxanthellae (*Symbiodinium*) from Coral. *PLoS ONE*, 9(12), pp.1–18.

Miller, J., H. Sweatman, A. Cheal, M. Emslie, K. Johns, M. Jonker, & K. Osbourne. (2015) Origins & Implications of a Primary Crown-of-Thorns Starfish Outbreak in the Southern Great Barrier Reef. *Journal of Marine Biology*, 2015, pp. 1–10.

Haraway, D. (1995) Foreword. In G. A. Olson and E. Hirsch (Eds.) *Women Writing Culture* (pp. x–xii). Albany: State University of New York Press.

Haraway, D. (2016) *Staying with the Trouble: Making Kin in the Chthulucene*. Durham and London: Duke University Press, pp. 30–58.

Haraway, D., N. Ishikawa, S.F. Gilbert, K. Olwig, A. Tsing, & N.O. Bubandt. (2016) Anthropologist are Talking about the Anthropocene. *Ethnos*, 81(4), pp. 535–564.

Hastrup, K. (2012) Scales of Attention in Fieldwork: Global Connections and Local Concerns in the Arctic. *Ethnography* 14(2), pp. 145–164.

Hayward, E. (2010) Fingeryeyes: Impressions of Cup Corals. *Cultural Anthropology*, 25(4), pp. 577–599.

Helmreich, S. (2010) How Like a Reef – Figuring Coral 1839–2010. In *Party Writing for Donna Haraway*, a webfestschrift, curated and edited by Katie King (originally commissioned by Sharon Ghamari-Tabrizi).

Hoegh-Guldberg, O. (2019) Coral Reefs in a Changing World. In P. Hutchings, M. Kingsford, O. Hoegh-Guldberg (Eds.) *Great Barrier Reef – Biology, Environment and Management*. Clayton: CSIRO Publishing.

Hoegh-Guldberg O. & S. Dove. (2019) Primary Production, Nutrient Recycling and Energy Flow through Coral Reef Ecosystems. In P. Hutchings, M. Kingsford, O. Hoegh-Guldberg (Eds.) *Great Barrier Reef – Biology, Environment and Management*. Clayton: CSIRO Publishing.

Hopley, D. & S. Smithers. (2019) Geomorphology of Coral Reefs with Special Reference to the Great Barrier Reef. In P. Hutchings, M. Kingsford, O. Hoegh-Guldberg (Eds.) *Great Barrier Reef – Biology, Environment and Management*. Clayton: CSIRO Publishing.

Hughes, T. P., J.T. Kerry, A.H. Baird, S.R. Connolly, T.J. Chase, A. Dietzel, T. Hill, A.S. Hoey, M.O. Hoogenboom, M. Jacobson, A. Kerswell, J.S. Madin, A. Mieog, A.S. Paley, M.S. Pratchett, G. Torda, & R.M. Woods. (2019) Global Warming Impairs Stock–Recruitment Dynamics of Corals. *Nature* 568, pp. 387–390.

Jacobsen, R. (2016) *Obituary: Great Barrier Reef (25 Million BC-…)*. Retrieved from www.outsideonline.com/2112086/obituary-great-barrier-reef-25-million-bc-2016

Latour, B. (2015) Telling Friends from Foes at the Time of the Anthropocene. In C. Hamilton, C. Bonneuil & F. Gemenne (Eds.) *The Anthropocene and the Global Environment Crisis – Rethinking Modernity in a New Epoch* (pp. 145–155). London: Routledge.

Latour, B. (2017) Anthropology at the Time of the Anthropocene – a personal view of what is to be studied. In M. Brightman & M. Lewis (Eds.) *The Anthropology of Sustainability*. Palgrave Studies in Anthropology of Sustainability. New York: Palgrave Macmillan.

Malm, A. & A. Hornborg. (2014) The Geology of Mankind? A Critique of the Anthropocene Narrative. *The Anthropocene Review*, 1(1), pp. 62–69.

Monastersky, R. (2015) The Human Age. *Nature: The Weekly Journal of Science*, 519(7542), pp. 144–147.

Muller-Parker, G., C.F. D'Elia, & C.B. Cook. (2015) Interactions between Corals and their Symbiotic Algae. In Charles Birkeland (Ed.) *Coral Reefs in the Anthropocene*. Netherlands: Springer.

Ogden, L., N. Heynen, U. Oslender, P. West, K-A. Kassam, & P. Robbins. (2013) Global Assemblages, Resilience, and Earth Stewardship in the Anthropocene. *Frontiers in Ecology and the Environment*, 11(7), pp. 341–347.

Pratchett, M., C.F. Caballes, J. Rivera-Posada, & H. Sweatman. (2014) Limits to understanding and managing outbreaks of crown-of-thorns starfish (ACANTHASTER Spp.). *Oceanography and Marine Biology*, 52, pp. 133–200.

Reef 2050 Long-Term Sustainability Plan – July. (2018) Commonwealth of Australia 2018.

Rivera-Posada, J., M.S. Pratchett, C. Aguilar, A. Grand, & C.F. Caballes. (2014) Bile salt and the single-shot lethal injection method for killing crown-of-thorns sea stars (*Acanthaster planci*). *Ocean and Coastal Management*, 102, part A, pp. 383–390.

Roosht, H.S. (2010) Introduction. In *Crafting Life: A Sensory Ethnography of Fabricated Biologies*. PhD Dissertation from Massachusetts Institute of Technology. Program in Science, Technology and Society.

Sapp, J. (1999) Green Island. *What is natural? Coral Reef Crisis*. Oxford and New York: Oxford University Press.

Steffen, W., P.J. Crutzen, & J.R. McNeill. (2007) The Anthropocene: Are Humans now Overwhelming the Great Forces of Nature? *Ambio*, 36(8), pp. 614–621.

Zalasiewicz, J., M. Williams, W. Steffen, & P. Crutzen. (2010). The New World of the Anthropocene. *Environmental Science and Technology Viewpoint*, 44(7), pp. 2228–2231.

Swanson, H., A. Tsing, N.Bubandt, & E. Gan. (2017) Introduction: Bodies Tumbled into Bodies. In A. Tsing, H. Swanson, E. Gan and N. Bubandt (Eds.) *Arts of Living on a Damaged Planet* (pp. 1–12). Minneapolis: University of Minnesota Press.

Szmant, A.M. (1986) Reproductive Ecology of Caribbean Reef Coral. *Coral Reefs* 5(1), pp. 43–53.

Seary, S. (2015) Annual Review of Anthropology, Climate Change, Anthropocene. *Anthropologies #21. Savage Minds*. Available online: savageminds.org/2015/08/31/anthropologies-21-annual-review-of-anthropology-climate-change-anthropocene/

Sydney Morning Herald. (2016) Australia, welcome to your new climate change policy. Retrieved from www.smh.com.au/opinion/pauline-hanson-says-the-barrier-reef-is-fine-welcome-to-our-new-climate-change-policy-20161208-gt6tpk.html.

Sweatman, H. (2018) *Long-term Reef Monitoring Program - Annual Summary Report on coral reef condition for 2016/17*. Townsville. Australian Institute of Marine Science.

Tsing, A. (2010) Worlding the matsutake diaspora. Or, can actor-network theory experiment with holism? In T. Otto and N. Bubandt (Eds.) *Experiments in Holism* (pp. 47–66). Oxford: Blackwell.

Tsing, A. (2014) Wreckage and Recovery: Four Papers Exploring the Nature of Nature. Department of Culture and Society, Aarhus University. *Wreckage and Recovery: exploring the nature of nature, More than Human*. AURA Working Papers, 2, pp. 2–14.

Tsing, A. (2016) Earth Stalked by Man. *The Cambridge Journal of Anthropology*, 34(1), pp. 2–16.

Tsing, A., A.S. Mathews, N. Bubandt. (2019) Patchy Anthropocene: Landscape Structure, Multispecies History, and the Retooling of Anthropology. In *Current Anthropology*, 60(suppl 20), pp. 186–196.

37

WHY HAPPINESS STUDIES OUGHT TO INCLUDE QUALITATIVE RESEARCH COMPONENTS

Cathrine V. Jansson-Boyd and Anke Plagnol

Introduction

Healthcare has long relied on self-reports, for instance, to assess patients' levels of pain and fatigue. However, in other research fields, subjective assessments have a much shorter tradition – one example is the study of societal and individual well-being, which has traditionally relied on objective measures, such as GDP and personal income (Sirgy, Michalos, Ferriss, Easterlin, Patrick, & Pavot, 2006). However, subjective well-being research has gained increased importance over the past decades with more governments and international organisations acknowledging the need to consider well-being in formulating new policies and assessing societal progress (Krueger & Stone, 2014). The Sarkozy commission recommended in 2009 that governments adopt subjective well-being measures to supplement traditional indicators of societal progress to be better able to put well-being at the heart of policymaking (for a summary, see Easterlin, 2010). However, conceptualisations of well-being – for instance, what is meant by the elusive concept of happiness – have changed over time and even now often differ between disciplines and researchers. In 2013, the OECD published a comprehensive guide on measuring subjective well-being (OECD, 2013) which combines findings from different approaches to studying individual well-being.

In this chapter, we will present different interpretations of happiness, one of the evaluative components of SWB as described in the OECD guide. We will further focus on two approaches to understanding and interpreting happiness that are also part of the OECD definition – namely the hedonic and eudaimonic approach. Finally, we will argue that well-being research would benefit from incorporating qualitative approaches to further refine our understanding of the determinants of individual well-being.

Defining happiness

Over 2000 years ago, Aristotle presented his theory of happiness and by doing so introduced the idea of a science of happiness in terms of a new field of knowledge. He proposed that happiness is the aim of all our actions and that it is thus the key purpose of human life (Aristotle, trans.

1934, Book I, Section VII; see Kolak & Thomson, 2016). Whilst happiness may be instrumental to many life goals, it is not fundamental to all actions. More recent definitions of happiness align better with the modern approach of the psychology of happiness in that they broadly focus more on well-being. According to the Merriam-Webster (2020) dictionary, happiness is "a state of well-being and contentment" and "a pleasurable or satisfying experience". This is similar to the American Psychological Association's (APA) definition of happiness that simply states that it is "an emotion of joy, gladness, satisfaction, and well-being" (APA, 2020). The similarity is in that they both include satisfaction and well-being. However, whilst the Merriam-Webster definition describes a satisfying experience, the APA focuses on the emotions experienced rather than the applicability to a specific event. The two definitions in turn differ from one postulated by Lyubomirsky (2008), who states that happiness is "the experience of joy, contentment, or positive well-being, combined with a sense that one's life is good, meaningful, and worthwhile" (p. 32). Here the difference is in the fact that happiness requires consensus with a good and meaningful life.

In psychological research, "happiness" has often been used as an umbrella term for subjective states of hedonic and eudaimonic well-being and it is thus a rather nebulous concept. Subjective well-being and happiness are often used interchangeably in the literature, especially in older publications, and the definition of what is captured by the term "happiness" can also vary by field and authors. The aforementioned OECD report proposes a broad definition of subjective well-being in which SWB is considered to capture: "Good mental states, including all of the various evaluations, positive and negative, that people make of their lives and the affective reactions of people to their experiences" (OECD, 2013, p. 10). The OECD definition thus encompasses both evaluations and experiences which contribute to a person's sense of well-being. Furthermore, the guidelines describe that subjective well-being encompasses three distinct components: "Life evaluation – a reflective assessment on a person's life or some specific aspect of it. Affect – a person's feelings or emotional states, typically measured with reference to a particular point in time. Eudaimonia – a sense of meaning and purpose in life, or good psychological functioning" (OECD, 2013, p. 10). More recent publications usually refer to subjective well-being as an umbrella term encompassing various well-being measures while older publications may refer to happiness as the umbrella term for subjective well-being states. According to the OECD definition, however, happiness is a component of subjective well-being and it would be misleading to conflate subjective well-being with happiness. While most well-being researchers now largely agree that subjective well-being includes different aspects of subjective states, some researchers focus mostly on hedonic states (e.g., Kahneman & Krueger, 2006) while others advocate for the consideration of psychological flourishing in well-being definitions, i.e., eudaimonic well-being (e.g., Huppert & So, 2013). To better understand the differences between the hedonic and eudaimonic approaches, it is useful to consider their ancient origins, which we will do further below.

In the following, we will focus on happiness as one component of subjective well-being; however, we acknowledge that many of the researchers cited in this chapter conflate happiness with subjective well-being. Some researchers believe that happiness means the same thing to all individuals (e.g., Layard, 2005; Myers & Diener, 1995), whilst others suggest that happiness is highly subjective. Thus, postulating that happiness means different things to each individual (Gilbert, 2006) and people might reflect on different aspects of their lives when they answer happiness questions in surveys. Because definitions of the word "happiness" are inconsistent and can be perceived as ambiguous, many researchers prefer more clearly defined research concepts such as "life satisfaction". However, it is important to note that life satisfaction and happiness, though they are two evaluative well-being components, are two distinct measures of subjective well-being.

Why research happiness

Research findings support the notion that it is an important research topic in that it has been found that most people think about how happy they are at least once a day (e.g. Diener, Suh, Smith, & Shao, 1995; Freedman, 1978). Investigating what factors are important for happiness also provides insights about general well-being and can help to clarify misconceptions. For example, lay people can be under the impression that material goods and extrinsic aspirations will be a path to happiness. However, neither has been found to satisfy psychological needs (Kasser & Ryan, 1996), as the acquisition of positional goods does not lead to long-term improvements in well-being due to psychological processes of hedonic adaptation and social comparison (e.g., Frank, 1997). Many also strive for fame and fortune, something that is usually contingent on engaging in specific controlled activities that tend to detract from a sense of authenticity and as a result can lead to lower psychological well-being (Ryan, Chirkov, Little, Sheldon, Timoshina, & Deci, 1999).

In short, if researchers can truly conceptualise and understand happiness, it can help create a better, healthier, and stronger society. As most people appear to believe that happiness is a desirable and worthy goal and it is closely aligned with how we feel, it is undoubtedly an important research area.

Two approaches to researching happiness

There are two distinct approaches; the hedonic and eudaimonic perspectives. The two approaches have their origins in different philosophical traditions that explain why these two perspectives are quite distinct (Keyes, Shmotkin, & Ryff, 2002).

The hedonic approach has its origins in Greece, during the fourth century BC, and concerns the pursuit of sensation and pleasure (Ryan & Deci, 2001). Some definitions of subjective well-being, usually definitions that were postulated before the OECD guidelines were published, only include hedonic components and encompass three core components: life satisfaction, the presence of positive mood, and the absence of negative mood (e.g., Diener, Suh, Lucas & Smith, 1999). The other approach, the eudaimonic perspective, has its roots in Aristotle's postulations (Ryan & Deci, 2001) which focused on the path of well-being and happiness as the realisation of one's true potential.

The hedonic approach

The hedonic approach is effectively looking at happiness as pleasure, comfort, and enjoyment. Even though there are many ways in which pleasure can be assessed, researchers who adhere to the hedonic approach have commonly used evaluative and affective measures of well-being as a means to tap into peoples' well-being and happiness levels. According to Diener (2009), SWB can be characterised as the extent to which people evaluate their lives in a positive way; i.e., in this view SWB encompasses the evaluative component of the OECD definition – often in the form of life satisfaction, and also incorporates positive and negative affect as a means to measure how people evaluate their lives (e.g. Diener, 1984; Diener, Suh, Lucas, & Smith, 1999). This tripartite structure has since been widely used. However, the psychology-based literature does not take a unified stance on what SWB really is; some believe that happiness is one of the key components of SWB and others that SWB is synonymous with happiness; however, recent contributions usually treat happiness as a component of SWB. Today, scientists in the field of SWB recognise that there are many other approaches to measure a good life (Diener, Oishi, & Tay, 2018) and that happiness is just one possible measure.

How is SWB measured?

Usually, SWB is assessed through quantitative measures of happiness, life satisfaction, negative and positive affect, or flourishing. The questions span from specific and concrete factors such as momentary experiences to global and abstract ones that take global judgements about respondents' entire lives into account. SWB measures have been found to be reliable and valid (e.g., Kahneman & Krueger, 2006), and they are now included in a number of large-scale, nationally representative surveys such as the UK Household Longitudinal Study and the European Social Survey. SWB has been extensively studied in relation to a wide range of factors, including marriage (Lucas, Clark, Georgellis, & Diener, 2003; Zimmermann & Easterlin, 2006), physical health (Okun, Stock, Haring, & Witter, 1984), and income (Diener & Biswas-Diener, 2002, for a review). However, in some domains, such as health, a complex pattern has emerged in that people with poor health report high SWB whilst others with low well-being have no signs of physical illness related symptoms. Such differences may come down to individual differences (Ryan & Deci, 2001). Most studies are correlational, which means that the direction of causality cannot be clearly established. However, it appears that health is generally positively associated with SWB; i.e., on average, those who report better health also report higher levels of subjective well-being (for an overview see Dolan, Peasgood, & White, 2008; Plagnol & Macchia, 2018). People appear to partially adapt to changes in health with respect to subjective well-being (Brickman, Coates, & Janoff-Bulman, 1978; Oswald & Powdthavee, 2008).

Are SWB measures good measures?

SWB measures have been found to be reliable and valid (for reviews, see Di Tella & MacCulloch, 2006; Kahneman & Krueger, 2006; Lane, 2017). For instance, self- reported well-being correlates with objective measures of well-being, such as cortisol levels (Steptoe, Wardle, & Marmot, 2005) and the frequency of Duchenne smiles (Ekman, Davidson, & Friesen, 1990), which are also known as smiles that cannot be faked. However, it has been suggested that there are issues to be resolved in regards to measuring SWB in its current format (e.g., Busseri & Sadava, 2011; Schimmack, 2008).

As many studies are correlational, it is often not possible to establish whether a change in life circumstances caused a change in SWB or vice versa. For example, health and illness can influence SWB just as SWB can affect them (Diener et al., 2018). However, some long-term studies suggest that raised levels of SWB in turn lead to improved health (De Neve, Diener, Tay, & Xuereb, 2013), thus suggesting that the relationship between health and SWB can be one-directional.

The suitability of SWB measures across all cultures can also be questioned as most research to date has been conducted within the Western world (Diener et al., 2018). Research has found cultural variations in the predictors of SWB; for instance, financial satisfaction is more strongly correlated with life satisfaction in poor countries than in richer nations (Diener & Diener, 1995;

Oishi, Diener, Lucas, & Suh, 1999). Whilst such findings may be relatively easy to explain, further exploration may be required to explain why self-esteem is a predictor of life satisfaction in American but not in Indian women (Diener & Diener, 1995). Such findings could benefit from more individual-based research whereby researchers use qualitative data to enrich our understandings of cultural differences that may play a role in self-esteem.

Eudaimonic well-being

Eudaimonia is traditionally translated as "happiness" though the alternate translation used in much of contemporary philosophy is "flourishing". In modern philosophy, many interpretations of – and commentaries on – Aristotle's eudaimonia have been offered (Annas, 1993; Haybron, 2008; Kraut, 1979; Norton, 1976; Tiberius, 2013). Shared among these is the notion that eudaimonia is a reflection of virtue, excellence, and the development of one's full potential (Huta & Waterman, 2014). Rooted in these philosophical origins, eudaimonia refers to that which is worth pursuing in life – an objective standard of goodness (Huta & Waterman, 2014). Effectively, the focus of the approach is on peoples' ability to set sophisticated goals that provide meaning on an individual and societal level.

There has been a lot of debate about whether the hedonic approach to happiness is the best when it comes to tapping into what makes people happy. Presumably, this is because hedonic happiness is easier to achieve than eudaimonic happiness in that it requires little effort such as "sitting on the couch watching TV, one hand on the remote, and the other in a bag of chips" (King, Eells, & Burton, 2012, p. 37), whilst eudaimonia is more complicated in that it relates to an individual's functioning in relation to opportunities to grow as well as commitment.

Lack of agreement on conceptualisation

The different eudaimonic approaches and theories all share the view that happiness is an ongoing process. They also all stress the importance of personal goals that have deeper meaning and that not all paths to happiness are equally good (Ryan & Deci, 2001; Veenhoven, 2003). In this view, it is important to avoid pursuits for sheer self-related pleasure as it can be detrimental to a person as well as society at large in that it advances the depletion of resources. Meaningfulness is a crucial part of the eudaimonic approach (Baumeister & Vohs, 2002), and thus researchers seek to identify how personal goals can lead to a greater good and thus be conducive to happiness. There is little agreement among scholars in this area regarding any one conceptual definition of eudaimonia (Huta & Waterman, 2014). This may not be too surprising considering the broad philosophical angles that underpin it. Waterman suggested an action that expresses virtue and used self-realisation and personal expressiveness as the core for defining eudaimonia (Waterman, 1993). A few years on, Ryan and Deci (2001) suggested that eudaimonia captures living a life in full accord with one's potential. Keyes (2002) included a component of social well-being into his conceptualisation of eudaimonia whilst Seligman (2002) claims that it is a product of one's characteristic personality traits or strengths. Bauer, McAdams, and Pals (2008) considered it in terms of psychosocial integration, ego development, and personal growth; meanwhile Ryff & Singer (2008) think of it in a broader trait-like manner, that is to be fully functioning and successful regardless of life's challenges that people may face. Moreover, Delle Fave and colleagues (Delle Fave, Brdar, Freire, Vella-Brodrick, & Wissing, 2011) conceptualise eudaimonia as flow experiences and long-term meaning-making, while Huta (2015) treats it as a motive to develop the best possible self.

Methods used for measurement

Just as there is no clear consensus on how to define eudaimonic well-being, there is also a lack of a shared methodological approach to measure it (Huta & Waterman, 2014). Ryff's (1989) Scales for Psychological Well-Being have been widely used to measure eudaimonia at the trait level. Additionally, the Questionnaire for Eudaimonic Well-Being (Waterman et al., 2010) has been used to measure traits as it taps into six different dimensions: self-discovery, perceived development of one's best potential, sense of purpose and meaning in life, investment of effort in pursuit of excellence, intense involvement in activities, and enjoyment of personally expressive activities.

Other scales used to tap into eudaimonic happiness include the "Mental Health Continuum" which assesses psychological, social, and emotional well-being (Keyes, 2002), and the "Personally Expressive Activities Questionnaire" (Waterman, 1993), which assesses engagement in self-defining activities. The aforementioned scales are constructed to target different aspects of eudaimonic well-being and are thus not comparable. There are also scales that include a broader range of eudaimonic related concepts such as the "Flourishing Scale" aimed at measuring aspects such as positive relationships, feelings of competence, and meaning and purpose in life (Diener et al., 2010).

Criticism

Kashdan, Biswas-Diener, and King (2008) have commented on the use of eudaimonia in furthering the science of well-being and happiness. They argue that the philosophical distinction between hedonic and eudaimonic well-being does not carry over well into the psychological science of well-being. Kashdan et al. believe that the definitions and measurements that are currently used fail to capture the concept of eudaimonia as postulated by Aristotle. Furthermore, they consider it problematic that the field of eudaimonic well-being lacks concise conceptual and operational definitions. Thus, it does not provide clear directives that researchers can follow. The vagueness of these definitions has also been debated elsewhere (e.g., Huta & Waterman, 2014; Waterman, 2008), however, without offering a solution in regards to how a robust theory can be created.

In addition, Kashdan et al. (2008) question whether it is appropriate to draw comparisons between hedonic and eudaimonic well-being. Partially, they view this as difficult because the study of eudaimonic well-being is more about *why* someone is happy rather than an accurate subjective assessment of *whether* someone is happy. This, they believe, conflates the experience of happiness with the common sources of this experience (Kashdan et al., 2008). However, there are those who think it is too early in the history of the psychological science of eudaimonia to engage in such pointed critiques regarding the shortcomings of this work in the first place (Waterman, 2008).

Two distinct approaches of happiness?

Originally, researchers did not distinguish between hedonic and eudaimonic approaches to happiness (Argyle, 1987; Easterlin, 1974; Wilson, 1967). However, over time, the two approaches have come to be thought of as distinctly different.

There are clear differences in what the two approaches represent. Hedonia is focused on personal achievement and fulfilment of needs (Veenhoven, 2003). This is different from the eudaimonic view, which, according to some, focusses on the happiness of the community with no place for self-interest. Instead, it supports harmonisation of an individual's happiness with societal well-being (Nussbaum, 1993) so that collective welfare is prioritised. Specifically, Delle Fave & Bassi (2007) proposed that there are three major polarities that set hedonic and eudaimonic happiness apart, namely state versus process, feeling versus functioning, and personal fulfilment versus "integrated fulfilment".

Even though there are clear differences in the two approaches to happiness, it has been proposed that the eudaimonic research should be incorporated into the hedonic view as the two approaches overlap conceptually (Kashdan et al., 2008). There are arguments in support of such a view, especially as the approaches have been found to be highly correlated even though they are separate constructs (Linley, Maltby, Wood, Osborne, & Hurling, 2009; Gallagher, Lopez, & Preacher, 2009).

There is evidence to suggest that people's experience of eudaimonic and hedonic well-being is related. For example, it has been found that an indicator of eudaimonia, the personal expressiveness reported for activities, is significantly correlated with the hedonic enjoyment of that activity (Waterman, 1993, 2008). However, other studies show a clear distinction between hedonic and eudaimonic measures. For example, Keyes et al. (2002) analysed Diener's (1984) model of subjective well-being and Ryff's model of psychological well-being and found that the two concepts are correlated and fit nicely into a two-factor structure. Thus, the authors concluded that hedonic and eudaimonic measures are "related but distinct conceptions of well-being" (Keyes et al., 2002, p. 1017). Similarly, exploratory factor analyses conducted by Linley et al. (2009) identified two-factor loadings for hedonic and eudaimonic measures of well-being.

In contrast, Disabato, Goodman, Kashdan, Short, and Jarden (2016) found that a one-factor model of hedonic and eudaimonic well-being worked equally well as a two-factor model. Moreover, in the two-factor solution, the factors were strongly correlated and had a high shared variance, thus supporting the closeness of the two concepts, as there is substantial overlap. These findings complicate the discussion on whether there are two independent approaches to happiness and suggests that more research is required to settle the question. Recent definitions of subjective well-being, like the one proposed by the OECD (2013), acknowledge that both approaches form an integral part of a comprehensive conceptualisation of individual well-being.

Some of the differences found are most likely due to the multiple conceptualisations of eudaimonia which complicates any comparisons made to hedonic happiness. As there currently is no systematic evaluation taking each of the different conceptualisations into account, the findings are unclear.

A unified approach

Recently, there have been shifts towards a unilateral approach of examining psychological well-being and happiness (e.g., Kashdan et al., 2008; Waterman, 2008). This has resulted in the proposition of integrated frameworks. For example, an "orientations to happiness framework" has been developed (Peterson & Seligman, 2004; Seligman, 2002), which proposes that there are three paths to happiness, namely: pleasure, engagement, and meaning. A life that includes high levels of all three components leads to the highest level of life satisfaction as opposed to a life with low levels of the three components. However, engagement and meaning contribute more significantly when it comes to happiness that is associated with pleasure (Peterson, Park, & Seligman, 2005; Vella-Brodrick, Park, & Peterson, 2009).

There have also been attempts at unifying the eudaimonic and hedonic perspectives. For example, Keyes (2002, 2005, 2007) introduced the concept of flourishing and subsequently developed a corresponding measure, the Mental Health Continuum, that assesses emotional, social, and psychological elements of well-being. *Emotional well-being* measures the presence of positive emotions and satisfaction with life (Diener et al., 1999). *The social aspect* indicates how well an individual functions in their social life in the context of larger society (such as social integration, Keyes, 1998). Whilst *psychological well-being* incorporates aspects of individuals' psychological functioning (such as sense of personal growth, Ryff, 1989).

Trying to integrate the hedonic and eudaimonic perspectives has not only triggered a general debate within the happiness field but it also opens up discussions on the importance of incorporating individual perspective into the research domain.

Where is the "individual" in happiness studies?

With the frequent use of questionnaires to investigate happiness or related concepts, there is little focus on the individual. The use of subjective well-being measures to inform policy requires large, nationally representative datasets; preferably longitudinal studies which allow better insights into the determinants of societal subjective well-being. Whilst there is a broader understanding of averages, we lack knowledge about the nuances in individual experiences that contribute to the experience of happiness. Thus, there is an argument to be made that by incorporating more idiographic approaches, a better understanding can be gained about the factors that underpin happiness. Qualitative research can help with this in that it has the ability to uncover novel and deeper understandings of happiness that may not be revealed by relying solely on quantitative techniques (Hefferon, Ashfield, Waters, & Synard, 2017). Currently, there are not many qualitative methodologies used within happiness research. A quick Google scholar search reveals how infrequently they are used. Using broad search terms, such as "psychology and happiness", between 2015 and the present date produces 16,900 results if one excludes book chapters, patents and reviews. Of those, 5,340 articles mention or include a qualitative component. Thus, less than a third of psychology papers take a qualitative approach to happiness. Albeit small in number, qualitative and mixed-method approaches have added value by demonstrating how individual circumstances and social environments can impact people (e.g., Csikszentmihalyi, 2000; Reynolds & Lim, 2007). In order to create a clearer picture of how qualitative studies can help inform our understanding of happiness as a science, it is important to extend the current epistemologies and methods used.

Are current happiness measures precise enough?

In 2018, an annual UN report that measures subjective well-being suggested that Finland was the happiest place in the world (BBC News, 2018). However, statistics across a number of health-related aspects within the Finnish population may raise some doubts in regard to whether these reports on Finnish happiness are entirely correct. For example, the population in Finland is approximately 5.5 million (Eurostat, 2019), but in 2014 there were 2.4 million visits to mental healthcare outpatient units in Finland (Nordic Centre for Welfare and Social Issues, 2019). Over 50% of the Finnish workforce experienced symptoms of burnout, and approximately 165,000 employees suffered from severe burnout (ILO, 2000). These are staggering figures considering the small number of people that live there. Furthermore, the Finns' relatively high suicide rates should also be considered. In fact, the World Population Review (2019) ranked Finland as the 24th country with the most suicides in the world. It is also a place where excessive alcohol use is common (NordAN, 2018) and there is a high prevalence of heavy episodic drinking (World Health Organisation, 2016).

Naturally, there are going to be individual differences within each country in regard to how happy people are. Cross-country happiness comparisons that report country averages often do not discuss the distribution of happiness scores within each country. However, there appear to be more than a few inconsistencies in the aforementioned factors as they suggest that people may not be so happy after all. This begs the question: how come the Finns are reportedly so happy?

It is difficult to determine exactly what components in peoples' lives form the foundations for or generate happiness. Some people base their happiness evaluations on larger domains in their lives such as marriage, work, or social relationships. Whilst others may be more specific in their approach in that they focus on the emotions felt during a particular event, such as meeting a person for the first time. Alternatively, people also focus on the here and now in that they trust what they are feeling at any point in time. The fact that there are different components to consider may account for differences in happiness reports.

However, another explanation may be found in how "happiness" has been measured. As most large surveys make use of quantitative self-report measures, it may cast some doubt on how precisely they actually measure happiness and whether there are gaps in that they don't include all the encompassing factors that contribute to happiness. For instance, happiness questions may elicit answers based on a temporary mood rather than general feelings of well-being, and indeed this is one of the reasons that large scale surveys often include measures of life satisfaction rather than happiness. Nevertheless, the incorporation of more qualitative research could help explain supposed happiness puzzles such as the concurrent high happiness ratings and high suicide rate in Finland.

The benefits of using qualitative research techniques

Qualitative research is not used to answer the same sort of questions that one may ask in quantitatively based research. Instead, it is a form of inquiry that analyses information conveyed through language and behaviour, mostly in natural settings. It has the ability to capture expressive information not conveyed in quantitative data about beliefs, values, feelings, and motivations that underlie peoples' behaviours and thoughts. Often, respondents are able to disclose their thoughts and feelings without limitation. Something that can be done by using techniques such as interview methods (Davis, Nolen-Hoeksema, & Larson, 1998) or the narration of life stories (Bauer et al., 2008).

When using qualitative research, it is more likely that the researcher can tap into "why" a participant is experiencing happiness. Something that can be left out when looking at quantitative data. The method is undoubtedly dynamic in that a researcher has the ability to follow up on answers given in real time; something that cannot be done with questionnaire-based methods.

Although the topic of happiness has been extensively researched, the data collected does not always get to the heart of this "ultimate human experience" (Lu, 2001). Instead, it would seem that we know more about the correlates of SWB than the individualistic experiences of happiness to plug the gaps required to fully understand human happiness (Lu, 2001). The hedonic approach has exerted great influence on western-based researchers dominating the field. Thus, it begs the question how applicable it is to non-western cultures that do not share the westernised individualistic perspective. Perhaps qualitative methodologies can help broaden our understanding of individual well-being.

The role of negative emotions

Pleasant emotions have been found to be positively associated with self-reported happiness (Tamir, Schwartz, Oishi, & Kim, 2017; e.g. Diener, 1984; Kahneman, Diener, & Schwarz, 1999;

Kuppens, Realo, & Diener, 2008; Lucas, Diener, & Suh, 1996). However, it can be difficult to tap into how people feel without deeper self-reflection – something that is achievable through use of in-depth interviews – i.e., by using a qualitative approach. Traditionally, happiness studies were based on the assumption that happiness and well-being require the experience of pleasant emotions. However, Tamir et al. (2017) proposed that one does not have to feel good in order to pursue happiness. They tested this idea by studying responses from over 2000 people from 8 countries and they did indeed find that participants were generally happier if they experienced the emotions they wanted to experience regardless of whether they felt good or bad.

Understanding negative emotions is particularly important as most people are, at some point in their lives, faced with adverse life events. Making sense of such events and attributing meaning to them can help a person understand why it happened and make them feel better in that it contributes to a sense of efficacy and self-worth (Baumeister & Vohs, 2002). Unemployment is one example of such a negative life event for which researchers have failed to address possible positives (McKee-Ryan, Song, Wanberg, & Kinicki, 2005). Because there is not much focus on the negative emotions experienced in the context of well-being, there have been calls for more qualitative research to address this gap (Blustein, 2008; Blustein, Kozan, Connors-Kellgren, 2013; Delle Fave, Massimini, & Bassi, 2011). By focusing on individuals' subjective experiences, a more complex understanding of well-being correlates and their role in negative life experiences could be developed.

Concluding remarks

Happiness research has been dominated by quantitative approaches. Bearing in mind that both the hedonic and eudaimonic approach usually rely on quantitative methods, it stands to reason that qualitative research has a place in happiness research. The key argument here is not that qualitative research is "better" than quantitative research but simply that it can assist in providing more nuance to what it is that makes people happy. It is more likely to provide insight into "why" a person is experiencing happiness, which is something that is currently lacking in the literature. The fact that qualitative methods give researchers the ability to follow up on answers provided by participants is a clear advantage when trying to gain individual insight. Hence, it can overcome the gaps that researchers are faced with using quantitative techniques.

The inclusion of qualitative studies would ultimately provide a more in-depth perspective on peoples' life experiences in relation to happiness that could be particularly helpful to clinical practitioners working on helping those with a negative outlook on life. Thus, it is concluded that there is clear value in incorporating qualitative research methods to supplement quantitative approaches to understanding happiness.

References

Annas, J. (1993). The morality of happiness. Oxford, UK: Oxford University Press.

APA. (2020). *APA dictionary of psychology*. dictionary.apa.org/happiness

Argyle, M. (1987). *The psychology of happiness*. Routledge.

Bauer, J. J., D.P. McAdams, & J.L. Pals. (2008). Narrative identity and eudaimonic well-being. *Journal of Happiness Studies, 9*(1), 81–104. doi.org/10.1007/s10902-006-9021-6

Baumeister, R. F. & K.D. Vohs. (2002). The pursuit of meaningfulness in life. In C. R. Snyder & S. J. Lopez (Eds.), *Handbook of Positive Psychology* (pp. 608–618). Oxford University Press.

BBC News. (2018). *Happiest report: Finland is world's 'happiest country'- UN*. www.bbc.co.uk/news/world-43414145

Blustein, D.L. (2008). The role of work in psychological health and well-being: A conceptual, historical, and public policy perspective. *American Psychologist, 63*(4), 228–240. doi.org/10.1037/0003-066X.63.4.228

Blustein, D.L., S. Kozan, & A. Connors-Kellgren. (2013). Unemployment and underemployment: A narrative analysis about loss. *Journal of Vocational Behavior, 82*(3), 256–265. doi.org/10.1016/j.jvb.2013.02.005

Brickman, P., D. Coates, & R. Janoff-Bulman. (1978). Lottery winners and accident victims: is happiness relative? *Journal of Personality and Social Psychology, 36*(8), 917–927. www.ncbi.nlm.nih.gov/pubmed/690806

Busseri, M.A. & S.W. Sadava. (2011). A review of the tripartite structure of subjective well-being: Implications for conceptualization, operationalization, analysis, and synthesis. *Personality and Social Psychology Review, 15*(3), 290–314. doi.org/10.1177/1088868310391271

Csikszentmihalyi, M. (2000). *Beyond boredom and anxiety.* Jossey-Bass.

Davis, C.G., S. Nolen-Hoeksema, & J. Larson. (1998). Making sense of loss and benefiting from the experience: Two construals of meaning. *Journal of Personality and Social Psychology, 75*(2), 561–574. doi.org/10.1037/0022-3514.75.2.561

De Neve, J.-E., E. Diener, L. Tay, & C. Xuereb. (2013). The objective benefits of subjective well-being. In J. Helliwell, R. Layard, & J. Sachs (Eds.), *World Happiness Report 2013.* UN Sustainable Development Solutions Network.

Delle Fave, A. & M. Bassi. (2007). *Psicologia e salute. L'esperienza di utenti e operatori* [Psychology and health. The experience of patients and professionals]. Torino: UTET Università.

Delle Fave, A., I. Brdar, T. Freire, D. Vella-Brodrick, & M.P. Wissing. (2011). The eudaimonic and hedonic components of happiness: Qualitative and quantitative findings. *Social Indicators Research, 100*(2), 185–207. doi.org/10.1007/s11205-010-9632-5

Delle Fave, A., F. Massimini, & M. Bassi. (2011). Hedonism and eudaimonism in positive psychology. In *Psychological Selection and Optimal Experience Across Cultures. Cross-Cultural Advancements in Positive Psychology, vol 2* (pp. 3–18). doi.org/10.1007/978-90-481-9876-4_1

Di Tella, R. & R. MacCulloch. (2006). Some uses of happiness data in economics. *The Journal of Economic Perspectives, 20*, 25–46. American Economic Association. doi.org/10.2307/30033632

Diener, E. (2009). Positive Psychology: Past, Present, and Future. In C.R. Snyder & Shane J. Lopez (Eds.), *Oxford Handbook of Positive Psychology.* Oxford: Oxford University Press.

Diener, E. (1984). Subjective well-being. *Psychological Bulletin, 95*(3), 542–75.

Diener, E., Diener, M., & Diener, C. (1995). Factors predicting the subjective well-being of nations. *Journal of Personality and Social Psychology, 69*, 851–864.

Diener, E. & R. Biswas-Diener. (2002). Will money increase subjective well-being? *Social Indicators Research, 57*, 119–169. doi.org/10.1023/A:1014411319119

Diener, E., S. Oishi, & L. Tay. (2018). Advances in subjective well-being research. *Nature Human Behaviour, 2*(4), 253–260. doi.org/10.1038/s41562-018-0307-6

Diener, E., E.M. Suh, R.E. Lucas, & H.L. Smith. (1999). Subjective well-being: Three decades of progress. *Psychological bulletin, 125*(2), 276–302.

Diener, E., E.M. Suh, H. Smith, & L. Shao. (1995). National differences in reported well-being: Why do they occur? *Social Indicators Research, 34*, 7–32.

Diener, E., D. Wirtz, W. Tov, C. Kim-Prieto, D.W. Choi, S. Oishi, & R. Biswas-Diener. (2010). New well-being measures: Short scales to assess flourishing and positive and negative feelings. *Social Indicators Research, 97*(2), 143–156.

Disabato, D. J., F.R. Goodman, T.B. Kashdan, J.L. Short, & A. Jarden. (2016). Different types of well-being? A cross-cultural examination of hedonic and eudaimonic well-being. *Psychological Assessment, 28*(5), 471.

Dolan, P., T. Peasgood, & M. White. (2008). Do we really know what makes us happy? A review of the economic literature on the factors associated with subjective well-being. *Journal of Economic Psychology, 29*(1), 94–122. doi.org/10.1016/j.joep.2007.09.001

Easterlin, R.A. (1974). Does economic growth improve the human lot? Some empirical evidence. In P. A. David & M.W. Reder (Eds.), *Nations and Households in Economic Growth: Essays in Honour of Moses Abramovitz* (pp. 89–125). Academic Press. doi.org/10.1007/BF00286477

Easterlin, R.A. (2010). Well-being, front and center: A note on the Sarkozy report. *Population and Development Review, 36*(1), 119–124. doi.org/10.1111/j.1728-4457.2010.00320.x

Ekman, P., R.J. Davidson, & W.V. Friesen. (1990). The Duchenne smile: Emotional expression and brain physiology: II. *Journal of Personality and Social Psychology, 58*(2), 342–353. doi.org/10.1037/0022-3514.58.2.342

Eurostat. (2019). *Population: Statistics illustrated*. ec.europa.eu/eurostat/en/web/population-demography-migration-projections/statistics-illustrated

Frank, R.H. (1997). The frame of reference as a public good. *The Economic Journal, 107*(445), 1832–1847. doi.org/10.1111/j.1468-0297.1997.tb00086.x

Freedman, J. (1978). *Happy people: What happiness is, who has it, and why*. Harcourt Brace Jovanovich.

Gallagher, M.W., S.J. Lopez, & K.J. Preacher. (2009). The hierarchical structure of well-being. *Journal of Personality, 77*(4), 1025–1050.

Gilbert, D. (2006). *Stumbling on Happiness*. New York: Knopf.

Haybron, D. (2008). Happiness, the self and human flourishing. Utilitas, *20*, 21–49.

Hefferon, K., A. Ashfield, L. Waters, & J. Synard. (2017). Understanding optimal human functioning–The 'call for qual' in exploring human flourishing and well-being. *Journal of Positive Psychology 12*(3), 211–219. doi.org/10.1080/17439760.2016.1225120

Huppert, F.A. & T.T.C. So. (2013). Flourishing across Europe: Application of a new conceptual framework for defining well-being. *Social Indicators Research, 110*(3), 837–861. doi.org/10.1007/s11205-011-9966-7

Huta, V. & A.S. Waterman. (2014). Eudaimonia and its distinction from hedonia: Developing a classification and terminology for understanding conceptual and operational definitions. *Journal of Happiness Studies, 15*(6), 1425–1456. doi.org/10.1007/s10902-013-9485-0

Huta, V. (2015). *An overview of hedonic and eudaimonic well-being concepts*. In L. Reinecke & M. B. Oliver (Eds.), *Handbook of media use and well-being*. Chapter 2. New York: Routledge. Manuscript accepted for publication on November 11, 2015.

ILO. (2000). *Mental health in the workplace - situation analysis Finland*. International Labour Office. www.ilo.org/wcmsp5/groups/public/@ed_emp/@ifp_skills/documents/publication/wcms_108222.pdf

Kahneman, D. & A.B. Krueger. (2006). Developments in the measurement of subjective well-being. *Journal of Economic Perspectives 20*(1), 3–24. doi.org/10.1257/089533006776526030

Kashdan, T.B., R. Biswas-Diener, & L.A. King. (2008). Reconsidering happiness: The costs of distinguishing between hedonics and eudaimonia. *Journal of Positive Psychology, 3*(4), 219–233. doi.org/10.1080/17439760802303044

Kahneman, D., E. Diener, & N. Schwarz. (Eds.). (1999). *Well-being: Foundations of hedonic psychology*. Russell Sage Foundation.

Kasser, T. & R.M. Ryan. (1996). Further examining the American Dream: Differential correlates of intrinsic and extrinsic goals. *Personality and Social Psychology Bulletin, 22*(3), 280–287. doi.org/10.1177/0146167296223006

Keyes, C.L.M. (2002). The mental health continuum: From languishing to flourishing in life. *Journal of Health and Social Behavior, 43*(2), 207–222. doi.org/10.2307/3090197

Keyes, C.L.M. (2005). Mental illness and/or mental health? Investigating axioms of the complete state model of health. *Journal of Consulting and Clinical Psychology, 73*(3), 539–548. doi.org/10.1037/0022-006X.73.3.539

Keyes, C.L.M. (2007). Promoting and protecting mental health as flourishing: A complementary strategy for improving national mental health. *American Psychologist, 62*(2), 95–108. doi.org/10.1037/0003-066X.62.2.95

Keyes, C.L.M., D. Shmotkin, & C.D. Ryff. (2002). Optimizing well-being: The empirical encounter of two traditions. *Journal of Personality and Social Psychology, 82*(6), 1007–1022. doi.org/10.1037/0022-3514.82.6.1007

King, L.A., J.E. Eells, & C.M. Burton. (2012). The good life, broadly and narrowly considered. In P. A. Linley & S. Joseph (Eds.), *Positive Psychology in Practice* (pp. 35–52). John Wiley & Sons, Inc. doi.org/10.1002/9780470939338.ch3

Kolak, D. & G. Thomson. (2016). *The Longman Standard History of Ancient Philosophy*. Routledge.

Kraut, R. (1979). Two conceptions of happiness. *Philosophical Review, 88*, 167–197.

Krueger, A.B. & A.A. Stone. (2014). Progress in measuring subjective well-being. *Science, 346*(6205), 42–43. doi.org/10.1126/science.1256392

Kuppens, P., A. Realo, & E. Diener. (2008). The role of positive and negative emotions in life satisfaction judgment across nations. *Journal of Personality and Social Psychology, 95*(1), 66–75.

Lane, T. (2017). How does happiness relate to economic behaviour? A review of the literature. *Journal of Behavioral and Experimental Economics, 68*, 62–78. doi.org/10.1016/J.SOCEC.2017.04.001

Layard, R. (2005). *Happiness: Lessons from a new science*. Penguin.

Linley, P.A., J. Maltby, A.M. Wood, G. Osborne, & R. Hurling. (2009). Measuring happiness: The higher order factor structure of subjective and psychological well-being measures. *Personality and Individual Differences, 47*(8), 878–884.

Lu, L. (2001). Understanding happiness: A look into the Chinese folk psychology. *Journal of Happiness Studies, 2*(4), 407–432. doi.org/10.1023/A:1013944228205

Lucas, R.E., A.E. Clark, Y. Georgellis, & E. Diener. (2003). Reexamining adaptation and the set point model of happiness: reactions to changes in marital status. *Journal of Personality and Social Psychology, 84*(3), 527–539.

Lucas, R.E., E. Diener, & E. Suh. (1996). Discriminant validity of well-being measures. *Journal of Personality and Social Psychology, 71*(3), 616–621.

Lyubomirsky, S. (2008). *The how of happiness: A scientific approach to getting the life you want.* Penguin.

McKee-Ryan, F., Z. Song, C.R. Wanberg, & A.J. Kinicki. (2005). Psychological and physical well-being during unemployment: A meta-analytic study. *Journal of Applied Psychology, 90*(1), 53–76. doi.org/10.1037/0021-9010.90.1.53

Merriam-Webster. (2020). *Happiness.* www.merriam-webster.com/dictionary/happiness

Myers, D.G. & E. Diener, E. (1995). Who is happy? *Psychological Science, 6*(1), 10–19. doi.org/10.1111/j.1467–9280.1995.tb00298.x

NordAN. (2018). *Alcohol consumption in Finland has decreased, but over half a million are still at risk from excessive drinking.* nordan.org/alcohol-consumption-in-finland-has-decreased-but-over-half-a-million-are-still-at-risk-from-excessive-drinking/

Nordic Centre for Welfare and Social Issues. (2019). *Mental health among youth in Finland.* nordicwelfare.org/wp-content/uploads/2017/10/finland_webb-1.pdf

Norton, D.L. (1976) Personal destinies. Princeton, NJ: Princeton University Press.

OECD. (2013). *OECD guidelines on measuring subjective well-being.* OECD Publishing. www.oecd.org/statistics/oecd-guidelines-on-measuring-subjective-well-being-9789264191655-en.htm

Oishi, S., E. Diener, R.E. Lucas, & E. Suh. (1999). Cross-cultural variations in predictors of life satisfaction: Perspectives from needs and values. *Personality and Social Psychology Bulletin, 25*(8), 980–990.

Okun, M.A., W.A. Stock, M.J. Haring, & R.A. Witter. (1984). Health and subjective well being: A meta-analysis. *International Journal of Aging and Human Development, 19*(2), 111–132. doi.org/10.2190/QGJN-0N81-5957-HAQD

Oswald, A. J., & Powdthavee, N. (2008). Does happiness adapt? A longitudinal study of disability with implications for economists and judges. *Journal of Public Economics, 92*(5–6), 1061–1077. doi.org/10.1016/J.JPUBECO.2008.01.002

Peterson, C. & M.E.P. Seligman. (2004). *Character strengths and virtues: A handbook and classification.* Oxford University Press.

Peterson, C., N. Park, & M.E.P. Seligman. (2005). Orientations to happiness and life satisfaction: The full life versus the empty life. *Journal of Happiness Studies, 6*(1), 25–41. doi.org/10.1007/s10902-004-1278-z

Plagnol, A.C. & L. Macchia. (2018). Economics of subjective well-being: Evaluating the evidence for the Easterlin Paradox. In A. K. Uskul & S. Oishi (Eds.), *Socioeconomic Environment and Human Psychology.* Oxford University Press.

Reynolds, F. & K.H. Lim. (2007). Turning to art as a positive way of living with cancer: A qualitative study of personal motives and contextual influences. *Journal of Positive Psychology, 2*(1), 66–75. doi.org/10.1080/17439760601083839

Ryan, R.M., V.I. Chirkov, T.D. Little, K.M. Sheldon, E. Timoshina, & E.L. Deci. (1999) The American dream in Russia: Extrinsic aspirations and wellbeing in two cultures. *Personality and Social Psychology Bulletin, 25*, 1509–1524.

Ryan, R.M. & E.L. Deci. (2001). On happiness and human potentials: A review of research on hedonic and eudaimonic well-being. *Annual Review of Psychology, 52*(1), 141–166. doi.org/10.1146/annurev.psych.52.1.141

Ryff, C.D. (1989). Happiness is everything, or is it? Explorations on the meaning of psychological well-being. *Journal of Personality and Social Psychology, 57*(6), 1069–1081.

Ryff, C.D. & B.H. Singer. (2008). Know thyself and become what you are: A eudaimonic approach to psychological well-being. *Journal of Happiness Studies, 9*(1), 13–39. doi.org/10.1007/s10902-006-9019-0

Schimmack, U. (2008). The structure of subjective well-being. In M. Eid & R. J. Larsen (Eds.), *The Science of Subjective Wellbeing* (pp. 97–123). Guilford.

Seligman, M.E.P. (2002). *Authentic happiness: Using the new positive psychology to realize your potential for lasting fulfillment*. New York: Free Press.

Sirgy, M.J., A.C. Michalos, A.L. Ferriss, R.A. Easterlin, D. Patrick, & W. Pavot. (2006). The Quality-of-Life (QOL) research movement: Past, present, and future. *Social Indicators Research, 76*(3), 343–466.

Steptoe, A., J. Wardle, & M. Marmot. (2005). Positive affect and health-related neuroendocrine, cardiovascular, and inflammatory processes. *Proceedings of the National Academy of Sciences of the United States of America, 102*(18), 6508–6512. doi.org/10.1073/pnas.0409174102

Tamir, M., S.H. Schwartz, S. Oishi, & M.Y. Kim. (2017). The secret to happiness: Feeling good or feeling right? *Journal of Experimental Psychology: General, 146*(10), 1448–1459. doi.org/10.1037/xge0000303

Tiberius, V. (2013). Recipes of a good life: Eudaimonism and the contribution of philosophy. In A. S. Waterman (Ed.), *The Best Within us: Positive Psychology Perspectives on Eudaimonia* (pp. 19–38). Washington, DC: American Psychological Association.

Veenhoven, R. (2003). Hedonism and happiness. *Journal of Happiness Studies, 4*(4), 437–457.

Vella-Brodrick, D.A., N. Park, & C. Peterson. (2009). Three ways to be happy: Pleasure, engagement, and meaning - Findings from Australian and US samples. *Social Indicators Research, 90*(2), 165–179. doi.org/10.1007/s11205-008-9251-6

Waterman, A.S. (1993). Two conceptions of happiness: Contrasts of personal expressiveness (eudaimonia) and hedonic enjoyment. *Journal of Personality and Social Psychology, 64*(4), 678–691. doi.org/10.1037/0022-3514.64.4.678

Waterman, A.S. (2008). Reconsidering happiness: A eudaimonist's perspective. *Journal of Positive Psychology, 3*(4), 234–252. doi.org/10.1080/17439760802303002

Waterman, A.S., S.J. Schwartz, B.L. Zamboanga, R.D. Ravert, M.K. Williams, V. Bede Agocha, S.Y. Kim, & M. Brent Donnellan. (2010). The questionnaire for eudaimonic well-being: Psychometric properties, demographic comparisons, and evidence of validity. *Journal of Positive Psychology, 5*(1), 41–61. doi.org/10.1080/17439760903435208

Wilson, W.R. (1967). Correlates of avowed happiness. *Psychological Bulletin, 67*(4), 294–306. doi.org/10.1037/h0024431

World Health Organisation. (2016). *Finland - Alcohol consumption: Levels and patterns*. www.who.int/substance_abuse/publications/global_alcohol_report/profiles/fin.pdf?ua=1

World Population Review. (2019). *Suicide rate by country 2019*. worldpopulationreview.com/countries/suicide-rate-by-country/

Zimmermann, A.C. & R.A. Easterlin. (2006). Happily ever after? Cohabitation, marriage, divorce, and happiness in Germany. *Population and Development Review, 32*(3), 511–528. doi.org/10.1111/j.1728-4457.2006.00135.x

38

A WHOLE-SCHOOL APPROACH TO HEALTH AND WELL-BEING

An auto-ethnographic account of a primary school

Jonathan Glazzard

Introduction

This chapter provides an auto-ethnographic case study of a primary school in England. The school is referred to as Marshlands. It is situated in an area of social deprivation and included a large number of children with social, emotional, and mental health needs as well as other special educational needs. Over several years this had resulted in declining attainment and consequently the school was designated as a school that was at risk of failing its inspection. Due to the needs of the children, the leaders focused on developing a whole school approach to well-being by prioritising the holistic needs of the learners and developing the skills of social and emotional regulation. This chapter tells the story of the school's inspection from both the perspective of one school leader (Jane) and my perspective as a school governor. The account illustrates the tensions between the standards agenda and the school's emphasis on pupil well-being and inclusion.

The inspection: Jane's account

"The room is empty but full of people. Silence surrounds me yet people speak. Friends are near but seem so far away. Aware of every single heartbeat thumping in my chest, my breathing is becoming ever shallower; my head thumps and my palms are clammy. I feel distant from the frightened faces around me. There is so much to say and yet I do not have the strength to verbalise my thoughts. I clearly recognise the physical symptoms of fear and my mind and body swiftly respond to them in preparation for fight or flight. The next hour will be life changing. It will confirm my greatest fears. The events of the last forty-eight hours play repeatedly and vividly through my mind. I re-live every word I have spoken, every decision I have made and every explanation I have offered. I am briefly distracted by a high pitched ringing in my ears and a deep sigh from a distant corner of the room. I swiftly return to my thoughts. How could we have averted this devastating outcome? How could we have changed the course of events which has unfolded and will now impact on the lives of so many for many months to come? I search deep inside my mind but no answers are forthcoming.

Forty-eight hours earlier life had been full of optimism, which was now crushed and broken like fragments of shattered glass. The buzz of excitement and energy was silenced. Smiles and laughter had quickly turned to pain and confusion etched on the faces of those around me. We sought comfort by staying in close proximity to one another as the predator advanced towards its prey. I had been lost in my thoughts and the realities of life had dawned on me as I looked up to view the unfolding reactions of my companions. Each reacted in their own unique way, and I carefully studied each and every response as I sat quietly on the edge of this picture of undeniable disbelief. Young and old, we were together, each feeling the other's pain. Some sat deep in thought, others chatted, and there were those who calmly offered words of comfort and advice. Every response was intended to offer us hope but we all knew that both hope and time had run out.

The door opened and I knew the time had come to face reality. I made eye contact with no one and left the room with my head held high. I was now devoid of any emotions as I walked resolutely towards our destiny, ready to absorb the injustice of the predicament with which we were now confronted. The strength to face the next few minutes of my life came from within as I resolved to deny myself any opportunity to demonstrate regret or denial of my long held views and deep-rooted beliefs.

Another school year has come to a close. A year filled with challenges which we have continued to face with determination. More children, and their accompanying needs, have joined the school, including two pupils demonstrating the behaviours of attachment disorder, one young child with epilepsy and considerable developmental delay and a statement of special educational needs. There is a child with Turner's syndrome who also has a statement of special educational needs and an eight-year-old with significant speech difficulties. This is not an exhaustive list but merely gives an indication of some of the significant needs we support in our day-to-day work. Each of them is fully and successfully included in a mainstream classroom. We have also continued to enjoy the rewards of working with a wonderful mix of children. So why am I so disillusioned, why am I so frustrated, why am I so angry, and why am I questioning my strong desire to work with the day-to-day challenges that I have thrived on for the entirety of my teaching career?

The reality is that my greatest fears have become a reality. Inspectors recently visited, prompted by one complaint from a parent. A parent who does not share my views in relation to inclusive education. A parent whose own child has achieved much success from beginning her education at our school and attaining level five at the end of her primary school education. Her own child, Sophie, began her education in my early years class seven years ago. She was an extremely timid child who found the experience of coming into full-time education extremely traumatic. Every minute of every day was a genuine difficulty for her. She clung tightly to my trouser leg and held my hand as she faced each and every new experience. When it rained she screamed, when it was playtime she screamed, when another adult came into the classroom she screamed. Her mother was understandably very anxious and would cry uncontrollably when the time came to leave her daughter each morning. With patience and understanding we supported both the mother and the child and both eventually grew in confidence. As the years went by, Sophie continued to find other aspects of school life difficult. She was, without doubt, a worrier, and each time she worried she could clearly see the distress she was causing her mother who needed and received the understanding and support we gladly offered. This aside is far from irrelevant to my current feelings of dismay. This same parent is also related to a member of the teaching staff who has recently resigned from their post rather than face capability proceedings against them. Revenge has become their reason for existing and the school leadership team has consequently faced an extremely challenging year. The aforementioned parent has logged several complaints against the school. Initially to the Headteacher, followed by the governing body and then the local authority. All complaints were formally and quickly addressed and no actions were taken against the school. Finally, she complained to the inspectorate. A telephone interview followed and then several weeks of silence. The silence was broken by a phone call informing us of a school inspection the following day in response to her complaint. Her complaint focused on her concerns in relation to her daughter being educated alongside more difficult children as well as her disbelief that her own daughter's attainment was as high as the school claimed (although Sophie's final test results at the end of her primary education have confirmed the school's judgements on her attainment).

And so, the inspector came to call and almost two weeks later I am of the opinion that she ripped the heart out of the school. As a teacher with much experience of school inspections I have never encountered an inspector who had seemingly made her decision before she had even set foot in the school. Our fate, it seems, was sealed. All cohorts but one had made at least good progress whilst one cohort had made above expected progress. Good progress was entirely disregarded. All attempts to demonstrate the good progress the school has made, in so many respects, were ignored. The focus of this inspection became the shortcomings of the school. We felt that there was so much to celebrate, though we know that much work still needs to be done. As a school we are not in denial and we are fortunate in having a staff that is totally committed to school improvement. Each and every one of them has worked tirelessly to bring about that change. They have worked with determination to enhance their practices and the improvement has been visible and has had clear and positive impact. This impact has been confirmed by those who have worked with us and who have shared and toiled alongside us to overcome the challenges. They too were celebrating with us. It seemed that the tide was turning and that the data confirmed this upward trend.

Based on the one complaint the inspectors had received, the focus of the inspection was the behaviour in school. In all previous inspections this had been identified as good. Because of the needs of some of our children, we would not deny that the behaviour of some children can be very challenging from time to time. It is for this reason that systems are frequently evaluated and the need for staff training is identified. Systems are well considered to ensure that the education of our children is not disrupted by the occasional responses of some troubled individuals. De-escalation strategies are effectively used by all staff. Triggers for individuals have been identified. Individuals are able to take "quiet time" when they recognise that they are becoming distressed, and many now independently and appropriately access this opportunity, recognising their own needs. The leadership team always carry walkie-talkies and can immediately respond to calls for additional support to remove particularly distressed individuals from classrooms. This is usually achieved without disruption when the identified child is invited to leave the classroom to have quiet time and then discuss the reasons behind their distress. This strategy has proved to be very effective and they are usually able to return to their class in a calm manner, ready to continue with their learning. All such incidents are of course recorded and parents are invited to meet with senior managers to discuss these events. The school log shows that nineteen such events have taken place in the last school year. The log clearly identifies four children. These children have very specific needs. Two are displaying behaviours clearly linked to attachment disorder; one has a statement of special educational needs for behaviour, emotional, and social development, and one is receiving support, with his family, from the school for behaviour, social, and emotional needs. Systems ensure that their behaviours are dealt with swiftly. In the two days that the school was inspected there was no evidence of poor behaviours. The behaviour log was however the evidence used against us. Nineteen incidents were deemed a concern. There was no opportunity to discuss the needs of the children involved or the ways in which we had supported them to successfully access their education with their peers for the larger part of each school week. The children have been placed in our school because the local authority special school is full. The inspector ignored our responses as we fought in vain to explain how we had developed systems to ensure that the learning needs of all children had been met. All attempts to show the improvements and successes of the school were completely disregarded. She had the bit between her teeth and she relentlessly focused on her perceived weaknesses of the school resulting in small holes quickly becoming craters. To her there was a simple solution. The four children in the behaviour log should have been excluded. Three of the children have previously been excluded from other schools. Their parents have frequently expressed their gratitude for the work we do. Unfortunately, they never took the time to convey their views to the inspector.

The school is situated in an area of social deprivation. The culture of many of the families it serves can be a challenge. Teachers are perceived, by many, to be figures of authority and authority has to be challenged. There are, however, many families who acknowledge and value the work we do. These are the families who never considered that their voices should be heard by the inspector. They are the families who remained silent. The voices heard were those who have relentlessly challenged our systems. Those who refuse to work with us to support their children but have always been quick to condemn us and seemingly challenge every initiative we introduce from healthy eating to the completion of homework. They are undeniably a very small minority of the families we serve but they were the voices that the inspector heard as these same parents circled like vultures on their prey. The school was swiftly deemed as inadequate. The entire staff, the governing body and the local authority have been left in a state of disbelief. Only one person who has worked closely with the school has expressed a degree of understanding of the judgement made. There is no time to be lost and the work to quickly move forward has already begun. There is no opportunity to contest the decision that the inspector made and as a school we must now pool all our energies into moving the school out of special measures. The next twelve months, at least, will be filled with challenge and the staff will face it with dedication and resilience. I have spent my entire career truly believing in and developing inclusive practices. My views and practices are deep-rooted and on a very personal level I must now question them. Do I respond by going against my strong beliefs which will result in ticking boxes to alleviate the current pressure or do I accept that I am simply out of step with current measures of success in education? That is the dilemma I must now resolve. Fighting the system is futile whilst believing in it is "impossible".

The inspection: my account

As a governor it was my duty to support Marshlands throughout its recent inspection. Luckily my own students had finished their studies for the year and I had the flexibility to be able to base myself in the school. I received an e-mail from the school secretary in July of that year to notify me of the inspection and to ask me to attend a meeting with the inspectors at 3.30 pm the following day.

I immediately telephoned Jane and told her that I would be in school at 8am the following day to support both her and the school through the inspection. It was the least I could do. She had supported me throughout my Thesis by giving me access to her life and her most private thoughts and experiences. I wanted to stand up for the school and tell the inspectors what a great job my colleagues there were doing. In particular I wanted to highlight to them the inclusive nature of the school and its commitment to learners with diverse needs.

Of course, we knew that there was a lot of explaining to do. The school data was not good. But then we had a very real story to tell behind that data. Many of the pupils had significant social, emotional, communication, and cognitive needs. Progress was being made but often the steps were too small to register in any "meaningful" way. I wanted to draw the inspectors' attention to the school's commitment to inclusion and emphasise the exclusionary practices that I was aware other local schools were demonstrating. Marshlands had developed a local reputation for inclusion and this had become the reason for its demise. Whilst other schools were excluding children with diverse needs, Marshlands was accepting them, working with them and keeping them. But it was also paying the price for doing so. I was determined to highlight the injustices to the inspectors and to draw attention to all the positive developments that had taken place in the school.

Jane called to collect me on the Tuesday morning. She was visibly anxious, smoking several cigarettes to calm her nerves. We travelled to school together in the car. We rehearsed what we wanted to say to the inspectors but we both knew deep down that the stories of the pupils and the school's successes in relation to inclusion would not interest those judging our school. The school's data would be the focus of the inspection. Still, we were determined to show them what a fantastic place Marshlands was.

It was all systems go when we arrived in school at 7am, an hour earlier than planned. Teachers were already in school and were busily preparing their lessons but this was not new. Most of them consistently arrive at this time. I tried to help by getting resources out for them and talking through with them their lesson ideas. I am a governor but also a teacher and teacher trainer. They value my opinion and want me to work with them. I felt no sense of panic and a positive vibe filled the air. I was impressed with what they had planned to do. Providing they could hold their nerve I felt they would do well.

Jane rallied the troops for the morning briefing. I joined them. The Head was already in the office with the inspector. It was 8 am: "You're doing a great job" she said. "Let's show ourselves at our best!" There was a sense of optimism, commitment and determination.

Jane and I then worked in her office together. It is a small, stuffy room and it was a very hot day, although the stress of an inspection could have raised the temperature. However well prepared one is for an inspection, there is always more to do during the process. We looked at the data for pupils with special educational needs. Their attainment was below national expectations but they were making good progress. Then we looked at the data for all pupils. It was the same picture. Attainment was below national expectations but progress from their starting points was good. We felt confident that this justified that the school was "good value for money", a term that inspection reports frequently cite. We just needed to show them that teaching was good and that our pupils were making good progress.

The story of the next few hours then unfolded. Jane and the Head were called into various meetings with inspectors. Lessons were observed in a cursory fashion. Jane dipped in and out of lessons with the inspectors, spending only a few minutes in each class. In Jane's view all of the lessons were good. However, some teachers who expected to be observed for full lessons expressed their disappointment to me. They had not been visited and they had had some great lessons. Instead, the inspectors spent their time behind a closed door trawling through the school data.

Then it was my time. At 3.30 pm precisely the governors went to meet an inspector. There were no introductions. The inspector went straight into interrogation mode about the data and more specifically about the low attainment of our pupils. We tried to explain the story behind the data. We talked about the diverse needs of our pupils and their very low starting points. We stressed how we effectively supported pupils with autism and those with challenging behaviour. We talked about inclusion. However, during these explanations there was no eye contact. The inspector looked down at her paper, scribbled notes, and continued with her own agenda. The pupil behaviour logs were raised. She questioned why four pupils with challenging behaviour had not been excluded. In response, we reiterated our commitment to inclusion and highlighted evidence that their behaviour over time had improved. We knew it had not gone well. At the end of the meeting there was a consensus of opinion that our voices had not been listened to. She was not interested in inclusion but it was clear that she was interested in exclusion. It is fascinating how policy changes over time and education simply becomes a political football.

On day two at the feedback meeting we were told quite simply that Marshlands was inadequate. I requested an explanation for this judgement. I was told that because the school had included pupils with challenging behaviour it had not fulfilled its duty to safeguard the rest of the pupils. Strange, because it certainly feels like a safe school when I walk around it. It is calm and pupils are generally courteous to each other. The other explanation offered was that teaching was inadequate because the data over time demonstrated that pupils were not performing in line with national expectations. Again, this demonstrated no recognition that lessons had been consistently good in the seven months leading up to the inspection. Certainly, the lessons I had observed as a governor were very impressive. Why had no consideration been given to the pupils' starting points or to their very specific and diverse needs? It all seems so unfair, especially when other local schools exclude pupils and do well in inspections. Why were the teachers left to feel as though they had failed when they had worked so hard not only during the inspection but also in the months prior to the inspection?

I am left feeling disgruntled with education. I question my role as a teacher trainer. What sort of education system am I preparing my students to enter in my role as a university lecturer? What will I say to them when they tell me that they want to work in a school like Marshlands? It certainly does not feel to me that the education system is socially just, not just for the teachers and other professionals who work at Marshlands but also for the pupils. They are the real losers because it is a system which ultimately fails those learners who are not able to demonstrate achievement in the dominant sense. "I am appalled that we are subjected to this regime".

The backstory: Jane's account

Stevie and his older brother had come into foster care with a local family who were anxious to eventually adopt the two boys. Stevie and his brother, I recall, had been found by social services in the south of England living in an attic. Their young mother had twins, only twelve months younger than Stevie. The history of Stevie and his brother was that some food was placed in the attic most days although with no regularity. His older brother had ensured that this was shared between them. Stevie had very poor language skills, demonstrated behaviour which was challenging and did not understand or adhere to most expectations. From the very first day Stevie proved to be a major challenge. He ran around the classroom, knocking things as well as other children over. He frequently left the classroom and ran amok in the school. This time there was no supportive Head Teacher. He did not challenge Stevie; he did not remonstrate with him. He simply ignored him. He would put his head round my classroom door to ask me: "Do you know that Stevie is running around out here?" Then he simply left. With thirty young children in my class and no additional support I would leave my classroom door ajar, enabling me to hear but certainly not see my class and go in pursuit of Stevie. With sole responsibility for my class and for Stevie I had no choice but to ensure that I quickly re-captured Stevie and took him back to the classroom where I could at least keep a watchful eye on him and the other children. This often meant that I had to keep a firm hold on Stevie's hand. As I again attempted to teach the other children Stevie would begin to pull against me. I would "hold firm" but was often gradually dragged around the classroom as I taught. I was, however, determined that his negative behaviours would be ignored. The weeks went by and Stevie continued to be a challenge. I recall one Friday when I simply found the whole ordeal too much. I spoke to my Head

Teacher, explaining that I needed him to support me rather than ignore me. His response was to ring Stevie's foster parents and ask them to remove Stevie from the school for the remainder of the day. Stevie's mother was very obliging, very apologetic and acknowledged that she didn't really know how I coped with Stevie. However, his father was nowhere near as understanding. This view was conveyed to me by Stevie's mother who explained that her husband did not understand. He felt that I was a poor excuse for a teacher if I was unable to control a five year old. Without really thinking this through I immediately suggested that we should invite Stevie's father to come and work with him in the classroom. Her response was amazing: "Now I think that's a bloody good idea." She responded. "He's coming. Don't worry I'll make sure of that."

To my utter amazement Stevie's father was in my classroom with Stevie at 9 o'clock on the following Monday morning. He spent the day working alongside Stevie and all credit was due to him in that he admitted that he had not realised how challenging Stevie's behaviour was and additionally he acknowledged the need for me to educate Stevie's peers too. Stevie's father was unemployed and Stevie and I enjoyed his support on several occasions during the coming weeks. This was the beginning of a strong school/parent partnership which greatly benefited Stevie. Not once in that first term did it ever occur to me that I did not wish to support Stevie. I often thought about his early childhood and knew that his difficulties were not of his own making. Again, I had no desire to completely change Stevie. I simply wanted to find ways of ensuring that he could be educated with his peers, that we understood him, and more over that his "differences" were accepted by staff and other children alike. After the first term his mother approached me with a complaint. She had received information that Stevie had a learning assistant to support him in his previous setting. Why was this not the case in our school? This was complete news to the school in which I was working. The school pursued this information and within two weeks I too began to enjoy the benefits of working with support for Stevie in my classroom. The difference was incredible but by no means surprising. In collaboration with his support assistant, I set and conveyed boundaries and expectations to Stevie. Unsurprisingly he spent much of the first month challenging those boundaries. With additional support I was now able to ensure that Stevie adhered to my expectations. There were tantrums and he often needed to be withdrawn from the classroom for periods of time. However, I was able to meet the need of his peers while his support assistant was able to focus on ensuring that he did not return to the classroom until he had met our expectations. Slowly the situation improved. Within three months we enjoyed, initially, a full day when Stevie was not withdrawn from class, followed by several days without the need to withdraw him. Eventually the days turned into weeks. The need to never withdraw Stevie was never realised, but he did love school. He made friends, yet there were disputes and challenges and from time to time his occasional outbursts continued. Stevie stayed with me for the next three years. Again, because of the bond I had apparently developed with him. Maybe this was in reality not the reason. He left my class at the age of seven and I knew that I had made a difference. His next teacher was determined to continue the work I had started. Stevie went on to successfully complete his primary education in our school. Many years later I encountered Stevie and his mother one afternoon in town. His mother flung her arms round me in the middle of a pedestrian crossing. "You know who this is, don't you?" she said to Stevie. Stevie looked me up and down before replying, "Not a clue." He shrugged his shoulders and walked on. He did not remember me, but of course I did remember Stevie. I made huge mistakes with him but above all else I learned so much.

The last fifteen years of my career have been spent in this school. It is here that I have again supported many children with many diverse needs. It is also in this school that I have learned so much more about supporting children to accept the differences and needs of others. We have focused relentlessly on pupil well-being. In this respect this school is so successful. I have encountered many more children with a range of diverse needs. Amongst these there have been several other children who have challenged us with behavioural issues, many far more challenging than Stevie. Additionally, on a daily basis I work with children with autistic spectrum conditions. The school hosts a specialist resource unit for these children and some of them are included in and access mainstream provision on a daily basis. Most of our children readily accept the needs of others and support one another. We deal firmly with those who torment the children in the unit. Sometimes we have caught children standing outside the unit upsetting the children inside. However, the vast majority accept their differences and take care of them. This is frequently evident to me when I visit children in other schools and compare their responses to children with additional needs. Such visits highlight the successes of our school and I return with an enormous sense of pride in our achievements. In so many respects I should now be a round peg in a round hole. However, in reality, although I thoroughly enjoy and believe in supporting and educating these children in a mainstream setting, wherever possible, there is a new challenge. It is the challenge of the standards agenda.

I am now charged with the responsibility of identifying, supporting, and tracking those children who, for a range of different reasons or for no apparent reasons whatsoever, are not meeting national expectations in terms of their progress and/or attainment. As a teacher of children in the early years I am acutely aware of child development. Children are not machines, they develop at varying rates and this is, to me, very evident and supported by specialists in the early years. So why do I face the insatiable pressure of justifying what are deemed as poor results each time I discuss progress with the powers that be? Individual education plans and intervention programmes support children's learning but further reinforce a sense of failure. Our reputation for supporting children with mental health needs, amongst other local schools, is celebrated and acknowledged. So much so that many of them now recommend us to parents of children with special needs. In discussions with these parents, it has become evident that they have not been made welcome in our neighbouring schools. These schools claim inexperience and parents have been assured that a move to our school is in the best interests of the child. We apparently have the expertise needed. This celebration and acknowledgement of our skills and understanding is that indeed parents frequently decide to place their children in our school. Today almost half of children on roll have special educational needs status. The result is that the attainment data of neighbouring schools results are good whilst our own data fluctuates from year to year and rarely meets national expectations. Some parents have not welcomed the heavy weighting of children with special educational needs, and many children have been withdrawn from the school resulting in small cohorts. In small cohorts each child obviously carries a high percentage in terms of data. One child can literally make a huge difference. This year there were only thirteen children in Year 6. Of those children nine had special educational needs and four of those children have complex mental health needs. On paper our attainment data is currently deemed as a huge cause for concern. A school inspection is imminent and under the new inspection criteria the school improvement partner has recently moved the school into a category of high risk of failure. Many of the children face challenges at home; their parents show little interest in school and it is a huge challenge to engage them in supporting their children. I recount these details only as a means of broadly illustrating that I know why the children in my class have not demonstrated attainment in line with nationally expected standards. Data for my class indeed does effectively demonstrate that the children have made extremely good progress. However, armed with this information I recently spoke to the School Improvement Partner. Her attitude was totally dismissive. I provided her with the contextual information related to these children. She merely focused on measuring them against national norms and my data was simply deemed as very disappointing. This response does anger me but above all else I am so upset for the children I have had the responsibility of teaching.

As a new academic year approaches I am already aware that four children with complex mental health needs will be included in my class next year. I have visited them in their current settings in local schools. One child in particular has already been labelled as "naughty." He has a diagnosis of autism. During a recent visit to meet him I was approached by another child as I observed my new pupil:

> "What are you doing?" he asked
> "I've come to see your lovely new classroom. I am a friend of Mrs T's (Head Teacher)." I replied.

The child was excited and quickly began to show me round his newly built classroom and to name some of the other children. At this point my new pupil went by on a bike.

> "That's Robert," explained my young companion. "He's a naughty boy."

I was standing with the Head Teacher at this moment in time and waited for her response. Her comments horrified me:

> "Yes, but you're a good boy aren't you?" was all she replied.

This was the Headteacher who, according to Robert's parents, had made them feel so unwelcome in her school and who had said that if he had to stay in her school she would do her best. Instead our school was recommended. Apparently her staff had little experience of dealing with "children like Robert." It seemed to me that her children may also have little experience or support in accepting the needs of others.

I make no apologies for my cynical view of aspects of the current system of judging schools and teachers. I continue to believe in a world in which success is celebrated and where there is a need to identify and support children in any aspect of their learning or life skills. It is the narrow measure of success and school effectiveness that I vehemently question. Success for all we hear again and again. No! Success in maths and English is the reality. Little else seems to be of any consequence. My belief is that such a measure of success is narrow and damages many children, and that their confidence is shattered in its wake. Despite this, I have the confidence to challenge such measures with the knowledge and understanding I hold about the children I teach, to support my views. I will continue to value the development and achievements of the whole child and I will continue to celebrate these. Already the battle to do so is becoming harder to fight. I will, however, continue that fight until maybe the unfortunate day arrives when there is no one who is prepared to listen. Sadly, I feel that such a day is fast approaching.

Conclusion

As the reader you will draw your own interpretations from this auto-ethnographic account. I have attempted to illustrate the need for schools to prioritise well-being, particularly in schools like Marshlands. However, the accounts illustrate the tensions which exist between focusing on well-being and raising academic standards within a discourse of performativity. It is now seven years since Marshlands experienced the inspection which ultimately resulted in its demise. I still believe in the approach that the school adopted, irrespective of the inspection outcome.

Without a focus on inclusion and well-being, children and young people will continue to experience marginalisation. They need to feel valued; they need to believe that they matter and they need to be immersed in a pedagogy of care. Many years after leaving school, young people will quickly forget curriculum knowledge but they will never forget how teachers made them feel. Jane was committed to a pedagogy of care which focused on prioritising pupils' well-being. As the reader it is up to you to ultimately decide whether this was the right course of action.

PART XVI

Conclusion

39

CONCLUSIONS AND THE FUTURE OF ETHNOGRAPHY IN HEALTH-RELATED RESEARCH

Challenges and innovations

Paul M.W. Hackett and Christopher M. Hayre

Introduction

Twenty minutes earlier, as she had walked across the lawn of the vicarage at St. Mary Mead, her feet had crunched upon the freshly fallen snow. It was not snowing now and as she stood near the wall at the rear of the garden, Jane Marple could see the body lying on the snow. She had been standing unmoving for a while now and she shivered slightly. The exclusion tape had already been set in place and there were a host of people moving around the body, all were dressed in protective suits, shoe covers, hair covers, and face masks, in order to avoid contaminating the crime scene. This made identifying them individually virtually impossible.

"Excuse me madam, please don't come any closer," a rather zealous young officer said to the aged spinster. "Don't worry young man," she crisply retorted, "I am aware of the procedures you know, and in fact I have been to more murder scenes than you have had hot dinners." Somewhat abashed, the young officer grinned at the old lady, but did not yield his ground. "Don't worry about Miss Marple, I'll take care of her." This was inspector Slack speaking.

"Now what are you doing here, Jane?" he asked in a kind manner. "You can't go rummaging about around bodies like you used to, you know." "Of course I am aware of that, Inspector," she said with a dismissive tone, "but I do live in the village and I am sure I can be of some help." "I think we can cope with this without your help Jane," Slack said, kindly but firmly. "Is that so, then do you know that the body is of Colonel Lucius Protheroe who is a wealthy magistrate from the village?" "We did know that, thank you, Jane." "Yes, but did you also know that he was in town this morning? When I got here a few minutes ago I recognised who the dead man was and I checked his Facebook and Instagram accounts on my iPhone, we are Facebook friends and close friends on Instagram you see. Anyway, there is a photograph he posted on Instagram from lunch-time today of him sitting with a group of people outside the Old Bell public house."

Table 39.1 Information type by method used

Method	Information type
Focus group	primary
Interview	primary
Netnography	Primary or secondary

Slack had not been aware of this fact and made a mental note to have this looked into. However, he was not going to let Jane Marple know that she was ahead of them. "We are aware of Colonel Protheroe's Instagram activity, thank you, Jane." "Yes, but are you aware that the man sitting immediately to the right of our dead man is James McIntire, a convicted cybercriminal of a particularly nasty type." "Go on, tell me more," said the detective. "He specialises in identity theft and ideas around identity being a contestable commodity which is both virtual and fluid. He has been pursued, but never prosecuted, for creating data-doubles for terrorists, internet paedophiles and other disreputable individuals. He wears a traditional suit but operates within the world of cyberpunks, trading DNA profiles and committing other genetic crimes."

Inspector Slack was not about to admit this, but, whilst he recognised a few of her words, he had little idea exactly what it was the old lady was on about. However, he did understand enough to realise that this James McIntire chap was a thoroughly disreputable sort and that this raised some serious questions. For instance, exactly what was a renowned magistrate doing in the pub with McIntire? Slack was also wondering if this meeting had anything to do with the magistrate being found dead shortly after posting a picture of himself and McIntire together. Furthermore, why would Colonel Protheroe advertise his meeting with McIntire in such a public way?

Miss Marple has obviously kept up with the times and has realised the usefulness and the importance of the internet and online activity in contemporary society. This is a lesson that healthcare researchers have similarly learnt. As more and more of everyday life moves online, from entertainment to commerce and from communication to social group participation, it is inevitable that the healthcare researcher should have also embraced this platform. In the section that follows, we will start to consider some of the implications of the move online of healthcare research.

The move online

Over the last two-decades, the internet has had a major impact upon healthcare research that has taken two broad forms. The first of these are enquiries that gather both primary and secondary material that can only be found online and that involves the researcher investigating online activity (blogs, internet for a, etc.) that are concerned with the health issue or practice of interest. This form of ethnographic research has several names, such as netnography, cyber anthropology, webnography (Kausel & Hackett, 2016; Kozinets, 1998), and digital anthropology (Horst & Miller, 2012). In this chapter we will refer to these approaches as netnography. The second broad class of online research involves the researcher conducting one or more online versions of the usual types of research to generate primary information. These include: online focus groups (Jervaeus, Nilsson, Eriksson, Lampic, Widmark & Wettergren, 2016; Reisner et al., 2018), online interviews (Hamama-Raz, Palgi, Leshem, Ben-Ezra, Lavenda, & Seedat,

Table 39.2 Synchronicity by interview types used

Timing	Interview type
Synchronous	Online or Face-to-face Focus group
	Online or Face-to-face Interview
Asynchronous	Online Focus group
	Online Interview
	Netnography

2017), and video interviews, including Skype interviews (Janghorban, Roudsari, & Taghipour, 2014) etc.

When considering online research, one important feature that must be kept in mind when designing research is whether the data is gathered synchronously or asynchronously.

Synchronous research

Synchronous research involves studies that gather data or information where the researcher is present in some way when the participants is providing their information, that is to say the procedure is conducted by the researcher in real time. An example of real time research is an interview that is conducted on Skype or Zoom, which enables researchers and participants to chat in a manner similar to a face-to-face interview. An example of this type of research in a health-related enquiry is provided by Wilson (2012), who used a semi-structured synchronous approach in an investigation into climate and health. Real time online focus groups are conducted with all participants simultaneously online, allowing participants to interact with each other and with the group moderator. The advantage of being able to see the participant is that the researcher may note non-verbal behaviours, such as facial expressions, that are usually not available in asynchronous research or in chat rooms that rely on the use of text. Due to the logistics of the situation and controlling the online focus group, these will tend to be of up to 8 participants (this is, fewer participants than is usual in a focus group), and will last one to one and a half hours.

Asynchronous research

In asynchronous research, interviews or focus groups are conducted when the participants and researcher are not online simultaneously. The asynchronous focus group is one that may run across a protracted period of time, usually a few days, and are also known as bulletin or message board focus groups. In this format, questions and answers are posted as written text along with images, videos, etc. Participants and moderators do not need to be online at the same time. In the situation of an interview with an individual, asynchronous interviews take place via email, through websites in which participants may give their responses, etc. Asynchronous focus groups use software that is very different from that used in synchronous focus groups as it usually does not include live interactions between the participants group or with a moderator. They also do not require a small number of respondents to be manageable and therefore may include twenty or thirty participants. Asynchronous approaches benefit from allowing respondents to reflect upon their responses (see, Dowling, 2012). Another obvious strength of this type of research is that participants and researchers do not have to occupy the same time zone and interviews can be completed when the participant wishes. However, on the negative side, some have noted that in asynchronous interviews it may be hard to keep interviews going and, especially in longitudinal research, maintaining motivation may be a problem (e.g., Rezabek, 2000). Having explained synchronous and asynchronous methods, we will next consider online focus groups and interviews in greater detail.

Online focus groups

Focus groups have long been a staple of many forms of research into human behaviour and experience. Such research has included a range of aspects of healthcare research. There is also growing usage of the online focus groups as methodologies to investigate health-related issues, for example, De Jong et al. (2012); Tuttas (2015). Online synchronous focus groups have a procedure that is similar to the in-person setting of a focus group, and software allows similar interactions and group exercises to be performed. There are several advantages of using online travel groups rather than their face-to-face counterparts. Benefits include the reduction of pollution that is caused by traveling to a focus group setting and the reduction of costs associated with this travel. Using an online format also allows a wider range of group members that may be drawn from a variety of regional, national, and international locations. A research project that includes an online focus group may be completed quicker due to respondents being recruited from existing lists and their not having to travel a large distance to undertake the online focus group.

As well as background and logistical advantages, the online session may be more likely to produce open and less-guarded responses than the traditional form of group research. This is especially useful for health-related groups as these are often concerned with embarrassing or sensitive issues. This point was noted by Reisner et al. (2018) who studied 29 female to male trans masculine transgender adults using 4 asynchronous online focus groups. They found the online format provided an anonymous setting in which participants were able to explore stigmatised or sensitive issues. They also found them beneficial when patient populations were spread across a wide geographical range.

Woodyatt, Finneran, and Stephenson, (2016) compared the online versus the traditional forms of focus group. These researchers noted how online focus groups were increasing in popularity and they investigated the quality of data yielded by both forms. They compared two focus groups of each type in a study of sensitive material involving intimate partner violence using a sample of gay and bisexual men. The themes that were generated were similar between the two focus group types, with an additional theme emerging in the online group. Traditional focus groups resulted in a lower word count than online, but were longer in time. In traditional, in-person focus groups, in-depth stories were shared less, however discussions of sensitive topics were less guarded. Woodyatt and colleagues (2016) concluded that the content of the data were very similar between the two forms of focus group, even though the data generated differed.

In another comparison study, Zwaanswijk and van Dulmen (2014) used a questionnaire to gather the opinions of individuals towards online and face-to-face focus groups in a group 284 child, adolescent, and adult participants. They found differences in strength of reaction between the three age groups but all appreciated the convenience to them of being able to participate at a time that suited them and from their own homes when completing the online focus group. Some respondents also valued the online group for being more anonymous and an easier place to discuss personal issues. Face-to-face were however seen as being better at facilitating whole group, fluid discussions.

Online interviews

Interviews are another commonly used research method that is employed within healthcare research and which may be readily adapted to be used online. When used in face-to-face research, the interview allows interviewers to probe deeply into the understandings that participants have about a healthcare issue and to discover how they feel and why they feel as they do. Conversations form the basis for revealing insight into a healthcare issue or practice. In what is perhaps their simplest form, online interviews are synchronous interviews between and interviewer and interviewee conducted in real time via a video link software such as Skype. As with focus groups, online interviews may also be conducted in an asynchronous format in non-real time via email, instant messaging, etc. Online interviews are similar to face-to-face interviews as the interviewer asks a question and the interviewee responds to this. However in email- and messaging-based research there is no visual contact and visual clues are not present to help in the interpretation of what is written. Whatever form the online interview takes the researcher will have to decide on whether to use a structured, semi-structured, or unstructured design, all of which may employ a synchronous or asynchronous presentation. However, some form of computer-mediated communication is common to all online interviews.

As with online focus groups, online interviews have many, often similar, pros and cons. For example, online interviews breakdown geographical and time zone restrictions and allow access to people who may otherwise be hard to interview due to being socially isolated or not being physically mobile. As with focus groups, online interviews reduce the pollution and costs associated with travel to an interview location, and the cost of hiring the location. Online interviews also allow participants the ability be in their own living area and to keep this location private from the interviewer. Privacy is also a consideration in online healthcare research – where email or messaging software helps to facilitate privacy, discussions in forum, left on a bulletin board, etc., are publicly available. However, asynchronous online interviews that are conducted over extended time periods allow researchers to think and plan any follow-up questions and to look back at the interview history before they respond to what an inter-viewee offers. It may also be beneficial to the health researcher to use online interviews as the subjects investigated in healthcare research are often sensitive, and being online may allow the interviewee to remain anonymous and to hide their race, age, gender, etc., all of which may have associated negative stereotypes attached. In these situations, disclosure about sensitive issues may be facilitated and the interviewee may also be less likely to attempt to appear in a good light to the interviewer. There are also benefits with online interviews in terms of analysing the arising data. If using synchronous methods, such as Skype, the interview may be easily recorded and then later transcribed. Asynchronous methods are essentially transcribed by the software itself.

The ability of the interviewer to establish rapport and trust with participants may be lessened in the online format of interview (Mann & Stewart, 2005). However, as we become ever more an online society, online rapport may become more readily facilitated, although it may still be difficult for the researcher to bring about closure at the end of a longer-term interview. Another difficulty in asynchronous interviews is that it is difficult to establish whether a respondent is taking a long time to reply or if they have withdrawn from the interview, and the role of other people on the interviewer cannot be assessed. Not all participants will possess the knowledge or ability to use a device-based piece of software or may not own a device. The typing skill of both the interviewer and interviewee may slow the rate at which a text-based interview progresses and, along with the need for emojis or typed expressions to be inserted to convey emotion, may cause the research to take much longer.

Ethical issues

In 2019 the Association for Internet Researchers issued their third edition of the Internet Research: Ethical Guidelines (Franzke et al., 2020). This document sets out the current state of ethics in the evolving understanding of internet based research ethics. The document contains some of the usual aspects of research with human subjects along with a consideration of the multiple perspectives on ethics and aspects that are particular to online human subject research. Ethical considerations vary due to such things as the norms of a particular social group, culture or nation. Exploration of ethical practice is beyond the remit of this chapter, and the interested reader is guided to this document. However, brief mention of a basic aspect of "netiquette" is appropriate here as this relates to online interviews. Online interviews require different ethical considerations than face-to-face interviews. For example when an interviewer in an online interview approaches an interviewee, he or she should probably first approach the forum moderator. Doing this is minimally disruptive compared with initially posting directly to the forum.

Netnography

The other form of online research mentioned earlier is that of netnography, which has been used in the area of healthcare research to garner and make understandable qualitative healthcare-related information (e.g., Germain, Harris, Mackay, & Maxwell, 2018; Schuman, Lawrence, & Pope, 2019). Netnography has also been used for some time within marketing and consumer research (e.g., Kozinets, 2002). Social media communities (blogs, the blogosphere, microblogs, vlogs, podcasts, social networking sites, fora, etc.) are arenas within which participants exchange information and influence each other (Muniz & O'Guinn, 2001; Almquist & Roberts, 2000). Netnography systematically analyses the content of social media of all kinds. Netnography is both the fieldwork that is undertaken to study an online community and the investigation of a community along with its artefacts and their meanings. Netnography is a research technique that typically gathers asynchronous primary and secondary information from social media websites. The traditional and very longstanding research technique in anthropology of participant observation, usually undertaken over a longer-term is called ethnography. Netnography is a reworking of this research approach in a manner that makes it suitable for the study of online culture. The methodology is qualitative and interpretive in its examination of the human behavioural activities that happen on social media. The approach gained a foothold in the study of consumer behaviour, marketing and business. Robert Kozinets (2010), in his seminal book on netnography, notes how research into social media has similar biases to other forms of research and that, like other qualitative research methods, netnography is concerned with the understanding of symbolic meaning, online behavioural patterns and digital-located cultural information. In netnography research, exactly how a researcher participates and becomes immersed within an online community is carefully planned and may involve full or light levels of participation.

On social media websites, information is usually freely exchanged and is assumed to be unmediated to a large extent, and the expression of participants' is generally honest and open. Netnography studies this form of open sociability and information exchange. Furthermore, such exchanges may be tracked and patterns within these communication patterns may be studied within their social context by the researcher over time. Through the use of participant and non-participant observation and rigorous planning and analysis, netnography is well placed to reveal cultural insights and understandings.

Using netnography in healthcare research

Over the last decade netnography has been increasingly embraced by fields outside of consumer research (see, for example, Hackett & Koval, 2016). Netnography in healthcare research is a relatively new but growing approach to qualitative research, and below we provide some examples of this research. However, the use of netnography in areas of research that are related to healthcare is increasing in number and subject matter.

Examples of netnographic studies related to healthcare include, Chretien, Tuck, Simon, Singh, and Kind (2015) investigated the ways that medical students informally use social media for education and career development. Another illustration of netnography in health research is by Nicole Bromfield (2016). She conducted research into commercial gestational surrogacy – a surrogacy undertaken for commercial recompense which is more than simply reimbursing the surrogate mother her medical expenses. This form of surrogacy has increased over the last few years even though many condemn this as dehumanising, exploitative commodification and treating a baby as a saleable asset. However, globally the US has some of the most lenient laws in this regard and this was where her research was located. This is, again, a sensitive subject, and commercial surrogates may be difficult to interview, yet Nicole Bromfield wanted to understand the experiences of surrogate mothers. She used blogs kept by gestational surrogate mothers to explore these experiences.

Sendler and Lew-Starowicz (2019) demonstrate one of the strengths of netnography, the approach's ability to reach marginalised communities and to analyse responses that are less socially sanitised. Their investigation was into zoophiliacs; individuals who have sex with animals. They analysed the anonymous forum postings of 953 participants. The researchers analysed descriptions of participants' living situations, their sexual activities, their beliefs and attitudes, and also how they felt about being socially branded. They identified themes which spoke about the concerns that they felt when chatting within online communities. Themes were also discovered that were related to their living situation, their sex lives, the acceptability of their practices in society, and their ability to get help.

In another example of netnography associated with well-being and health, Nimrod (2011) conducted research into the online communities of seniors. They found that fun online was the most common content present in seniors' online communities. They employed a netnographic analysis of 50,000 posts across one year from six leading seniors' online communities. They discovered that most posts were part of cognitive, associative, and creative social games. "The main subjects in all contents were sex, gender differences, aging, grandparenting, politics, faith, and alcohol. Main participatory behaviors were selective timing, using expressive style, and persolisation of the online character." (Nimrod, 2011, 226). They also found in the dialogues they collected that active participants fostered community relationships and norms. They concluded that online communities for seniors offered a matchless type of informal leisure that varied between different participant groups and provided the chance for individuals to exercise and show their abilities, helping them cope with aging and positively affecting their well-being.

In another example of heath-related netnography, Lee (2017) investigated the effects of infertility in women from different socio-economic sectors. Lee was interested in the differences that were present in infertility rates ("income, race, and education in infertility prevalence, access to infertility services, and success rates after receiving infertility treatments" Lee, 2017, 341) and how these were related to the lived experiences of women with infertility issues. Lee noted, however, that few studies had considered inequalities in the ability of these women to access psychological support. In an attempt to investigate this, Lee conducted a netnographic exploration of the patient forum, "Finding a Resolution for Infertility," which is hosted by the National Infertility Association RESOLVE. Fifty-four women were recruited from the forum and interviewed about their infertility. The research investigated the language used and the values and norms of the forum in order to examine how social support functions in this online environment. What they found in their research was that the forum's discourse contained narratives about infertility that they labelled "persistent patient." They described the narrative thus: the patient conducts comprehensive research into treatment options. In spite of multiple failures in their attempts to have a healthy baby, the patient undertakes repeated cycles of treatment. During this time, little, if any, discussion is provided about the costs, both financial and social, and the patients' possessing these resources in order that they may perform within the script strictures. Mihan Lee concluded that women who did not have the requisite resources often found themselves alienated from, silenced by, and even denied mental health support by the online community.

Interestingly, infertility, but this time the relatively less researched area of male infertility, has also been studied using netnography, by Esmee Hanna and Brendan Gough (2016). The experiences of men with fertility problems are of emotional distress associated with stigma, threats to masculinity, and the belief that they should not sow their emotions. Thematic analyses of men's online emoting on men-only infertility discussion boards were performed and produced the themes of: "the emotional rollercoaster," "the tyranny of infertility" and "infertility paranoia." The authors continue to offer insight into how men negotiate diagnosis, treatment outcomes, their intimate relationships, and their patterns of sharing with other men in the same situation.

Conclusions and the future

In the writings above, some potential opportunities of going digital for healthcare research have been presented. What has been written is in no way supposed to be definitive or comprehensive. Instead, what is being offered are illustrations of how the virtual world has been exploited to the ends of researchers in a health and well-being settings. There is much more that could have been included in this chapter, including the integration of other ethnographic research practices with virtual research using mapping sentences (Hackett, 2016). Telemedicine is an area of growing health-related practice, and an obvious area within which healthcare research is needed in terms of its practice and patient reactions.

COVID-19 pandemic

The Coronavirus/COVID-19 pandemic is starting to hit the world at the time of writing this, and will have unknown impacts upon health globally and the research undertaken around the pandemic and how we will recover from this. Instead of including a section on this in this chapter we have decided to include an extra chapter in this book that addresses research methods that may improve understanding of healthcare related to the pandemic.

References

Almquist, E. & K.J. Roberts. (2000) A 'Mindshare' Manifesto, Mercer Management Journal, 12, 9–20.
Bromfield, N. (2016) Surrogacy Has Been One of the Most rewarding Experiences in my Life: A Content Analysis of Blogs by U.S. Commercial Gestational Surrogates, International Journal of Feminist Approaches to Bioethics, 9(1): 192–217.
Chretien, K., M. Tuck, M. Simon, L. Singh, & T. Kind. (2015) A Digital Ethnography of Medical Students Who Use Twitter for Professional Development, Journal of General Internal Medicine 30(11): 1673–680.

De Jong, I.G.M., H.A. Reinders-Messelink, W.G.M. Janssen, M.J. Poelma, I. Van Wijk, C.K. Van Der Sluis, E.A. Fridman. (2012) Mixed Feelings of Children and Adolescents with Unilateral Congenital Below Elbow Deficiency: An Online Focus Group Study (Mixed Feelings of Children/Adolescents with UCBED), PLoS ONE 7(6): E37099.

Dowling, S. (2012) Online Asynchronous and Face-to-Face Interviewing: Comparing Methods for Exploring Women's Experiences of Breastfeeding Long Term, in, Salmons, J. (ed.) (2012) Cases in Online Interview Research, Thousand Oaks, CA: Sage Publishers. pp. 277–302. dx.doi.org/10.4135/9781506335155.n11

Franzke, A.S., A. Bechmann, M. Zimmer, C. Ess, & the Association of Internet Researchers (2020). Internet Research: Ethical Guidelines 3.0. aoir.org/reports/ethics3.pdf

Germain, J., J. Harris, S. Mackay, & C. Maxwell. (2018) Why Should We Use Online Research Methods? Four Doctoral Health Student Perspectives, Qualitative Health Research, 28(10): 1650–657.

Hackett, P.M.W. (2016) Integrating Ethnographic Consumer Research Using Facet Theory and the Mapping Sentence, in, Hackett, P.M.W. (ed.) (2016) Qualitative Research Methods in Consumer Psychology: Ethnography and Culture, London: Routledge. pp. 1–15.

Hackett, P.M.W. & E. Koval. (2016) Ethnography 2: Field Observations, Questionnaires and Focus Group Interviews at a Water Park, in, Hackett, P.M.W. (ed.) (2016) Qualitative Research Methods in Consumer Psychology: Ethnography and Culture, London: Routledge. pp. 91–104.

Hackett, P.M.W., J.B. Schwarzenbach, & U.M. Jurgens. (2016) Consumer Psychology: A Study Guide to Qualitative Research Methods, Opladen, Berlin, Toronto: Barbara Budrich Publishers.

Hamama-Raz, Y., Y. Palgi, E. Leshem, M. Ben-Ezra, O. Lavenda, O. & S. Seedat. (2017) Typhoon Survivors' Subjective Wellbeing: A Different View of Responses to Natural Disaster, PLoS ONE, 12(9): E0184327.

Hanna, E. & N. Gough, N. (2016) Emoting infertility online: A qualitative analysis of men's forum posts, Health, 20(4): 363–382.

Horst, H.A. D. Miller. (eds.) (2012) Digital Anthropology, London: Berg Publishing.

Jewkes, Y. & M. Yar. (2013) Handbook of Internet Crime, London: Routledge.

Jervaeus, A., J. Nilsson, L.E. Eriksson, C. Lampic, C. Widmark, & L. Wettergren. (2016) Exploring Childhood Cancer Survivors' Views about Sex and Sexual Experiences -findings from Online Focus Group Discussions, European Journal of Oncology Nursing, 20: 165–172.

Kausel, C.L. & P.M.W. Hackett. (2016) Netnography: Possibilities and Resourcefulness, in, Hackett, P.M.W. (ed.) (2016) Qualitative Research Methods in Consumer Psychology: Ethnography and Culture, London: Routledge. pp. 252–261.

Kozinets, R.V. (1998) On Netnography: Initial Reflections on Consumer Research Investigations of Cyberculture, in Alba, J.W., and Wesley, H.J. (eds.) NA -Advances in Consumer Research, volume 25, Provo, UT: Association for Consumer Research. pp. 366–371.

Kozinets, R.V. (2002) The Field Behind the Screen: Using Netnography for Marketing Research in Online Communities, Journal of Marketing Research, 39(February), 61–72.

Kozinets, R.V. (2010) Netnography: Doing Ethnographic Research Online, Thousand Oaks, CA: Sage Publishers.

Janghorban, R., R.T. Roudsari, & A. Taghipour. (2014) Skype Interviewing: The New Generation of Online Synchronous Interview in Qualitative Research, International Journal of Qualitative Studies on Health and Well-being, 9(1): 24152.

Lee, M. (2017) Don't Give Up! A Cyber-ethnography and Discourse Analysis of an Online Infertility Patient Forum, Culture Medicine and Psychiatry, 41: 341–367. doi.org/10.1007/s11013-016-9515-6

Mann C. & F. Stewart. (2005) Internet Communication and Qualitative Research: A Handbook for Researching Online, London: Sage Publishers.

Muniz, A.M., Jr., & T.C. O'Guinn. (2001) Brand community, Journal of Consumer Research, 27(4): 412-432. doi.org/10.1006/319818

Nimrod, G. (2011) The Fun Culture in Seniors' Online Communities, The Gerontologist 51(2): 226–37.

Reisner, S.L., R.Z. Randazzo, J.M. White Hughto, S. Peitzmeier, L.Z. Dubois, D.J. Pardee, E. Marrow, S. Mclean, & J. Potter. (2018) Sensitive Health Topics With Underserved Patient Populations: Methodological Considerations for Online Focus Group Discussions, Qualitative Health Research, 28(10): 1658–673.

Rezabek, R. (2000). Online focus groups: Electronic discussions for research, Forum Qualitative Sozialforschung / Forum: Qualitative Social Research, 1(1). www.qualitative-research.net/fqs-texte/1-00/1-00rezabek-e.htm

Schuman, D.L., K.A. Lawrence, & N. Pope. (2019) Broadcasting War Trauma: An Exploratory Netnography of Veterans' YouTube Vlogs, Qualitative Health Research, 29(3): 357–70.

Sendler, D. J. & M. Lew-Starowicz. (2019) Digital Ethnography of Zoophilia – A Multinational Mixed-Methods Study, Journal of Sex and Marital Therapy, 45(1): 1–20.

Tuttas, C.A. (2015) Lessons Learned Using Web Conference Technology for Online Focus Group Interviews, Qualitative Health Research, 25(1): 122–33.

Wilson, L. (2012) Integrated Interdisciplinary Online Interviews in Science and Health: The Climate and Health Literacy Project, in, Salmons, J. (ed.) (2012) Cases in Online Interview Research, Thousand Oaks, CA: Sage Publishers. 239–260. dx.doi.org/10.4135/9781506335155.n12

Woodyatt, C.R., C.A. Finneran, & R. Stephenson. (2016) In-Person Versus Online Focus Group Discussions: A Comparative Analysis of Data Quality, Qualitative Health Research, 26(6): 741–49.

Zwaanswijk, M. & S. van Dulmen. (2014) Advantages of Asynchronous Online Focus Groups and Face-to-Face Focus Groups as Perceived by Child, Adolescent and Adult Participants: a Survey Study, BMC Res Notes 7, 756. doi.org/10.1186/1756-0500-7-756

40

CORONAVIRUS AND COVID-19

Qualitative healthcare research during and after the pandemic

Paul M.W. Hackett and Christopher M. Hayre

Introduction

As I sit here in my home in Massachusetts, my movement and the activities that I am able to engage in outside of the house have been restricted. In Asia, the Coronavirus pandemic has been extant for some three months (it was first reported to the World Health Organisation on December 31st, 2019) and is now hitting the whole world. Moreover, it is unknown exactly what form and extent the devastation will cause upon global health. The pandemic will also have profound and unpredictable effects upon the research that is undertaken by academics who are concerned with peoples' health and how we, as individuals, families, communities, countries and, indeed, as a global population, will address the pandemic and recover from this. Given the severity of the situation we have decided to include an extra chapter in this book that addresses research and methods for undertaking such research that may improve understanding of health, well-being, and healthcare related to the pandemic. It is likely that we will need to conduct healthcare-related research that answers different questions at different stages of the pandemic, however, the timing of such stages is obviously unknown.

We are at present in the Spring of 2020 and much of the world has suspended a significant degree of its citizens' activities. Economies and production have, to some extent, been put on hold. The term lockdown, instead of curfew, which is usually of a shorter time period and also has negative civil control associations, is used to describe this state of social isolation and is being employed to describe what is happening in our societies. Recent restrictions have been implemented by governments in the United Kingdom, Australia, Massachusetts and many other regions, which severely restricts personal movement in some communities to only going out to buy essential pharmaceutical products, food, and other essentials. There is a need for information and guidelines to be issued about the present state of the pandemic and its trajectory as it heads towards its first predicted peak around the world. Not all countries are developing the virus at the same rate, and a shared and coordinated international response, as called for by the secretary general of the United Nations, António Guterres, is not in sight but would surely help.

Even though we are only at the start of this pandemic, there have already been seismic changes in the world we live in, and many thousands of people have already died. In Britain, how people work as well as behaviours related to health have been radically changed. Indeed, Britain, and many other countries, has gone through a social revolution of the kind that has previously been associated with the effects of a world war. Flights are grounded around the world and borders are closed. However, in Britain and Europe there is evidence of a war-time spirit and a sense of solidarity. Maybe this camaraderie will only be temporary, but gone are the divisions between Brexiteers and remain voters, and whether these divisions return or whether Britain and other countries are heading for a lasting social change is probably dependent upon how hard the pandemic hits and how long it will last, which in turn are associated with how long we take to find a treatment and/or a vaccine. Social distancing, which has been implemented to mitigate against the transmission of the virus, along with the regular and vigorous washing of hands, may have to remain for over a year.

We are also developing new ways of buying online and having things delivered to our door and these new shopping behaviours may become hard to shake-off. A vaccine is expected to be some 18 months away and given the extent of changes that have happened over a few weeks, the world may be unrecognisable by that time. Here in the US, President Trump has stated that he will re-open the country for business, because that is what America does. This seemed a thin, unlikely and dangerous promise that he later rescinded. Indeed, it appears almost certain that in the next few months, restrictions around the world will become stricter with businesses closed and travel almost eliminated.

Perhaps one of the greatest of the social changes we have witnessed is that many more people are working from home. However, the big challenge in society will be associated with how people who cannot work from home, such as those in the gig economy and low-paid unskilled workers, are going to be able to earn an income? The gig worker is going to become more and more crucial to our way of life as they are often the ride share driver who also doubles as a local delivery driver for the stores that we are attempting to avoid because of the virus. These workers in the US typically have no health benefits and little security. As the virus progresses, more and more essential workers are likely going to become ill, including such gig workers and medical staff. Vulnerable and poorly paid workers, such as delivery drivers, shelf fillers, packers in distribution centres, etc., are putting themselves at risk for the rest of us and there may be pressures to better reward these workers. Scientists suggest that the increases in the incidence of infection and mortality in the first wave of infection should come around three months after the first reports of the virus in a region with both indicators slowing, and at this point some restrictions may be eased. When this happens, some economic activities may be resumed, although social distancing and protective gloves and masks will be needed to stave off a resurgence of cases.

It is interesting to speculate upon what impact our working from home for several months and our becoming accustomed to not traveling will have upon our behaviour both now and later. We will hopefully have developed new ways to work remotely and these may prove to be less costly in many ways and even harder to relinquish. For instance, I am now both conducting research and lecturing from home and I am also rarely venturing out of the house except to take exercise around the area in which I live. I have started having a shopper shop for my food and then deliver it to my house. Having become used to buying increasing numbers of things online from Amazon, clothes stores, eBay, etc., this has been a relatively easy transition. I have also, in the last week, used a telemedicine service to have a tick bite diagnosed by my local emergency care centre and then had the requisite drugs delivered. Getting used to this sort of consultation, ordering, and delivery service will likely have a profound effect upon the high street and shopping mall. It is also likely to cause a large number of people who are at present employed in these locations lose their jobs or to have them changed.

For many decades, Green politicians and activists have called upon us to act locally and think globally. The virus will force us to think more in this way and may make transporting anything internationally a very different prospect to how it was before the pandemic. It is a possibility and perhaps a probability that we will grow and manufacture more locally to the place of consumption. In China, where the virus was first identified around 3 months ago, authorities are starting to see a levelling off of new infections from the virus and are beginning to lift some of the more severe restrictions that have been in place. However, if the removal of restriction has been enacted too soon then it is likely that a resurgence of cases will happen. We do not know the way in which this new disease will progress and it may be that we will have further outbreaks and these will soon have a severe impact upon the economy. It is also likely that we will all be feeling the effects of a global recession with high levels of both unemployment and benefit payments. There could well be many health implications of the changes that have and will happen as we will further develop our sedentary lifestyles as we work from home and call into the office as needed. Many social gathering places may also stay closed for a long time and when universities re-open there may be fewer international students as they may be unable or reluctant to travel a distance to their educational institution. Furthermore, having broken down resistance towards remote learning there may be some reluctance to abandon these forms of education. Moreover, there will have been a drastic cut in carbon emissions during the pandemic, and it is likely that there will be a call to not return to pre-pandemic levels of emissions, which may produce new opportunities for a non-carbon based economy.

The Coronavirus pandemic will hasten many of the changes that were underway prior to its occurrence. With such a rapid change, however, we will have to decide how long-term transformations are incorporated into societies and are funded, including deciding on how those that no longer have jobs make a living and how we allocate health and well-being services both associated with the pandemic and those that are not. There may be an enduring sense of looking after each-other, but there may also be a more fractional response when those people with jobs and opportunities are asked to look after those without. Medical professionals will have learnt to work in different ways to how they did before the outbreak and we will have to be training professionals for their new or modified roles and the implementation of a treatment and/or vaccination programme. Coronavirus will have become a part of our lives and may well be here to stay. In the US we will have to decide if we still think that it is efficient to have a market-based health system, and funding for the NHS in the UK will have to be reviewed.

From political leaders to the next-door neighbour, we all want to help, both now and later, but we must be careful not to assume our existing knowledge will apply in this new situation. Many professional organisations are issuing guidelines about the way their members may react to the virus. For example, my professional organisation, the British Psychological Society, has issued guidelines (BPS, 2020) that cover the following areas of practice:

- Keeping psychological services and psychological therapies services open through the immediate crisis
- Maintaining psychological professions training programmes
- Remote delivery of psychological therapies and interventions
- Maintaining a psychological approach to prevention, care, and treatment
- Supporting the well-being of NHS organisations, teams, and staff

Virtual groups for health and other professionals have also been initiated to provide a discussion forum and to provide support.

Another area that will need to be addressed is that of the services that a society can put into place to assist with treating the virus and later the services that will be needed for a society to recover. Research in this area will be especially varied across different societies due to the different ways in which health services are provided in the public and private sectors in different countries. Many suggestions have and will be made by governments. For example: the UK government in terms of the pandemic itself (GovUK, 2020a) and Public Health England in terms of how to cope with the effects of the virus upon public health and the changes to our daily lives (GovUK, 2020b). Other agencies (such as the NHS in the UK, (NHS, 2020)) are also suggesting how we can best cope with the effects of the pandemic, as well as how to best deal with self-isolation. These include suggestions such as avoiding news that you find stressful and distressing, and when you do search for information try to concentrate on finding information about protecting yourself. Moreover, when seeking information it is probably a good idea to avoid constant news feeds and to expose yourself to news at specific, limited, times.

Establishing new routines will take some time but we should attempt to do this and we should be in regular email and phone contact with friends and family. We should also do our best to have differentiated days and variety in what we do in isolation. In the UK, the mental health charity MIND has issued extremely thorough recommendations for how we can attempt to keep mentally well (MIND, 2020). Their suggestions include making sure we have time off from work and, when possible, going into nature and the sunlight as well as exercising and eating and drinking well. AnxietyUK (AnxietyUK 2020) have put forward the APPLE technique that we should practice.

- **Acknowledge:** Notice and acknowledge the uncertainty as it comes to mind.
- **Pause:** Don't react as you normally do. Don't react at all. Pause and breathe.
- **Pull back:** Tell yourself this is just the worry talking, and this apparent need for certainty is not helpful and not necessary. It is only a thought or feeling. Don't believe everything you think. Thoughts are not statements or facts.
- **Let go:** Let go of the thought or feeling. It will pass. You don't have to respond to them. You might imagine them floating away in a bubble or cloud.
- **Explore:** Explore the present moment, because right now, in this moment, all is well. Notice your breathing and the sensations of your breathing. Notice the ground beneath you. Look around and notice what you see, what you hear, what you can touch, what you can smell. Right now. Then shift your focus of attention to something else – on what you need to do, on what you were doing before you noticed the worry, or do something else – mindfully, with your full attention (AnxietyUK 2020).

A list of sub-topics for classifying research into understanding mass communication associated with COVID-19 has been suggested for submissions to a Frontiers special edition (Arriaga, Esteves, Pavlova, & Picarra, 2020) that addresses the impact and the role of the mass media during the pandemic may be usefully included here as a framework for research into this area:

- Effective health communication for the adoption of sustainable preventive measures and curtailing misinformation;
- Public health communication to increase psychological resources and resilience in distinct age groups and socioeconomic conditions;
- Effective strategies for helping individuals in dealing with social and physical distancing;
- Reduction of stigma, prejudice, discrimination, and inequalities.

I do not wish to make the statement that all academic research should now be directed towards the virus as that would be ridiculous. However, I do think we should think about the research we are doing and ask ourselves if we could, at least at this time, be directing our efforts towards assisting in treating and coping with the pandemic in some way. As academics, we are often in a peerless position in regard to the knowledge we possess. Being well-informed we are therefore able to provide advice from a position of research-based knowledge rather than anecdote, supposition or opinion. Having such a knowledge base also puts us in a position where we can use our research and knowledge to fight xenophobic and racist accusations that arise in association with the pandemic. Unfortunately, there have been attacks, blame, and prejudice expressed towards Chinese and other Asian people. These are based on notions that COVID-19 is a Chinese or Asian virus. It is our responsibility to use our research-based knowledge to interrupt misinformed and inhumane attacks that are especially unhelpful at a time when the world needs to unite to fight the virus. More specifically, we must speak out if we encounter defamatory comments and provide information about COVID-19 that is based on scientific knowledge (the circumstances of how the virus arose will need careful investigation at a later date). We can counter opinions that are not based upon the knowledge we have about the virus and stand with all people as we experience the effects of a non-discriminating global pandemic. As academics in healthcare we are in a position to write to the media, whether this is traditional newspaper, radio, or on television or social media, when we become aware of nationalistic, racist, or xenophobic comments that are being made and founded upon misinformation about the virus. If we are conducting research that is directly associated or relevant to the virus then our comments about the virus and its effects may be extremely valuable in providing an insight into the true nature of the virus and our attempts to deal with this. It is also incumbent upon us to become more aware of how activities that spread xenophobia are practiced to ensure that we do not ourselves add to these.

Thus far a background to the virus has been given as this is related to the need and usefulness of qualitative healthcare related research. In the next section, details are provided of a few qualitative research methods that may be used to garner primary data at this time.

Appropriate qualitative research methods

An example of the way in which healthcare research has already felt the effects of the virus is demonstrated in the following example. In the UK, the first death of a prisoner was reported in March and all primary research in prisons that involved researcher and participant contact has been prohibited by the home office. This had a large impact upon master students at the University of Suffolk, Department of Criminology who are now looking to move their research project from face-to-face data gathering to some other form of information collection. These restrictions will affect the ability to gather knowledge regarding the lives, activities, and experiences of inmates, staff, and others associated with prison life. I mention this situation as it exemplifies some of the difficulties that researchers will have during the pandemic. As a supervisor of research projects at the University of Suffolk I have been making suggestions as to how students may change their research approach. I do not want to concentrate upon research in prisons as I have mentioned this form of research simply as an example of the problems that exist and will be faced in conducting safe primary research. Any form of research that involves either traveling to a site to access people or other forms of data is now problematic in many countries. Furthermore, it is not possible for a researcher and participant to be closer than two-metres from each other and even this distance may be too close to be totally safe and should not be maintained for more than a few minutes. These are drastic restrictions that may not endure for long, but it is likely that some form of restriction will persist for a more protracted time and may have a longer-term effect upon research practice with human subjects.

My initial response to the cutting of the above types of primary research was to suggest to my students the use of secondary sources of information. However, this often does not answer the questions that are pertinent to contemporary research. Consequently, it appears to me that the use of netnography is an appropriate research orientation at this time (see, Germain, Harris, Mackay, & Maxwell, 2018; Kausel and Hackett, 2016; Kozinets, 1998). In aforementioned chapters we spent some time discussing the use of netnography as a procedure in healthcare research and we will not repeat this content. Notwithstanding the above comment, at the time of this virus, netnography offers a research approach to healthcare issues that is particularly suited to investigations in closed communities such as prisons or those that exist at present in many communities around the world. In these types of settings, and in all other situations, netnography is a safe approach to research that has the ability to garner much information about the lived experiences of people with the virus or who are affected by the virus. It is easily appreciated that at this current time, and for the immediate future, people will be out of contact with each other and will use social media to "have a social life". This being the case, the investigation of social media communications will tell us much about the experiences that surround the virus. Anthropologists employ the use of digital platforms to study online communities (Horst & Miller, 2012), where the American Anthropological Association have a special interest group, the Digital Anthropology Group, which is concerned with research that involves the internet as a site for the observation and interpretation of social interactions. In this type of research the researcher is able to either simply analyse postings and conversations that are present in social media or to immerse themselves and participate within an online community. When participating in a deeply engaged sense and forming observations, the researcher is also able to use these as the basis for online interviews and the gathering of secondary information. Netnography or digital ethnography can also be combined with offline observations and other types of data gathering. This form of research facilitates the establishment of what have become traditional forms of behaviour, norms, histories, stories, practices, conflicts within the group and outside, and much more. Netnographic research within healthcare has the potential to provide information that will enable the modification and improvement of services during and after the pandemic.

Allied to netnography is visual ethnography which may also be performed online. In this procedure, participants may be asked to gather a number of images together that, to them, represent the virus, official responses to the pandemic, how their lives have been impacted by the virus, or any other specific topic. The use of images may produce responses that are less under the conscious editing of participants and may reveal deeper understanding about the issues surrounding the virus than simply asking people what they think, feel, or do. A variation of this approach is to ask participants to gather images, none of which are directly associated with the virus (images cannot be of medical people treating people with the virus, police enforcing virus lockdowns, streets in London empty because of the lockdown, etc.), but instead must express how they are thinking or feeling about the virus. All visual approaches offer the ability to use participants' pictorial responses as a lever for delving into deeper levels of understanding and for facilitating subsequent discussion with participants. If participants are asked to arrange images in a way that is meaningful to them in relation to the virus, participants' descriptions of such configurations may allow us to access the deep metaphors that are being used to understand a variety of aspects and issues associated with the virus (see the ZMET approach of Gerald Zaltman, (Zaltman & Zaltman, 2008)).

The keeping of diaries is also another research method that is an appropriate tool to be used at this time (Hyers, 2017). The qualitative research diary is of particular usefulness and pertinence at this time as it focusses upon the events that happen in a person's life whilst appreciating its temporal context. By emphasising the time-related aspects of a person's life, the diary is able to chart and track the experiential progression of the disease. Diary research may involve asking participants to keep diaries or the analysis of diaries that were kept for reasons other than for research purposes. Another important and unique aspect of the research diary is ita applicability for use in longitudinal research into the experiences of people with the virus or associated carers and medical staff (Bolger & Laurenceau, 2013).

Diary-keeping has a long tradition in health research in the form of both traditional and electronic diaries. The term "diaries" is being used here in a generic sense to denote a type of information gathering that requires a person to keep a record of their activities, thoughts, feelings, etc. The actual medium of the record keeping can be extremely varied and may include: writing in traditional diaries, recording thoughts into a mobile phone, writing a blog or making a vlog, collecting images to represent a specified phenomenon, etc. The content of the diary can either be closely specified by the researcher, left entirely to the participant's discretion, or some mix of these approaches. The frequency of what is written or collected may also vary from brief answers to specific questions provided at specified time intervals to free text, the content and frequency of which is entirely determined by the participant.

An early example of the use of digital diaries in health research is Hyland, Kenyon, Allen, and Howarth (1993) who compared both traditional and digital forms of patient diaries in their investigation into asthma patients. Diaries have also been used to look at patient's experience of well-being. For example, Travers (2011) investigated diary keeping as a methodology through which she explored the accounts of thirty young people. Her focus was upon the experiences of this cohort's ability to cope with the stress associated with the exams and other life changes that were occurring at the end of their undergraduate university life. More recently, Herron, Dansereau, Wrathall, Funk, and Spencer (2019) allowed participants to choose whether they would keep a diary on a computer, tablet or on paper and they also allowed the entry content to be determined by the participant (whether this was textual, drawings, or photographs). In doing this, they demonstrated the potential and benefits of a flexible use of the digital diary.

The ability for diary research to be conducted online is obviously a great asset at the present time and has the potential to yield extremely interesting and useful information about living with the Coronavirus for those who have the disease, who are supporting someone with the virus, who are part of a medical staff concerned with treating virus patients, and many other types of people affected by the pandemic. The use of diary research may yield insights that could be used to improve the lives of individuals and to allow services aimed to mitigate the effects of the virus to be responsive to the needs of patients and professionals.

Online focus groups (Abrams & Gaiser, 2017) may also be conducted with benefit at this time. Reisner and colleagues (2018) used online focus groups because they provided, they claimed, an anonymous setting in which sensitive issues associated with participants' health may be discussed. They said that the anonymity provided by online focus groups better allowed an open discussion than traditional focus groups, especially when used with marginalised populations such as transgender individuals. Their article reviewed the pluses and minuses of online focus groups with other sensitive populations and with geographically dispersed, rare, and stigamatised conditions. They concluded by making suggestions regarding ways of conducting online focus groups in order to increase the comfort of those taking part, to maximise the engagement of participants and to stimulate rich, qualitative information, all of which are important points when working with those affected by the pandemic.

According to Tuttas (2015), Web conference is a form of synchronous audio-visual technology that can allow researchers a new way to conduct focus groups. She reviewed the literature on both synchronous and asynchronous focus groups along with other online data collection methods, such as chat rooms, discussion boards and emails. In her qualitative research into job integration experiences of US travel nurses geographically dispersed across the country, she employed Web conferencing software for conducting online focus groups. She evaluated the usefulness of the online focus group as a research technique and considered how responses can be transcribed using software and claimed the online focus group to be a useful technique in qualitative health-related research. In another piece of qualitative health- and well-being-related research, Woodyatt, Finneran, and Stephenson (2016) noted that by the middle of the last decade online focus groups were becoming a widely used method in qualitative research. These researchers compared the two methodologies of traditional and online versions of the focus group in terms of the quality of the data that arises out of the two approaches. Their study was of a sensitive nature regarding violence between intimate partners within a sample of gay and bisexual men. They found that whilst online focus groups were usually shorter in time than traditional face-to-face focus groups, they yielded a larger word count. The themes that emerged between the two focus group modalities were overlapping but an additional theme was present in the online focus group design. Furthermore, they discovered that in-depth stories were shared less in face-to-face settings and sensitive topics were also discussed less. They concluded that overall the information that was generated in both focus group types was similar but with some differences. It would therefore appear that the online focus group is a research method that would sensitively gather experiential information within the context of COVID-19.

Ethical and other issues

All research has to observe guidelines to ensure ethical practice. Online research, such as conducting netnographies, visual ethnographies, online interviews of different types, etc., have ethical standards that are similar to their in-person counterparts and which must be maintained. Additionally, and dependent upon the precise type of research being conducted, the researcher will need to be engaged and active in the research to an even greater extent than may be the case with traditional research. Online researchers will have to become aware of ethical practices in an online setting and will have to keep in mind that we are at present conducting research with respondents who are particularly vulnerable. In this chapter I am suggesting some ways in which we may be able to conduct research that addresses the individual and social needs that have arisen from COVID-19. With this being the case, the research we are conducting is into a particularly sensitive and distressing subject. It is therefore important that researchers establish clear expectations of the participant and that they create a supportive environment within the research procedure. As well as standard good ethical practice such as obtaining informed consent, allowing unquestioned and easy participant withdrawal from the study with no penalty, ensuring psychological and physical safety, etc., the researcher should be especially sensitive to the needs of the participant and encourage participants to express these.

When conducting research associated with the pandemic, the researcher should introduce participants to the research as a collaborative setting and process. The virus may be a challenging subject matter for the participant and it is important that the researcher provides stability and support especially in difficult or emotional parts of the research. To these ends, the researcher must be well prepared for such possibilities. In emotionally charged online research, it is probably a good idea for the researcher to progress more slowly through the research process than they would in a face-to-face setting. If the research is asynchronous then extremely full and precise instructions and guidance must be provided to mitigate against the lack of opportunity for participants to ask questions in real-time. It should also be remembered that some participants will have considerable experience with digital technology whilst others will have very little.

Participants will also vary in terms of their familiarity with and ability to understand complex written medical and other information. They will also have a wide variety of health and other life circumstances. It may help, when encountering challenging points in the research, if the researcher provides rest periods for the participant and leads the session with gentle questions and offers responses that embody subtlety in their understanding of the participant in a way that enables participants to express shades of meaning in their responses. De-briefing after the research may help to alleviate some of the anxieties that respondents have about the virus, but researchers must have the contact details of services that could support a respondent who experiences distress. It is important that we attempt to infuse our research approach with compassion whilst emphasizing that in our research we are attempting to discover useful information about the circumstances surrounding the virus.

Other factors that arise from conducting online research include that your respondents will be in a wide variety of physical locations that are experiencing the pandemic in different ways. These physical differences will influence participation and the responses you receive. If synchronous research is conducted with participants in a variety of global locations the quality of online connection may be variable and it may be problematic for multiple respondents to participate at a specific time.

Conclusion

This is the stage that we are at at the present time. There is a lot of information that is being spread about the virus by word of mouth, social media, and many other sources. Unfortunately, much of this is misinformation which is coming from the same sources and unfortunately it is also coming from some of our political leaders. Of course, websites and other forms of communication about the virus do exist that are reputable and provide trustworthy information. However, academics have both the facilities, training, and skills to take an important part in promoting understanding about COVID -19, its treatment, and a future with and after the pandemic. Moreover, academics have a social responsibility to use their skills for the good of others at this time. All of the writing in this chapter is to some extent speculative, however, as thinking about what comes after the virus, relies to a great extent, upon gazing into a crystal ball. There is no way of knowing what will happen after the virus but it seems likely that there will have been many changes in societies across the globe and that at least some of these changes will be profound. The findings from well thought out research can help us all to re-build our lives and establish a healthy life with a sense of well-being.

References

Abrams, K.M., & T.J. Gaiser. (2017) Online Focus Groups, in, Fielding, N.G., and Lee, R.M. (eds.) (2017) The SAGE Handbook of Online Research Methods, Thousand Oaks, CA: Sage Publishing.

Anxiety UK. (2020) Health and Other Forms of Anxiety and Coronavirus, www.anxietyuk.org.uk/blog/health-and-other-forms-of-anxiety-and-coronavirus/ accessed April 12, 2020.

Arriaga, P., F. Esteves, M.A. Pavlova, & N.G. Picarra. (eds.) (2020) About This Topic:Coronavirus Disease (COVID-19): The Impact and Role of Mass Media During the Pandemic, special edition Frontiers in Psychology, Lausanne, Switzerland: Frontiers Media SA.

BPS. (2020) New guidance for psychological professionals during the COVID-19 pandemic, www.bps.org.uk/news-and-policy/new-guidance-psychological-professionals-during-covid-19-pandemic?utm_source=BPS_Lyris_email&utm_medium=email&utm_campaign= accessed March 28, 2020.

Bolger, N. & J-P. Laurenceau. (2013) Intensive Longitudinal Methods: An Introduction to Diary and Experience Sampling Research (Methodology in the Social Sciences), New York: The Guilford Press.

Frontiers. (2020) Coronavirus Knowledge Hub: A Trusted Source for the Latest Science on SARS-CoV-2 and COVID-19, https://coronavirus.frontiersin.org/ accessed April 12, 2020.

GovUK. (2020a) Coronavirus (COVID-19): what you need to do, www.gov.uk/coronavirus accessed April 12, 2020.

GovUK. (2020b) Guidance for the Public on the Mental Health and Wellbeing Aspects of Coronavirus (COVID-19) updated March 31, 2020, www.gov.uk/government/publications/covid-19-guidance-for-the-public-on-mental-health-and-wellbeing/guidance-for-the-public-on-the-mental-health-and-wellbeing-aspects-of-coronavirus-covid-19

Germain, J., J. Harris, S. Mackay, & C. Maxwell, C. (2018) Why Should We Use Online Research Methods? Four Doctoral Health Student Perspectives, Qualitative Health Research, 28(10): 1650–657.

Herron, R., L. Dansereau, M. Wrathall, L. Funk, & D. Spencer. (2019) Using a Flexible Diary Method Rigorously and Sensitively With Family Carers, Qualitative Health Research, 29(7): 1004–015.

Horst, H.A. & D. Miller. (eds.) (2012) Digital Anthropology, London: Berg Publishing.

Hyers, L.L. (2017) Diary Methods: Understanding Qualitative Research, Oxford: Oxford University Press.

Hyland, M.E., C.A. Kenyon, R. Allen, & P. Howarth. (1993) Diary Keeping in Asthma: Comparison of Written and Electronic Methods, BMJ: British Medical Journal, 306(6876): 487–489.

Kausel, C.L. & P.M.W. Hackett. (2016) Netnography: Possibilities and Resourcefulness, in Hackett, P.M.W. (ed.) (2016) Qualitative Research Methods in Consumer Psychology: Ethnography and Culture, London: Routledge, pp. 252–261.

Kozinets, R.V. (1998) On Netnography: Initial Reflections on Consumer Research Investigations of Cyberculture, in Alba, J.W., and Wesley, H.J. (eds.) NA –Advances in Consumer Research Volume 25, Provo, UT: Association for Consumer Research, pp. 366–371.

MIND. (2020) Coronavirus and your wellbeing, www.mind.org.uk/information-support/coronavirus/coronavirus-and-your-wellbeing/ accessed April 12, 2020.

NHS. (2020) Advice for everyone-Coronavirus (COVID-19), www.nhs.uk/conditions/coronavirus-covid-19/ accessed April 12, 2020.

Reisner, S.L., R.K. Randazzo, J.M. White Hughto, S. Peitzmeier, L.Z. DuBois, D.J. Pardee, E. Marrow, S. McLean, & J. Potter. (2018) Sensitive Health Topics With Underserved Patient Populations: Methodological Considerations for Online Focus Group Discussions, Qualitative Health Research, 28(10): 1658–673.

Travers, C. (2011) Unveiling a Reflective Diary Methodology for Exploring the Lived Experiences of Stress and Coping, Journal of Vocational Behavior, 79(1): 204–216.

Tuttas, C.A. (2015) Lessons Learned Using Web Conference Technology for Online Focus Group Interviews, Qualitative Health Research, 25(1): 122–33.

WHO. (2020) Global Research on Coronavirus disease (COVID-19), www.who.int/emergencies/diseases/novel-coronavirus-2019/global-research-on-novel-coronavirus-2019-ncov accessed April 12, 2020.

Woodyatt, C.R., C.A. Finneran, & R. Stephenson. (2016) In-Person Versus Online Focus Group Discussions: A Comparative Analysis of Data Quality, Qualitative Health Research, 26(6): 741–49.

Zaltman, G. & L.H. Zaltman. (2008) Marketing Metaphoria: What Deep Metaphors Reveal About the Minds of Consumers, Cambridge, MA: Harvard Business Review Press.

41

BLACK LIVES MATTER

Birdwatching in Central Park and the murder of George Floyd

Paul M. W. Hackett and Jessica Schwarzenbach

Introduction

Racism has deep implications upon the health and wellbeing of minorities. Within the Coronavirus pandemic alone there is a correlation between a high incidence of COVID-19 and being Black. Gould and Wilson state, "Black workers face the two most lethal preexisting conditions for coronavirus – racism and economic inequality. … ..Black Americans make up 12.5% of the US population but account for 22.4% of COVID-19 deaths" (2020). Within days of the incident in Central Park, a Black Birder's movement developed with online discussions of what it means to be Black in the outdoors and within what are traditionally thought of as White spaces. The intent of the group is to encourage ongoing conversations "to boost recognition and representation of Black people enjoying and studying the natural world" (Mock, 2020).

This chapter has been added to the Handbook at the last moment due to the universal outrage instigated by the murder of George Floyd and the expanding influence of the Black Lives Matter global network. The fact that this chapter is an addition, an after-thought, says much about how we, as white academics, have neglected the matter of racial inequality. All scholarly authors, especially ethnographers, or any disseminators of knowledge, must attempt to identify possible detrimental preconceptions which might influence their perspectives before, and while, pursuing a research project or publication. This process of self-examination is called bracketing in qualitative research and is an ongoing process of studying one's own motives, personal characteristics, and behavior.

The authors of this chapter acknowledge that we are two persons who are both white and middleclass and that this background impacts our appreciation of racism and how we write about racist issues. Before the latest attacks on Black people in the US and the worldwide Black Lives Matter protests that followed, the editors of this volume did not think to include a chapter on racial inequality and its effects upon healthcare. However, the issue of racism was just as important, and the acts of violence and abuse were just as disgusting and prevalent the day before George Floyd was killed as they are now.

Human beings are not good at planning ahead or implementing change until forced to do so. For example, most people know of a road junction that they feel is tricky to maneuver. They will curse every day as they negotiate their way through it saying, "This junction is so dangerous, somebody should do something about it". Yet, only after a fatal crash takes place at the junction, (or even two), do we actually implement the redesign of its layout and bring in the road construction crews. To extend this situation analogously to the killing of Black people in our communities we can ask the question: How many *fatal crashes* have there been in our society, and by fatal crashes we mean how many deaths have been caused by prejudice and racial discrimination? Yet, we, in America, have not made changes to the way in which our society is laid out. How many more fatal crashes are needed to bring about change?

Some years ago, through legislation and changing societal norms, the United States and many other western nations pronounced the use of abusive racial slurs unacceptable language in public life. The "N" word could no longer be used by whites in decent company. The use of the "N" word is known to fan emotions of hatred in perpetrators, as well as invoking painful suffering in those who share a history of sub-human treatment. This word should never be used and the same is true of many other terms of racial abuse. Although a vital step, modifying our language and deleting particular words from our vocabulary is merely a pat on the back for making certain vocal behavior superficially unacceptable. But we all know that more Black persons and other non-Whites are stopped by police at a vastly disproportionate rate from White persons. We know that people of color occupy more prison cells than White people, that African Americans are almost three times more likely to be killed by a police officer than are Whites and the sixth most common cause of death amongst young Black men is by the hands of the police (Economist, 2020). People of color occupy many of the jobs that White people do not want and are paid less than their White counterparts. People of color have fewer life opportunities, and consequently, poorer health. The White status quo has ignored this pervasive situation while committing smugly to the tokenism of the restricted use of language. As we write, the COVID-19 pandemic is hitting minority communities much harder than white communities.

Pertinent to the first author's own experience is the incident of Christian Cooper, the bird watcher. The first author has been a birdwatcher for almost five decades and has walked and looked at birds in places all over the world. He admits that occasionally he has felt conspicuous when using his binoculars and even nervous about how he may be perceived by others. When birdwatching in the former Eastern Bloc, many decades ago, he remembers being wary and on the lookout for the secret police and he was careful not to watch birds near airports and other sensitive locations. Today, while watching birds near people's homes, he is always careful to avert the gaze of his binoculars so as not to intrude on the residents' privacy. While wandering the woods of Central Park he has felt cautious, not because he is white, but due to movies depicting the antics of cops and robbers racing through the undergrowth. In Central Park, he has never been afraid of being labeled a White man; a person who is "not of color". His color is transparent. He has no color. He is just a male birdwatcher. His situation is dissimilar to the birdwatcher Christian Cooper who was labelled an African American male by an irate dog owner. This politically correct epithet was utilized by his accuser to describe Cooper to the police, to label him with a term of difference, a term of racial abuse.

However, in this chapter the authors do not intend to continue listing the egregious ways in which people of color are treated in our society but rather will attempt to clarify various methods which can be used by ethnographers to address the all-pervasive yet often unrecognized forces of racism. We start by offering a very brief and crude netnographic study which looks at the experiences of Black bird watchers.

Using netnography to explore the experiences of Black bird watchers

Netnography is a method used in ethnography to conduct online research in order to understand social interaction within the contexts of contemporary digital communications. An example of how a netnography can be used to provide a voice for Black experience is demonstrated by Axelson (2020). On June 6th of this year, a few days after the Christian Cooper incident, the Cornell Lab of Ornithology published an article online called, "5 Key Lessons To Take Home From The First #BlackBirdersWeek" (Axelson, 2020). The page was written by Gustave Axelson who is an editorial director at the Cornell Lab with a background in journalism. His writing is a netnographic exploration (also known as a digital ethnography) of posts on Twitter and other social media outlets that arose from the verbal attack by the irate dog owner upon Christian Cooper under the hashtag, #BlackBirdersWeek.

Axelson introduces his article by noting that Christian Cooper described New York City's Central Park in spring as his "happy place". Axelson goes on to set the scene for his review of social media posts by noting how Mr. Cooper's right to watch birds in the Park was assaulted on May 25th and that this came in the midst of other assaults on people of color. Axelson commented on how the verbal attack and false accusations were recorded and posted by Christian Cooper on social media, which then went viral and received wide media coverage. Soon after this incident, approximately 30 young Black birders, scientists, and nature lovers organized a #BlackBirdersWeek to provide a place in which they were able to discuss their experiences as Black bird watchers and researchers. This resulted in almost "9 hours of Instagram and Facebook Live events, thousands of questions, at least 7 hashtags, and more than 50,000 viewers" (Axelson, 2020). Axelson continued by noting how the discussions were on topics that included how safe the group members felt when birdwatching to mnemonics for remembering bird songs. He also noted that there were several themes that came up across the week. The themes that Axelson identified were: a. The cooper incident wasn't unusual; black birders often feel unwelcome; b. Happy places are essential; c. Please don't dismiss talk about the black birding experience as "political"; d. Representation matters.

We will now briefly consider each of these themes.

The cooper incident wasn't unusual; black birders often feel unwelcome

Axelson cited comments from online platforms that can be subsumed under this heading. For example, during a livestream on June 4th, Christian Cooper was quoted as saying "I think it's important for us to discuss it specifically in the birding community, because there are so many places where I think we [as Black birders] are vulnerable and perhaps feel unwelcome". On the YouTube series Birds of North America, host Jason Ward commented how birds all come out at once to feed after hunkering down during heavy rain. Ward described how after a storm in north Atlanta he was watching birds in parking lots when he noticed that he was being followed: "That police SUV follows me … and parks about 100 feet from me. So now I'm raising my binoculars, looking at nothing, just raising the binoculars up, like 'Don't shoot.' [So] they can see that I'm here birding". Ward also claimed that his ability to travel in order to watch birds had been negatively impacted. For example, he claimed, "There are certain counties that I am hesitant in visiting. A lot of times we're by ourselves. We are wearing binoculars (dark objects) and don't want them mistaken for other objects". Jeffrey Ward (Jason's brother) is also quoted as remembering when he and his brother were looking for grasshopper warblers in the Georgia countryside and they called into a fast food restaurant, "a pickup truck swerved in front of me and rolled down the window, and [they] screamed, 'Jesus isn't Black!' So, I wouldn't go there alone".

Axelson also quotes a North Carolina State University graduate student in urban ecology who claims that she has been followed whilst she was undertaking fieldwork, "I've had an individual come outside with her dog and follow me around. I've had the cops sit across the street.

I don't want to have to rush to get done with my fieldwork. No one should feel like they can't do their job because of the color of their skin".

Happy places are essential

Under this heading Axelson noted that the places that were special came from across the US. He also commented upon how participants in livestream discussions described their personal happy places. For example, a graduate student in natural resources at the University of Georgia, stated that she preferred "a porch in the Appalachian Mountains, [where] miraculously all the birds fly by, red and purple, in a beautiful rainbow". Jason Ward, nominated the Lower Rio Grande Valley: "Seeing birds like Green Jays and Plain Chachalacas, and just the huge diversity of birds that can be found in South Texas". A wildlife biologist said that for her it was birding near Tucson, Arizona, "seeing hummingbirds, and maybe an Elegant Trogon or two". However, Axelson includes under this heading a statement by a person who was professionally involved in bird conservation. The man said that for him birdwatching provided much happiness in a world that is often painful, "When I'm in [a] cynical mindset the only thing that gets me out is the joy and unapologetic strength and style of Black birders". Perhaps this quote does not describe a "happy place" but of many places made more joyful by the presence of Black birders.

Please don't dismiss talk about the black birding experience as "political"

The third theme that Axelson identified was slightly different in its nature to the previous two themes. The author notes that on social media posters frequently raise an objection to #BlackBirdersWeek on the grounds that this is politicizing birdwatching, something to which those posting object. It is also claimed in some posts that white birders don't "see color". To such posts, Axelson provides an example to counter such claims: "I think putting that [political] label on it is dismissive and putting a blanket over it, because you don't want to see it anymore. 'Political' is just a cop-out".

Representation matters

One of the organizers of the #BlackBirdersWeek event stated how representing Black birders within the broader birding community was one of the events main aims: "BlackBirdersWeek really aims to create a space where Black people can be visible, and to let everyone out there know that there are systematic barriers, especially racism, that can prevent Black people from utilizing these spaces and enjoying birds, like everyone else who isn't Black might be enjoying them. We hope that this event will start a movement to change that narrative".

Axelson also looked at social media meetups and found a lot of discussion about how Black bird watchers can be supported. One person suggested: "If you see a Black person or a person of color ... and you consider yourself an ally, try to make [them] comfortable. Go talk to them. Not with the condescending tone of 'Why are you here?' But start with something like, 'What's the last cool bird you've seen?' Just an icebreaker". Christian Cooper made the following suggestion regarding the best thing that birdwatchers can do: "help each other out, regardless of race, creed, color, sexual orientation. The birds don't care. Why should we?"

Axelson also noted other comments that were made aimed at welcoming Black birdwatchers. These were: acknowledge Black bird watchers, smile, and be friendly; establish sincere conversation, as one birder to another; don't make assumptions about a birder's skill based on their appearance; speak up for Black birders in the field if you witness others being disrespectful or intolerant; expand those you invite to others to join your bird walk.

Finally, it was noted that two basic obstacles that got in the way of Black birdwatchers were the availability of binoculars and problems accessing safe, local, urban greenspaces.

Neither the article by Axelson (2020) nor the research that underpins this writing appear to have been conducted for academic purposes or in an academically stringent manner, i.e., no sampling details or analysis methods are stated. The present authors provide Axelson's work as an example, not as a recipe for the methodological approach of netnography, but as an illustration of how the qualitative research technique of netnography may form a voice for Black people. Some may not think the discussions of #BlackBirdersWeek are directly related to health and healthcare research, however examining ways to make the outdoors a safer and more welcoming place for Black people by Black people is essential for all of our wellbeing. Again, this example is intended to illustrate possibilities through which ethnographic research may possess a Black voice.

Declarative mapping sentence

In an earlier chapter (Hackett, 2020a) and elsewhere (Hackett, 2020b) the first author advocated the use of declarative mapping sentences as templates for designing qualitative research. Below we offer a declarative mapping sentence for the area of understanding acts of racism. The aim behind developing this sentence is to provide a template that may be used in qualitative research in order to ensure that the important aspects of an act of racism are incorporated into the research.

Box 41.1 Declarative mapping sentence for understanding acts of racism

A specific person or group of people (x) commit the:

Intent

intentional
unintentional
unthinking

Type of action

verbal
physical
mixed

racist act, which is targeted against:

Target

an individual
specific group

---

wider culture

and has the consequence of causing:

Consequence

death
physical injury
psychological injury
mixture of the above
social segregation/unrest

to a person or persons, and which is perceived by a person who is:

Person viewing

Black
not Black

The above declarative mapping sentence is offered as an initial template that may be used when designing a qualitative research project into racist acts and their consequences. Within this framework we offer our initial thoughts regarding the pertinent features of racist action. The emboldened words are called facets and they denote the main aspects of the racist action as being the intent of the perpetrator, the type of racist action committed, the target of the racist action, the consequence of the action and also who is viewing or interpreting an act of racism. We believe that it is important to consider these aspects of the situation when designing or interpreting a piece of qualitative research into racism.

Under each of the facets we have listed elements, which are specific forms of each of the aspects of a racist action. However, these elements may be changed and adapted to suit any particular piece of research. The elements we propose in the mapping sentence are initial suggestions for modification.

Initially, the mapping sentence states that racist acts are committed by people, either individually or in groups. The sentence specifies that such an act may be thought of in terms of the type of action committed and we have suggested these may be verbal, physical, or acts that are a mixture of these. We then think it important to consider the intention behind such an action, which may be intentional, unintentional, or unthinking. Who is the action targeted against is of importance and we suggest that the targets may be individual, specific groups, or wider culture groups. The consequence of the action is also important to keep in mind when designing and interpreting research. We suggest the elements of death, physical injury, psychological injury, a mixture of these, and social segregation/unrest. Finally, we note in the sentence that the person who is viewing and interpreting the action is an important component of the research in terms of whether they are Black or not Black. We believe that by using the mapping sentence to design research into racist actions will help the researcher keep all of the important aspects of such actions in mind. Of course, this is an initial suggestion for the content of the mapping sentence and this may change with usage.

Another point that the authors wish to make is that institutions of qualitative research can take an active role in addressing racism. An example of such action is provided in an announcement published by the Society for Applied Anthropology in response to the George Floyd killing.

Ways ethnographers can combat racism

The Society for Applied Anthropology (SfAA), an American organization, issued a statement which emphasizes the sadness and frustration felt over the death of George Floyd and for the many others who have been the victims of racial prejudice. The society emphasizes that such discrimination can no longer be tolerated and reiterates that, "As a professional society of applied social scientists committed to respect for human diversity, cultural understanding, and empowerment of all people, we repudiate all forms of hatred in our neighborhoods, communities, and world" (SfAA, 2020). Having made this assertion, the society goes on to say that it is not enough to be outraged, that everyone must be active in creating an inclusive, safe, and just world. The statement pledges the society's role in using "action-oriented social science to catalyze change (through) … personal and professional commitment, active listening, advocacy, teaching, training, policy work and more" (SfAA, 2020). Vital to the SfAA's commitment to change are collaborations at the grassroots and community-based level where the Society proffers its role as a hub of "meaningful conversation and sharing knowledge, resources and networks (SfAA, 2020)". Such activities, the Society claims, add to the establishment of social justice work at many scales. Suggestions are listed below of areas through which the Society and other researchers can effect positive social change:

- conducting applied research into areas that are directly relevant to understanding and fighting racism such as: education, employment rights, issues of poverty, police activities, immigration, and the climate
- conducting research into COVID-19 as this pandemic reveals the disparities in health and health care provision
- working collaboratively on human rights initiatives with other professional organizations
- providing instruction about systemic racism and structural violence and conducting training that allows people to build what they call their "activist toolkits" which includes learning skills such as performing public advocacy and working with the media and, perhaps of prime importance, using anthropological knowledge and skills in rapid response to emergencies
- finally, the SfAA pledges that the Society's membership will reflect global diversity

These are laudable aims from a Society based in a country that is reeling from racist murder after racist murder and the swelling turmoil that has followed.

When thinking about how we, as ethnographers, can respond to racism, perhaps the first step is to confront our own self-awareness, our biases, and personal history. Both authors, although involved in a myriad of multicultural projects, have largely carried out research in areas of their own European heritage. This is likely to be the case with many ethnographers who often come from countries that are predominantly white and have white ancestry. Even though as individuals the authors believe in racial equality and enjoy meeting people of color, we move in white circles and work in a predominantly white academia. People of color do not form a significant part of our lives. We teach at private universities in undergraduate and post-graduate courses on qualitative research, ethnography, and global cultures, yet people of color are vastly under-represented in our classes. Thus, as authors, we must ask ourselves the question: Do we look at Black culture through similar lenses or even with the same level of interest as we do when we are considering white cultures? There seems to be a disconnected, yet, selective focus in our lives and in the direction of our gaze.

The small number of Black students in our classes have alerted the authors to the severe need for Black researchers who can act as role models. Of course, there are Black ethnographers. Yet, as we have heard it said many times before that there are no Black birdwatchers, the truth is: there are some Black birders out there but African Americans are certainly underrepresented in the world of outdoor exploration and appreciation. The authors, therefore, ask the question, How might we encourage more Black people to become involved in ethnography and in other activities in which they are underrepresented?

Conclusion

In the previous chapter of this volume the first author spoke about the need for researchers to respond to the COVID-19 pandemic. This virus represents an ongoing dramatic event that is killing many thousands of people and disrupting the global economy. The pandemic is a discrete event and whilst it may change the world, most likely at some point the world will move on. The murder of George Floyd is a similar discrete event but his death is part of systemic racism that is ever present. We have seen the written phrase "pandemic racism", which the authors do not like as the expression seems to miss the point about prejudice. We agree with the motive of stressing discrimination as serious a health threat to individuals and societies as the COVID-19 pandemic. However, racism is not a disease but a form of volitional behaviour and cannot be treated with medicine or guarded against through the development of a vaccine. Racism is something that we encounter every day, whether directly or indirectly. In America almost 1000 Black men are murdered by White police officers every year. George Floyd is part of this flagrant and horrific American phenomena as were the false accusations made against Christian Cooper. The lessons learned from these two and all other racial attacks are that no individual, society, or country can stand back and dismiss these events as being of little relevance: we all must act. We must strive to listen, to understand these feelings that come from within as well as from without and to learn how to build more inclusive and welcoming societies. Black lives matter.

References

Axelson, G. (2020). 5 Key Lessons To Take Home From The First #BlackBirdersWeek, All About Birds: The Cornell Lab of Ornithology, June 6th 2020, www.allaboutbirds.org/news/5-key-lessons-to-take-home-from-the-first- blackbirdersweek/

Economist. (2020). Police violence, race and protest in America, www.economist.com/leaders/2020/06/04/police-violence-race-and-protest-in-america?utm_campaign=racial-injustice-special-edition&utm_medium=newsletter&utm_source=salesforce-marketing-cloud&utm_term=2020-06-09&utm_content=header_image

Gould, E. & V. Wilson. (2020). Black workers face two of the most lethal preexisting conditions for coronavirus-racism and economic inequality, www.epi.org/publication/black-workers-covid/

Hackett, P.M.W. (2020a) The declarative mapping sentence as a framework for conducting ethnographic health research, in Hackett, P.M.W., and Hayre, C. (eds.) (2020) Handbook of Ethnography in Healthcare Research, London: Routledge, Taylor and Francis.

Hackett, P.M.W. (2020b) Declarative Mapping Sentences in Qualitative Research: Theoretical, Linguistic, and Applied Usages, London: Routledge.

Mock, J. (2020, June 1) 'Black birders week' promotes diversity and takes on racism in the outdoors, *Audubon Magazine*. www.audubon.org/news/black-birders-week-promotes-diversity-and-takes-racism-outdoors

Society for Applied Anthropology. (2020). Statement on Global Violence, Systemic Racism, June 5th, 2020, www.appliedanthro.org/about

#BlackBirdersWeek. https://twitter.com/hashtag/BlackBirdersWeek

INDEX

interdependence in 142; internal locus of control 143; limits of knowledge, clinicians admitting 147–148; loneliness of patient, communication by clinician and 145–146; power relations 141; professional knowledge/patient autonomy 144; psychotherapist-client relationships and 141–142; questions, explaining purpose of 146; routine (clinician's)/emergency (patient's) 146–147; transparency in clinician communication 149; trust 141–143; *see also* doctor-patient relationship

coaching, clinician-patient relationships and 142

coding 20; computer-assisted qualitative data analysis software (CAQDAS) 418, 419, 422; descriptive 418; example 428–429; field notes 315; text 83; topic 418

Coffey, A. 48, 228, 262

cognitive toolkits 393–394

Colaizzi, P. 431

Colatruglio, A. 370

Cole, J. 430

collaging 334

Collip, D. 278

colonization 69–70

Common Rule 34–35

community-based participatory research (CBPR): accompaniment, principle of 236; African American church as initiator 235–236; ALIVE! project 235; challenges of 251; divine readings with wellness themes 247–248; factors contributing to success 251; feedback from church members 252–254; fieldwork 239; inside/outside ethnographers *238*, 238–239; interactions, faith and wellness defined by 244–245; internal validity 242–243; lay leaders 242; *lectio divina* 241, 247–248; limitations 254–255; methods 236–239, *237*, *238*; needs assessment (NA) 236, 238, 240–241, 251; pastor as role model 248–249; principles of 235; racism as collective reality 249–250; reflection on observations 242–243; soul food as love 245–247; *Soul Food Junkies* (Hurt) (documentary) 241–242, 250; teams 239; wellness as faith experienced with community 243–244

community building at playgrounds 118–119

community consent to research participation 38

community relations, NHS as broker of 191–192

comprehensibility, dimension of 301, 303–304

computer-assisted qualitative data analysis software (CAQDAS): advantages/disadvantages of computer use 434; amounts of data collected 414–415; cloud-based 417; coding 418, 419, 420–421, 422; creeping featurism 416; data analysis with 418–419; data management with 415, 416–417, 419–420; defined 415; export functions 421; fears about using 421–422;

flexibility in using 421; format of data 416; functions of 415; health ethnographies using 419–421, **420**; history and development 415–416; initial set up of files 417; memos 418; mixed methods research and 418–419; organization of data 417; portability 416–417; purpose of 415; reasons for use of computers in research 433–434; separation/distance issue 422; storage of data 417

condition-, meanings-, and reasoning analysis: action possibilities following 410–411; challenges of 412; character and quality of empirical material 403; choice of analysis method 403; conditions **407**, 408–409, 409–410; Conduct of Everyday Life (CEL), concept of 404; course of analysis 405; critical psychology 404; different meanings of conditions 410; Greenland as context for research 406; John, example of 406–410, **407**; Julie, example of 410; meanings **407**, 409; purpose of 407; reasonings **407**, 409; self-reflection by researcher 411–12; social practice, analysis of 405

Conduct of Everyday Life (CEL), concept of 404

confidentiality: focus groups 355–356, 371; medical education, ethnography of 157

consent: ethics 27; *see also* informed consent

consideration(s), use of term 11

constant comparative method of data analysis 428–429

constructionism 5

consumer culture, rise of 390–391

container of the field 380

content analysis: declarative mapping sentences 81–87; diaries 287n3; thematic analysis 20

context: contextualization of research 73–74; research findings and 21; visual ethnography, contextualizing in 177

control: locus of 143; narrative 297

conversational analysis 287n3

Cooper, C. 514, 515, 516

coproduction of knowledge 169, 171, *171*, *172*, 173

coral-like ethnography: emergency, emergence and immersion 456; ethics of earthly survival, studying the 461–463; noticing 458–461; tracing patchy stories 458–461, 464; transcending scale 457–458, 464

Coronavirus *see* Covid-19/Coronavirus

corporate setting and language: author and 388–389; big data 397–398; consumer culture, rise of 390–391; design research 392–393; ethnography as part of 391–392; field books 391–392; problems, need to understand 394–395; proof of problem/concept 394–395; struggles going on 398; trend research 395–397, 398n2

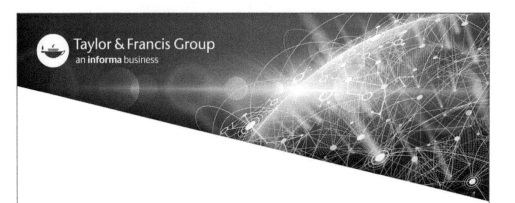
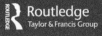
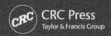

For Product Safety Concerns and Information please contact our EU
representative GPSR@taylorandfrancis.com
Taylor & Francis Verlag GmbH, Kaufingerstraße 24, 80331 München, Germany

www.ingramcontent.com/pod-product-compliance
Ingram Content Group UK Ltd.
Pitfield, Milton Keynes, MK11 3LW, UK
UKHW031042080625
459435UK00013B/554